Essentials of
CLINICAL
ONCOLOGY

Essentials of
CLINICAL
ONCOLOGY

Editors

Robert de W. Marsh
MD FACP
Professor of Medicine and Director
Clinical Trials Office
University of Florida Shands Cancer Center
Gainesville, Florida, USA

J. Samuel
MD FRCS FACS
Surgical Consultant, 'Hospice', Cochin, India

Associate Editors

George Jacob
MD D Ortho
Assistant Director, Clinical Trials Office
University of Florida Shands Cancer Center
Gainesville, Florida, USA

Jame Abraham
MD FACP
Medical Director and Assistant Professor of Medicine,
Division of Hematology/Oncology Mary Babb Randolph
Cancer Center, West Virginia University, Morgantown, USA

K. Pavithran
MD DM (Onco) FICP
Department of Medical Oncology
Rajiv Gandhi Cancer Institute, New Delhi, India

Shirley George
MSc PhD
Lecturer, Liggin's Institute, Faculty of Health
and Medical Sciences, University of Auckland, New Zealand

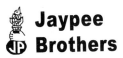

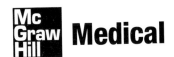

QZ
200
E78
2007

© 2007 Robert de W. Marsh, J Samuel

First published in India by
Jaypee Brothers Medical Publishers (P) Ltd
EMCA House, 23/23B Ansari Road, Daryaganj
New Delhi 110 002, India
Phones: +91-11-23272143, +91-11-23272703, +91-11-23282021, +91-11-23245672
Fax: +91-11-23276490, +91-11-23245683   e-mail: jaypee@jaypeebrothers.com
Visit our website: www.jaypeebrothers.com

First published in USA by The McGraw-Hill Companies, 2 Penn Plaza, New York, NY 10121-2298. Exclusively worldwide distributor except South Asia (India, Nepal, Sri Lanka, Bhutan, Pakistan, Bangladesh).

NOTICE

Medicine is an ever-changing science. As new research and clinical experience broaden our knowledge, changes in treatment and drug therapy are required. The authors and the publisher of this work have checked with sources believed to be reliable in their efforts to provide information that is complete and generally in accord with the standards accepted at the time of publication. However, in view of the possibility of human error changes in medical science, neither the editors nor the publisher nor any other party who has been involved in the preparation or publication of this work warrants that the information contained herein is in every respect accurate or complete, and they disclaim all responsibility for any errors or omissions or for the results obtained from use of the information contained in this work. Readers are encouraged to confirm the information contained herein with other sources. For example and in particular, readers are advised to check the product information sheet included in the package of each drug they plan to administer to be certain that the information contained in this work is accurate and that changes have not been made in the recommended dose or in the contraindications for administration. This recommendation is of particular importance in connection with new or infrequently used drugs.

ISBN   0-07-148580-5
ISBN 13 9780071485807

Dedicated

To the doctors, nurses and health workers

Serving patients selflessly in cancer hospitals across India

under difficult conditions

and

To the Holy Cross Sisters who started the first

Hospice 'Avedan' at Mumbai, in India

Na jayete mriteye va vipychinnayam
Kuthachhinna bhafuva kachhit
Ajonithyam swaswatho ayam purano
Na hanyate hanyamane sareeram

Kattha Upanishad
B.C.5000 Circa

(Kattha Upanishad is a discourse between a father and his son. The father is well versed in the Vedas and the son asks his father for a gift. The father says, "My dear son, I am giving you the gift of death.")

The intelligent self is neither born nor does it die
It did not originate from anything
Nor did anything originate from it
It is birthless and eternal, undecaying and ancient
It is not injured even when the body is killed

Kattha Upanishad
B.C.5000 Circa

Contributors

Jame Abraham MD
Medical Director and Assistant
Professor of Medicine, Division of
Hematology/Oncology, Mary Babb
Randolph Cancer Center, West Virginia
University, Morgantown, USA

Mohan Abraham MS MCh
Department of Pediatrics, Amritha
Institute of Medical Sciences and
Research Center, Cochin, India

Ramin Altaha MD
Division of Hematology/Oncology, Mary
Babb Randolph Cancer Center, West
Virginia University, Morgantown, USA

C. Balachandran MS MCh
Lakshmy Group of Hospitals
Cochin, India

Mathew Dominic MS FRCS
Department of Ear, Nose and Throat
Medical Trust Hospital
Cochin, India

P. Gangadharan MSc MS (Stat) (Pitt)
Amritha Institute of Medical
Sciences, Cochin, Kerala, Formerly
Retired Associate Professor Emeritus
Medical Scientist (ICNR), Regional
Cancer Center, Trivandrum
Kerala, India

Alice George MD MRCOG
Department of Obstetrics and
Gynecology, Christian Medical College
Vellore, India

Shirley George MSc PhD
Lecturer, Liggin's Institute, Faculty of
Health and Medical Sciences
University of Auckland, New Zealand

T.K. Jayakumar MS MCh
Department of Cardiothoracic Surgery
Medical College, Kottayam
Kerala, India

Pamela Jayaraj MD
Department of Oncology, Reader in
Radiotherapy, Christian Medical College
and Hospital, Ludhiana, India

Sanjay Joseph MD MRCP
Worcester Royal Infirmary
Worcester, UK

Abraham Kurian MS
Lecturer, Department of Urology
Christian Medical College and Hospital
Ludhiana, Punjab, India

Mohan Kurian MS
Retired Lecturer, Medical College for
Women, Dubai, UAE

Kim Mammen MS MCh
Professor, Department of Urology
Christian Medical College
Ludhiana, India

Rachel Mathai FRCP (Glasgow)
Consultant Dermatologist, Muthoot
Medical Center, Kozhencherry
Kerala, India. Formerly Professor
Department of Dermatology, Christian
Medical College, Vellore, India

Aleyamma Mathew PhD
Division of Epidemiology and Clinical
Research, Regional Cancer Center
Trivandrum, Kerala, India

Bhagyam Nair MD
Pathologist, Medinova Diagnostic
Center, Dubai, UAE

K. Pavithran MD DM (Onco) FICP
Head of the Department of Medical
Oncology, Amritha Institute of Medical
Sciences and Research Center
Cochin, Kerala

Abraham Peedicayil MD MRCOG
Department of Obstetrics and
Gynecology, Christian Medical College
Vellore, India

Paul Puthuran MD
Department of Medicine, Lourde's
Hospital, Cochin, India

B. Rajan MD
Director and Professor of Clinical
Oncology, Regional Cancer Center
Trivandrum, Kerala, India

M. Nageswara Rao MCh
Department of Neurosurgery, Medical
College, Guntur, India

J. Samuel FRCS FACS
Surgical Consultant, Hospice
Cochin, India

N.V. Seethalakshmy
DCP Dip NB (Pathology)
Associate Professor of Pathology
Amritha Institute of Medical Sciences
and Research Center, Cochin, Kerala

Iqbal S. Shergill
BSc (Hons) MRCS (Eng)
Clinical Research Fellow, Institute of
Urology and Nephrology
London W1W, 7EJ, UK

A.R. Rama Subbu MS FACS
Professor and Head of General Surgery
Raja Dental College, Vadakangulum
Tamil Nadu, India

S. Sudhindran MS FRCS FRCS (Gen)
Department of GI Surgery
Amritha Institute of Medical Sciences
and Research Center
Cochin, India

Venugopala Rao Tanneru MD
Professor, Department of
Anesthesiology, Medical College
Guntur, India

Antony Thomas MD
Pathologist, Prime Medical Center
P.O. Box 5239, Deira
Dubai, UAE

M. Thomas
R.N., Indian Medical Services
New Delhi, India

Narayanan Kutty Warrier
MD (Int Med) DM (Med Onco)
Consultant Medical Oncologist
Department of Medicine, Division of
Medical Oncology, Medical College
Calicut, Kerala, India

Babu Zachariah MD
Associate Professor of Radiation
Oncology, H.Lee Moffitt Cancer Center
University of South Florida
Tampa, Florida, USA

Preface

This is an attempt to share our experiences in dealing with the problems of cancer with practitioners of modern medicine, medical students, interns, nurses and especially those who work in oncology services and hospices. India has a large population of 1 billion (1000 million) and attempts are made, in many regional centers for cancer, to develop Cancer Registries, which are regularly updated. The National Cancer Registration program has evolved strategies to collect data from urban and rural areas and hospital records. The epidemiological study is also undertaken with new perceptions of prevention of common cancers in India. The readers must note that there are different medical systems in this country like Ayurveda, Siddha, etc. and the villagers still have not lost faith in these systems for the treatment of common ailments. At the same time, particularly in urban and semi-urban areas, people are conscious of cancer and they approach the doctors when they feel a lump in the breast, irregular vaginal bleeding or an unhealed ulcer in the mouth. It is true that the patients who keep their faith in alternative systems of medicine may be late when they attend the cancer centers for diagnosis and therapy.

The problem of cancer is universal. To the uninitiated, cancer means painful and slow death. But the scenario is changing rapidly. Most of the patients with early diagnosis of cancer live for many years with proper treatment. In a number of cases, the cancer is cured. In the majority, the cancer is controlled for some time. In India, there is also an active interest among physicians to develop both domiciliary and hospital-based palliative care centers. There is optimism among the physicians, the surgeons, the radiotherapists and the chemotherapists who treat these cases. This book is meant to give hope and show the positive side of cancer therapy. It is meant to instill confidence in the physicians and health workers that slowly but surely, we shall conquer cancer as we have conquered other infectious diseases or control it as we control hypertension or rheumatoid arthritis. This book is meant to create an awareness in medical students, physicians and health workers who may pass on this optimistic information to the Indian millions through their personal approach, by word of mouth and electronic media. The people in different parts of India, both in villages and towns, should know that if they approach a doctor early, that is, in the early stage of the disease, it could be cured. The problem must be approached with a sense of objectivity tempered with modern scientific outlook.

The etiological factors are many. Recent research has shed light on the role of genes in the origin of cancers. We are not unfamiliar with the familial cancers developing in certain families, particularly in the gastrointestinal tract, the breast and the ovary.

The role of environment on initiating cancer by smoking, chewing tobacco and imbibing spurious alcohol is also well documented.

Environmental causes have become a serious problem in the 21st century. There are many carcinogens in the industrial waste. The automobile exhaust fumes, pesticides and other chemicals are incriminated in the initiation of cancer. Our rivers, lakes, paddy and wheat fields, cities and towns have become polluted with chemicals and industrial waste. Radiation too has become a serious etiological problem. The story of Hiroshima and Nagasaki still haunts the minds of research workers. Frequent deaths in these cities by non-leukemic cancer still occur, 55 years after atomic bombing. The Chernobyl disaster too has cast a pall of gloom among the scientists involved in the role of nuclear fission in the production of energy. The problem of disposal of nuclear waste is still not solved. The health officials in many developed countries have still not found an answer to the growing hazards of radiation in the major cities in the West.

The task of writing a book on this subject is a strenuous one. Consider merely the vast amount of material available as research papers being published from different centers in the world. The Internet will provide a large number of publications but to choose the necessary information therefrom is a laborious task.

This book is divided into three sections with 56 chapters. The first one deals with general discussion about cancer like its etiology, molecular basis of cancer, investigations, the cancer metastases, enigma of unknown primary, etc. The second section deals with system or organ specific cancer like that of the breast and the alimentary system, tumors of male and female genital tracts, leukemia, lymphoma, etc. The third and final section deals with the treatment of cancer such as radiation, chemotherapy and palliative care. Even though the book is on oncology, which includes both benign and malignant tumors, throughout the book, the authors have given more stress on the diagnosis and treatment of malignant neoplasms.

The adult cancer patients go through the following 5 phases once a competent physician diagnoses cancer:
1. The phase of disbelief
2. The phase of anger and resentment
3. The phase of bargaining with God
4. The phase of acceptance
5. The phase of peaceful death

In the case of children, the first 3 phases are not present. They accept the diagnosis without any emotion, they are not angry towards anyone; nor do they bargain with others or God. They accept the diagnosis, they all want to live but hardly challenge fate and succumb to death quietly. One boy of 17 told a few minutes before his death, "Doctor, I am all right." and became deeply unconscious.

Lastly a chapter has been included in which the care of the terminally ill patient is discussed. This chapter on the care of the terminally ill patients is to help those who have dedicated themselves to the service of these unfortunate men and women in our country. We intend to tell doctors and nurses that death, after all, is not a painful experience but the final and true freedom. All the aspects of palliative care, the drugs used and the counseling for the terminally ill patients shall be discussed in this chapter. The readers are advised to read books on these subjects by Kubler-Ross, Dame Cicely Saunders, Ms Satyavathy Sirsat and Fr Louis Pereira.

It is our attempt to keep the discussions as simple as possible. A book like this, with multidisciplinary approach on cancer edited by international editors, is not available in India. Many biochemists and oncologists are spending their whole lives in different parts of the world to find answers to many vexing problems. Oncology is one of the fast advancing fields in medicine and things are changing almost everyday. A few questions are answered but the challenge lingers on.

Robert de W Marsh
J Samuel

Acknowledgements

It is hardly possible for two or three individuals to write a book on cancer in modern times. The vast amount of researches in molecular changes in genes, newer concepts of tumor suppressor genes, etc. different modalities of investigation and treatment demand the help of many men of excellence to complete such a book. We have sought the help of many such outstanding teachers, clinicians and research workers around the world who have come forward in writing different chapters in this book.

They have come forward with great enthusiasm, as this is one of the few books in India on cancer edited by international authors. Their names appear on page VII in the list of contributors. We know that most of them are busy with their clinical work, teaching and research, and yet they found time to write excellent chapters. To each of them, we are deeply grateful.

Some others too, seeing our enthusiasm, helped us in many ways—some of them reading the manuscript as well as giving valuable suggestions and others checking the language errors.

They principally include:

Dr M Krishnan Nair, MD, Director, The Regional Cancer Center, Trivandrum, Kerala, India.

Dr J Jacob, FRCP, Formerly Director, Christian Medical College, Ludhiana, India.

Dr Aleyamma Mathew, MD, FRCP (Path), Cheshire, UK.

Dr Rejoo Daniel, MS, FRCS, Department of Paediatric Surgery, Hull Royal Infirmary, Hull, UK.

Dr Sunil Mathai, MD,DM (Gastroenterology), Medical Trust Hospital, Cochin, Kerala, India.

We are grateful to the staff of the Department of Radiology and Pathology of Christian Medical College, Vellore, India for providing the CT scan pictures and histological pictures respectively which appear in the chapter on cancers of female genital organs.

Mr MT Thomas, Professor, Department of English, Bharata Mata College, Thrikkakara, Cochin, Kerala, India has always been rendering his services as an efficient orthographer and language consultant. To him we are ever so grateful for the careful shepherding of the manuscript.

To Mrs Aley Jacob, MA and Ellen Samuel, we offer our sincere gratitude for reading through a few sections of the manuscript.

Mr MG Rajan of Chaithanya Computer Center, Cochin, India was responsible for the typing and page layout. To him we are deeply indebted.

To Mr M Antony who designed the cover pages, we offer our sincere thanks.

To Ms Shali Joseph, the secretary, we remain indebted for the preliminary job of typing the manuscript.

Contents

Central Nervous System Tumors

Hematologic Malignancies

Endocrine Tumors

Other Malignancies

Section I

General Principles in Cancer

- *Introduction*
- *Etiology of Cancer*
- *Biology of Cancer*
- *Cancer in India—Data Sources and Statistical Relevance*
- *Epidemiology of Cancer and Prevention of Cancer in India*
- *Screening and Prevention of Cancer*
- *Investigations in Cancer*
- *Cancer Metastases*
- *Carcinoma of Unknown Primary*
- *Paraneoplastic Syndromes*
- *Oncologic Emergencies*

Introduction

1

J Samuel

The incidences of malignant disease vary with sex, age and geographic locations. Both females and males have almost the same proportion of cancer. The common cancers that affect the women are those of the breast, colon, cervix, ovary, and skin while men are more prone to develop cancer of the lungs, gastrointestinal tract, skin, prostate, oral cavity, pharynx, larynx, bladder and testis. In fact the gap is closing with respect to cancer of the lung in most of the western countries where males and females are equally prone to lung cancer. In fact there is decrease in cancer of the cervix in the west but in India, the problem of cervical cancer is still a serious one. Pediatric cancers are far less than what is seen in adults, but it is growing in importance in terms of mortality. Cancer is the leading cause of death in children up to 14 years, except for accidents, in the developed world. Acute leukemia of both myeloid and lymphatic variety and the solid pediatric tumors of different types like nephroblastoma, retinoblastoma, medulloblastoma, hepatoblastoma and embryonic sarcoma are a few of them. Both Hodgkin's and non-Hodgkin's lymphomas develop in male and female patients in equal proportion at any age.

HISTORY OF CANCER

In a historical sense, mention about tumors, particularly about bone and soft tissue tumors, has appeared in the Ramayana, an Indian epic written 2000 years before Christ. References are also available in Susrutha Samhitha (circa 5th BC), a textbook on operative surgery and the surgical removal of tumors. Descriptions about human tumors have appeared in Egyptian papyri (circa1500 BC). In the ancient library in Nineveh in Babylon, in the cuneiform inscriptions, the tumor of the breast is described. Hippocrates of Cos (460-375 BC) coined the word 'carcinomas' for malignant tumors and 'karkinos' for benign lumps and chronic ulcers. Interestingly, this term 'cancer' originated from the Greek word 'karkinos' meaning 'crab'. There is also a Latin word 'cancrum' that meaning 'crab'. There is also a Latin word 'cancrum' that means 'crab' and it is possible that the word cancer had its origin from the Latin word.

Galen (131-201 AD) wrote about cancer in his prolific writings on medicine. He was also aware of the tumors of the breast and the problem of metastasis and he was the first to coin the word sarcoma (Gr.sarkoma– fleshy growth) under which he included many fleshy tumors. Paul of Aegina (625-690 AD), a well-known Byzantine physician wrote, "Cancer is particularly frequent in the breasts of women." Hardly any medical or scientific writing was available during the dark ages between the 7th and 17th centuries. The Renaissance, which extended through Europe in the 17th century, brought fresh light on the different facets of medicine including cancer. The invention of microscope by Anton van Leeuwenhoek (1638-1723 AD) and the establishment of histology by Marcello Malpighi (1628-1694 AD) were notable events in the study of cancer. These events led to the discovery by Virchow of the division of cells and from these events, the modern concept of pathology was born.

THE OCCUPATIONAL CANCER

Sir Percival Pott in 1775 incriminated soot, which by its contact on the skin of the scrotum of the chimneysweeps, functions as an etiological factor in the cancer of the scrotal skin, and the concept of occupational cancer became a matter of concern to public health officials. It was found later that these compounds were capable of producing skin cancers in different types of industrial workers. It was noted that workers in Lancaster mills had developed cancer of the abdominal wall skin due to the splash of lubricant oil. In leather industry, the use of isopropyl alcohol is found to be a carcinogenic agent.

In 1884, a German surgeon Rein noticed an outbreak of bladder cancer in workers in the aniline dye industry. It was found that, of the nitrophenols, the dangerous ones are the 2-naphthylamine and 4-dimethylaminoazobenzene. Well-water mixed inadvertently with arsenic was used by people in Taiwan a few decades ago particularly in villages and now a few of them are attending the urology centers with bladder tumors (personal communication). It must not be forgotten that there is usually a lapse of many years between the exposure of a carcinogen and the development of urothelial cancers.

When reports started pouring in from Germany about the urothelial cancers in chemical and dye workers, attention was also drawn to the cluster of workers who developed a peculiar type of lung cancer in the Jochimsthal mines. Bronchogenic cancer of tobacco smokers is yet another example of polycyclic hydrocarbon causing cancer.

More recently, workers in polyvinyl chloride industry have been seen to develop angiosarcoma of the liver and Raynaud-like syndrome due to constant contact with polyvinyl chloride. In India, the chemical industries came into being in the middle of the 20th century but the authors are unable to give statistical data about the etiology of these compounds in the production of cancer.

EXPERIMENTAL CARCINOGENESIS (CHEMICAL AND VIRAL)

Attempts to produce cancer in experimental animals started by the end of the 19th century and the earliest work by Imagiwa and Ichikawa concerning the role of polycyclic hydrocarbon gave conclusive evidence of chemical compounds that induce neoplasm. The original work was done on the skin of the ear of a rabbit, which was painted, with a coal tar product for a few years that ultimately produced skin cancer and their results were published in 1924. The role of polycyclic hydrocarbon has been intensively studied on animals as inducers of neoplasia.

In the case of chemicals that cause cancer, the work of Somervelle in a small Christian hospital, in Kerala, India cannot be forgotten. The incidence of oral cancer, which is high even today, was prevalent among his patients. His inference is that the betel chewing where tobacco and lime (calcium hydroxide) are used initiates mucosal changes in oral mucosa and causes cancer of the oral region.

The role of viruses producing cancer in animal struck the attention of research workers as early as 1910. The experimental work was carried out in rodents and fowls. Ellerman and Bang in 1908, discovered fowl leukemia as the first virus induced tumor. Rous in 1911, Shope in 1932, Lucke in 1934 and Bittner in 1936 are some of the earliest workers in the field. Among them, Rous identified in 1911 a filterable virus producing neoplasm in animals. It was seen that this filterable agent is a virus capable of producing nonlethal mutations in normal stable cells that ultimately develop into a neoplasm. Later this virus was identified as RNA virus. He was awarded the Nobel Prize for this pioneering work on the role of virus in cancer in 1966.

Nigerian and Harris isolated a microorganism, which they thought, was of viral nature from cases of human leukemia but it has been shown that this is in fact a mycoplasma, and its etiological connection with leukemia is very doubtful. The occurrence of patients with leukemia in clusters would support the hypothesis that an infective agent, possibly a virus, was responsible for the initiation of leukemia.

Another important landmark in the study of oncogenic viral tumors is the work of Gross in 1951. He was able to isolate the virus producing leukemia in a mouse and by 1953; he isolated another virus from the cell filtrate that can cause tumors in mice, rats and hamsters. This is polyoma virus, which specifically causes salivary gland tumors in the above-mentioned animals. The research workers in this field accepted the concept that the virus alters the genetic code in the DNA and from a normal cell, a mutated cell that ultimately produces a clone of malignant cell is developed.

THE MOLECULAR BASIS IN CANCER

Even though the scientists knew about the role of virus in animal cancer, they found it difficult to pinpoint the sites at which these changes take place. The pathologists working with a light microscope found that the structure of a malignant cell was different from that of normal cell. Walter Sutton in the year 1903, while an undergraduate student at Columbia University, discovered the chromosomes and its pattern in the cells. It was difficult to evaluate the role of chromosome in certain familial diseases and the search for some other factors in chromosomes that would give an answer to these genetic diseases. Working on these hypotheses, Thomas Morgan and his associates at the Columbia University mapped the position of different genes in the chromosomes for which he was awarded the Nobel Prize for medicine in 1933. In 1934, Bovril suggested that cells become malignant either by the overexpression of genes that promote replication or the inhibition of genes that control cell division.

"What is the mechanism of the perfect replication of cells?", was a question the scientists wanted an answer to. Is there a code that can be transferred from one cell to its progeny? James Watson and Frances Crick, who identified the structure of DNA, and opened a gate to the new universe of scientific discoveries, provided the answer to this question. This discovery gave the concept of transferring the genetic information through genetic sequence that controls the division of cells and expression of nucleoprotein, which is unique for each cell. With Wilkins, Watson and Crick received the Nobel Prize for this epoch-making discovery in the year 1962. The next step was to find out why certain cells escape from normal growth control and permit uncontrolled replication. It was thought, the uncontrolled replication is due to mutations in the DNA by carcinogen.

The next discovery of great merit was by two American physiologists Michael J. Bishop and Harold E. Varmus who discovered that the sequences of the genetic codes of RNA virus and animal cells are identical. Bishop and Varmus coined the terms protooncogene and virus oncogene. These two scientists received the Nobel Prize for medicine in 1989.

The readers interested in the study of cancer cannot forget the other Nobel Prize winners in medicine and physiology for their lifelong contribution to the search for the cause of cancer. They are Fritz A. Lipton and Hans A. Koreas (1953) for the study of living cells, J. Lederberg, George W. Beadle and E.L. Tatum (1958), for their work in the genetic transmission of hereditary characteristics, Robert W. Holley, Har Gobind Khorana and Marshal W. Nirenberg (1968) for their contribution to further studies in genetic code. In 1975 David Baltimore and Renato Dulbeccobo received the Nobel Prize for medicine and physiology in recognition of their masterly work on interaction between the cells and their replication.

In the field of cancer chemotherapy, many scientists in different centers in Europe, the UK and the US have contributed significantly to evolve a therapeutic protocol by animal experiments and phase trials. For the introduction of monoclonal antibodies as a chemotherapeutic agent for the first time in 1975, Kohler and Milstein won the Nobel Prize for medicine in 1984.

Five years prior to the AIDS era, research workers of different centers in big cities in the US, were trying to find the relation between AIDS and microbes, especially the ones targeting T4 helper cells. In 1981, Dr Robert Gallo, the central figure in the discovery of AIDS discovered 3 retroviruses as the causative factors in AIDS. (The term 'retrovirus' arises from the fact that in this type of virus the DNA is produced 'backwards' from RNA while normally the RNA is produced in a direction 'forwards' from the DNA). In the year 1978, Dr Gallo also isolated for the first time, a type of retrovirus HTLV1 causing a rare type of cancer in man known as T cell leukemia. Interestingly, this virus too has tropism for T4 helper cells as in the AIDS virus. The virus can destroy the T helper cells once it gains entry, and by destroying the immunocompetence of the body, can cause T cell leukemia.

The worldwide appearance of acquired immunodeficiency syndrome (AIDS) has given a new dimension to the problems of rare malignancies like Kaposi's sarcoma and B-cell non-Hodgkin's lymphoma occurring in the man, woman and child infected with AIDS virus. The type of retrovirus HIV-1 identified in 1978 has profound influence on body's protective immune system. It also damages the protective immunological surveillance that inhibits the tumor suppressor genes and activates, in turn, the tumor producing genes.

The discovery of the tumor suppressor gene p53 has gone a long way in the advancement of knowledge on control of cell cycle. It is called 'the guardian of the genome'. With the other genes such as cyclins and growth hormone receptor, p53 is involved in the control of cell cycle with the gene products. It came to prominence in the early 1980 as a tumor antigen (tumor protein 53) and in the late 1980, it was realized that this gene in its mutated form has the ability to produce tumors. Further work on the property of gene unfolded its critical step in the majority of human and rodent tumors. It lies on chromosome 17p and encodes 2.8 kb mRNA. It works in close relation with another gene p21 through its encoded proteins. The loss of normal p53 protein facilitates the emergence of malignant traits in the normal cell.

THE CANCER PATTERN IN INDIA

The problem of cancer is universal. Cancer in all forms causes 12 percent of deaths throughout the world that includes the developed and developing countries. In developed countries, cancer is ranked as the second commonest cause of death (2.5 million), while in developing countries; it is ranked third (3.8 million), next to infectious diseases and cardiovascular diseases.

India is one of the developing countries with a population of 1000 million, and most of the people are engaged in agricultural work and living in villages (700 million). The rest are in the cities and towns engaged in different types of jobs including industrial work. There are nearly 2.5 million persons suffering from cancer at any given time. Around 7,00,00 new cases are added each year. The age-adjusted incidence rate of all cancers varies from 44 to 122 men per 100,000 males and 52 to 128 per 100,000 females in the different urban and rural registries. The age adjusted mortality rate is 61 per 100,000 males and 58 per 100,000 females (Mumbai Cancer Registry 2001). The lifetime cumulative risk indicates that on an average one in 10 to 13 people develops cancer in urban areas. The author (J.S.) admits that the populations covered by these registries in the urban and rural areas are small–nearly 5 percent of the total population. It gives some idea of the extent of the problem of cancer in India.

The incidence of cancer in men in the order of the frequency of occurrence is oropharynx, esophagus, stomach, trachea, bronchus and lungs. Tobacco is widely used in India both for chewing and smoking and is thought to be the single major cause of initiating cancer of the oral cavity, pharynx, lungs and the stomach. Added to this poor oral hygiene, inadequate intake of wholesome food and unhygienic environment also contribute to the development of cancer. In the case of women, the occurrence of cancer in the descending order is of the cervix, breast, oral cavity, pharynx and esophagus. Among Indian women the cancer of the breast and cervix forms a large group of 60 percent of all cases. The etiological factors are poor genital hygiene, early marriage, multiple pregnancy and sexual contact with more than one partner.

In India, more people are stricken with cancer in this decade when compared to the earlier decades of the last century. The reasons are many: There is longer life expectancy (It was 27 years in 1930 and now it is around 65), different types of vegetables treated with pesticides, increased use of tobacco, and inhaling noxious fumes expelled from automobiles, heavy industries and chemical factories.

The pattern of cancers is different in different countries. There is a high incidence of gastric cancer in Japan and a lower one in the US and it would be somewhere in the middle in India. The incidence of cervical cancer is high in India and in Colombia (South America) and low in Japan. In south Asian countries, the oral and uterine cancers top the list of malignant tumors especially the uterine cervical cancers. In spite of the fact, that these anatomical regions are accessible for easy and quick physical examination and exfoliative study, the patients come unusually late for treatment in general hospitals. The use of tobacco is more prevalent in men and the cancers related to this habit are seen more in men than in women.

India too is emerging as a great industrial force using nuclear fission for energy. The Atomic Energy Commission has taken steps to guard against any mishaps like the one at Chernobyl and other atomic plants in different parts of the world. The problem of the disposal of atomic waste worries our public health officials.

We have achieved a lot in controlling cancer and treating it. More has to be done. The cancer research has to be taken up with more dedication and vigor. The carcinogens specific in India have to be identified. It is true that there is a lot of suffering among the people in the fringes of our society. Early screening for cervical, breast and colon cancers has to be undertaken on a national level. The major issues like the cost and the patient compliance have to be worked out by public health officials.

Etiology of Cancer

2

Antony Thomas, J Samuel

Sir Percival Pott in 1775 for the first time suggested an etiological factor in the development of neoplasm. He pointed out that coal dust might be an etiological factor in the scrotal skin cancer of chimney sweeps. The chimney sweeps climb through the chimneys in British homes and their clothes become soaked with tarry deposits that accumulate in the corrugated scrotal skin. After many years of work, a few of them developed squamous carcinoma of the scrotal skin. Ever since, various causative factors and agents have been described in the development of neoplasm. Two distinct time frames can be seen in these attempts, the earlier from the last decade of the 18th century to the middle of the 20th century and the second era from the middle of the 20th century till the present date. In the first era, the few remarkable developments include experimental induction of carcinoma over the skin of the ear of the rabbit in 1914 by the Japanese scientists Yamagiwa and Ichikawa, the evidence of viral oncogenesis provided by Danish veterinary surgeons in 1908 and the isolation of sarcoma virus by Peyton Rous in 1911. The second era is full of dramatic scientific discoveries, with understanding of chromosomes, genes, and molecular biology of cellular proliferation. With these studies, the etiological agents in carcinogenesis can be classified into two groups, namely, endogenous which includes the non-modifiable host factors and genetic make up of the individual, and exogenous which includes the acquired and environmental factors. However the concept of single etiological factor is not sufficient as most neoplasms are due to the involvement of both or are multifactorial. These factors induce the formation of a single virtually autonomous transformed cell, which proliferates to form a cancerous mass. Hence cancers are monoclonal.

ENDOGENOUS FACTORS IN CARCINOGENESIS

AGE

Neoplastic diseases are seen in any age, however, carcinomas are common in old age especially in the fifth to the seventh decade. This is due to the structural alterations associated with longer life, longer period of exposure to carcinogens and defective immune status. A few neoplasms common in infancy and childhood include retinoblastoma, Wilms' tumor, acute leukemia, lymphoma, Ewing's sarcoma and rhabdomyosarcoma.

SEX

In general, cancers outside the reproductive system are common in males. Tumors of thyroid, salivary gland, meninges and breast are more common in women. This implication of sex difference is probably related to hormone status. Sexual practice is also implicated in carcinogenesis, especially in relation with the promiscuity and spread of HPV and HIV.

RACE

Some carcinomas are common in certain races, and may be attributed to genetic and environmental factors. A few to name are carcinoma of stomach in the Japanese due to the consumption of smoked food items, of cervix in South Americans attributed to promiscuous sexual practices, hepatocellular carcinoma in Africans and the Chinese related to hepatitis B virus and oropharyngeal carcinomas in Indians due to tobacco chewing.

HEREDITY

Many neoplasms develop due to environmental influence in individuals with hereditary predisposition. Hence there can be familial clustering and cancer can run in families. Bonaparte family was affected with carcinoma of the stomach. The hereditary types of cancer can be classified as auto-somal dominant, autosomal recessive, X-linked inheritance and familial cancers. These are associated with specific genetic and phenotypic presentations and involve specific sites and tissues. The autosomal dominant and autosomal recessive familial neoplasms are briefly described in Table 2.1. The X-linked disorders like Bruton's agammaglo-bulinemia and Wiskott-Aldrich syndrome are associated with the development of lymphoma and leukemia. Familial cancers include a set of neoplasms whose mode of inheritance is not clear. Two recently described tumor suppressor genes BRCA-1 and BRCA-2 (breast carcinoma) are associated with familial cancers. BRCA-1 is mapped to 17q12, with the risk of developing breast cancer in females and ovarian cancers. BRCA-2 is mapped to 13q12, and is susceptible to male breast cancer as well as ovarian and prostate cancers.

HORMONES

A number of hormones can induce neoplasia in experimental animals, the chief among them being estrogens and androgens. Neoplasm can be

Table 2.1: Autosomal dominant and autosomal recessive inheritance in neoplasm

Inheritance	Features	Associated neoplasms
AUTOSOMAL DOMINANT	Inherited cancer syndromes	
Familial Adenomatous polyposis of colon	FAPC gene mapped to 5q21, a cancer suppressor gene. Loss is associated with multiple polyps of colon (colon carpeted with polyps)	Carcinoma of colon
Familial retinoblastoma	Cancer suppressor gene mapped to chromosome 13q14.	Retinoblastoma and Osteogenic sarcoma
Neurofibromatosis types 1 and 2	Cancer suppressor gene. NF-1 mapped to 7q11 NF-2 on 22 q12	Multiple neurofibromatosis (Von Recklinghausen disease) Acoustic neurofibromatosis
Multiple endocrine neoplasia	A group of familial neoplasms	Multiple neoplasms affecting the various endocrine organs
Von Hippel-Lindau syndrome	Characterized by hemangioblastoma of cerebellum and retina. VHP gene is a cancer suppressor gene 3p25	Renal cell carcinomas and pheochromocytoma
AUTOSOMAL RECESSIVE	DNA instability syndrome or syndromes associated with defective DNA repair	
Xeroderma pigmentosum	Deficiency of endonuclease enzyme resulting in defective DNA repair. Characterized by extreme photosensitivity	Skin cancers in sun exposed region
Ataxia-telangiectasia	Hypersensitivity to ionizing radiation	Lymphoid malignancies
Bloom syndrome	Characterized by cerebral ataxia and cutaneous telangiectasia	Lymphoid malignancies and skin cancers
Fanconi anemia	Hypersensitivity to ionizing radiation. Associated with developmental defects Defective DNA repair to DNA cross-linking agents and associated aplastic anemia	Leukemia

induced by hormone (hormone induced neoplasm) or can be hormone dependent. Classical hormone induced neoplasm seen in association with hyperestrogenism includes carcinoma breast, endometrium, leiomyoma of uterus and carcinoma breast in males. Developments of carcinoma breast in sex transformed persons and clear cell vaginal adenocarcinoma in young women, who were in their fetal life exposed to administration of diethyl stilbesterol to their mother, are also hormone induced. Use of anabolic androgens is known to induce hepatocellular carcinoma and oral contraceptives in the development of hepatic adenoma.

Some tumors are dependent on hormones for their growth and withdrawal of these hormones can control their development. Some types of prostate carcinoma are androgen dependent and can be controlled either by orchidectomy or by administration of estrogen. Many of these tumors show specific hormone receptors and estrogen receptors in breast carcinoma and progesterone receptors in meningiomas signify hormone dependence.

Apart from hormones, some chemical carcinogens are also implicated in the development of neoplasm of sexual organs. This includes smegma, which is probably carcinogenic in penile and cervical cancers.

IMMUNITY

Immunodeficiency states, whether primary or secondary is more prone to the development of leukemia and lymphoma. The roles of HIV and induced immunosuppression as in transplant recipients are well implicated in the development of various neoplasms, including Kaposi's sarcoma.

EXOGENOUS FACTORS IN CARCINOGENESIS

Environmental and various acquired factors in carcinogenesis include physical, chemical and biological agents. These agents cause genetic alteration to create a transformed cell, which grows to a neoplasm. The role of physical agents such as nucleate energy, chemical carcinogens and biological agents such as certain viruses are well documented.

PHYSICAL CARCINOGENS

These include mainly radiation carcinogenesis, and in addition, persistent trauma and chronic diseases.

RADIATION CARCINOGENESIS

Radiant energy in the form of ionizing radiation, UV rays and even in thermal form is carcinogenic. Ionizing radiation whatever its origin— electromagnetic (X-rays, gamma rays) or particulate (alpha particles, beta particles, protons, neutrons)—induces cancer. The excess of cancers and excess of death from non-leukemia, non-Hodgkin's lymphoma, thyroid and skin cancers in the Japanese population even 58 years after the atomic bomb attack on Hiroshima and Nagasaki prove beyond doubt the role of ionizing radiation as an etiological factor in causing cancer. The ionizing radiation produces chromosomal mutation that either excites the tumor-producing oncogenes or inhibits the tumor-suppressor genes. The initiation and the propagation of the tumors have considerable latent period and become evident many years after initial exposure.

Ultraviolet rays are derived from the sun and have long wavelengths, low frequencies and penetrate only skin. They induce squamous cell carcinoma, basal cell carcinoma and melanoma of skin. These cancers are more common in white people than the blacks, since melanin absorbs the UV rays and prevent nuclear damage. Solar spectrum of UV rays including, UVA (320-400 nm) is considered harmless, UVB (280-320 nm) induces skin cancers, and UVC (200-280) is highly mutagenic; however it is filtered by ozone layer (hence the concern about global ozone depletion) and humans are spared.

The development of neoplasm in undescended testis, carcinoma of the lip in pipe smoking and carcinoma cheek and palate in chutta smoking (reverse smoking with fire end inside the mouth, common in Andhra Pradesh, S.India) could be related to thermal radiation. Development of cancer in scars (Marjolin's ulcer), carcinoma colon in ulcerative colitis, cheek cancers with ill fitting dentures, squamous cell carcinomas in association with lithiasis of gall bladder or urinary bladder etc. could be related to persistent irritation and cytokines are blamed for it.

CHEMICAL CARCINOGENS

John Hills, who related development of nasal polyps in snuff users, noted the association of chemical agents in carcinogenesis as early as 1961. Sir Percival Pott in 1975 suggested a single agent-coal dust-for the development of scrotal skin cancer in chimney sweeps. Ever since, various agents associated with atmospheric pollution, habits, occupation, pesticides and even medicines were found to be carcinogenic. Depending upon the mode of action, the carcinogen could be direct acting or could be a pro-carcinogen, which requires in vivo chemical transformation to be carcinogenic. In terms of transformation of a normal cell into neoplastic cell, a chemical could be an initiator or a promoter. Initiators are capable of inducing permanent DNA damage (mutation) in a cell and promoters promote additional mutations in an initiated cell. Neither initiator alone nor promoter alone is sufficient for the development of tumor, and exposure of promoter in an initiated cell is the prime factor in chemical carcinogenesis. This may play a role in the development of cancer in some and spare a few fortunate ones, who are exposed to the same carcinogen. The major chemical carcinogens depending upon the mode of action and type of exposure are given below: direct acting carcinogens in Table 2.2, procarcinogens especially aromatic hydrocarbons, aromatic amines, naturally occurring carcinogens and nitrosamines in Table 2.3, and carcinogens acquired in relation to habit in Table 2.4.

Table 2.2: Direct acting carcinogens

Alkylating Agents B-Propriolactone, Dimethyl-sulfate	These are weak carcinogens and they interfere with the DNA. This action renders them carcinogenic (induces lymphomas and leukemias) as well as makes them potent anticancer agents
Anticancer drugs (cyclophos-phamide, Chlorambucil) Others-Acetylating agents like Acetyl-imidazole and Dimethyl-carbamyl chloride	

Table 2.3: Procarcinogens

Aromatic Hydrocarbons Benzanthracene, Benzopyrene, Dibenzanthracene, 3-methylcholanthrene	First chemical carcinogen identified as causing the scrotal skin cancer in chimney sweeps. Hydrocarbons are formed by burning of any material containing carbon and are present in cigarette smoke, petroleum products and in charred or smoked meat and fish
Aromatic amines, Amides and Azo dyes B-Naphthylamine, Benzidine, 2-Acetylaminofluorene, Dimethylaminoazobenzene (butter yellow)	These are widely used in plastic, paint, rubber and textile industries, and also in medical laboratories. They induce bladder cancer
Naturally occurring carcinogens Aflatoxin B1, Cycasin, Safrole, Pyrilizidine alkaloids, Griseo-fulvin	Aflatoxin is a mycotoxin derived from the fungus *Aspergillus flavus* that grows in stored grains and peanuts as a fibrillary blackish substance. Cycasin is a contaminant in food, Safrole in cinnamon and camphor, Pyrilizidine alkaloids in bush tea and griseofulvin. All these are known to cause hepatocellular carcinoma
Nitrosamines	Nitrates and nitrites are widely present in soil, vegetables and water, and are also used as preservative. They are converted into procarcinogen nitrosamines in GIT and are known to cause carcinoma of stomach and liver

BIOLOGICAL CARCINOGENS

The role of biological agents especially the viruses producing cancer in both animal and man caught the attention of research workers as early as 1910. They were called tumor-producing or oncogenic viruses. Ellerman and Bang in 1908 discovered fowl leukemia as the first virus induced tumor. Rous in 1911, Shope in 1932, Lucke in 1934 and Bittner in 1936 are some of the trail-blazers in the field. Among them, Rous identified a

Table 2.4: Habit Related Carcinogens	
Cigarette (Tobacco)	Contain the chemical carcinogens: aromatic hydrocarbons, NNK, naphthylamines and polonium 210, carcinogenic metals such as arsenic, nickel, chromium and cadmium, and various promoters such as acetaldehyde and phenol. In carcinogenesis, they leave no organs untouched.
Betel nuts	Directly acting on the buccal mucosa as an irritant.
Alcohol	Not a direct-acting carcinogen but its metabolite acetaldehyde may act as a tumor promoter. Its use is associated with an increased incidence of cancer of oral cavity, pharynx, esophagus and liver.

filterable virus associated with the production of neoplasm in animals. It was seen that this filterable agent is an RNA virus transfecting normal stable cells causing mutations that ultimately produce neoplasm. He was awarded the Nobel Prize for medicine in 1968, when he was 82 years old. Gross in 1951 isolated the virus producing leukemia in a mouse and by 1953; he isolated another oncogenic virus from the cell filtrate that can cause tumors in mice, rats and hamsters. This virus is known as polyoma virus, which specifically causes salivary gland tumors in the above mentioned animals. Now, both DNA and RNA containing viruses are identified in many tumors. In addition to viruses, bacterial agents like Helicobacter pylori and trematodes (blood flukes) like schistosoma hematobium also are identified.

The worldwide appearance of acquired immunodeficiency syndrome (AIDS) has given a new dimension to the problems of rare malignancies like Kaposi's sarcoma and B-cell non-Hodgkin's lymphoma. The HIV virus has the unique ability to destroy the CD 4 molecules in the T-helper-inducer cells and the monocyte-macrophage cells and thus it removes the protection against opportunistic infections in almost all body tissues. It also damages the protective immunological surveillance that inhibits the tumor suppressor genes and activates in turn the tumor - producing genes.

DNA ONCOGENIC VIRUSES

DNA viruses that are associated with oncogenesis in human beings include human papilloma viruses (HPV), Epstein-Barr virus (EBV), hepatitis B virus (HBV) and Kaposi's sarcoma herpes virus (KSHV).

THE PAPILLOMA VIRUSES

Human papilloma viruses (HPV) belong to the group of "Papova virus" which stands for the first two alphabets of papilloma, polyoma and vacoulating viruses. There are more than fifty types of papilloma viruses, known to cause both benign and malignant tumors in human beings. They are transmitted sexually or by close contact and hence induce tumors of genitalia, especially the cervix, penis and oral cavity. Viral types HPV 6 and HPV 11 (low risk types) induce dysplasia and carcinoma in situ; meanwhile high risk types like HPV 16 and HPV 18 induce invasive carcinoma. These viruses produce proteins, which excite viral oncogenes E6 and E7. These oncogenes encode proteins, which bind to the DNA and inactivate the tumor suppressor p53 and Rb genes. This is the initiation of cervical neoplasia. The virus is sexually transmitted. In women it causes severe dysplasia of the cervix, later leading to malignancy. In gays, the anal skin gets infected and later develops anal cancer. Compared to cervical cancer, genital warts are almost benign. It is also observed that these changes alone are not enough to produce cancer. There should be associated factors such as the activation of ras oncogenes, poor hygiene, low protein intake and promiscuity of the sexual partner.

EPSTEIN-BARR VIRUS

EBV belongs to the family of gamma herpes virus. It is found to be associated with lymphoid malignancies like the African form of Burkitt lymphoma, B-cell lymphomas in immunosuppressed individuals and a few cases of Hodgkin's disease and epithelial malignancies like nasopharyngeal carcinoma. Normal immunocompetent individuals develop antibodies against this infection and they either become asymptomatic or develop infectious mononucleosis. Infection in immunosuppressed individuals like those with HIV infection or following organ transplantation is prone to the development of lymphoid neoplasms. EBV infects the B-lymphocytes via the CD 21 molecule expressed on their surface. The viral particle remains in an episomal form in the nucleus of lymphocytes and prevents apoptosis or immortalizes the cell resulting in polyclonal proliferation of B cell. Such cells are prone to mutations like translocation between chromosome number 8 and 14, as well as additional mutation involving N-ras. Such transformed cell undergoes monoclonal proliferation to develop Burkitt lymphoma. The development of various lymphoid neoplasms suggests the role of various co-factors including genetic, immunological, environmental and associated infections.

KAPOSI'S SARCOMA HERPES VIRUS (KSHV)

KSH virus also known as human herpes type 8, is found in all cases of Kaposi's sarcoma both in HIV infected and non-infected individuals. The viral genes of KSHV resemble several human genomes that involve in cellular proliferation, and they activate the release of various cytokines and growth factors. These viral genes induce proliferation of mesenchymal cells and angiogenesis resulting in the development of neoplasm.

HEPATITIS B VIRUS (HBV)

HBV belongs to hepadnaviridae family, and is universally present. In case of HBV-associated liver cancer, the viral DNA is found integrated to the host cell genome. This integration induces genomic instability, and HBV X proteins activate various growths promoting genes. These promote the development of malignancy. The latent period in the development of hepatocellular malignancy is about 20 to 30 years after the original attack of viral hepatitis. Cirrhosis of the liver associated with both B and C hepatitis viruses as well as with alcoholism, hemochromatosis, and toxin in the food like Aflatoxin do contribute to the development of liver cancers.

RNA ONCOGENIC VIRUSES

Human T-cell Leukemic Virus

The only proven RNA oncogenic virus in man is the retrovirus, human T-cell leukemic virus -1 (HTLV-1), which is associated with T-cell leukemia/lymphoma. These tumors are widely seen in certain parts of the Far East, the Caribbean islands and certain southern parts of the United States. It has a few features in common with HIV. They infect by sexual intercourse, use of drug sharing needles and by blood products or by breastfeeding. In addition it involves the CD4 T-lymphocytes and by its specific oncogene tax, it induces polyclonal T-cell proliferation. The proliferating T-cells undergo transformation by mutation, resulting in the monoclonal proliferation of cells and neoplasia.

Non-Viral Agents

Among the many bacteria that infect man, only one, *Helicobacter pylori* is suggested to be the causative factor in the development of gastric lymphoma and gastric cancer. Chronic infection with *H. pylori* induces polyclonal proliferation of B-lymphocytes, prone to additional mutation and the development of monoclonal neoplasm. Similarly, chronic gastritis with intestinal metaplasia produced by this organism results in the development of gastric carcinoma later.

Among the trematodes (blood flukes), infection with *Schistosoma haematobium* (Bilharzia) which is a urinary tract fluke that produces chronic infection of the bladder wall and later granuloma, can initiate neoplastic changes in the bladder. The antigen present in the egg of the Schistosoma produces both early and delayed hypersensitivity with eventual granuloma formation. The infection with this trematode is considered an etiological factor in the development of carcinoma of the bladder. The infection with this fluke is seen in South America, Egypt, Saudi Arabia, the Middle East and the Far East.

The list of carcinogens is never ending and new agents have been added day by day and many are still unknown. The role of various agents used by alternative systems of medicine in carcinogenesis is still an unexposed field. Above all our behavior, approach to life, socioeconomic status, mental, religious and spiritual attitude may play a role. Finally, what about "Destiny"?

FURTHER READING

1. Brugge J, et al. Origins of human cancer : A comprehensive review. Cold Spring Harbor, Cold Spring Harbor Laboratory Press, 1991.
2. Bussey HJR. Familial polyposis coli. Family studies, histopathology, differential diagnosis and results of treatment. Baltimore: Johns Hopkins University Press, 1975.
3. Cavenee W, Ponder BAJ, Solomon E (Eds). Cancer Surveys Vol 9. Genetics and Cancer. Oxford: Oxford University Press, 1991.
4. De Bruin LS, Josephy P. Perspectives on the chemical etiology of breast cancer. Environ Health Perspect Suppl 2002;11:119-28.
5. Easton D, Peto J. The contribution of inherited predisposition to cancer incidence. In: Cavenee W, Ponder BAJ, Solomon E (Eds). Cancer Surveys Vol. 9. Genetics and Cancer. Oxford: Oxford University Press, 1991.
6. Grobstein C, et al. Diet, nutrition and cancer. Washington, D.C. Nutritional Academy Press, 1982.
7. Holleb A I, et al. American Cancer Society, Textbook of Clinical Oncology. Atlanta, American Cancer Society Inc., 1991.
8. Ott J. A short guide to linkage analysis. Ed. Human Genetic Diseases: A Practical Approach. Oxford: IRL Press, 1986.
9. Ponder BAJ. Prospects for genetic diagnosis of inherited predisposition to cancer.Trends Biotechmol 1990;8:98-102.
10. Quirk JT, Kupinski JM. Chronic infection, inflammation, and epithelial ovarian cancer. Med Hypotheses 2001;57(4):426-28.

Biology of Cancer

3

Antony Thomas, J Samuel

From the previous chapter on etiology, it has been learnt that in addition to the inherited and endogenous factors, man is exposed to various physical, chemical and biological hazards, from the time of conception and these contribute to the development of cancer. This occurs in a multistep sequence, which includes initiation (irreversible mutation resulting in the formation of a transformed cell), monoclonal proliferation of the single transformed cell into tumor mass and progression by local invasion and metastasis. This biology of cancer includes the molecular pathogenesis, progression of tumor and the properties of cancer cells.

THE MOLECULAR PATHOGENESIS OF CANCER

Carcinogenesis occurs in a multistep process. Nonlethal genetic damage of a single cell to a transformed cell and its monoclonal proliferation results in tumor formation. Monoclonality of tumor can be assessed by polymorph X-linked markers like G6PD isoenzymes A or B in females or by X-linked restriction fragment length polymorphisms (RFLP). Genes with DNA and its product the RNA, hold the key of cell replication and the production of amino acids, which are the building blocks of new cells. Five classes of genes are involved in normal growth, and they include:

1. Protooncogenes,
2. Tumor suppressor genes,
3. Genes that regulate apoptosis,
4. Genes that regulate DNA repair, and
5. The genes that act on proofreading enzymes. They act as an eternal vigilant force. This results in very accurate proofreading of the replication of the DNA, and the new DNA similar to the parent DNA is formed.

As mentioned, these genes are involved in normal growth, and their nonlethal damage is associated with the development of cancer. The role of the first four genes in carcinogenesis is better understood now and their role is recapitulated here:

PROTOONCOGENES AND CARCINOGENESIS

Protooncogenes are normal cellular genes whose products are associated with normal growth and differentiation. The mechanism behind normal growth and differentiation is a complicated process and can be compared to that of the activities of a postal department where the letter passing through various hands reaches your mailbox and then your hands for appropriate action. The message for normal growth is triggered by the growth factor, which binds to growth factor receptor on cell membrane. The message is transduced to the cytoplasm by signal transducing proteins. Ultimately the message is carried to the nucleus by the nuclear transcription proteins. These proteins activate nuclear regulatory factors like cyclins and cyclin-dependent kinases, and induce cell growth.

Protooncogenes are converted to oncogenes or cancer causing genes, whose products are associated with tumor growth. This conversion is mediated by transforming retroviruses. V-onc is the viral growth-promoting gene and resembles protooncogene. Retroviruses convert protooncogenes to oncogenes by transfer of V-onc sequences to proto-oncogenes called *retroviral transduction.* V-onc in *f*eline *s*arcoma virus is named V-*fes*, in *s*imian *s*arcoma virus V-*sis* and in *r*at *s*arcoma virus V-*ras*, and the protooncogenes that resemble them are designated fes, sis and ras. The RNA viruses that do not contain V-onc sequences insert their proviral DNA near protooncogene and induce structural change converting them to oncogenes, by the process called *insertional mutagenesis.* Human T-cell leukemic virus-1 (HTLV-1) induces T-lymphocyte neoplasm by a separate mechanism. It activates the genes that encode the cytokine, interleukin-1 and its receptor and thus results in the proliferation of T-cells. Ultimately the conversion of protooncogenes to oncogenes takes place by any of the three structural changes— point mutation, chromosomal translocation or gene amplification.

1. **Point mutation** In this one junction of the DNA gets broken and gets attached to another gene at some other junction, as if one cross- step of the ladder is changed and a new step of different material is placed. The point mutation of ras oncogenes is seen in many tumors as pancreatic carcinoma, colon, thyroid, lung and leukemia. Mutation involving K-ras is associated with carcinomas and N-ras mutations with leukemias.

2. **Chromosomal translocation**, wherein a segment of the chromosome is transferred to another. In Philadelphia chromosome t(9:22), abl protooncogene from chromosome 9 is transferred to the bcr on chromosome 22. The resultant abl-bcr hybrid gene on chromosome 22 encodes a chimeric protein that has tyrosine kinase activity. This is classically associated with chronic myeloid leukemia where the molecular weight of chimeric protein is 210kD and is also seen in acute lymphoid leukemia, where the molecular weight of chimeric protein is 180kD. In Burkitt's lymphoma [t (8:14)], myc protooncogene

on chromosome 8 is translocated very close to the Ig site on the long arm of chromosome 14, resulting in persistent stimulation of myc gene.

3. **Amplification of genes** is characterized by multiplication of proto-oncogenes and the resultant overexpression of products. Amplification is characterized by double minutes or by homogenous staining region. Amplification of N-myc in neuroblastoma and c-erb-B2 in carcinoma of the breast is associated with poor prognosis.

From the above discussion, it is clear that protooncogenes are involved in normal growth, and the mutations in it like point mutation, chromosomal translocation or gene amplification induced by retroviruses convert them into oncogenes. Oncogenes encode proteins called oncoproteins, which resemble normal products of protooncogenes and they are involved in cancer formation. Figure 3.1 depicts the role of protooncogenes in normal cell growth; its conversion to oncogenes and tumor formation.

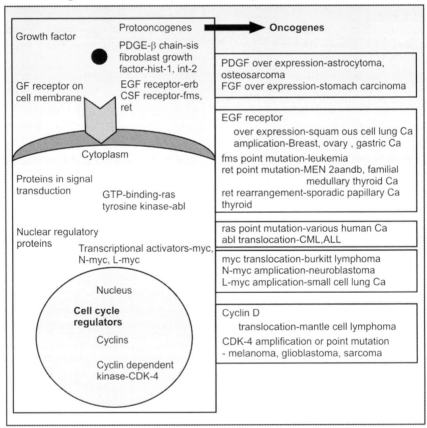

Figure 3.1: On the left side, normal cellular growth with role of protooncogenes at cell membrane, cytoplasmic and nuclear level, and on the right side, mechanism of conversion to oncogenes and the tumors associated with it, is depicted
PDGF- Platelet derived growth factor, EGF-Epidermal growth factor, CSF- Colony stimulating factor

TUMOR SUPPRESSOR GENES

One of the fascinating discoveries in recent times is the identification of this unique gene, the tumor suppressor gene or antioncogene. The physiologic function of this gene is to regulate cell growth or to prevent unregulated cell growth that occurs in tumor. The transformation of a normal cell to a malignant one takes place not only by activation of oncogenes but also by inactivation or deletion of tumor suppressor genes. Similar to protooncogenes that regulate cell growth at varying cellular level, the protein products of tumor suppressor genes also function at varying cellular location. In recent years, many tumor suppressor genes are discovered acting at different cellular levels, namely, Rb, p53, WT-1, p16, BRCA-1 and BRCA-2 at nucleus, APC in cytoplasm, NF-2 at cytoskeleton, NF-1 under the plasma membrane and TGF-b receptor and E-cadherin at cell surface.

Rb Gene

This is the first of its kind discovered. This gene is located on the long arm of chromosome 13 (13q14) and is found in association with the childhood neoplasm, retinoblastoma. The protein product of Rb gene, pRb is a nuclear phosphoprotein that involves in the regulation of cell cycle. Normally there are two alleles of this gene, and it is necessary to inactivate both of them to produce neoplastic transformation as proved by "two hit" hypothesis of Knudson. In familial cases, one of the alleles is hit in the germ line itself and the other is lost as a result of somatic mutation to complete the "two hit". In sporadic cases, both Rb alleles are hit as a result of somatic mutation. Mutations involving this gene are associated with retinoblastoma, osteosarcoma as well as carcinomas of the breast, colon and lung.

P53 Tumor Suppressor Gene

It is located on the short arm of chromosome 17 (17p13). This gene is called the molecular policeman, since it is involved in the repair or apoptosis of genetically damaged cells, as a policeman who maintains law and order. The genetic damage induced by radiation or by chemicals causes a rapid increase in the p53 level and its activation. This activation of p53 induces cell cycle arrest by p21, a CDK inhibitor and this interval in cell cycle allows the cells to induce repair. In case of irreparable genetic damage, p53 induces apoptosis by activation of proapoptotic gene bax. In the cell with mutations or homozygous loss of p53, there is no repair or apoptosis of genetically damaged cells. This results in the formation of transformed cell and the development of neoplasm. Homozygous loss or mutation of this gene is found to be associated with many types of cancers and sarcomas. Individuals with inheritance of a single mutant allele are said to have Li-Fraumeni syndrome, and the somatic "hit" of other genes makes them prone to the development of a malignant tumor at a very young age. Hence p53 can be called the protector of genome.

Other Tumor Suppressor Genes

BRCA-1 and BRCA-2 (breast carcinoma) genes, have already been mentioned in the previous chapter on etiology. The function of these genes is not clear and may be associated with DNA repair. Individuals with inherited mutation of these genes are associated with development of cancer of breast as well as various other organs including ovary. BRCA gene mutations are associated with inherited cancer syndrome and hence familial clustering.

APC (adenomatosis polyposis colon) genes (5q21) are involved in the regulation of signal transduction. Individuals with inherited mutation of single allele develop hundreds of polyps of colon by their early youth. With the "hit" of other allele and with additional mutations including that of p53, one or more of these polyps undergo malignant change leading to the development of colon cancer.

NF-1 and NF-2 Gene

NF-1 is located under plasma membrane and its mutations are associated with schwannomas and sarcomas. NF-2 is located in cytoskeleton and the mutations are associated with acoustic schwannoma and meningiomas.

Development of cancer is a multistep process. The normal cell is transformed to a neoplastic cell. This transformation is induced by DNA damaging agents, physical, chemical and viral factors etc. The transformed cells are characterized by activation of oncogenes, inactivation of cancer suppressor genes and the involvement of DNA repair and proapoptotic genes. Such a single transformed cell proliferates to form the tumor. This growth depends on the various factors and is discussed next.

BIOLOGY OF TUMOR GROWTH

Growth of tumor depends on the growth of the transformed cell, capability for local invasion and distant spread. Growth of transformed cell to a neoplasm depends on the mitotic activity, time required for each proliferation or the doubling time, tumor cell loss by necrosis or apoptosis, stromal support and the blood supply, hormone dependency and the availability of growth factors.

Local invasion and distant spread (metastasis) are the features of malignant tumors. Malignant cells infiltrate into the surrounding tissues and induce tissue destruction. For metastasis, cells first detach from the primary mass due to the loss of intercellular adhesion molecules like epithelial (E) cadherin. Such loose cells penetrate into extracellular matrix by receptor-mediated attachment of tumor cell to laminin and fibronectin, and they migrate through extracellular matrix by proteolytic enzymes like collagenase. Using the same mechanism, they migrate through the basement membrane of blood or lymphatic vessels and intravasate. Within the circulation, they are covered by platelet aggregates and form a tumor embolus. Embolus is carried to a distant site, deposits and proliferates and forms the metastasis.

THE PROPERTIES OF A TUMOR CELL

The tumors are divided into two main types, benign and malignant. There is also an intermediate type, which does not fit into the classical definition. The cells of the benign tumor resemble the parent tissue and hence are well differentiated. As the cells in these types of tumors divide slowly, there are only a few mitotic progeny. In case of malignant tumors, there is loss of differentiation and orientation of cells and the normal cellular pattern seen in the epithelial or glandular tissues are absent. The loss in the uniformity of cells and in their architectural orientation is referred to as *dysplasia*. The cells of malignant tumor show characteristics that range from well differentiated to poorly differentiated or undifferentiated. Such lack of differentiation is termed *anaplasia*. It was Hansmann who, in 1880, first suggested that anaplasia is one of the common signs of malignancy. The cells show pleomorphism (variation in size and shape). These cells have a large nucleus when compared to the cytoplasmic volume and there would be hyperchromatism. This is due to the increased amount of chromatin in the cell nuclei resulting in increased amount of stain with hematoxylin. In all malignant cells, there is considerable mitotic activity as the DNA is the seat of brisk replication. Normal mitosis is biradiate; while in malignancy it may be triradiate and this feature may go on to daughter cells. Another interesting feature in anaplasia is the appearance of multinucleate giant cells, and the important reason for its formation is endonuclear mitosis without cell division. The cytoplasm of the tumor cell may resemble the normal counterpart or show variation depending upon the differentiation.

The presence of anaplasia and dysplasia along with presence of abnormal or atypical mitosis limited to epithelium and with intact basement membrane is called *carcinoma in situ*. This is considered to be pre-invasive state of malignancy.

In addition, the tumor cells can show functional differentiation, and a well developed tumor cell elaborates the functions by its normal counterpart, as in the production of keratin by well differentiated squamous cell carcinoma or mucin by adenocarcinoma, hormones by endocrine tumors or production of immunoglobulins by myeloma cells. They can also perform abnormal functions like the production of ectopic hormones discussed with paraneoplastic syndromes or the various oncofetal antigens discussed with tumor markers. The various genetic changes like ploidy (variation in chromosomal number), translocations and deletions, have already been discussed. Electron microscopic changes are also important aspects of tumor cells and at times evaluated for diagnostic and prognostic purpose. An equally important part of the tumor is the stroma composed of connective tissue and blood supply and it provides supportive framework, on which the tumor cells grow and receive nourishment.

CELL KINETICS

The cell kinetics was the subject of study in many of the cancer research centers. It was found that the replication of cells is faster in the early period of the growth. Later, even in the rapid growing tumors the cell turnover is slower than in normal tissues as in hematopoietic and gastrointestinal systems. The difference is explained by the fact that the cell removal system is inadequate or they escape the genetically programmed cell death—the apoptosis. It is also noted that most of the cells in a progressive tumor are outside the replicate phase and the growth index is only 20 percent of the total cellular pool. High growth factor is seen in some of the lymphomas. The clinical implication of the study of cell kinetics is that most of the chemotherapeutic agents act on the dividing cells, and tumors with high growth index are more susceptible to chemotherapeutic agents. Another concept that has been evolved in the study of cell kinetics is the latent period of the progression of tumors. If all the cancer cells are in the replicate pool, a tumor will be clinically noticeable in its early period of initiation. Usually it does not happen that way. The early dividing cells after a time move to the resting phase and only after many months and years the tumor becomes manifest.

HOST RESPONSES TO NEOPLASTIC CELLS

The antigenic make-up of tumor cells as shown in experimental rodents undergoes simplification. They may lose some of the antigens of the cells from which they were derived. This phenomenon may explain the fact that certain tumors can be successfully transplanted into more than one genetically distinct host. However, there is also evidence that neoplastic cells provoke an immune reaction in the animal in which they arise; the most convincing evidence comes from experiments in which a chemically induced tumor is transplanted into mice belonging to a pure cell line, with the same genotype.

Nearly all the animal tumors that have been tested, whether provoked by a chemical carcinogen or by a virus, or arising spontaneously, have been shown to contain antigens, which produce specific immune responses. Chemical carcinogens produce tumors, which possess antigens specific to each individual tumor and not to the chemical, whereas in virus-produced tumors the antigen is specific for the virus. Tumor cell antigens could be tumor specific or could be expressed or shared in various tumors, or it could be derived from oncogenic virus, like the E-7 proteins of HPV-16. CALLA antigen or CD 10 is yet another type of antigen seen in B cell leukemia and lymphomas. This is called a differentiation antigen, as it is normally seen in immature B cells.

Clinical and pathological findings in man are consistent with the presence of immune responses to neoplastic cells. Many tumors induce a cellular reaction of T and B cells and natural killer cells, which infiltrate the tissue at the edge of the advancing mass of malignant cells. These cells may be said to be troops in retreat. Had they been victorious, it is unlikely that the tumor would have come to the pathologist's attention. Another hypothesis, is the concept that neoplasm occurs in the tissues and organs of the body much more frequently than is generally supposed. The cells so formed are recognized as 'foreign' by the body's immuno-logical mechanisms and are destroyed before they become sufficiently numerous to form a tumor. Only an occasional lesion 'gets away' and develops to form a clinical tumor.

Suppression of the immune response by drugs used to alter the response to organ transplantation is associated with an increased incidence of tumors of the reticuloendothelial system and higher incidence of malignant neoplasms in the elderly may be related to impaired immunity mechanisms. The appearance of Kaposi's sarcoma and lymphomas in HIV patients is an example of malignancy in immunocompromised patients. The possibility exists of utilizing the immune reaction as a means of bringing about rejection of tumors in humans although the problem is fraught with ethical and practical problems.

Secondary growths occur predominantly in certain organs. Other organs and tissues in the body are only rarely involved. Frequent sites of secondary tumor growth are lymph nodes, lungs, liver, brain and skeleton, while the spleen and the skeletal muscles are usually spared. Some of this distribution may be attributable to the arrangement of the vascular and lymphatic circulation. From a primary tumor in any part of the body, mobile cancer cells that enter the venous system are carried to the lungs; cells from primary tumors of the gastrointestinal tract entering the portal vein must reach the liver. However, it is difficult to explain why certain tumors show a tissue predilection of their secondary growth; thus carcinoma of the lung metastasizes frequently to the adrenal glands and the brain, and carcinoma of the prostate shows a marked tendency to metastasize to bone. Lacking any real understanding of the factors involved which cannot be explained on such simple grounds as distribution of circulation, we take refuge in a 'seed and soil' theory. This suggests that the differences are in part explicable on the basis of the varying degree of local tissue immunity.

Now let us pause. The whole of this chapter is used for giving the readers all the negative and positive factors that converge on the nuclei for transformation from a friendly cell to a killer cell. The last word is still obscure but oncologists are moving closer in their understanding of the different ways in which human cancer is caused. There are many checks and counterchecks to prevent the development of a mutant gene. These checks are built in every genetic code of a normal gene. The normal cell may be bombarded with DNA damaging agents such as ionizing radiation, chemicals, and viruses or inherited familial tumor producing gene at different times in its life. If the external physical agent is capable of causing damage to the genetic code, the damaged DNA undergoes repair successfully particularly with an efficient proofreading gene so that cancer-producing gene is removed. If by any chance the genetic damage is not repaired, mutations can occur leading to a further step in carcinogenesis. If these changes go uncontrolled, a cancer-producing clone appears which ultimately becomes a clinical cancer. It must not be forgotten that most of us are saved by the onslaught of the dreaded disease by body's own protective mechanism. Biology of carcinogenesis is a complicated subject and we do not intend to make it more complicated by giving too many details. However well we describe the subject, it is still incomplete. For further details on carcinogenesis, we advise the students to refer detailed textbooks on pathology.

FURTHER READING

1. Birchmeier W. E-cadherin as a tumor (invasion) suppressor gene. BioEssays 1995;17:97.
2. Chang F. Implications of the p53 tumor suppressor gene in clinical oncology. J Clin Oncol 1995;13:1009.
3. Cossman J. Molecular genetics in cancer diagnosis. New York, Elsevier, 1990.
4. Horowiz JM, Park SH, et al. Frequent inactivation of the retinoblastoma anti-oncogene is restricted to a subset of human tumor cells. Proc Natl Acad Sci USA 1994;87:2775-79.
5. Klein G. Epstein–Barr virus strategy in normal and neoplastic B cells. Cell 1994;77:791.
6. Levine AJ, Momand J, et al. The p53 tumor suppressor gene. Nature 1991; 351:453-56.
7. Mac Donald F, Ford CHJ (Eds). Molecular Biology of Cancer. Bios Scientific Publishers Ltd, Oxford, 1997;73-97.
8. Ruoslahi E. How cancer spreads. Sci Am 1996;275:72.
9. Terdiman JP, Conrad PG, Sleisenger MH. Genetic testing in hereditary colorectal cancer: indications and procedures. Am J Gastroenterol 1999;94:2344-56.
10. Weinberg RA. How cancer arises. Review on the molecular basis of cancer. Sci Am 1996;275:62.

by several registries. Survival rate compilation and end result analysis are being done by Actuarial Method, Kaplan Meier method, and Relative Survival Rate estimation is being increasingly utilized for assessing survival. Statistical techniques like Age Adjusted Rate, Risk Ratios etc have been developed for effective comparison of cancer occurrence among populations.

CANCER REGISTRIES

Cancer registries provide systematically collected essential data for all study activities and in cancer control. A cancer registry can be defined as an organization for the collection, storage, analysis and interpretation of data on persons with cancer on a continuing basis'.

Three basic types of registries may be identified.

The hospital based registry is organized in a hospital or a group of hospitals for systematic cancer case recording for studies of cases seen in the hospital.

The population based registry is organized for a well defined population and records all newly diagnosed cancer cases occurring among the residents in the population ('Resident' here is defined as a person who has lived in the defined population area for at least 1 year prior to diagnosis of cancer) (ICMR–NCRP).

The special purpose registry addresses issues related to a specific cancer type or of specific exposure e.g. lymphoma registry, bone cancer registry, pediatric cancer registry and exposure related registry like the Bhopal Cancer Registry associated with exposure to MIC gas, or the Karunagappally Cancer Registry (Kerala, India) to study the problems of chronic exposure to high natural radiation respectively.

All these special purpose registries collect data on biologic and prognostic factors or exposure levels. This may require periodic updating. A cohort approach for observation and analysis is required in these studies. Various statistical methodologies have been used for collection and analysis of data obtained from the above mentioned registration systems.

In India and in several developing countries cancer is not a noticeable disease and due to this cancer registries collect information on cancer by an active cancer registration method by visiting patients in hospitals, homes and other locations where cancer patients are seen.

REGISTRY STANDARDS

Apart from these, any cancer registration process has to define and strictly observe a reference date of registry i.e. (a) the date of onset of registration, (b) list of reportable neoplasms and (c) provision for strict annual follow-up of cases.

The registry should develop in-house methods to enhance data quality, viz. high percentage of microscopic verified cases, duplicate elimination, a low mortality to incidence ratio, consistency checks and strict norms for inclusion or exclusion of cases and for obtaining complete information on every patient.

MEASURES OF DISEASE OCCURRENCE

A universally accepted standard measure of occurrence of cancer in a population is the 'Incidence rate'. This is provided only by a Population Based Cancer Registry.

This rate is defined by WHO as follows

$$\text{Incidence Rate} = \frac{\text{The number of new cases of cancer occurring in a defined population in a year} \times 100{,}000}{\text{Total population at risk during the year}}$$

Generally when a registry collates data of a few years, the denominator i.e. population at risk is multiplied by the number of years of registration and denoted as 'Person years' at risk.

CRUDE INCIDENCE RATE

This is always expressed as an annual rate per 100,000 population and the word 'incidence rate' is used only in this context.

To obtain this rate, knowledge of a well defined population and a mechanism to record continuously all cancer cases arising in this defined population during the year are essential along with the necessary methods for data scrutiny and processing. The population study should be defined as that residing in a certain geographic area or a group of people with known age and gender distribution. The cancer cases recorded are checked for consistency etc. and tabulated according to age and gender and then related to the base population similarly tabulated. This ratio is multiplied by 100,000. As the proportion of cancer cases occurring in any population is low, the ratio is multiplied by 100,000 to obtain a workable number.

Crude incidence rate can thus be calculated if the numerator and denominator are known and in relation to a period which as mentioned above, is a year. The rate is obtained for males and females separately and for each 5 year age group and site/type of cancer. When the number of new cancer cases in a particular age group during one year is divided by the population in that age group and multiplied by 100,000, the rate is identified as 'age specific incidence rate'. Age specific incidence rates are obtained for each 5-year age groupings and there can be 17 or 18 such 5-year age grouping covering 0-80 years of age in a given population. Similar tabulation is done for each cancer site.

The crude incidence rate in a population is the appropriate measure of the cancer occurrence in the studied population and is most essential for planning patient services, epidemiologic studies and for implementing control programs.

However, for identifying risk differences in relation to life style etc, comparison of incidence rates between the experiences of two populations is resorted to. By such comparisons, the hypothesis is developed and in-depth statistically designed studies especially case-control studies are employed. While comparing the incidence rates of two population groups, it is important that the data capture methods and processing are similar and comparable.

AGE ADJUSTED INCIDENCE RATE (AAR)

It will be seen from the age specific rates that cancer incidence increases with age. Due to this, populations, which have high proportion of old age people, will have high crude incidence rates. The summary index–Crude Incidence Rate–is thus seen to be compounded with the age structure of the population. While comparing the incidence rates of the disease with other population groups, age specific rates are the best. At the same time, when there are 18 age groups to be compared it is almost impossible to comprehend or summarize the differences. To facilitate such comparisons the age standardized or age adjusted rates are obtained.

The population based cancer registry data obtained for a population is made comparable to other population based cancer data only after eliminating the age disparities between the populations. This is done by estimating cancer incidence in a standard population with an assumed age distribution based on the data from the population study. This process is known as age standardization and the estimated rates are known as Age Adjusted Rates (AAR). The IARC-WHO has defined the standard population now identified as World Standard Population (WP). This was first described in 1960 by Mitsuo Segi from Japan. The age specific rates obtained by a Cancer Registry is applied to the age distribution of the Standard Population (WP) and the incidence rate. World Population (WP) is constructed by pooling data of age adjusted population rate with predominantly older age group as in the US and with younger age group as in developing countries. AAR is estimated for the standard population. The AAR is thus made comparable to other population-based reported rates which are similarly converted to AAR. Calculation of AAR is shown in Table 4.1.

The US Connecticut white males had an all cancer crude rate (1993-1997) of 571.8 and females had 523.8 per 100,000 population. Compared to this, the Mumbai males had a rate of 68.8 and females had 80.4 per 100,000 population (1993-1997). The higher rate seen in the US is partly due to the higher proportion of the population in old age groups in the US compared to the population of Mumbai. This is demonstrated by the AAR. The AAR (WP) for US Connecticut for 1993-1997 was 378.6 for males

Table 4.1: Calculation of crude, age adjusted and truncated adjusted rates, Karunagappally Cancer Registry, 1993-97 (5 years)

Age	No. of cases	Population	Age specific rates	World population	Expected cases in WP	TAR
	(A)	(B)	(C)	(D)	(E)	(F)
0 – 4	11	16546	13.3	12000	1.6	
5 – 9	10	17129	11.7	10000	1.2	
10 – 14	6	19631	6.0	9000	0.5	
15 – 19	10	19005	10.8	9000	1.0	
20 – 24	14	20718	13.8	8000	1.1	
25 – 29	13	18795	14.1	8000	1.1	
30 – 34	16	16246	19.6	6000	1.2	
35 – 39	32	16800	38.3	6000	2.3	$\underline{55.8 \times 100{,}000}$
40 – 44	36	11858	60.9	6000	3.7	31,000
45 – 49	76	9813	154.3	6000	9.3	= 180/100,000
50 – 54	77	7703	200.1	5000	10.0	
55 – 59	119	7243	328.8	4000	13.2	
60 – 64	138	6390	431.9	4000	17.3	
65 – 69	137	5340	512.7	3000	15.4	
70 – 74	111	2770	801.2	2000	16.0	
75 +	89	4570	389.9	2000	7.8	
Total	895	2,00,557	89.5	1,00,000	102.7	

(Data Source–P. Gangadharan, P. Jayalekshmi. Cancer Morbidity & Mortality in Karunagappally 1993-97, Regional Cancer Centre, 2000.

WP- World Standard Population).

and 304.3 for females-much lower than the crude incidence rates. In Mumbai, the AAR were 116.3 and 122.4.

Using different standard populations one can obtain different Age Adjusted Rates. By this, it is to be noted that AAR is a fictitious rate and can be used mainly for comparison with data from other registries.

CUMULATIVE RATE

The Crude Incidence Rates and the Age Adjusted Incidence Rates offer summary indices of cancer occurrence. Another summary measure of cancer occurrence is the cumulative rate and cumulative risk.

The cumulative rate is an approximation for cumulative risk. The cumulative rate has several advantages over Age-Standardized Rates. Firstly as a form of direct standardization, the problem of choosing an arbitrary reference population is eliminated. Secondly as an approximation to the cumulative risk, it has a greater intuitive appeal, and is more directly interpretable as a measurement of lifetime risk, assuming no other cause of death is in operation.

The cumulative rate is not in fact a rate but a dimensionless quantity. It is not expressed in units of 'per annum' but simply as a number. It is expressed as a percentage. The methodology for obtaining this value is quite simple.

Cumulative rate 0-80 years = 5 × Sum of Age Specific (5-year age groups) Incidence Rates in the 0-80 age groups.

TRUNCATED AGE STANDARDIZED RATE (TASR/TAR)

Doll and Cook (1967) suggested a truncated age range 35-64 years for comparison between population experiences. The argument was that the rates observed at old ages, which are presumably due in part to a state of affairs that existed in the more distant past and may now be altered are less relevant than the rates at younger ages. Further, the number of cases reported in older ages are liable to be less accurate than those at younger ages. The deficiencies in reporting the cause of death in old ages, provision of medical care and diagnosis in old ages are factors that influence the cancer case identification. A good proportion of the causes of death reported in old age groups is observed to be non-specific–'cardiorespiratory failure' or 'old age'-especially in developing countries. In many developing countries death registration is not undertaken for all deaths even though it is made mandatory for disposal of the body. The age specific rates in the truncated age period 35-64 is standardized using the World Population Standard of 35-64 years, and the Truncated Age Standardized Rates are obtained (Calculation shown in Table 4.1).

HOSPITAL REGISTRY DATA

Hospital cancer registries (HCR) record all cancer cases seen in a hospital and information is collected and analyzed regarding the stage or extent of the disease, treatment, survival and for each cancer site. The NCRP-ICMR has developed procedure norms and code manuals for recording cancer cases in Hospital and Population Cancer Registries. Patient care evaluation is the major thrust area of the HCR. HCR data does not provide incidence of cancer but it provides an efficient data set to plan and conduct etiological and epidemiological studies, case-control studies, clinical trials, studies on therapy outcome, prognostic factors etc. The ten year consolidated report of the Hospital Based Cancer Registries 1984-1993 of NCRP-ICMR published in 2001 presents several aspects of cancer patient management.

From a hospital-based or institution-based data one can get the relative frequencies e.g. if in a hospital 3500 cancer cases are seen annually of which 350 had oral cancer, the frequency ratio of oral cancer seen in the hospital is 10 percent. This is not the incidence rate. This signifies the importance of the problem as seen in the particular hospital only. The patients in a hospital are very sensitive about the policy and facilities in the hospital and several other known and unknown factors. The NCRP-ICMR has 5 hospital based registries and the data from these registries indicate that only about 10 percent of all cancer is seen in initial stages when first seen. If control program has to be effective a much higher percentage of cases should be made to undergo treatment in the earlier stages of the disease.

Incidence rate is an absolute measure whereas hospital based data gives only relative ratios and hence is unstable. Conclusions derived from comparison between two hospital series can be misleading. This is shown in Table 4.2.

In the two series of cases A and B, the relative frequencies are shown as percentage. Incidence rates are calculated with A having a population of 400,000 and B 250,000 people. The Crude Incidence rates obtained are shown as CI. Lung cancer was 15 percent of total in A, but B had higher percentage viz. 20 percent. However, the incidence rate was similar in both the populations being 11 per 100,000. Oral cancer had almost similar relative frequencies, with a slight excess in series B but incidence rate was lesser in B than in A. Breast cancer relative frequency and incidence rates were both increased in series A. Similar inconsistencies are found between the relative frequencies and incidence rates which make them non-comparable.

The following are some of the rates and ratios used in Cancer Epidemiologic Studies.

$$\text{Point Prevalence} = \frac{\text{No. of existing cancer cases in a defined population at any one point in time}}{\text{No. of people in the defined population at the same point in time}}$$

Table 4.2: The comparison of cancer types between two series of cases A & B are shown and discussed					
Site	*A*	*%*	*CI*	*B*	*%*	*CI*
Lung	45	15.0	11.3	29	20.7	11.6
Oral Cancer	60	20.0	15.0	30	21.4	12.0
Breast	75	25.0	18.7	24	17.1	9.6
Cervix	90	30.0	22.5	42	30.0	16.8
Others	30	10.0	7.5	15	10.7	6.0
Total Cases	300	100.0	75.0	140	100.0	56.0
Population:	A – 400,000		B – 250,000		CI – Crude Incidence	

$$\text{Risk} = \frac{\text{No. of new cases of diseases arising in a defined population over a given period of time}}{\text{No. of disease free people in that population at the beginning of that time period}}$$

$$\text{Odds of Disease} = \frac{\text{No. of new cases of diseases arising in a defined population over a given period of time}}{\text{No. of people in that population who remain disease free during that time period}}$$

Prevalence = Incidence rate × Average duration of diseases.

$$\text{Risk Ratio} = \frac{\text{Risk in the exposed group}}{\text{Risk in the unexposed group}}$$

$$\text{Rate Ratio} = \frac{\text{Incidence rate in the exposed group}}{\text{Incidence rate in the unexposed group}}$$

$$\text{Odds Ratio} = \frac{\text{Odds of the disease in the exposed group}}{\text{Odds of the disease in the unexposed group}}$$

GLOBAL CANCER INCIDENCE DATA

Cancer Incidence in 5 Continents (Ref Ch 5 Vol VIII–IARC)

Among all diseases, it is unique that only on cancer, statistical data have been gathered from populations uniformly and repeatedly across the 5 continents. Volume VIII of CI 5 published in 2002 by IARC contains population based cancer incidence data from 214 population groups living in 60 countries. From India, 9 population groups have reported the incidence data in this. These data have been collected, standardized, uniformly scrutinized and processed and remain the single largest compiled data set on cancer across the 5 continents.[11]

CANCER REGISTRIES IN INDIA

Cancer data collection has been undertaken in India by several workers since the past 6 to 8 decades. The first Population Cancer Registry was established by the Indian Cancer Society in 1963 covering the Greater Mumbai population. Mumbai had several large well-equipped hospitals and further, all the deaths needed medical certification before dispensing the body. After the National Cancer Control Program was initiated in 1974, the National Cancer Registry Programme (NCRP) was started by ICMR in 1981 and the Mumbai Cancer Registry became a part of it. Under NCRP, 6 population based cancer registries are now functioning. They cover the population in Mumbai, Chennai, Bangalore, Bhopal, Delhi and Barshi. Simultaneously Hospital based cancer registries were started in Tata Memorial Hospital Mumbai, Kidwai Institute of Oncology Bangalore, Cancer Institute (WIA) Chennai, Medical College Dibrugarh, Regional Cancer Centre Trivandrum and PGI Chandigarh. Cancer registries under ICMR network have well programmed review meetings and the functioning is highly standardized to International Standards. There are registries outside this ICMR-NCRP network. They are PBCR (population based cancer registry) at Ahmedabad, Pune, Nagpur, Aurangabad, Kolkata, Trivandrum, Karunagappally and Ambilikkai. Most of them are rural registries. Lack of cancer data from rural populations in India is thus a major obstacle in collecting true data of cancer patients. The difficulties for organizing a rural cancer registry especially in areas where there are no cancer diagnostic and treatment facilities are enormous. The poor death registration system additionally contributes to the difficulties. The rural area in Karunagappally and Trivandrum in Kerala cannot be considered as typically rural as the Kerala rural area would appear only as an extension of an urban area. The available incidence rates from different registration areas are shown in Table 4.3. There are site-wise variations in incidence rates and these will have to be continuously monitored. Further, populations hitherto not covered by registry operations will have to be brought under registry set up. Wider collection of data for the rural areas is necessary to build up a more valid database for cancer in India.

CANCER PATIENT SURVIVAL DATA

The ultimate objective of cancer control is to reduce deaths from cancer. This is almost the same as increase of survival rate from cancer. Programs for prevention, early detection, successful treatment etc. can reduce morbidity and thus mortality. Survival rate is related to appropriate and timely treatment. Hence survival rate assessment is a major function of any cancer control program. In a hospital setting patients get selective treatment and optimal outcome can be expected. However, the cancer survival experience in a population reflects the overall delivery of care of the cancer patient also, hence it is a measure of control efforts.

Survival rate estimation is resorted to because the survival time of all cases of cancer seen in a population is not available. Some are censored due to loss in follow-up or death due to intercurrent illness. Actuarial method of survival estimation utilizes the information regarding maximum survival time and to obtain probability of survival in a given period. Kaplan Meier estimate also utilizes such censored information. A third method is to estimate relative survival rate. This gives a survival rate as percentage of normal life expectancy (refer Cancer Survival in Developing Countries–IARC Technical Report No. 145).

Table 4.3: Age adjusted cancer incidence in various registry areas in India

Source	Registry population	AAR Male	AAR Female	Registry organization
CI5 Vol VIII	Ahmedabad 93-97	107.2	82.9	Gujarat Cancer and Research Institute, DD Patel, PM Shah et al.
CRAB*	Aurangabad 94	61.7	56.8	Indian Cancer Society, BB Yeole, DJ Jussawala et al.
CI5 Vol VIII	Bangalore 93-97	88.3	110.7	Kidwai Memorial Institute, PS Prabhakaran, Aruna Prasad et al.
ICMR**	Barshi 90-96	46.2	57.7	Nargis Dutt Memorial Cancer Hospital, B.M. Nene, A.M. Budukh
ICMR**	Bhopal 90-96	100.4	92.2	Gandhi Medical College, S. Kanhere, S. Surange et al.
CI5 Vol VIII	Chennai 93-97	108.0	118.0	Cancer Institute (WIA), V. Shanta, V. Gajalekshmy et al.
CI5 Vol VIII	Delhi 93-96	123.7	135.6	Rotary Cancer Hospital, Kusum Verma, B.B. Thyagi et al.
CI5 Vol VIII	Karunagappally 93-97	102.6	76.0	Regional Cancer Centre, P. Gangadharan, P. Jayalekshmi
CRAB*	Kolkata@ 90-97	68.4	82.0	Chittaranjan National Cancer Centre, M. Siddiqi, Urmi Sen et al.
CI5 Vol VIII	Mumbai 93-97	116.3	122.4	Indian Cancer Society, B.B. Yeole
CI5 Vol VIII	Nagpur 93-97	118.4	118.8	Indian Cancer Society, B.B. Yeole, Varsha Sagadev
CI5 Vol VIII	Pune 93-97	103.9	115.3	Indian Cancer Society, B.B. Yeole, Asha Prathinidhi
RCC	Trivandrum R 98-99	85.5	70.2	Regional Cancer Centre, A. Mathew, Vijayaprasad
RCC	Trivandrum U 98-99	93.8	90.8	Regional Cancer Centre, A. Mathew, Vijayaprasad
CCC	Ambilikkai 96-98	89.3	122.3	Christian Fellowship Community Health Centre, R. Rajkumar, R. Sankaranarayanan et al.

CI–Cancer international 5 continents
CRAB–News letter of the National Cancer Registry Project of India, Vol. VIII, 2001
RCC Regional cancer centre. Trivandrum
CCC–Jl of Cancer, Control and Causes
** Consolidated Report of the Population Based Cancer Registries 1990-1996, Prepared by Dr. A. Nandakumar, ICMR, August 2001.
@ Deaths are not included. Hence minimum rates.   R–Rural U–Urban
Note: The AAR is high in women at Ambilikkai, a village in S.India, compared to other areas in India.

Table 4.4. Five year relative survival rates

Cervical cancer		Breast cancer	
Barshi (88-92)	33.3%	Bangalore (82-89)	45.1%
Bangalore (82-89)	40.4%	Mumbai (82-86)	55.1%
Mumbai (82-86)	50.7%	Chennai (84-89)	49.5%
Chennai (84-89)	60.0%		

		5-Year relative survival rates - Other sites			
Chennai	%	Chennai	%	Bangalore	%
Lip	46.1	Hodgkin's disease	40.2	58.0	
Tongue	25.8	NHL	21.1	34.5	
Oral Cavity	32.8	Lymphatic leukemia	25.4	30.7	
Oropharynx	20.9	Myeloid leukemia	17.0	21.5	
Hypopharynx	17.5	All leukemias	21.6	23.4	
Esophagus	6.8				
Stomach	7.8				
Pancreas	5.0				
Larynx	39.0				
Lung	7.5				
Bladder	22.8				

Cancer survival in developing countries – IARC Scientific Publication No. 145 gives a well systematized survival analysis from 10 population based cancer registries in India. The data presented from the Indian registries are tabulated in Table 4.4.

FURTHER READING

1. Armitage P, Berry G. Statistical Methods in Medical Research (3rd ed). Oxford: Blackwell Scientific Publications, 1994.
2. Breslow NE, Day NE. Statistical Methods in Cancer Research Vol. I, IARC Scientific Publications, 1980;32.
3. Breslow NE, Day NE. Statistical Methods in Cancer Research Vol. II, IARC Scientific Publications, 1987;82.
4. Cancer Epidemiology, Principles and Methods. Isabel dos Snatos Silva. International Agency for Research on Cancer, Lyon, France, 1999.
5. Cancer Incidence in Five Continents, Vol. VIII. Parkin DM, Whelan SL, et al. IARC Scientific Publication 155, IARC, 2002.
6. Cancer Registration and Its Techniques. Robert Maclennan, Calum Muir, Ruth Steinitz, Ali Winkler. IARC Scientific Publication 21, IARC, 1978.
7. Cancer Registration, Principles and Methods. Jensen OM, Parkin DM, et al. IARC Scientific Publication 1996;95.
8. Cancer Survival in Developing countries, Sankaranarayan R, Black RJ, Parkin DM, IARC Scientific Publications 145,2000.
9. Cutler SJ, Ederer F. Maximum utilization of the life table method in analyzing survival. Jl Chronic Dis 1958;8:699-712.

10. Doll R, Cook P. Summarizing indices for comparison of cancer incidence data. Int J Cancer 1967;2:269-79.
11. Evergreen Problems in Epidemiology. Leena Tankamen (Ed). Publications – 3 University of Tampare, School of Public Health, Finland, 1999.
12. Kaplan EL, Meier P. Non parametric estimation from incomplete observations. J Am Stat Assoc 1958;53:457-81.
13. Mathe A, Vijayaprasad B. Population based cancer registry, Thrivandrum 1997-1998.
14. Michel P, Coleman J, Esteve P. Trends in Cancer Incidence and Mortality. IARC Scientific Publications 121, IARC, 1993.
15. Nandakumar A,Thimma Shetty KT. National Cancer Registry Programme (ICMR), Two years report of the population based cancer registres 1997-1998, ICMR, 2002.
16. National Cancer Registry Programme (ICMR), Consolidated Report of the Population Based Cancer Registries 1990-96. Prepared by Nandakumar A. ICMR, New Delhi, August 2001.
17. National Cancer Registry Programme (ICMR), Ten years consolidated Report of Hospital Registries 1984-1993 Prepared by Nandakumar A, Muralidhar. ICMR, New Delhi, December 2001.
18. Nicholas Day. Cumulative Rate and Cumulative Risk. Cancer Incidence in 5 Continents Vol. V. Calum Muir, John Waterhouse, Tom Mack et al. IARC Scientific Publication 88, IARC, 1987.
19. Ray FB, Parkin DM, Whelan SL, et al. Age Standardization Cancer Incidence in Five Continents Vol. VIII. IARC Scientific Publications 2002, 155:87-89.
20. The Role of the Registry in Cancer Control. Parkin DM, Wagner G, Muir C. IARC Scientific Publication 66, IARC, 1985.

Epidemiology of Cancer and Prevention of Cancer in India

5

Aleyamma Mathew, B Rajan

INTRODUCTION

Cancer is increasingly being recognized as a global public health problem and the outcome still remains gloomy despite advances in diagnosis and treatment. Epidemiological studies provide compelling evidence that many cancers are preventable. It is widely held that 80-90 percent of human cancers are attributable to environment and life-style factors such as tobacco, alcohol and dietary habits. Cancer prevention includes primary prevention (avoiding carcinogenic substances in the environment or known high-risk dietary factors) and secondary prevention (detection and removal of benign neoplasm and early detection of oral, cervical and breast cancers). An international agency for research on cancer estimated that over 10 million new cases of cancer occurred in 1996 (nearly two thirds from developing countries) and over 7 million people died of cancer.

CANCER EPIDEMIOLOGY IN INDIA

In India, the absolute number of new cancer patients is increasing rapidly, due to the growth in size of the population, and increase in the proportion of elderly persons as a result of improved life expectancy following control of communicable diseases. The life expectancy has steadily risen from 32 years for males and 31 years for females in 1947 to 63 years and 64 years respectively in 1996, indicating a shift in demographic profile. Such changes in the age structure would automatically alter the disease pattern associated with aging and increase the burden of problems such as cancer, cardiovascular and other non-communicable diseases in the society.

CANCER REGISTRIES IN INDIA

Population-based cancer registry (PBCR) is the source of data in estimating the incidence and mortality as it records data on all cancer cases occurring in a defined region. Data on cancer incidence has been available since 1963 from the Bombay Cancer Registry (now Mumbai Cancer Registry), the first PBCR established in India. Realizing the paucity of data on the magnitude of cancer problem in India, the Indian Council of Medical Research (ICMR) initiated a national cancer registry program in 1982 to set up cancer registries in different regions of India. The ICMR-based registries have expanded over the years and now consist of 6 PBCR (5 urban and 1 rural-based). There are some other PBCRs in Kerala, West Bengal, Ahmedabad and Maharashtra (excluding Mumbai) that are not under ICMR. Although the population covered by these registries is very minimal (5% of Indian population), they give some idea of the extent of the cancer problem in the country.

CANCER INCIDENCE AND MORTALITY RATES IN INDIA

The age-adjusted incidence rates of all cancers vary from 46 to 122 per 100,000 males (Figs 5.1 and 5.2) and 57 to 136 per 100,000 females (Figs 5.3 and 5.4) in the various urban and rural registries. The incidence rates were quite low for men and women in rural population compared to the urban counterparts.(Figs 5.3 and 5.4). However, in terms of the absolute number the incidence per se is very large. In 1992, NCRP gave an estimation that the number of new cancer patients in the country would be around 0.8 million by the turn of the century. The lifetime cumulative risk indicates that an average of one out of 10 to 13 people in the urban areas is stricken by cancer during their lifetime.

In India, cancer mortality rates are under-reported due to poor recording of the cause of death. Mumbai cancer registry has reported that the age-adjusted mortality rate (AAMR) is 61 per 100,000 males and 58 per 100,000 females. The AAMR per 100,000 population for males and females in Bangalore is 35 and 29 and in Chennai 42 and 30 respectively.

CANCER INCIDENCE PATTERN IN DIFFERENT REGIONS IN INDIA

Lung, esophagus, stomach, oral and pharyngeal cancers are the predominant cancers in men. In women, cancers of the cervix and the breast (these two cancers together account for nearly 40 percent of all female cancers) are the predominant ones followed by those of the stomach and the esophagus (Tables 5.1 to 5.4). There is variation in the site-wise distribution within the various population groups. Esophageal cancers are often found in the Southern states of India such as in Bangalore and Chennai and also in Mumbai and Ahmedabad. Stomach cancers are more common in Southern India with the highest incidence in Chennai. Cancers of oral

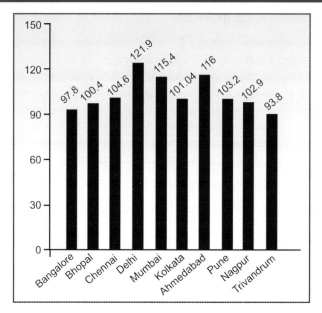

Figure 5.1: Cancer incidence rates in India per 100,000 males (Urban)

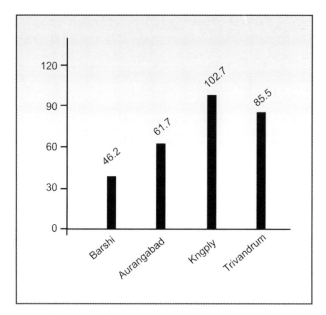

Figure 5.2: Cancer incidence rates in India per 100,000 males (Rural)

cavity are high in Kerala (Southern India) and pharyngeal cancers in Mumbai (western India). Thyroid cancers among women are more common in Kerala. Gallbladder cancer is high in northern India, particularly in Delhi area.

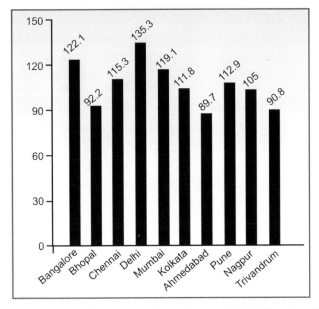

Figure 5.3: Cancer incidence rates in India per 100,000 females (Urban)

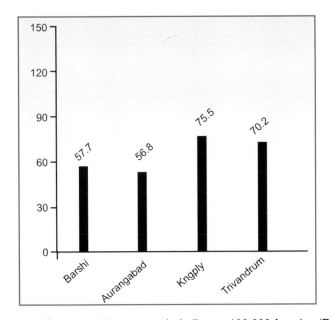

Figure 5.4: Cancer incidence rates in India per 100,000 females (Rural)

TRENDS IN INCIDENCE RATES OF COMMON CANCERS IN INDIA

Trends in the risk of cancer with time are of particular interest since they imply changes in exposure to environmental factors. Trend analysis of

Table 5.1: Age-adjusted (World-population) incidence rates (AAR) of 10 leading cancers in the southern states in India (Male)

Trivandrum (U)		*Trivandrum (R)*		*Karunagappally*		*Bangalore*		*Chennai*		*Pune*	
Site	*AAR*	*Site*	*AAR*	*Site*	*AAR*	*Site*	*AAR*	*Site*	*AAR*	*Site*	*AAR*
Mouth	8.8	Mouth	8.9	Lung	19.4	Stomach	9.5	Stomach	13.6	Esophagus	8.3
Lung	8.4	Lung	8.5	Mouth	6.8	Esophagus	9.1	Lung	11.2	Lung	7.7
Prostate	7.8	Tongue	4.8	Esophagus	6.3	Lung	7.4	Esophagus	8.8	Mouth	7.1
Tongue	3.6	Stomach	5.4	Stomach	5.1	Hypopharynx	5.8	Mouth	6.4	Larynx	6.3
Stomach	3.9	Larynx	4.5	Tongue	4.5	H.Lymphoma	4.6	Hypopharynx	5.2	Stomach	5.4
Lymphoma	4.4	Esophagus	3.6	H.Lymphoma	4.4	Prostate	4.3	Hypopharynx	5.1	Hypopharynx	4.6
Larynx	4.2	Prostate	3.0	Liver	3.9	Larynx	4.2	Tongue	5.1	Tongue	4.3
Leukemia	4.7	Leukemia	3.6	Leukemia	3.8	Tongue	3.5	Larynx	4.5	Brain	4.2
Oropharynx	3.5	Brain	2.7	Larynx	3.7	Leukemia	3.4	Rectum	3.0	Lymphoma	4.2
Brain	3.1	Rectum	2.3	Urinary Bladder	3.0	Bladder	3.1	NHL	4.6		
								Prostate	3.8		

H.Lymphoma: Hodgkin's lymphoma

Mathew A, Vijayaprasad B. Cancer incidence and mortality in Trivandrum (1998-1999), Population based cancer registry, Regional Cancer Centre, Trivandrum, Kerala, India, 2002.

2. NCRP (National Cancer Registry Programme). Consolidated report of the population based cancer registries 1990-1996. Indian Council of Medical Research, New Delhi, 2001.

AAR - Age Adjusted Rate.

Table 5.2: Age-adjusted (World population) incidence rates (AAR) of 10 leading cancers in the northern states in India (Male)

Mumbai		Kolkata		Aurangabad		Nagpur		Bhopal		Delhi	
Site	AAR	Site	AAR	Site	AAR	Site	AAR	Site	AAR	Site	AAR
Lung	12.0	Lung	10.1	Lung	6.3	Esophagus	13.3	Lung	13.1	Lung	12.9
Esophagus	8.5	Mouth	3.0	H.lymphoma	5.1	Larynx	10.0	Mouth	7.1	Larynx	9.3
Hypopharynx	6.3	Pharynx	2.9	Tongue	4.8	Lung	7.2	Tongue	8.8	H. lymphoma	6.9
Larynx	6.9	Larynx	4.6	Hypopharynx	4.7	Tongue	5.2	Esophagus	7.5	Esophagus	6.2
Prostate	7.1	Stomach	2.5	Esophagus	4.5	Leukemia	4.9	Hypopharynx	7.3	Tongue	6.0
Stomach	6.4	Esophagus	3.1	Larynx	3.9	Mouth	4.8	Prostate	5.1	Urinary bladder	6.1
Tongue	5.7	Tongue	2.6	Mouth	3.3	Stomach	4.8	Larynx	3.9	Prostate	6.5
Mouth	5.7	Prostate	2.9	Leukemia	2.2	Prostate	3.4	Stomach	3.4	Leukemia	5.3
Bladder	4.6	Bladder	2.4	Brain	1.9	HD lymphoma	3.4	Brain	2.9	Mouth	4.1
NHL	5.4	Hypopharynx	2.2	Pancreas	1.7	Colon	2.7	Urinary bladder	2.9	Brain	4.4

Sources: Cancer Registry Abstract (2001); Parkin et al. (1997); Mathew and Vijayaprasad 2002.

Table 5.3: Age-adjusted (world population) incidence rates (AAR) of 10 leading cancers in the southern states in India (Female)

Trivandrum (U) Site	AAR	Trivandrum (R) Site	AAR	Karunagappally Site	AAR	Bangalore Site	AAR	Chennai Site	AAR	Pune Site	AAR
Breast	31.7	Breast	16.5	Cervix	15.0	Cervix	26.1	Cervix	30.8	Breast	26.3
Cervix U	9.7	Cervix U	11.3	Breast	14.9	Breast	22.1	Breast	21.7	Cervix	21.1
Ovary	6.3	Mouth	4.5	Thyroid	5.0	Mouth	8.1	Mouth	6.0	Esophagus	7.4
Thyroid	4.5	Thyroid	3.0	Mouth	3.4	Esophagus	8.3	Esophagus	6.1	Ovary	6.8
Mouth	1.9	Thyroid	3.5	Ovary	3.0	Stomach	5.1	Stomach	6.5	Lung	4.0
Leukemia	1.8	Tongue	1.8	Lung	2.9	Ovary	5.0	Ovary	5.5	Mouth	3.9
H. lymphoma	2.4	Thyroid	3.0	Esophagus	2.6	Thyroid	3.0	Rectum	2.4	Stomach	3.0
Body of uterus	4.8	Leukemia	3.9	Leukemia	2.0	Leukemia	2.8	Lung	2.4	Colon	2.7
Lung	2.8	HD Lymph	1.8	Tongue	1.7	Rectum	2.8	Hypopharynx	1.9	Rectum	2.7
Tongue	2.3	Body of Uterus	1.4	Brain	1.7	H. Lymphoma	2.9	Corpus uteri	2.0	Brain	2.5

Table 5.4: Age-adjusted (world population) incidence rates (AAR) of 10 leading cancers in the northern states in India (Female)

Mumbai Site	AAR	Kolkata Site	AAR	Aurangabad Site	AAR	Nagpur Site	AAR	Bhopal Site	AAR	Delhi Site	AAR
Breast	28.6	Breast	18.4	Cervix	12.7	Cervix	22.4	Cervix	21.7	Breast	28.1
Cervix	17.2	Cervix	21.8	Breast	9.7	Breast	22.3	Breast	19.9	Cervix	26.6
Esophagus	6.7	Gallbladder	3.7	Ovary	4.2	Esophagus	9.1	Ovary	5.6	Ovary	8.3
Ovary	7.3	Ovary	3.9	Esophagus	2.7	Ovary	6.6	Esophagus	4.9	Gallbladder	8.9
Mouth	4.2	Lung	2.8	Mouth	2.2	Mouth	3.3	Mouth	5.0	Esophagus	4.4
Stomach	3.2	Esophagus	2.9	Tongue	2.1	Leukemia	3.1	Lung	2.6	H. lymphoma	3.8
Lung	3.4	Body of uterus	2.1	H.D lymph	2.1	Rectum	2.3	Gallbladder	2.5	Leukemia	2.4
Colon	3.0	Tongue	1.5	Colon	1.7	Lung	2.3	Rectum	1.6	Brain	3.1
Rectum	2.4	NHL	1.7	Leukemia	1.7	Stomach	2.1	Skin	1.4	Lung	2.8
Gallbladder	2.5	Rectum	1.5	Rectum	1.2	Liver	1.0	Stomach	2.5		

Sources: Cancer Registry Abstract (2001); Parkin et al (1997); Mathew and Vijayaprasad 2002.

cancer incidence data during 1982-1996 in Mumbai showed that the overall rates are increasing with greater increase among females (Table 5.6). The largest increase among females is seen for cancer of the breast and among males for cancer of the prostate. Increasing trends are observed for lymphoma, cancers of the urinary bladder and gallbladder and brain tumors in both sexes. Cancer of the colon is increasing in females and kidney cancers in males. Esophageal and stomach cancers are decreasing in both sexes. Cervical cancer is showing a declining trend. In Chennai, the overall cancer incidence rates in males during 1982-97 are increasing with the highest increase noted in prostate cancer followed by lung cancer. In females, the highest increase was noted for lung cancer followed by cancer of the corpus uteri. Cancer of the cervix and penis showed declining trends (Tables 5.3 and 5.4).

CANCER INCIDENCE PATTERN BY RELIGION IN INDIA

The religion-wise incidence rates vary for common cancers (Table 5.5). In Mumbai, the overall incidence is high, particularly of breast and ovarian cancers among Christian and Parsi populations. Cervix cancer incidence is low among Muslims. In Chennai also, breast cancer incidence is highest among Christians (26.1 per 100,000 females) and lowest among Muslims (17.9 per 100,000 females) as compared to Hindus (20.6 per 100,000 females).

Marked geographical variations, time trends of cancer incidence and analytical epidemiological studies suggest the importance of risk factors in the etiology of cancer. Tobacco and alcohol consumption, dietary practices, occupational hazards, environmental factors, sexual history and reproductive history are identified as major risk factors for cancer.

MAJOR RISK FACTORS FOR CANCER IN INDIA

Tobacco

Indians use tobacco in a variety of ways. The habits of tobacco chewing (15-70%) and smoking (23-77%) vary considerably from area to area. Globally, the cancer risks of tobacco use have been extensively investigated. The principal impact of tobacco smoking is seen in the higher incidence of cancers of the lung, larynx and esophagus. *Bidi*, the common method of tobacco smoking in India, also confers high risk for cancer of the oropharynx as well as of the larynx. Cigarette smoking has been associated with cancers of the pancreas, bladder, ureter, and pelvis of the kidney. Smoking has been associated with an increased risk of squamous cell carcinoma of the cervix.

The chewing of quids containing tobacco as well as other substances such as arecanut, betel leaf, and lime (the common method of tobacco chewing in South India) is closely associated with cancer of the mouth. It

Table 5.5: Incidence rates (IR) per 10^5 person-years of five most common cancers in different religions by sex, Mumbai, 1996

	Male			*Female*		
	Site	No.	IR	Site	No.	IR
Hindus	Lung	295	6.1	Breast	701	21.8
	Esophagus	190	5.5	Cervix	481	13.9
	Prostate	177	3.8	Ovary	194	6.6
	Leukemia	173	4.2	Esophagus	148	3.9
	Larynx	167	4.7	Leukemia	88	3.3
Muslims	Lung	85	9.5	Breast	163	19.6
	Hypopharynx	41	3.9	Cervix	69	8.3
	Larynx	38	3.9	Ovary	36	4.8
	Tongue	38	4.0	Mouth	26	2.6
	Oropharynx	38	3.9	Lymphoma	16	2.2
Christians	Lung	28	11.1	Breast	78	32.5
	Esophagus	25	8.4	Cervix	20	9.5
	Prostate	24	6.4	Ovary	22	8.7
	Larynx	19	5.6	Brain	10	3.6
	Tongue	17	4.4	Stomach	7	5.9
Parsies	Prostate	6	14.9	Breast	29	67.6
	Esophagus	5	8.5	Colon	9	15.0
	Stomach	5	8.5	C Uteri	7	12.5
	Rectum	4	8.5	Endometrium	5	10.0
	Lung	4	8.5	Lymphoma	4	10.0
Buddhists	Hypopharynx	7	1.5	Breast	10	1.0
	Tongue	5	1.2	Cervix	8	9.1
	Colon	5	1.2	Uterus	3	1.0
	Larynx	5	1.8	Ovary	2	0.6
	Lymphoma	3	1.2	Tongue	1	0.6
Jains	Lung	10	2.5	Breast	15	9.0
	Brain	9	2.0	Esophagus	7	0.5
	Hypopharynx	8	2.0	Ovary	6	3.0
	Esophagus	6	2.0	Cervix	4	2.5
	Larynx	4	2.0	Stomach	3	0.5

Kavarna et al. 2001

has been estimated that 90 percent of oral cancers in India are directly attributable to chewing and smoking of tobacco. In house-to-house surveys of over 150,000 individuals in rural India, the habits of tobacco chewing

Site	Male			Female		
	Rate 1982	Rate 1994	APC**	Rate 1982	Rate 1994	APC
Mouth and pharynx	30.0	26.7	-0.7a	11.7	10.9	0.5
Esophagus	11.2	9.4	-0.9a	8.4	6.9	-0.7
Stomach	7.4	7.4	0.3	5.4	3.8	-2.4a
Colon	2.5	5.3	4.7a	2.3	4.0	3.1a
Rectum	4.0	3.3	0.7	2.4	2.6	0.9
Liver	3.8	3.7	1.5	2.7	1.9	-0.9
Gallbladder and biliary ducts	0.7	2.0	9.8a	1.0	2.9	8.3a
Pancreas	2.2	2.7	2.1	1.4	1.7	3.8a
Nasal cavities, sinuses	1.1	1.2	0.8	0.8	0.7	-0.1
Larynx	7.0	8.5	0.3	1.2	1.3	-0.1
Lung	13.7	14.7	0.5	3.3	3.9	2.4
Breast	—	—	—	21.4	31.5	3.2a
Cervix uteri	—	—	—	18.5	18.0	0.2
Corpus uteri	—	—	—	2.1	3.5	3.5a
Uterus, unspecified	—	—	—	1.5	1.3	-1.9
Ovary	—	—	—	5.9	8.2	2.9
Prostate	5.4	8.5	3.4a	—	—	—
Bladder	3.4	6.1	5.0a	0.7	1.4	10.1a
Kidney	1.1	2.5	6.1a	0.5	0.9	4.8a
Thyroid	0.6	0.9	1.8	1.5	2.1	4.0a
Hodgkin's disease	1.1	0.8	-1.2	0.6	0.6	-2.7
NHL	2.6	6.1	4.9a	1.8	4.1	5.3
Leukemia	3.7	4.3	1.8	3.0	3.3	1.4a
ALL SITES	119.9	138.3	1.2A	111.2	132.0	1.7A

Table 5.6: Trends in incidence rates* of common cancer in Mumbai

Per 100,000 person-years, directly age-adjusted using the world standard. – Annual percent change. P <0.05-

National Cancer Registry, Draft report. Indian Council of Medical Research, New Delhi (1997); Jin et al. (1999) {3767;3774}

a. Statistically significant at 5 percent liver

* Per 100,000 person-years, directly age-adjusted using world standard

** Annual percent change

Source: Yeole et al. (1999)

and smoking were found to be strongly associated with oral cancer and pre-cancer.

It is estimated that in India, cancer incidence related to tobacco habits, per year, is 151,900 (48%) in men and 66,400 (20%) in women with an overall estimate of 218,300 (34%) for the two sexes. The estimates are based on the occurrence of cancers of the mouth, pharynx, larynx, esophagus, lung, bladder and pancreas. Of the 218,300 tobacco related cancers, 75 percent were seen in the mouth, pharynx, larynx and esophagus. Lung cancer alone accounts for 15 percent of all tobacco related cancers. Tobacco control thus assumes a very important role in all primary cancer control measures.

Alcohol

Generally, alcohol intake is low in south Asian populations (less than 2 ml/day). Hence the risks associated with alcohol intake per se are not as high as those associated with tobacco for cancer. Epidemiological studies carried out in India have shown that increased alcohol consumption is positively associated with cancers of the mouth, pharynx (excluding nasopharynx), larynx and esophagus. Heavy alcohol drinkers are frequently heavy smokers as well. A multiplicative effect has been suggested for alcohol and tobacco smoking, i.e. the cancer risk in a drinker who smokes is much higher than the sum of the risks incurred by a non-drinking smoker and a non-smoking drinker. Global results from several case-control and cohort studies indicate that excessive alcohol consumption is responsible for the incidence of primary liver cancer. Studies have shown an association between alcohol consumption and increased risk of cancer of the colon, rectum and breast.

Diet

Scientific evidences from epidemiological, experimental, clinical/metabolic and intervention studies in the past two decades positively suggest the role of diet in human cancers. These studies indicate that increased intake of fat is associated with a higher risk of cancers of the colon and the prostate. High intake of food rich in animal fat can lead to cancer of the breast, uterus (body) and ovary. The declining trend of stomach cancer in most countries is related to changes in dietary patterns, particularly lesser use of salting and pickling for food preservation. High consumption of fruits and vegetables is associated with reduced risk of colorectal and other cancers (especially stomach and esophageal cancers). The inverse relationship between dietary fiber and cancer especially colon cancer and Vitamin A and lung cancer has been demonstrated. The consumption of diets high in various micronutrients lowers the incidence of certain cancers, especially those of the breast, colon, and uterus.

In India, the National Nutrition-Monitoring Bureau has been conducting diet/nutrition surveys from ten states since 1972. The nutrition scenario in India indicates that chronic energy deficiency and deficiencies of vitamin A, folate, riboflavin, iodine and iron are rampant. Diet-cancer relationships from Indian studies are summarized in Table 5.7. Epidemiological studies focusing on relationship of diet and nutritional factors with various types of cancers are few. It is essential therefore to develop appropriate dietary assessment methods to assess more accurately the past intake of food groups/ nutrients to arrive at causal relations.

Occupation

Occupation is responsible for 5-10 percent of cancers and factors in the environment for 1-2 percent although the public overemphasize the adverse impact. There is sufficient evidence to suggest arsenic exposure, radiation exposure, asbestos and metal mining as carcinogenic particularly for lung cancer. Benzene exposure can lead to leukemia. Exposure to soot and certain forms of mineral oil have been found to be associated with cancer of the scrotum, and chemicals used by dye workers with bladder cancer.

Table 5.7: Diet-cancer relationship from Indian studies. Based on quality/ frequency of intake and computed nutrient intakes or measured blood levels

Cancer site	Dietary constituents	Nutrients
Oropharynx	Decreased intake of vegetables, fruits, fish, buttermilk and groundnut oil. Increased intake of millets (ragi), red chillies, tea	Decreased intake of beta carotenes, vitamin A, vitamin B complex and vitamin C; zinc and selenium
Larynx	Decreased intake of vegetables, fruits, fish, butter, milk, pulses and groundnut oil Increased intake of tea, red chillies, egg	
Esophagus	Decreased intake of vegetables, fruits, fish, butter, milk and groundnut oil Increased consumption of very spicy foods, chillies, high temperature foods and beverages	Decreased intake of vitamin A, folic acid, zinc and selenium
Stomach	Increased consumption of chillies high temperature food, fried food, salty food	
Uterine cervix		Decreased intake of vitamin C and E

Sources: Notani and Jayant (1987), Siddiqui and Preussmann (1989), Siddiqui et al. (1988), Krishnaswamy et al. (1993), Prasad et al. (1992), Phukan et al. (2001); Mathew et al. (2000).

Infections

Chronic active infection with hepatitis B virus and hepatitis C virus can lead to hepatocellular carcinoma (HCC). Case control studies from all over the world have consistently shown a higher prevalence of HBsAg in causing HCC. Another virus-cancer relationship is between Epstein-Barr virus and Burkitt's lymphoma affecting mainly children. Evidence indicates that sexually transmitted human papilloma virus is associated with a variety of malignancies. These include esophageal carcinoma, anal cancer, penile cancer, and oral cancer. However, most of the research has focused on the association of HPV and carcinoma of the cervix. Studies carried out in India also have confirmed the role of HPV in cervical cancer.

Sexual and Reproductive Factors

Global results from several epidemiological studies indicate that sexual and reproductive factors affect the incidence of cervical and breast cancer. Epidemiological data strongly implicate sexually transmitted agents in the etiology of cervical cancer. Studies carried out in India show that late age at first childbirth and nulliparity increase the risk of breast cancer. Early age at first intercourse and multiple sexual partners add to the risk of cancer of the cervix. Women presenting with sexually transmitted diseases and HIV infection have 3 times more likelihood to have abnormal Pap smear compared to HIV sero-negative women presenting without STDs.

CANCER PREVENTION PROGRAMS IN INDIA

The Government of India launched a National Cancer Control Program in 1975-76 based on scientific principles to maintain uniformity in practice for the whole country to tackle the increasing incidence of cancer. This was later revised in 1984-85 with the objectives of primary prevention of cancer particularly tobacco related cancers and early diagnosis as well as treatment of cancer of the uterine cervix. These services were to be distributed through Regional Cancer Centers as well as Medical and Dental colleges. Primary prevention focuses on health education regarding hazards of tobacco consumption, genital hygiene, and sexual and reproductive health. Secondary prevention aims at early diagnosis of cancers of the uterine cervix, breast and oropharynx by various screening methods. A national cancer control board was set up to guide the activities of the program. On the recommendations of the control board, the Government of India has requested various states in India to formulate State Cancer Control Board for the proper coordination of activities.

Tobacco related cancers such as oral, pharyngeal and lung are mainly amenable to primary prevention programs. Results of an eight-year primary prevention follow-up study of oral cancer among Indian villagers have shown that through extensive and persuasive health education program, it is possible to control/reduce the tobacco habits in the community.

PRIMARY PREVENTION

Prospects for the primary prevention of cervical cancer are good as they are related to certain defined risk factors involving life-style and behavior. Raising the age of marriage beyond 18 years, observing small family norm, maintaining sexual and obstetric hygiene, containment of genital infection by controlling sexual promiscuity and use of barrier contraceptives have achieved results in reducing the risk for developing cervical cancer as shown by various studies carried out in India. In the absence of organized mass screening programs, primary prevention would be the most cost-effective and feasible strategy for uterine cervical cancer.

SECONDARY PREVENTION

Cervical Cancer Screening Programs

Cervical cancer screening programs practiced in different parts of the world have shown that the disease has a detectable pre-clinical phase and hence it is amenable for secondary prevention. Pre-invasive disease has virtually 100 percent cure rate if adequately treated as compared to less than 35 percent if diagnosed in advanced stages.

For the purpose of detecting cancer of the cervix at an early stage, early cancer detection centers in different medical colleges and Pap smear testing units under a postpartum program in 105 medical colleges in the country have been established.

During the period 1990-91 a demonstration project named District Cancer Control Program was initiated in selected districts of the country for the early detection of cervical cancer at the doorsteps of the rural community of the country. The district projects are linked up with Regional Cancer Centers and Medical College Hospitals having the infrastructure for the treatment of cancer. These centers supervise and monitor the program in collaboration with the state governments concerned. Under this project, medical and paramedical staff of the district hospitals and primary health centers are trained in the visual examination of the cervix, collection of Pap smears and they refer the suspected cases to the district hospital for further evaluation.

Cervical Cytology Screening Programs Based at Institutions such as Cancer Hospitals and General Hospitals

Several hospital-based cervical cytology-screening programs have been reported from India highlighting the load of cervical pre-cancerous and cancerous lesions. In cervical cytology screening studies carried out at 16 hospitals in different parts of the country, the frequency of mild or moderate dysplasia per 1000 women screened varied from 2.5 to 13.72. For severe dysplasia or carcinoma *in situ*, the range has been reported to vary from 1.4 to 4.9. In an early cancer detection program conducted in south India, cytological abnormalities in 3,602 women were correlated with age, gynecological complaints, number of years of married life and parity to identify if pre-selection for cytology screening was possible. The results suggest that asymptomatic women below the age of 40 years with a married life of less than 20 years and parity below 3, may be excluded from screening campaigns, and that pre-selection for cytologic screening is possible by introducing a program of clinical and speculum examination of the cervix.

Cervical Cancer Screening by Visual Inspection

Visual inspection of the cervix through a speculum in good daylight by medical or paramedical personnel has been proposed for the early detection of cervical cancer, as an alternative to routine cytology screening in developing countries. It is hoped that when asymptomatic women undergo this test, cancer could be detected in earlier stages with reduced case fatality rate. Although downstaging by visual screening is inferior in comparison to cervical cytology, this approach is more realistic in situations where necessary resources, manpower and facilities are not available for routine cytology screening. A study was carried out among women attending gynecological outpatient departments in eight hospitals of Delhi to define a high-risk group of women for selective cytology. All women attending gynecologic outpatient departments were subjected to visual examination of cervix followed by a Pap smear. Of the 67,416 women examined clinically and cytologically 13.7 percent had unhealthy, suspicious looking cervix or cervical erosions bleeding on touch.

In a community study in Delhi, Luthra et al. (1988) demonstrated that it is possible to train paramedical staff to distinguish referable lesions from non-referable lesions to an extent of 80 percent. In another community study in the villages of Tamil Nadu, 6,459 women were screened by trained village health nurses (VHN). The agreement between the gynecologists and the VHN in identifying cancer among those with abnormal cervix was 95 percent. However the study involving 2,843 married women in Kerala to evaluate visual inspection in detecting precursor lesions and cancer were not very promising either as a pre-selection procedure for cytology or as low-technology measure for cervical cancer screening.

Oral Cancer Screening Programs

Oral cancer satisfies the criteria for screening and oral visual inspection is a suitable test for oral cancer screening. A community-based, randomized, controlled oral cancer screening trial in Kerala consisting of 59,894 subjects in the intervention group (given oral visual inspection by trained health workers) and 54,707 subjects in the control group yielded oral cancer incidence rates of 56.1 and 20.3 per 100,000 person-years in the intervention and control groups, respectively. The same screening trial indicated that it is possible to train persons to perform the oral cancer screening test as accurately as doctors, although experience appears to be a crucial component of the individual health worker's accuracy.

In another study to evaluate the feasibility of mouth self-examination (MSE), some 450 college students distributed to 9,000 households copies of a brochure describing the risk factors of oral cancer, with pictures of appearance of pre-malignant and malignant lesions of the oral cavity and the methods of MSE. All subjects with tobacco habits and/or aged 30 years or above were asked to read the brochure carefully and to report to the clinic conducted in their locality on fixed days, if they suspected an abnormality while practicing MSE. Of the 22,000 eligible subjects, 8,028 (36%) practiced MSE and 247 reported to the clinic. Of these, 3 percent had oral cancer and 85 (34%) had oral pre-cancerous lesions; the others had either benign lesions or normal anatomical variations. The detection rates of oral cancer compared favorably with the previously reported detection rates using trained health workers.

Breast Cancer Screening Programs

The incidence of breast cancer is rising in developing countries, and strategies for controlling breast cancer need to be defined taking into account the prevailing socio-economic realities. Mammography is unlikely to be a cost-effective approach to early detection. Since most breast cancers in developing countries occur in women below the age of 50, mammography is also likely to be less effective.

The model proposed for breast cancer in the country relies mainly on physical examination of the breasts by trained paramedical personnel in a primary healthcare set-up and referring those with palpable lumps to district/medical colleges for further evaluation. The use of aspiration cytology would cut down the cost of unnecessary biopsies. The studies carried out by Tata Memorial Hospital, Mumbai has shown that lesions up to 3 cm in size are compatible with better prognosis in terms of survival and that paramedical persons can detect these lesions easily. Breast self examination could pick up early lesions. Training of available human resource and health education should be undertaken towards this objective.

FURTHER READING

1. Block G, Patterson B, Subar A. Fruit, vegetables, and cancer prevention: a review of the epidemiological evidence. Nutr Cancer 1992;18:1-29.
2. Cancer Registry Abstract. Newsletter of the National Cancer Registry Project of India, 2001;8.
3. Das BC, Sharma JK, Gopalkrishna V, et al. A high frequency of human papillomavirus DNA sequences detected in cervical carcinomas of Indian women as revealed by Southern blot hybridization and polymerase chain reaction. J Med Virol 1992;36:239-45.
4. Doll R, Peto R. Cigarette smoking and bronchial carcinoma: dose and time relationships among regular smokers and life-long non-smokers. J Epidemiol Community Health 1978;32:303-13.
5. Gajalakshmi CK, Shanta V. Risk factors for female breast cancer. A hospital-based case-control study in Madras, India, Acta Oncol 1991;30:569-74.
6. Gupta PC, Metha FS, Pindborg JJ, et al. Intervention study for primary prevention of oral cancer among 36000 Indian tobacco users. Lancet, I, 1986;1235-38.
7. Juneja A, Murthy NS, Sharma S, Shukla DK, Roy M, Das DK. Selective cervical cytology screening: discriminant analysis approach. Neoplasms 1993;40:401-04.
8. Krishnaswami K, Prasad MPR, et al. Selenium in cancer—a case-control study. Ind J Med Res 1993;98:124-28.
9. Kavarana NM, Kamat MR, et al. Cancer morbidity and mortality in greater Mumbai, Annual Report, 2001.
10. Mathew A, Gangadharan P, et al. Diet and stomach cancer: A case-control study in South India. Eur J Canc Prev 2000;9:89-97.
11. Mehta FS, Gupta PC, Daftary DK, et al. An epidemiologic study of oral cancer and precancerous conditions among 101761 villagers in Maharashtra, India. Int J Cancer 1972;10:134-41.
12. Mittra I. Screening for breast cancer in India, Natl Med J India 1993;6:101-04.
13. National cancer control programme. Directorate general of health services, ministry of health and family welfare, Govt. of India, New Delhi, 1997.
14. NCRP (National cancer registry programme), Biennial report 1988-89, Indian Council of Medical Research, New Delhi, 1992.
15. NCRP (National Cancer Registry Programme): A consolidated study of population based cancer registries data, cancer statistics 1995-96, Indian Council of Medical Research, New Delhi, 2000.
16. National Nutrition Monitoring Bureau. Report of repeat surveys, 1988-90, National Institute of Nutrition, ICMR, Hyderabad, 1991.
17. Notani PN, Jayant K. Role of diet in upper aerodigestive tract cancers. Nutr Cancer 1987;10:103-13.
18. Parkin DM, Whelan SL, Ferlay J, Raymond L , Young J. Cancer Incidence in Five Continents. VII. International Agency for Research on Cancer, Lyon, France, IARC Scientific Publications, 1997.
19. Phukan RK, Chetia CK, et al. Role of dietary habits in the development of esophageal cancer in Assam, the north-eastern region of India. Nutr Cancer 2001;39:204-09.
20. PBCR (Population Based Cancer Registry), Report 1991-95; Regional Cancer Centre, Trivandrum, 1999.
21. Prasad MPR, Krishna TP, Pasricha S, Qureshi MA, Krishnaswami K. Diet and esophageal cancers- a case-control study. Nutr Cancer 1992;18:85-93.

22. Sankaranarayanan R, Duffy SW, et al. Risk factors for cancer of the buccal and labial mucosa in Kerala, Southern India. J Epidemiol Community Health 1990;44:286-92.

23. Shanta V, Gajalakshmi CK, Swaminathan R. Cancer incidence and mortality in Chennai Biennial Report: 1996-97. Cancer Institute (W.I.A), Chennai, India, 2000.

24. Siddiqui M, Tricker AR, Preussmann R. The occurrence of preformed N-nitroso compounds in food samples from a high-risk area of esophageal cancer in Kashmir, India. Cancer Lett 1988;39:37-43.

25. Siddiqui M, Preussmann R. Esophageal cancer in Kashmir and assessment. J Cancer Res Clin Oncol 1989;115:111-17.

26. Sujathan K, Kannan S, Pillai RK, et al. Implication of gynecological abnormalities in pre-selection criteria for cervical screening: preliminary evaluation of 3602 subjects in south India. Cytopathology 1995;6:75-87.

27. Trock B, Lanza E, Greenwald P. Dietary fiber, vegetables, and colon cancer: critical review and meta-analysis of the epidemiological evidence. J Natl Cancer Inst 1990;82:650-61.

28. Yeole BB. Trends and predictions of cancer incidence cases by site and sex for Mumbai. Indian J Cancer 1999;36:163-78.

Screening and Prevention of Cancer

6

J Samuel

It must be understood that by taking adequate public healthcare in prevention and early detection, a few of the cancers could be prevented or cured and all the pain and suffering associated with it could thus be eliminated. In the last few decades, the world population has got rid of many fatal infectious diseases such as small pox, anterior poliomyelitis, measles etc. by worldwide programs in immunization at the behest of the World Health Organization and through public healthcare.

The prevention of cancer is twofold—one is the primary prevention where there is correction of genetic abnormality and the other removal of environmental imbalances. The latter involves educating the people about the risk of smoking and chewing pan. They are instructed to use food with roughage and observe good personal hygiene. The industrial workers associated particularly in the production of asbestos, nickel, arsenic, pesticide and the manufacture of polyvinyl compounds must be subjected to regular screening of the tumor of the lungs, nasopharynx and the GI tract. They must be advised to use facemasks and overalls while working in mines which extract the above mentioned metals. The public must be advised either by lectures or visual media to avoid the substances, which are identified to be carcinogenic.

The change of dietary habits such as avoiding fat and polished cereals in the food, protects the persons from the development of cancer of the colon, breast, endometrium and prostate. Even if it is not proved statistically, low-fat diet with high fiber, has a protective effect against the above mentioned cancers. Vitamin supplementation and use of fresh vegetables and fruits help to prevent the development of colorectal cancer.

The reader must try to become familiar with the screening criteria published by the American Cancer Society and World Health Organization (WHO). The Indian Cancer Society has started working on these criteria.

The screening of an asymptomatic patient is the ideal way to control cancer by early detection of the disease. It is true that early detection will increase the chances of cure. It must be understood that screening is done for healthy individuals belonging to the high-risk group particularly with familial cancer. The advantage of screening lies in the fact that most of the sites are easily accessible for clinical examination. Exfoliative cells from these sites can be stained by Papanicolaou's stain (Pap smear) and studied by a pathologist. Most cancers begin as a localized lesion, which stays at the site for many years before the invasion takes place. (See chapter 5: Cancer epidemiology and prevention in Indian Ambience). Pap smear is used mostly in the identification of cervical cancer but occasionally used in other cases of suspected malignancy where there is exfoliation of the cell from its superficial mucosal surface, for example, endometrium, lung, stomach and bladder. It can also detect malignant cells in effusions such as pleural and peritoneal fluid. The physician must be concerned about the woman whose near relative had cancer of the ovary, breast or cervix. Similarly the man, whose near relative had carcinoma of the stomach, colon or prostate, must undergo screening for cancer in those organs. The public health officials must work out a protocol of inexpensive and quick procedures, which can be used in appropriate intervals. How far is the screening test accurate? Doubts have been raised by a few about those patients who at the time of screening did not show positive result but developed the disease later.

SCREENING FOR COLORECTAL CANCER

The cancer of the colon shows an increasing trend in India, particularly in the females. This may be due to the refined food particularly wheat and rice, used in different regions in India. There are more proteins, particularly animal proteins such as milk, curd, fish and egg in the food in urban areas. In many households, especially those belonging to cities, non-vegetarian food like meat and fish are used

It must not be forgotten that a few among the healthy persons belong to the high-risk group. They are considered high-risk if they

1. have a close relative, the parent, siblings or children with simple or multiple polyps,
2. have a family history of adenomatous polyposis,
3. have a family history of non-polyposis rectal cancer,
4. have undergone treatment for adenomatous polyps,
5. have been treated for colorectal cancer previously,
6. have a history of inflammatory bowel diseases like ulcerative colitis and Crohn's disease.

The screening criteria used are:

1. Screening test for occult blood is a quick and cheap test that could be done in an ordinary clinical laboratory and should be done at an interval of 12 months.

2. Rectal examination is mandatory for all examinations of any colonic pathology.70 percent to 89 percent of colonic malignancies are below the mid-sigmoid and rectal area. The anus is 2.5 cm long and the rectum is at an average, 12 cm long. The index finger of an average adult can reach up to 9 to 10 cm, and the anal and most of the rectal mucosa can be examined for any tumors or polyps by digital examination of the anorectal region.
3. Flexible sigmoidoscopy is yet another method of screening the ano-rectal and the sigmoid. If during the course of examination, a lesion is seen, it is studied carefully and multiple biopsies are taken for histological evaluation and this examination is done once in 4 years.
4. The whole length of the colon is examined nowadays with a total colonoscope. Video endoscopes have almost replaced the conventional fiberoptic colonoscope. In high-risk group, the total colonoscopy is done once in 24 months. The whole colon is visualized from anus to cecum. In case any lesion or growth is identified, detailed examination with multiple biopsies is done from the different areas of the surface of the lesion. In certain cases where a polyp is identified, it can be removed with polypectomy snare and the excised tumor examined for any malignant changes.
5. Barium enema is also used as a screening procedure alternative to flexible sigmoidoscopy and total colonoscopy. In evaluating colorectal cancer, barium enema is inferior but centers where there is no provision of the fiberoptic total colonoscopy, this method is used. This screening technique is used both in normal risk and high-risk groups once in 48 months as an alternative procedure.

SCREENING FOR PROSTATE CANCER

The diagnostic modalities that are used for screening the cancer of the prostate are digital rectal examination, transrectal ultrasound and PSA estimation. In suspicious cases, a transrectal ultrasound prostatic biopsy is also carried out. There is controversy amongst oncologists and the urologists about the efficacy of these modalities. A few of the cancers are slow growing which will not affect the patient's lifespan. To treat these cases with total prostatectomy and hormonal manipulation has not gained universal approval. Each case must be treated on its own merit.

SCREENING FOR SKIN CANCERS

The skin examination by the patient is all that is necessary as a screening method. If the patient finds an abnormal skin lesion as a pigmented mass or a growth, the public health nurse should be contacted for further examination.

The molecular changes in the DNA and the presence of oncogenes will certainly have a role in the identification of early changes in the different organs in healthy persons. It is hardly used as an early diagnostic tool in routine clinical work. At present, the role of oncogenes as screening criteria is still under scrutiny in many oncology centers.

THERAPEUTIC PREVENTION OF CANCER

Can cancer be prevented by therapeutic methods?

There is no straight answer to this question. The age-old concept that there are two stages in the development of cancer has been accepted by many, those of initiation and progression. The initiators and the promoters are different substances. The former produces genetic changes either by inheritance of a mutated gene in the germ line or by environmental causes. Once the initiation of cancer takes place, there are promoters like estrogen in the case of breast, ovary and endometrial cancers and androgen in prostatic cancer. In high-risk cases, the suppression of the promoters may be helpful to prevent cancer in those particular organs. The prevention of cancer is twofold—one is the primary prevention where there is correction of genetic abnormality and its removal. The secondary prevention comprises the regular examination of various organs such as breast, mouth, cervix, ovary, and colorectal areas.

As a general rule, the population must be informed by media, the most effective being the visual media. The use of tobacco in any form must be avoided, as tobacco is the common denominator in most of the aerodigestive cancers. Alcohol must be used only in moderation.

Chemoprevention is being tried in many forms of cancers and most of them are in national trials. They shall be mentioned below and the readers are advised to refer textbooks dealing with chemoprevention of cancer so as to get a clearer understanding.

1. In premalignant lesions in head and neck	Isotretinoin
2. Non-small cell lung cancer	13-cis- retinoic acid
3. Hepatocellular carcinoma	Use of hepatitis B vaccine Use of interferon Alpha in case of chronic hepatitis C for 14 weeks
4. Carcinoma of the colon	High fiber, low caloric, low meat intake. Daily intake of calcium 1 gm in patients with recurrent adenoma Daily intake of folic acid, vitamin D
5. Anal cancer	Recognizing high risk groups particularly in homosexual men and patients with cervical and vulvar cancer

6. Breast cancer   Tamoxifen in high-risk daily for 2
             years from the age of 35

The Prevention of Cancer (Refer Chapter 5 pp.55-58).

FURTHER READING

1. British Society of Gastroenterology: Colorectal cancer screening in the UK: Joint position statement Gut 2000;46:746-48.
2. Cooper J, Wamakulasuriya KAAS, et al. Screening for oral cancer. Europe against cancer, Report to the European Commission 1994.
3. Cuckburn J, Redman S, et al. Understanding of medical screening. J Med Screening 1995; 2:224-27.
4. Jacobs I, Skates SJ, MacDonald N, et al. Screening for ovarian cancer: a pilot randomised controlled trial. Lancet 1999;353:1207-10.
5. Rhodes JM, Campbell BJ. Inflammation and colorectal cancer: IBD-associated and sporadic cancer compared. Trends Mol Med 2000;8(1):10-16.
6. Terdiman JP, Conrad PG, et al. Genetic testing in hereditary colorectal cancer: indications and procedures. Am J Gastroenterol 1999;94:2344-56.
7. Whitemore AS, Gong G, et al. Prevalence and contribution of BRCA 1 mutations in breast cancer and ovarian cancer: results from three U.S. population based case control studies of ovarian cancer. Am J Hum Genet 1997;60:496-504.
8. Zhang YL, Zhang ZS, et al. Early diagnosis for colorectal cancer in China. World J Gastroenterol 2002;8(1):21-25.

Investigations in Cancer

7

Antony Thomas, Jame Abraham
J Samuel

A good clinical examination can never be replaced by even the most modern machines in the investigation of a malignant lesion. A small lump in the breast, progressively growing mass in the neck, unexplained bleeding from the orifices, a localized lesion in the skin, tongue or mouth, unexplained backache, headache and vomiting, anemia and loss of weight must warn the clinician that there is something amiss in the patient. Each physician must learn to do proper investigation in patients, particularly those past 40 years, if cancer is suspected in any organ as in the skin, lymph glands, uterus, mouth, breast, lungs, rectum, prostate and thyroid. Leukemia and lymphoma are always kept in mind as they can occur at any age.

Finding out answers to the following questions is a time consuming and expensive exercise:

1. Is the tumor clinically identified as a malignant one?
2. Which is the specific organ where the tumor is seen?
3. Is the tumor confined to the organ or has it extended to nearby tissues and regional lymph glands?
4. Has the tumor spread to distant specific or nonspecific sites?
5. Has the tumor shown signs of dissemination?
6. How far have the therapies like surgery, radiotherapy and chemotherapy helped the patient?

Different modalities used in the investigations of cancer cases are:

1. Routine blood studies including liver function tests, sugar, urea and creatinine. Commercial packs are available to detect BRCA1 and BRCA2 from leukocytes or oral swabs
2. Electrophoresis if multiple myeloma is suspected
3. Bacteriological, virus and parasites studies
4. Tumor markers
5. Laparoscopy for GI tract and female genital tract tumors and thoracoscopy for thoracic tumors

6. Bone marrow biopsy
7. Tissue biopsy for histological confirmation, fine-needle aspiration cytology, tissue blocks biopsy, frozen section biopsy etc. Ultrasound or CT guided needle biopsy is used in deeper structures
8. Endoscopy evaluation for intraluminal tumors in aerodigestive tract such as nasopharynx, pharynx, larynx, bronchus, GI tract, lower and upper urinary tract and female genital tract
9. Video assisted biopsy for thoracic tumors and laparoscopy biopsy for intra-abdominal and pelvic tumors
10. Immunohistochemistry for detecting estrogen receptor protein, progesterone receptor protein, etc.
11. Electron microscopy
12. Flow cytometry
13. Cytogenetic evaluation
14. Molecular genetic testing
15. Imaging studies

Although an experienced doctor can make a provisional diagnosis of malignant tumors, proper treatment cannot be started unless the oncologist is sure of accurate staging and grading of the tumors. The staging requires the data comprising the site, and size of the tumor, the local extent of lymph node involvement and near and distant metastases. Planned examination must be undertaken with modern imaging techniques. Surgical interventions to obtain representative malignant tissues are necessary for histopathological examination. Time honored X-ray examination will offer further diagnosis in tumors of the lung and bony tumors mainly in the long bones, pelvis and spine (primary or secondary). Different types of modern imaging techniques are now available such as X-ray, Ultrasound, CT scan, Magnetic Resonance Imaging and Radionuclide scan and they must be used with discretion.

The next attempt is to narrow down the search to the organ where cancer exists.

BLOOD TESTS

Complete Blood Analysis

If signs and symptoms suggest a patient may have cancer, CBC is done to determine the Hb, white cell and differential counts. Hemogram is a major element in the diagnostic protocol. Anemia is seen in malignant conditions especially of GI tumors, leukemia and myeloproliferative diseases. Polycythemia is not uncommon in renal tumors. The white cell count is invariably around 100,000 per cmm in leukemia in 90 percent of cases and in the rest 10 percent it is normal or around 10,000 per cmm. Immature white cells including the blast cells may be seen in the peripheral smear. No time should be lost in planning a bone marrow biopsy either from the sternum or the posterior superior iliac crest. In the marrow, there is increased cellularity with blast cells either of the lymphoid or the myeloid variety.

In leukemia the platelet count could be depressed but not always. Evidence of thrombocytopenic manifestations like skin ecchymosis or bleeding gums may be the earliest sign. In liver tumors particularly with a cirrhotic background, coagulation disorders can occur. The determination of the following tests such as bleeding time, clotting time, the prothrombin time and prothrombin index are useful in evaluating bleeding disorders. Any invasive procedure of the liver carries considerable risk when the coagulation process is deranged. Erythrocyte sedimentation rate (ESR) has a limited role in the investigation of cancer. It is high in most cases of Hodgkin's lymphoma and multiple myeloma in elderly people.

Isolation of Bacteria, Virus and Parasite Associated with Cancer

Among the bacteria *Helicobacter pylori* have caught the attention of epidemiologists as an etiological factor in initiating stomach cancer. Stomach cancer is the second most common cancer in males and the fourth among females. Among them the diffuse subtype has increased in frequency and this type is associated among other etiological factors, with *Helicobacter pylori*. Its identification and eradication are essential in preventing gastric cancer.

Individuals with AIDS infection are prone to three types of cancers - Kaposi's sarcoma, Non-Hodgkin's lymphomas (peripheral lymphoma and central nervous system lymphoma) and genital cancer.

Among the other viruses, human papilloma virus is associated with cervical cancer and oral cancers. Laboratory investigation for isolations of virus and serological studies will be helpful in identifying the human papilloma virus and planning definitive treatment.

Schistosoma haematobium, a genus of blood flukes is common in Africa and south western Asia. This parasite can cause bladder tumors in individuals working in farmlands in these countries. In suspected cases of bladder tumors, isolation of this parasite will help in planning proper therapy.

Serum Tumor Markers

Some types of cancer release certain substances into the bloodstream. If these substances are present in blood samples of patients with cancer, they can provide valuable clues to the origin of the cancer. For example, high prostate-specific antigen (PSA) levels suggest malignancy of the prostate gland. High CA 125 levels suggest ovarian cancer and high levels of human chorionic gonadotropin (HCG) suggest a germ cell tumor, a type of cancer that can begin in the testicles, ovaries, the mediastinum or the retroperitoneum. Alpha-fetoprotein (AFP) is produced by some germ cell tumors as well as hepatocellular carcinoma.

The serum markers are broadly classified into oncofetal antigens; tumor associated antigen, hormones and degradation products in neuro-endocrine tumor. In the recent years, considerable work has been done to discover ideal tumor markers. Only a few tumor markers are found useful for diagnosis, confirmation and treatment follow-up. By quantifying the amount of the tumor marker in the serum, clinicians identify the presence of residual tumor, its recurrence or metastasis after treatment. The ones that are generally used are in the detection of prostatic, colorectal, ovarian, hepatic, testicular and breast cancers. Tumor markers are widely used for screening purpose rather than diagnosis of tumors and to monitor the progress of the treatment. The higher or lower titer of tumor markers helps the oncologist to decide whether the therapy had been useful or should be discontinued, whether other modalities have to be tried. In certain cases, it may be necessary to perform imaging studies or surgery to detect the recurrence of the tumors. Persistence or rising titer of a specific tumor marker even after treatment suggests recurrence or metastasis.

ONCOFETAL ANTIGEN

The principle used in this tumor marker is that in cases of malignancy, the tumor cells revert to their fetal genetic structure. These antigens are developed from the placental-fetal complex. They could be either monoclonal or polyclonal. As the malignant cell traces back to its fetal form the levels of the antigens rise in the blood and can be detected by immunochemical investigations.

Carcinoembryonic antigen (CEA) is normally produced in the embryonic tissues of GI tract, pancreas and liver in the early fetal life. It is a complex glycoprotein and is widely used as tumor markers in the diagnosis of colorectal, pancreas, breast and gastric tumors. CEA is raised in 60 to 90 percent of colorectal, 50 to 80 percent of pancreas, and 25 percent of gastric and breast tumors. Nevertheless, in non-malignant conditions like alcoholic cirrhosis, ulcerative colitis and healthy cigarette smokers, the CEA levels are elevated. Thus this test lacks both sensitivity and specificity and needs to be clinically correlated.

AFP is raised in hepatocellular carcinoma and non-seminomatous germ cell tumors of testis. It is the first oncofetal antigen discovered and is a well-accepted tumor marker in carcinoma of the liver and yolk sac remnants of gonads. Serum levels greater than 500 ng per cc are present in hepatocellular carcinoma (HCC) and non-seminomatous testicular tumors. Significant elevation is also seen in gastric, pancreatic, colorectal and lung carcinoma, not to the level that is noted in HCC and non-seminomatous testicular tumors. It must not be forgotten that the serum AFP is normal in 30 to 50 percent of biopsy proved HCC, which shows the lack of specificity. Values more than 500 units in patients with cirrhosis are diagnostic of coexisting HCC. Frequently it is high in teratocarcinoma of testis, tumors of the ovary and extragonadal teratoma. Modest elevation is also seen in alcoholic cirrhosis, hepatitis and in pregnancy where there is fetal death.

Prostatic specific antigen (PSA) is used for screening and diagnostic evaluation of prostatic malignancy. This tissue marker is produced in the columnar epithelium and periurethral glands of the prostate. The enzyme is produced by normal prostatic cells in small quantities but in considerable amount in adenocarcinoma of the prostate and it spills into the bloodstream. The serum level in a normal patient is 4 ng/cc. This level is also elevated in prostatic trauma, prostatic infarct, benign nodular prostate and chronic prostatitis. It must not be forgotten that the level of PSA can be higher than normal in benign prostatic hypertrophy and can be within normal in prostatic cancer. A few more new tests are being used in research setting in recent times. They are PSA density, PSA staining and age-specific PSA. It is found that the PSA rises by 3.5 ng/cc per gram in cancer and 0.5 ng/cc per gram in benign prostatic hypertrophy. A special stain that stains the malignant tissues deeply is used to differentiate normal and malignant prostatic tissues. The assay of prostatic acid phosphatase has very limited role in the diagnosis of early carcinoma of the prostate.

CELL SURFACE ANTIGENS

Ca 125 is a mucin and is accepted as a tumor marker in ovarian adenocarcinoma. The normal value is less than 35 units per cc. Other type of carcinoma antigens is Ca19-9. Ca19-9 is a carbohydrate antigen identified by monoclonal antibodies raised against a colorectal tumor cell line. It is used as a tumor marker for pancreatic cancers mainly to evaluate the tumor burden after surgery. Kits are available to detect Ca 19-9 in the patient's sera and the normal values are less than 35 units per cc. In acute pancreatitis, the serum level is less than 100 units per cc but in pancreatic cancer it is well above 100 units per cc. Two tumor markers in carcinoma breast are Ca 27.29 and 15-3. Among the other cell surface antigens as tumor markers, increased presence of keratin is noted in carcinoma of the cervix also.

HORMONES

The hormone, human chorionic gonadotropin (HCG) is normally produced from the corpus luteum and the placenta. In gestational trophoblastic disease, the level of HCG rises 1000- fold in the serum and is filtered into the urine. There are three types of trophoblastic disease, the benign hydatidiform mole, the invasive mole and choriocarcinoma, and the titer of HCG progressively rise from the benign hydatidiform to the malignant choriocarcinoma. The rise and fall of HCG titer offer the clinician an opportunity to monitor the response to therapy. The value of estimation of HCG over a period of time is accepted as the specific and ideal tumor marker in gestational trophoblastic disease and in testicular tumors. In 70 to 80 percent of non-seminomatous tumors and in 20 percent of seminomatous tumors HCG shows marked elevation. Other hormones used as tumor markers include calcitonin, catecholamine and its metabolites and the ectopic hormones. Calcitonin is elevated in medullary carcinoma of thyroid and is used widely in its diagnosis. Catecholamine and its metabolite vanilyl mandelic acid are elevated in pheochromo-cytoma. Estrogen and progesterone receptor proteins are evaluated planning the therapy for carcinoma of the breast. Ectopic hormones are discussed with paraneoplastic syndromes.

The list of common tumor markers is given below:

a. Alpha fetoprotein (AFP)   hepatoblastoma and germ cell tumors
b. Carcinoembryonic   colorectal carcinoma, mesothelioma
   antigen (CEA)
c. Beta HCG (phCG)   benign hydatidiform mole, malignant choriocarcinoma, trophoblastic germ cell tumors (non-seminomatous tumors and seminomatous tumors)
d. CA 15-3   breast, ovary, lung, gastrointestinal tumors
e. CA 19-9   pancreas, gastrointestinal tumors
f. CA 125   ovary, uterine, breast, lung

Bone Marrow Aspiration and Biopsy

Bone marrow examination is now widely used in different types of cancers particularly in leukemia, lymphoma, myelofibrosis and multiple myeloma and secondary cancers. It is also useful in determining the prognosis of leukemia and staging of lymphoma. The marrow is aspirated from posterior iliac crest or from the manubrium or body of the sternum either by a bone marrow needle or a bone marrow trephine under local anesthesia. A bone biopsy is also used occasionally in case of failed marrow aspiration or in association with aspiration. The marrow study will provide with precision the cytology and cytogenetic, immunonological phenotyping of the cells in the aspirate. In leukemia the marrow is hypercellular with 20 percent or more of leukemic blast cells. In AML Auer bodies are seen within the cytoplasm of the myeloblastic leukemic cells. In aleukemic leukemia, all the mature forms may be reduced in peripheral blood but the bone marrow will be flooded with blast cells. Low white count and extensive involvement of the marrow is suggestive of poor prognosis. In multiple myeloma, malignant plasma cells are seen in marrow aspirate. In hairy cell leukemia, the study of bone marrow is most rewarding. The characteristic hairy cell is seen associated with severe neutropenia. The cell types are B-lymphocytes, which expresses CD 25.

In multiple myeloma, plasma cells can be seen in the marrow. Both in non-Hodgkin's lymphoma and in Hodgkin's lymphoma, bone marrow biopsy has to be carried out before and after chemotherapy to determine the response if the bone marrow is involved at the time of diagnosis.

HISTOPATHOLOGICAL EVALUATION

Even though proper clinical examination, the examination of regional glands, the assessment with tumor markers and the imaging would give the clinical oncologist a working diagnosis, the final court of appeal is the identification of the cells of the tumor with histopathological diagnosis. Most of the time it is not difficult but it must be realized that "this is a no man's land and the wise must tread cautiously." (Robbins, Cotran and Kumar).

The histological diagnosis determines the aggressiveness of cancer and predictability regarding the spread. Many different methods of obtaining tissue for malignant mass are available now. They can be broadly classified into cytological evaluation and tissue evaluation. In cytology, the attempt is to evaluate the nuclear hyperchromatism and increased cell-cytoplasm ratio. But in the evaluation of the tissue, the attempt is to determine the cytological appearance of the tumor cells, its nuclei, and the relation of the cells to the surrounding tissues.

CYTOLOGICAL METHODS

The exfoliative cytology and fine needle aspiration cytology (FNAC) have become important tools in the detection of tumors. Among the modern diagnostic techniques that have increased the cost burden, this is really a blessing as this is inexpensive, and requires very minimal technical skill and assistance. An experienced pathologist can often give information equivalent to that provided by a tissue biopsy.

THE PAP SMEAR

The practice of exfoliative cytology is almost 150 years old. Papanicolaou (1883-1962), a Greek pathologist working in New York, developed a stain by which abnormal dysplastic and malignant cells could be identified in cervical smears and sputum. The principle is that cancer cells lose adherence between nearby cells and are exfoliated from the tumor surface or from the lumen as in a cervical tumor or in bronchogenic carcinoma. The technique was later called Pap smear and the term is synonymous with cervical smear examination and has become a useful tool in early detection and screening for cervical cancer. The same technique was later used in the identification of dysplastic or anaplastic cells from tissue scrapings, sputum, urine, pleural, peritoneal exudates, and bronchial and gastric washings. A positive Pap smear should be followed by a tissue biopsy before planning further treatment.

FINE-NEEDLE ASPIRATION CYTOLOGY

In fine-needle aspiration cytology (FNAC), the cells are aspirated from the mass for cytological evaluation. This technique is applicable both for superficial and deep tumors, the latter usually done under guidance of imaging technique. It has become so popular that in case of tumors of the breast, thyroid, enlarged lymph glands, salivary tumors and any mass that lies below the skin, the clinician awaits the report of FNAC from a specially trained pathologist before planning further tests and treatment. The advent of CT scan has gone a long way in obtaining tissue samples from deep structures like those in the neck, lungs, mediastinum, liver, pancreas, and intraperitoneal lymph glands particularly the glands at porta hepatis. In fact, no tissue is beyond the tip of a fine long needle for accurate biopsy even though it entails a few risks. Occasionally the tissue so obtained may be inadequate. It is advised not to attempt FNAC in testicular growths. In renal tumors, FNAC can cause some problems such as bleeding from a vascular tumor or seedling along the needle tract. If the test is positive for malignancy, the surgeon must plan for biopsy for confirmation. It must be understood that negative FNAC does not rule out a malignant tumor of breast and if the mass is clinically suggestive of malignancy supported by mammography, the surgeon must proceed with frozen section biopsy to confirm the diagnosis.

In case of breast and superficial tumors, FNAC is done with a 21G needle attached to a 10-cc syringe. The mass is held between the thumb and the index finger and the needle is slowly advanced through the skin to the mass. Once within the mass, negative pressure is applied and the needle is moved in a different direction. The aspirated material is placed in 4 to 6 slides fixed with 95 percent alcohol and is forwarded for cytological evaluation. The samples are adequate when they have a rich collection of cells while it is inadequate when there are no cells or a poor harvest of cells. If necrotic or blood clot only is present, a repeat aspiration must be undertaken. It must be understood that a dry tap does not rule out malignancy. In good centers with a trained pathologist the yield is 95 percent positive. If clinically suspicious and with negative FNAC result, the surgeon must proceed with an open biopsy.

DIFFERENT TYPES OF TISSUE BIOPSY

Core Needle Biopsy

The core biopsy needle is slightly wider than the FNA needle and it removes more tissue, usually one or more cylinders of tissue about 3 to 4 mm wide and 1 to 2 cm long. Core biopsies can be done by touch or guided by imaging tests, depending on the tumor's location. With a core needle, tissues are taken from deeper organs such as the liver, lung, mediastinum, pancreas, prostate and the pelvic organs before planning a proper therapeutic regimen. In case of a liver tumor, it is identified with a real time ultrasound and the core of tissues taken from the center of the mass with the help of either a Vim Silverman, Chiba, Menghini or tru-cut needle. A prebiopsy scan is important to rule out hemangioma or post-traumatic hematoma. Biopsy must never be attempted in patients with coagulation defects. Before doing a needle biopsy of any internal organ, bleeding time, clotting time, prothrombin time and platelet count should be checked and appropriate treatment modalities are to be taken. Any form of coagulopathy can cause serious problems and in certain cases death with continuous bleeding. Transjugular aspiration needle 16-gauge 85 cm long is used to obtain liver tissue when there is reduced prothrombin time and this procedure is not free from the risk of bleeding within the hepatic tissues in cases of coagulopathy. In the case of the prostate, biopsy can be done transperineally or transrectally either by a Franzen needle or a tru-cut needle. In most of the centers, transrectal ultrasound is used for evaluation of the prostate and for biopsy using a needle fixed on to the ultrasound probe. Needle track spread can occur and may be the site of recurrence in later months.

Excision Biopsy

Excision biopsy is used both for diagnostic and curative purposes. Small skin or subcutaneous tumor or a small tumor in the breast is subjected to this type of biopsy. In case of melanoma or basal cell carcinoma wider excision may be necessary after the preliminary limited excision. The patient must be warned that there is such a possibility when the initial excision is planned. In case of breast tumor if the excision is complete and the edges are free from malignant cells, this could be considered as lumpectomy. Further excision may be done only after a joint consultation with the radiotherapist and chemotherapist.

Incision Biopsy

When excision biopsy is difficult or dangerous or when the treatment of choice is radiotherapy or chemotherapy, incision biopsy would be the correct choice. The surgeon should be careful to get adequate and representative tissue for histological examination. It goes without saying that the tissue obtained by the incision biopsy is bigger than a needle biopsy. Errors can creep in the incision biopsy particularly in tumors where the periphery of the mass emerges with normal tissue. The surgeon must be careful not to damage the vascular structures near the tumor lest uncontrollable bleeding should occur. In bigger tumors the center of the mass may be cellular and necrotic and may not be representative in nature.

Laparoscope Aided Biopsy

Laparoscope biopsy is getting popular in the diagnosis of intraperitoneal tumors. An abdominal ultrasound plays a key role in evaluating the site, the size and the necrotic area within the mass. The nature of growth is identified with the laparoscope and a piece of tissue is removed with a biopsy forceps. Multiple pieces of true representative tissue can be harvested for histological examination. This technique is well suited for intraperitoneal malignant growths. Video assisted transthoracic biopsy is done to take tissue samples from the lung and mediastinum.

Frozen Section Techniques

Frozen section biopsy can provide rapid diagnosis in ascertaining whether the tissue removed in the operation theater is malignant or not, particularly in a brain or breast tumor. The sample of the tumor obtained by excision or incision is frozen and evaluated by a pathologist and can provide with a diagnosis within minutes. The surgeon could proceed with radical excision or ablation of the mass on receiving the report from the pathologist. If the diagnosis is doubtful, the surgeon must not hesitate to take another piece of tissue from another area for the frozen section studies. The patient is then spared a second anesthesia and a second operation. It will also help him to find out whether the margin of the resected specimen is clear of any malignant growth.

Endoscopic Biopsy

This technique is popular with the wide use of different types of fiberoptic flexible endoscopes. It helps to visualize intraluminal tumors and collect adequate tissue for microscopic evaluation. It is regularly carried out when the oncologist suspects the presence of a tumor in nasal, pharyngeal, bronchial, esophageal, gastric, bile duct, colonic or anal regions. Total colonoscope is a useful tool in collecting samples of tumor tissue from anal region to the cecum.

The cystoscopy is regularly done to obtain tissue samples from the urinary bladder. Fiberoptic flexible biopsy forceps with the proximal lighting system is used to obtain tissues from the ureteric lumen from the bladder to the renal pelvis. The lower urinary tract and bladder.

A similar type of flexible fiberoptic stereotactic biopsy forceps is used to collect tissues from different areas in the brain particularly in a low grade glioma from the brain. This technique demands the availability of spiral 3 dimensional CT scan.

The tissue that has been secured by biopsy should be immediately transferred to 10 percent formalin and sent to the pathologist without delay. Certain units use micropore cellulose filter and it is then put in a fixative fluid before transferring to the Pathology Department.

Paracentesis

In patients with ascites, samples of the fluid can be removed through a needle for examination under the microscope. This is done to see if the fluid contains cancer cells, and if so, to determine the type of cancer that is present.

All types of biopsy samples are examined for histological evaluation. In some cases, the appearance of the malignant cells under the microscope after routine processing of the sample will be useful in predicting the origin of the cancer or in classifying the cancer into broad categories in order to guide treatment.

The reader must be aware that the final court of appeal in all cases of malignant tumors is the histopathological examination. There is loss of differentiation and orientation of cells, and the normal cellular pattern seen in the epithelial or glandular tissues is absent. The loss in the uniformity of cells and loss in their architectural orientation is referred to as dysplasia. The cells of malignant tumor show characteristics ranging from well differentiated to poorly differentiated or can be undifferentiated. Such lack of differentiation is termed anaplasia. It was Hansmann who in 1880, first suggested that anaplasia is one of the common signs of malignancy. The cells show pleomorphism (variation in size and shape), have large nucleus when compared with the cytoplasmic volume. There would be hyperchromatism also. There is increased amount of chromatin in the cell nuclei resulting in increased amount of stain with hematoxylin. In all malignant cells, there is considerable mitotic activity as the DNA is the seat of brisk replication. . Another interesting feature in anaplasia is the appearance of multinucleated giant cells, and one of the important causes for its formation is endonuclear mitosis without cell division. The cytoplasm of tumor cell may resemble the normal counterpart or show variation depending upon the differentiation.

If routinely processed biopsy samples do not provide adequate information to guide treatment, additional investigations mentioned below are undertaken:

Immunohistochemistry

Thin slices of tissue samples are treated with a special antibody designed to recognize a specific substance present only in some types of cancer cells. If the patient's cancer contains that particular substance, the antibody will attach to the cells. Additional chemicals are then added so that cells to which antibodies have attached change color. This color change can be seen on viewing the sample under a microscope. There are hundreds of antibodies used for immunohistochemical tests by laboratories on specialized cancer centers. Some are quite specific, meaning that they react only with one type of cancer. Others are non-specific and may react with different types of malignant tumors. By considering these results in the context of the cancer's appearance after routine processing, it is often possible to classify the cancer in a way that can help in diagnosing the type of tumor.

Immunohistochemistry (IHC) is a biological technique, which permits the identification and visualization of a tissue constituent (antigen), in situ by means of a specific antigen-antibody interaction. This technique allows (1) the localization of an antigen within the tissue, (2) identification of specific cells and the cell-types which express the antigen, (3) subcellular distribution of the antigen under study and, (4) detection of circulating autoantibodies. Estrogen receptors and progesterone receptors can be detected by IHC and special staining technique. IHC helps us to derive valuable information regarding the expression of various antigens in normal tissue as well as in a pathophysiological condition. IHC is carried out on wax embedded or free floating tissue sections. Binding sites of the antibody can be identified either by direct labeling of the antibody or by using a secondary labeling method and can be visualized using a light microscope or fluorescence microscope.

Electron Microscopy

The typical medical laboratory microscope uses a beam of ordinary light to view specimens. A much more complex, larger, and more expensive instrument called an electron microscope uses beams of electrons. The electron microscope's magnifying power is hundreds of times greater than that of an ordinary light microscope, and this sometimes helps find very tiny details of cancer cell structure that provide clues to the tumor type or origin.

Flow Cytometry

Flow cytometers are automated fluorescent detection devices which allow multiparametric recording of several cell properties as the cells are allowed to move in a single file in a liquid stream through a beam of laser light. The various cell properties which can be measured include cell size, viability, surface antigens, DNA and RNA content, etc.

The essential components of a flow cytometer include a laser light source, an optical system to focus the light to a point on the sample stream, a sample chamber which transports the sample through the laser light source, an electronic system that can convert light impulses to digital signals and a computer system for data collection and analysis.

The cells to be analyzed are made to react with fluorochrome-conjugated antibodies, which link to the antigens present on the cell surface or cyto-plasm. Multiple antibodies can be linked to differently colored fluoro-chromes to decrease cell number requirement and reduce technical time.

Only a certain cell population can be selected for analysis. This is referred to as "gating". Cell suspensions can be prepared from peripheral blood, bone marrow, lymph node and other tissues. As the cells pass through the laser beam they scatter light and emit fluorescence. The degree of light scattering depends on factors like cell size and the nuclear and granular contents of the cell.

Flow cytometry is an important technique in the evaluation of neoplasms of the hemato-lymphoid system, in the early detection, diagnosis and classification of leukemias and lymphomas. It helps in the determination of leukemic lineage (myeloid versus lymphoid) when morphological and cytochemical studies are inconclusive. In lymphomas it is useful in assessing the clonality of lymphoid proliferations, identification of lineage and detection of residual disease. Detection of even small populations of tumor cells is possible with flow cytometry because of its high sensitivity.

Cytogenetics

In recent times, molecular diagnostic techniques are employed in investigations of cancer. The common techniques that are employed include polymerase chain reaction (PCR), fluorescent in situ hybridization (FISH), and other recombinant DNA techniques. The scientists have developed very sensitive diagnostic probes so that the presence of chromosomal deletion and translocation from one chromosome to another, presence of an oncogene such as myc oncogene and deletion of tumor suppressor genes can be determined. Modern molecular techniques are used to identify benign polyclonal proliferation of B or T lymphocytes from malignant monoclonal proliferation. It has a role in the demonstration of various mutations including specific translocations, which helps in diagnosis as well as in prediction of prognosis.

Some types of cancer have characteristic abnormalities of their chromosomes. Recognizing these changes helps in identifying certain types of cancers. Several types of chromosome changes can be found in cancer cells.

Polymerase Chain Reaction (PCR)

Polymerase chain reaction (PCR) is a simple but clever method of amplifying segments of DNA, a million times in a few hours time without purification or the use of vectors such as bacteria or virus. With the availability of PCR, genetic analysis of tumors is more frequently conducted and has a dramatic impact on the study, analysis and diagnosis of tumors. PCR amplifies the specific DNA target and helps in the detection of point mutations, translocations, insertions and deletions associated with various neoplasms.

PCR is used in various clinical settings:

1. For the detection of genetic abnormalities in hematologic malignancies like chronic myelogenous leukemia, acute lymphoblastic leukemia, acute promyelocytic leukemia and in various lymphoma including anaplastic large cell lymphoma.
2. Presence of certain chromosomal abnormalities is indicative of prognosis of the tumor, e.g. the presence of Philadelphia chromosome associate with chronic myelogenous leukemia is a favorable factor meanwhile its presence brings unfavorable outcome in acute lymphoblastic leukemia.
3. Presence or absence of some chromosomal abnormalities is used to differentiate some malignancies – absence of Philadelphia chromosome is mandatory to differentiate chronic myelogenous leukemia from other chronic myeloproliferative disorders like chronic neutrophilic leukemia, chronic eosinophilic leukemia, polycythemia vera and essential thrombocythemia.
4. Soft tissue tumors with small round cell features, like Ewing's sarcoma, primitive neuroectodermal tumor and alveolar rhabdomyosarcoma are also amenable for detection of translocation by PCR.
5. Detection of minimal residual disease (MRD). A high percentage of patients with leukemia or lymphoma achieve a complete clinical remission after initial treatment. However, many of these patients will eventually relapse from residual tumor cells undetected by the common staging procedures. The focus of the study of minimal residual disease (MRD) is to redefine the concept of tumor remission by using more sensitive molecular techniques to detect the level of disease burden below the resolution threshold of conventional pathology. The PCR based qualitative detection of MRD is associated with a relative increase in relapse rate. However, even without relapse, some patients affected with hematological malignances will still test positive for the tumor marker using standard PCR.

Tests of the cancer cell's DNA by methods such as polymerase chain reaction (PCR) can find many translocations that are visible under a microscope in cytogenetic tests. DNA tests can also find some translocations involving parts of chromosomes too small to be seen with usual cytogenetic testing under a microscope. This sophisticated testing is available in certain centers in India.

FLUORESCENT IN SITU HYBRIDIZATION (FISH)

FISH is a method of cytogenetic analysis, in which chromosomes or parts of chromosomes are labeled with fluorochrome-bound oligonucleotides that are complementary to specific sequences on a chromosome. FISH is carried out by fluorescence microscopy and it is applied in both dividing and non-dividing cells, meanwhile it is limited to metaphase in classical cytogenetic analysis by banding technique. FISH is used in the following tumor associated conditions:

1. Detection of any inherited or constitutional abnormality like Down's syndrome (trisomy 21) in patients with acute lymphoblastic leukemia or acute myeloid leukemia.
2. Confirmation of an uncertain condition like myelodysplastic syndrome by detection of the various cytogenetic abnormalities associated with it.
3. Confirmation of specific conditions like chronic myeloid leukemia, lymphoma, soft tissue sarcoma, small round cell tumors and germ cell tumor.
4. In the determination of prognostic factors and monitoring response to treatment.

TELOMERE AND TELOMERASE

Telomeres are short repeated sequences of DNA that form the linear ends of chromosomes. This ensures complete replication of chromosomal ends and protects the chromosomal ends from fusion and degeneration. The telomere sequence is generated by a specialized ribonucleoprotein enzyme, telomerase. Telomerase activity is maximum in germ cells and actively dividing cells. Its activity is low in stem cells and somatic normal cells with subsequent mitosis, and the resultant telomere shortening. Once the telomeres are shortened beyond certain point, the loss of function of protection of chromosomal end occurs which leads to the cell death. This is an important factor in the cellular senescence. In cancer cells, telomerase is reactivated with telomere elongation. This is now recognized as an important step in tumor formation, "the horror that awaits us when the ends fail to meet the needs". The role of telomerase in tumor formation is still under scrutiny.

IMAGING STUDIES

X-rays

During diagnosis and evaluation of a cancer, a chest X-ray and bone X-rays may be obtained. These may show a mass in the chest or evidence of the cancer's invasion of the bone. But they are not useful in finding out what type of cancer is present or in what organ it started.

Mammography

Mammography is widely used soft tissue radiological study in breast tumors.

Ultrasound

This test uses sound waves to produce images of internal organs. It is a safe and quick diagnostic procedure and is widely used in the diagnosis of an abdominal or pelvic mass. It can help us to identify which organs have been affected by carcinoma of the unknown primary (CUP) and rarely, can help us in finding the organ where the tumor has originated.

Computed Tomography (CT Scan)

CT scans are often used in malignant intracranial, intrathoracic and intra-abdominal cases. It also helps to delineate the extent of cancer spread to various parts of the body. They can help us to find out tumors in the throat, sinuses, pancreas, ovaries, etc. CT scans are also very helpful in guiding placement of fine needle or core biopsy needle into cancers deep inside the body for biopsy.

Magnetic Resonance Imaging (MRI)

This procedure uses large magnets and radio waves instead of radiation to produce computer-generated pictures of internal organs. The pictures look very similar to a CT scan, but are more detailed. Unlike the CT scan, MRI cannot be used to guide a biopsy needle because of interactions between the scanner's magnet and the metal needles.

It must not be forgotten that in spite of all these different investigating modalities, and with the presence of a metastasis, it may not be able to identify the primary site. The term, cancer of unknown primary, is used in this context and would challenge the diagnostic ability of an oncologist.

Positron Emission Tomography (PET Scan)

With the emergence of positron emission tomography (PET) from research laboratories into routine clinical use, more and more oncologists are using this modern imaging modality in determining different stages in cancer therapy and evaluating its efficacy. It is a non invasive technique using a radiotracer such as fluorodeoxyglucose (FDG). The radiotracer will determine the cellular activities of normal and tumor cells and will show reduction in glucose uptake level of the tumors in response to the therapy.

1. **Breast cancer:** In the detection of involvement of the axillary lymph nodes. PET is a non-invasive and painless alternative to axillary lymph node dissection (ALND) for screening patients referred for partial mastectomy. Although PET is unlikely to replace current methods for screening certain populations of women-specifically, young patients with dense breasts, or those with strong family history of the disease, those with fibrocystic disease, those whose needle aspirations have been inconclusive, and those with negative needle aspirations who nevertheless warrant high suspicion of disease.

2. **Soft tissue sarcomas:** Although the most essential step in the diagnostic evaluation of soft tissue sarcomas is tumor biopsy, functional imaging technique is used in determining the molecular

and cellular activities of normal and tumor cells through the use of radiotracers that engage in cell metabolism. PET scan usefulness is not limited to its ability to differentiate benign from malignant lesions. The scan can detect intralesional morphologic variation which is especially true in soft tissue sarcomas, it can predict tumor grade, and it is of value in staging, restaging and assessing the prognosis.

3. **Lung cancer:** Traditionally, lung masses have been evaluated with chest X-rays, CT, and more recently, MRI invasive biopsy techniques and thoracotomy. PET has demonstrated extraordinary utility in diagnosing and staging this disease. Once a solitary pulmonary nodule has been identified, PET can determine its malignancy precisely and non-invasively. As a result, using PET can greatly reduce the number of benign nodules that are resected, thereby minimizing the number of thoracotomies performed and sparing patients needless cost and pain. PET also makes valuable contributions in staging patients for mediastinal or distant metastases.

4. **Hodgkin's and non-Hodgkin's lymphoma:** When used for this purpose, PET frequently results in a change in disease staging, and therefore treatment plans can be modified to improve their effectiveness. Furthermore, PET has demonstrated efficacy in monitoring therapeutic responses.

5. PET scan is also used in evaluating the efficacy of chemotherapy/radiotherapy in ovarian, head, neck, and thyroid cancers. The scan would identify minimal residual tumors in the metastatic sites and provide the physician adequate information for planning further therapy. The scan rapidly exhibits changes in response to chemotherapy and/or radiation therapy. It also quickly determines whether the patient is responding to the type of chemotherapy that has been used.

FURTHER READING

1. Bryson GJ, Lear D, Williamson R, Wong RC. Detection of the CD56+/CD45-immunophenotype by flow cytometry in neuroendocrine malignancies. J Clin Pathol 2002;55(7):535-37.

2. Braylan RC. "Lymphomas," Clinical Flow Cytometry: Principles and Applications, Bauer KD, Duque RE, Shankey TV (Eds). Baltimore, MD: Williams and Wilkins, 1993.

3. Creager AJ, Geisinger KR, Bergman S. Neutrophil-rich Ki-1-positive anaplastic large cell lymphoma: A study by fine-needle aspiration biopsy. Am J Clin Pathol 2002;117(5):709-15.

4. Grumbach Y, Baratte B. Screening and imaging guided biopsies of the breast. J Radiol 2002;83:535-50.

5. Jerusalem G, Hustinx R, Beguin Y, Fillet G. PET scan imaging in oncology. Eur J Cancer 2003;39(11):1525-34.

6. J N Wiig A1, A Berner A2, K M Tveit A3, K -E Giercksky A1. Evaluation of digitally guided fine needle aspiration cytology versus fine needlecore biopsy for the

diagnosis of recurrent rectal cancer. International Journal of Colorectal Disease Springer-Verlag Heidelberg 1996;11(6)17:272-75.

7. Kristoffersen Wiberg M, Aspelin P, Perbeck L, Bone B. Value of MR imaging in clinical evaluation of breast lesions. Acta Radiol 2002;43(3):275-81.

8. Lymphoproliferative Disorders Using Two-Color Flow Cytometric Analysis," Am J Clin Pathol 1991;96(1):100-08.

9. Ng SB, Chuah KL. Fine needle aspiration cytology of metastatic malignant granular cell tumor: A case report and review of the literature. Cytopathology 2002;13(3):164-70.

10. Positron emission tomography of soft tissue sarcomas.Israel-Mardirosian N, Adler LP. Curr Opin Oncol 2003;15(4):327-30.

11. Sapino A, Cassoni P, Zanon E, et al. Ultrasonographically-guided fine-needle aspiration of axillary lymph nodes: role in breast cancer management British Journal of Cancer 2003;88(5):702-06.

12. Thomas G, Pandey M, Jayasree K, Pradeep VM, Abraham EK, Iype EM, Krishnan Nair M. Parapharyngeal metastasis from papillary microcarcinoma of thyroid: report of a case diagnosed by peroral fine needle aspiration. Br J Oral Maxillofac Surg 2002;40(3):229-31.

Cancer Metastases

8

Antony Thomas, Jame Abraham
J Samuel

INTRODUCTION

Metastases, rather than primary tumors, are responsible for most cancer deaths. The metastasis is brought about by dissemination of cancer cells along the blood vessels, lymphatics and the celomic cavity. To prevent these deaths, improved ways to treat metastatic disease are needed. Blood flow and other mechanical factors influence the spread of cancer cells to specific organs, whereas molecular interactions between the cancer cells and the specific organ influence the probability of the cell growth in the new environment. The inhibition of the growth of metastases in secondary sites offers a promising approach for cancer therapy.

THE GROWTH OF CANCER CELLS IN METASTATIC SITES

The progressive nature of malignancy is an inevitable consequence of cancer. When cancer is detected at an early stage, before it has spread, it can often be treated successfully by surgery or local irradiation, and the patient will be cured or the growth of the tumor is controlled. However, when cancer is detected after it is known to have metastasized, treatments are much less successful. Furthermore, for many patients in whom there is no evidence of metastasis at the time of their initial diagnosis, metastases will be detected at a later time. It must be understood that the tumor becomes more aggressive, more invasive and prone to distant metastases with the passage of time.

Metastasis consists of a series of sequential steps, all of which must be successfully completed. Metastases arise following the spread of cancer from a primary site and the formation of new tumors in distant organs. As a primary tumor grows, it needs to develop a blood supply that can support its metabolic needs—a process called angiogenesis. These new blood vessels can also provide an escape route by which cells can leave the tumor and enter the body's circulatory blood system—known as **intravasation**. Tumor cells might also enter the blood circulatory system indirectly via the lymphatic system. The cells need to survive in the circulation until they can arrest in a new organ; here, they might **extravasate** from the circulation into the surrounding tissue. Once the cells reach the new site, cells must initiate and maintain growth to form pre-angiogenic micrometastases. This growth must be sustained by the development of new blood vessels so that a macroscopic tumor is formed.

ORGAN SPECIFIC METASTASES: THE CONCEPT OF 'THE SEED AND SOIL'

The metastases from a primary tumor site can show an organ-specific pattern of spread. Breast cancer frequently metastasizes to bone, *liver, brain* and *lungs*; prostate cancer preferentially spreads to bone. Patients with *colorectal cancer*, by contrast, often develop initial metastases in liver.

In 1889, Stephen Paget published an article in *The Lancet* that described the propensity of various types of cancer to form metastases in specific organs, and proposed that these patterns were due to the 'dependence of the seed (the cancer cell) on the soil (the secondary organ). This idea was later challenged in the 1920s by James Ewing, who suggested that circulatory patterns between a primary tumor and specific secondary organs were sufficient to account for organ-specific metastasis.

In fact, these theories are not mutually exclusive, and current evidence supports a role for both factors namely dependence of the organ and the vascular pattern. Experimental data from metastasis assays in laboratory mice also support the concept that both mechanical factors (how many cells spread to an organ?) and seed–soil compatibility factors (does the organ preferentially support or suppress the growth of the specific cancer-cell type?) contribute to the ability of specific types of cancer to spread to various target organs.

VASCULAR PATHWAYS AFFECT METASTATIC SPREAD

Figure 8.1 shows the blood-flow pathways for cancer cells from a primary site to secondary site, for example in a breast tumor. Breast cancer cells that escape from the primary site into the blood circulation will reach the capillaries of the lungs, where many would arrest. The cells that are able to escape from the tumor are carried by mechanical force to secondary sites, where they are arrested by size restriction in small capillaries in the new organ. The metastases within the lung can shed cells to the arterial flow, travel to different parts of the body and form microscopic nidus of

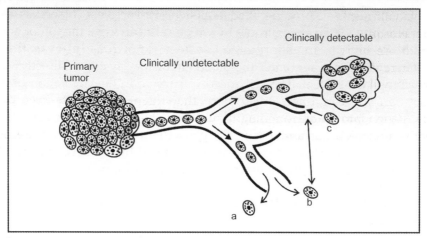

Figure 8.1: The diagram showing the escape of cancer cells along the vascular channel from a primary tumor and arrest in secondary sites. A few of them extravasate into the tissues. (a) Some of these cells die, (b) some will remain in a state of dormancy, (c) some of the cells in the state of dormancy may proliferate. After some time, the dormant cells intravasate into the vascular channels and find a new site of metastasis.
(a) Cells destined to die, (b) Dormant cells, (c) Cells that proliferate

new sites in remote organs like bone in course of time. The passage of malignant cells though a blood vessel from the primary tumor is not clinically detectable but the arrival of circulating cancer cells in an organ and its growth is clinically detectable at a later stage. Cancer cells are deformed to fit the vasculature in the new sites, depending on the blood pressure in the new organ. In fact, the biology of dissemination is an unknown or hidden process and inherently difficult to observe. A microscopic clone of malignant cells has many properties. It can infiltrate, invade into blood vessels and lymph channels and become autonomous in its progression outside the control of cellular homeostasis. After cells have arrested in an organ, their ability to grow is dictated by molecular interactions of the cells with the environment in the organ.

Alternatively, some breast cancer cells might invade lymphatics in the primary site and would be taken first to the draining lymph node, where they might grow. From the lymph nodes, however, there are no direct lymphatic routes to the sites where breast cancer metastases are often found–bone, liver, brain and lungs. So the cells in the lymphatic system would eventually need to enter the blood circulation to be transported to these sites. This could occur indirectly, through efferent lymphatic vessels that eventually flow into the venous system, or directly into newly formed blood vessels that serve lymph node metastases. Although lymph node metastasis is a negative prognostic factor for breast and other cancers, it is still not known whether metastasis to other organs proceeds sequentially from lymphatic spread or in a parallel line by a hematogenous route.

Possible fates of cancer cells in a secondary site, following the extravasation of cancer cells are as follows: 1) dormant solitary cell, 2) small pre-angiogenic metastases, 3) larger vascular metastases.

There is another set of cells or micrometastases outside these subsets, which will die or remain dormant for many years. Only a proportion of vascularized metastases is clinically detectable. Dormant solitary cells refer to cells that are undergoing neither proliferation nor apoptosis, whereas pre-angiogenic micrometastases refer to those in which active proliferation is balanced by active apoptosis, resulting in no net increase in the size of the metastases. This group can stay dormant for many years and then develop into vascularized metastases. Metastasis is an inefficient process. Microassay studies of the metastasis have led to the conclusion that early steps in metastasis are completed very efficiently. By contrast, later steps in the process are inefficient. Metastatic inefficiency is due primarily to the regulation of cancer-cell growth in secondary sites that is under control of local immunological factors, efficiency of neoangiogenesis and effects of cytokine activities.

MIGRATION OF CANCER CELLS TO SPECIFIC ORGANS

How efficient are capillaries at 'filtering' out these circulating cancer cells? Studies using *in vivo* video microscopy and quantitative cell-fate analyses indicate that both lung and liver are very efficient at arresting the flow of cancer cells and that most circulating cancer cells arrest by size restriction. Capillaries are small (typically 3-8 microns in diameter) and are designed to allow the passage of red blood cells—which average 7 microns in diameter and are highly deformable—whereas many cancer cells are quite large (20 microns or more in diameter). As the lumen narrows down the passage, arrest of the cells in vessels takes place.

The actual percentage of circulating cancer cells that arrest by size restriction in any given organ will be determined by physical factors, such as the relative sizes of the cells and the capillaries, the blood pressure in the organ and the deformability of the cell. However, it has been noted that the cancer cells can undergo adhesive arrest if the capillary endothelium is activated by cytokine interleukin-1. So the initial delivery and arrest of the cancer cells in the particular organ is primary mechanical. Once the cells have been 'seeded' to an organ future developments will depend on the compatibility of the 'seed' with 'soil'. The growth regulation is influenced by the molecular interaction between the cancer cells and the environment of the new organ. So, given the very high initial arrest of cancer cells in the first capillary bed they encounter, it is reasonable to propose that organ-specific adhesive interactions are indicative of organ-specific signaling, rather than factors that enhance the physical arrest of cancer cells in specific sites.

MOLECULAR FACTORS

It is seen that certain cytokines and their receptors can influence organ-specific metastatic growth of cancer cells. One good example is the chemokines in breast cancer cells, which express high levels of the CXCR4 chemokine receptor, and lung tissue expresses high levels of CXCL12, a soluble ligand for the CXCR4 receptor. At the same time, melanoma cells express high levels of the CCR10 receptor and lower levels of CXCR4 and skin tissue expresses high levels of CCL27, a soluble ligand for the CCR10 receptor (Fig. 8.2). Therefore, breast cancer cells that are taken to the lung by the blood flow would find a strong chemokine–receptor 'match', which would lead to chemokine-mediated signal activation. By contrast, breast cancer cells taken to skin would not find such a match. Melanoma cells, however, taken to skin by the circulation or by local invasion, would find a CCL27–CCR10 chemokine–receptor 'match' that would lead to the activation of chemokine-mediated pathways.

It is further seen that the activation of chemokine signaling can result in several changes in cells, including activation of RAS signaling pathways, polymerization of intracellular actin and cytoskeletal changes, formation of pseudopodia, and increased cell motility, migration and tissue invasion.

ACTIVATION OF RAS SIGNALING PATHWAYS

The activation of RAS signaling pathways can protect small metastases and promote their early growth. In the RAS activated micrometastases,

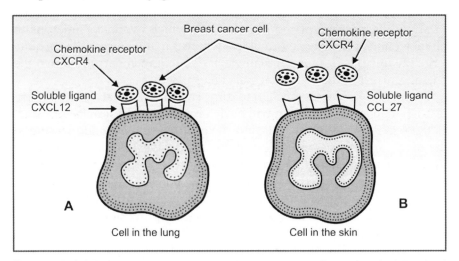

Figure 8.2: (A) The diagram shows that the breast cancer cells express high levels of the chemokine receptors CXCR4. A soluble ligand CXCL12 for the chemokine receptor CXCR4 is found at elevated levels in lung. A strong chemokine –receptor match which influences metastatic growth in lung results. (B) In the skin, the soluble ligand is CCL27 and no match is seen for CXCR4. No metastasis develops in the skin.
Adapted from Nature, Review Cancer, 2, 563-572 (2002)

the balance between apoptosis and proliferation was tipped to favor progressive growth. Any of these changes could contribute to the ability of cancer cells to survive and to initiate and maintain metastatic growth, and could therefore contribute to the regulation of organ-specific metastatic growth.

TUMOR METASTASIS TO REGIONAL LYMPH NODES

Tumor metastasis to regional lymph nodes is a crucial step in the progression of cancer. Detection of tumor cells in the lymph nodes is an indication of the spread of the tumor, and is used clinically as a prognostic tool and a guide to therapy. The mechanisms that underlie lymphatic spread and the role of lymphangiogenesis were unknown until recently, particularly its molecular mechanisms.

The proliferation of new lymphatic vessels (lymphangiogenesis) is controlled, in part, by members of the vascular endothelial growth factor (VEGF) family, namely, VEGFC and VEGFD and their closely related receptor on lymphatic endothelium, VEGFR3. These secreted growth factors are activated by proteolysis to form high-affinity ligands that activate VEGFR3 and stimulate lymphangiogenesis. Experimental studies with VEGFC and VEGFD have shown that they can induce tumor lymphangiogenesis and direct metastasis to the lymphatic vessels and lymph nodes. By contrast, angiogenic factors such as VEGF act to enhance the growth of tumors by promoting a more extensive blood vessel supply. The published patterns of expression of lymphangiogenic factors in human tumors, in general, support the hypothesis that these factors promote the lymphatic spread of human tumors.

In this context, it is well to remember that monoclonal antibodies, receptor bodies or tyrosine kinase inhibitors could be useful for anti-metastatic approaches to the treatment of human cancer as these agents inhibit tumor lymphangiogenesis directed to VEGFC, VEGFD or its receptor VEGFR3.

The walls of the lymph vessels are thin and there are numerous communication pathways between lymph channels and the vascular system. In fact the thoracic duct enters the confluence of the left internal jugular and the subclavian veins. The first filter of malignant cells from the primary site is the regional lymph glands. The tumor cells in the first stage, by periodic shower of malignant emboli into vascular channels, find their way to different predicted and unpredicted tissues.

Another type of dissemination is the transcelomic spread of mucin secreting tumors of stomach, colon, gallbladder and occasionally breast. Here too both mechanical and molecular forces have their roles to play, from the surface of these intraperitoneal organs, cancer cells are shed and they find their way to the peritoneal cavity and surface of the ovary. A well known but rare tumor of this type is the Krukenberg tumor of the ovary. The molecular factor is the presence of notching chemokine receptors and the matching ligands on the peritoneal and ovarian surfaces.

DORMANCY OF METASTASES

Metastases can arise long after the apparently successful treatment of a primary tumor. In breast cancer or melanoma, for example, metastases have been known to occur decades after primary treatment. Where are the cancer cells during this period of dormancy, and what awakens them? These questions are clinically important, but are largely unanswered at present.

Like the metastatic process itself, dormancy is a 'hidden' state, and is difficult to observe and study directly. Experimental studies, however, are now shedding some light on tumor dormancy. Judah, Folkman and his colleagues have provided evidence for the existence of pre-angiogenic micrometastases, in which cells actively divide, but at a rate that is balanced by the apoptotic rate because of failure of the micrometastases to become vascularized. Pre-angiogenic micrometastases could therefore be one source of tumor dormancy. If these small metastases subsequently acquire the ability to become vascularized, dormancy might cease and tumor growth would occur.

Another possible contributor to tumor dormancy is the persistence of solitary cells in secondary sites. Large numbers of solitary cells, which arrive in a secondary site but fail to initiate cell division, can persist for long periods of time in the organ. Furthermore, these cells can persist in a background of actively growing metastases, indicating that both dormant and non-dormant cells can be present in a secondary site. So, despite their apparent dormancy at a secondary site, the recovered cells still retained their tumorogenic phenotype. A better understanding of molecular factors that contribute to the maintenance and subsequent release from dormancy in secondary sites, both of solitary cells and pre-angiogenic metastases, will be important in treating this aspect of metastatic disease.

SYSTEMIC MANIFESTATIONS OF DISSEMINATED CANCER

One of the disabling problems in the treatment of cancer patients is the severe nutritional disorder. The term cachexia (Gr. kakos, bad, + hexis, condition) is used in wasting associated with malignancy. It is result of the so-called "systemic manifestations" of cancer or of the common host response to cancer. This type of wasting affects the skeletal muscles, fat and all organs with the exception of the liver and the brain. Wasting is due to many different factors, some hormonal, others being chemical transmitters. The hormones that are incriminated in malignant cachexia are adrenocorticotrophic hormone (ACTH), melanocyte-stimulating hormone (MSH) and chemical transmitters such as interleukin-1, serotonin and vasoactive amines. The cachexia cannot be strictly correlated to the size of the tumor or the rate of tumor growth.

a. Anorexia with diminished food intake
b. Hypermetabolism for the nutritional state of the individual
c. Wasting of body tissues or cachexia

Nausea and vomiting may be due to the inhibition of the satiety center in the brain. Intercurrent infection, malignant ulcers particularly of the cheek and the region of the neck too can produce nutritional imbalances.

MANAGEMENT OF A PATIENT WITH DISSEMINATED CANCER

The oncologist must find answers for the following questions. Which steps in the metastatic process are good targets for therapy? In theory, inhibition of any of the steps in the metastatic process — from the initial release of cells into the circulation at the site of the primary tumor, to the final stages of growth in the new organ — could offer therapeutic targets. In practice, however, two factors limit the potential success of targeting any phase of the metastatic process. First, is the step clinically accessible? Second, is the process a good biological target? Both of these factors indicate that the growth phase of the metastatic process is a promising therapeutic target.

The cancer cells can exist in two separate states :

1. Solitary cells that are not dividing; active pre-angiogenic micrometastases in which proliferation is balanced by apoptosis with no net increase in tumor size.
2. Vascularized metastases, which might be either quite small or clinically undetectable or larger and detectable by current technology. Furthermore, cells in all three states might be present in the same organ at the same time. Any therapy that prevents the progression of metastases to form clinically damaging tumors has the potential to benefit patients.

Systemic Therapy in Metastatic Cancer

Current anti-angiogenic strategies clearly meet the requirements of being both clinically accessible and biologically relevant, and would target both the growth of vascularized metastases and the progression of micrometastases to a vascularized state. These growth stages would also be targeted by anti-growth therapies, such as cytotoxic chemotherapeutic agents and molecularly based strategies that are designed to block specific growth pathways (for example, trastuzumab (herceptin), imatinib (glivec) and farnesyl transferase inhibitors). Also included in this category would be biphosphonate treatment to prevent the growth of metastases in bone.

Metastatic growth therefore offers a temporally broad target, which is both biologically and clinically appropriate. Any therapy that prevents the growth of metastases and the subsequent physiological damage caused by this growth has potential clinical utility. The search for 'anti-metastatic' agents must be broadened to include organ-specific growth as an appropriate target. The 'seed' and 'soil' compatibility that leads to organ-specific growth promotion of certain types of cancers in specific organs is itself a therapeutic target, if ways to interfere with the dependence of the cancer cell on factors present in the target organ can be identified. To achieve this aim, a better understanding of the factors that influence organ-specific metastatic growth of individual tumor types in various target organs is needed.

Surgery

The role of surgery is limited in a patient with metastatic malignant disease. When prominent symptomatology is obstruction, bleeding and ulceration over the skin and mucosal surfaces, surgery, whenever possible is done to alleviate the symptoms caused by the metastases. Surgery is also carried out to remove a solitary metastatic tumor, either symptomatic or asymptomatic, in the hope that it is the only metastatic site. It is not unusual to find a metastatic tumor in a proximal part or distal part of colon developing many years after the initial surgery. This tumor also has to be removed. Surgery is also indicated in these types of tumors.

Radiotherapy

Local metastases causing symptoms in such sites as bone, pleura and peritoneum frequently respond to palliative radiation therapy. Types of therapy used for specific areas are considered elsewhere.

FURTHER READING

1. Ann F, Chambers, Alan C Groom, Ian C MacDonald. Dissemination and growth of cancer cells in metastatic sites. Nature Reviews Cancer 2002;2:563-72.
2. Fidler IJ. Critical determinants of cancer metastasis rationale for therapy. Cancer chemother. Pharmacol 2002;43:503-10.
3. Fujimoto T, Zhang B, Minami S, Wang X, Takahashi Y, Mai M. Evaluation of intraoperative intraperitoneal cytology for advanced gastric carcinoma. Oncology 2002;62(3):201-08.
4. Steven A, Stacker, Marc G. Achen, Lotta Jussila, et al. Lymphangiogenesis and metastasis. Nature Rev Cancer 2002;2:573-83.
5. Woodhouse EC, Chuaqui RF, Liotta LA. General mechanisms of metastasis. Cancer 2002;80:1529-37.
6. Wyckoff JB, Jones JG, Condeelis JS, Segall JE. A critical step in metastasis in vivo analysis of intravasation of the primary tumor. Cancer Res 2001;60:2504-11.

Carcinoma of Unknown Primary

9

Antony Thomas, J Samuel

DEFINITION

Carcinoma of unknown primary (CUP) represents a hetero-geneous group of tumors first presenting with metastases for which detailed investigations as listed below fails to identify the site of origin at the time of diagnosis.

97 percent of patients complain of symptoms of metastatic sites, which become apparent on clinical examination. It must be understood that the primary sites of some of these cancers may be eventually determined by additional tests and they are no longer classified as cancers of unknown primary and they are renamed as newly discovered sites of origin.

For example, a patient with a metastasis to a lymph node on the side of the neck may be diagnosed with cancer of unknown primary. The appearance of the cancer under the microscope might suggest that the cancer started in the mouth, pharynx or larynx and later a detailed examination may prove that the primary lesion is in the pharynx. From then on, the patient has a pharyngeal cancer and not cancer of unknown primary.

In most cases of CUP, the source of the cancer is never discovered. Even when the primary site is not known, the histological studies with the information about the organs it has already affected, may help the clinician to plan the treatment.

THE SITES OF UNKNOWN PRIMARY

Carcinoma of unknown primary represents about 5 percent of all cancers diagnosed in the United States. Carcinoma of unknown primary (CUP) is more common among men than women. The average age of patients with these cancers is about 58 years.

Prognosis

When the spread of a CUP is limited to the cervical lymph nodes, between 30-50 percent of patients live for at least 5 years. When only the axillary lymph nodes are affected, about 25 percent of patients survive for 5 years after diagnosis. The 5-year survival rate is about 50 percent if spread is limited to inguinal lymph nodes and 30 percent when it is limited to the mediastinum or the retroperitoneum. The relatively good outlook for patients with limited spread to these areas depends on the effectiveness of local treatment.

The outlook is less favorable for patients with CUP that has spread more extensively and/or to other parts of the body. Among patients whose cancer of unknown primary has spread to multiple internal organs, about 5 percent remain alive 5 years after diagnosis. Most of the cancers in this group are fast spreading cancers and hence of poor prognosis.

Because the exact type of cancer is not known, it is more difficult to start any definitive treatment that is likely to help the patient. Among those cases with poor prognosis, male patients with adenocarcinoma histology, multiple number of organ sites and supraclavicular lymphadenopathy are worthy of mention.

Table 9.1 gives the reader an idea of the distribution of CUP. The cancers of the lung and pancreas top the list.

Table 9.1: The data is collected from a series involving a total of 1,453, which presented as CUP. (Diagnosed during life or at autopsy)	
Primary sites	%
Lung	23.7
Pancreas	21.1
Ovary	6.4
Kidney	5.5
Colorectal	5.3
Gastric	4.6
Liver	4.3
Prostate	4.1
Breast	3.4
Adrenal	2.2
Thyroid	2.2
Urinary tract/bladder	1.9
Esophagus	1.5
Lymphoma	1.5
Gallbladder/biliary tree	1.2
Testicular germ cell	1
Mesothelioma	0.5

With kind permission of Jame Abraham, Carmen J. Allegra.

Bethesda Clinical Oncology, Philadelphia, Lippincott, 2001.

CLINICAL FEATURES

Most of the patients complain of symptoms of CUP due to its presence in different presenting sites (Table 9.2).

Lymphoid Enlargement

The signs and symptoms of a cancer of unknown primary vary depending on which organs it has spread to. They include prominent, firm, non-tender lymph nodes on the sides of the neck or in the axilla or in the groin. These nodes are usually noticed by the patient or identified by the clinician during a routine check-up.

Abdominal Distension

Another metastatic site is within the abdomen that can be felt or produces a feeling of 'fullness'. This is often caused by liver metastasis or less often, the metastasis within the spleen. It is not unusual for multiple metastases to develop on the surface of many organs like intestine, small and large, omentum and peritoneum. This type of spread is usually associated with ascites.

Shortness of Breath

The patient experiences shortness of breath caused by cancer with involvement of lungs or by pleural effusion. Some of them complain of pain and discomfort in the chest and abdomen due to entrapment of nerves within these areas with malignant tissues.

Bone Pain

The bone pain can be severe when cancer has spread to bones. They may be weakened and fractures may result from minor injuries or even the normal stress of supporting the body's weight.

Skin Changes

One of the metastatic sites is the skin where CUP can be first seen. Certain cancers that start in the internal organs can spread through the blood stream to the skin. Because swelling or lump in the skin is easily seen, skin metastases are sometimes the first sign of spread from an internal organ and develop as cancer of the unknown origin.

Generalized Symptoms

The generalized symptoms of weakness, fatigue, poor appetite, and weight loss may be due to cancer spread to specific organs or systems such as the bone marrow or digestive system. It must be noted that half of the patients have multiple sites numbering more than 2 at the time of the first presentation.

Table 9.2: Common presenting sites		
Common presenting sites	%	*Range %*
Lymph node	26%	14-37
Lung	17%	18-19%
Bone	15%	15 - 30%
Liver	11%	4 –10%
Brain	8%	7-10%
Pleura	7%	2-12%
Skin	5%	0-22%
Peritoneal cavity	4%	1-4%

With kind permission of Jame Abraham, Carmen J.Allegra. Bethesda Clinical Oncology, Philadelphia, Lippincott, 2001.

Table 9.3 showing the metastatic site that was first apparent or first symptomatic in a total of 611 patients.

Risk Factors

Each type of cancer has distinct risk factors. Since the exact type of unknown primary is not known, it is difficult to identify the risk factors. Again, these cancers are a very diverse group, making this issue even more complicated.

Many of these cancers are known to start in the pancreas, lung, kidneys, throat, larynx or esophagus. Other cancers of unknown primary are eventually found to have started in the stomach, colon or rectum. Malignant melanoma is another source of cancer of unknown primary.

Table 9.3 where all principal metastatic sites in each patient were counted, the total number of patients being 1,051.

Table 9.3: Common metastatic sites	
Sites	%
Lymph node	41
Bone	29
Lung	27
Pleura	11
Peritoneum	9
Brain	6
Adrenal	6
Skin	4
Bone marrow	3

With kind permission of Jame Abraham, Carmen J.Allegra. Bethesda Clinical Oncology, Philadelphia, Lippincott, 2001

ETIOLOGY

The etiology of known cancers and cancers of unknown primary could be the same. Gene mutations which stimulate oncogenes and inhibit tumor suppressor genes have a role to play in the initiation of CUP. Usually DNA mutations related to CUP occur during life rather having been inherited before birth. Acquired mutations may result from smoking, dietary habits, exposure to ultraviolet light, radiation or cancer causing chemicals. Sometimes they occur for no apparent reason.

Many CUP can be prevented by lifestyle changes that reduce certain risk factors.

Smoking is by far the most significant risk factor that a person can control. One-third of all cancer deaths are estimated to be the direct result of smoking. Quitting or never starting offers the greatest opportunity for preventing cancers of many types, including those of unknown primary. Nutritional factors are estimated to be the cause of another third of fatal cancers.

Because the exact type and the origin of a CUP are unknown, it is not possible to say how that cancer might have been prevented. It is important to realize that many people with cancer have no apparent risk factors, and there is nothing they could have done to avoid the disease. On the other hand, other people have many risk factors but never develop cancer.

Screening Tests

The Indian Cancer Society has specific screening recommendations for early detection of oral, breast, prostate, cervical and colorectal cancer. The society also recommends a routine cancer-related checkup that can detect skin and thyroid cancers at an early stage. However, these cancers account for a relatively small fraction of cancers of unknown primary. There are still no screening tests that are effective in the early detection of the cancers that spread most rapidly and are likely to be diagnosed as cancer of unknown primary, such as lung, pancreatic, stomach and kidney cancer.

The problem of identifying an unknown primary with a positive cytological diagnosis of a metastatic gland or a visceral mass can be taxing to many physicians and oncologists. In most cases of cancer, the diagnosis of the primary lesion is made in the early period of the disease, while in some, the tumor presents in an advanced stage with metastases at the first consultation. But in a few cases, the oncologist becomes aware of the presence of a malignant lesion 'somewhere' in the body by the presence of a metastatic gland either in the neck, axilla, groin or metastasis in an organ such as the lung, liver or bone.

The two possible categories an unknown primary falls into are: metastatic involvement of lymph nodes and those with visceral involvement. The usual viscera that are involved are the lung and liver. The involvement of bone is also not unusual. The pleura, peritoneum, meninges too can be the seats of metastases.

This situation poses many challenges. The proper treatments either by chemotherapy or radiation demand an accurate histopathological diagnosis. In case, the primary is not easily recognized, proper pathological evaluation becomes mandatory.

GENERAL APPROACH TO DIAGNOSIS OF CARCINOMA OF UNKNOWN PRIMARY

The first step in evaluating a person with CUP is taking a detailed medical history and conducting a well planned clinical examination. In many cases, these simple steps will reveal, or at least strongly suggest, the source of the cancer. For example, during an interview, a patient with a lymph node enlargement with hoarseness will suggest a cancer of the larynx. Or, the physical examination may reveal a small tumor in the mouth that the patient had overlooked or assumed to be a benign condition. It is essential to undertake different laboratory tests and imaging studies to confirm the site of the CUP. *A* biopsy of the presenting site, whether it may be lymph gland, the liver mass or the skin tumor must be subjected to histology evaluation and the diagnosis of cancer must be confirmed before undertaking any other tests. Choice of tests would depend on which cancers are likely to occur in the patient's age and gender. Metastases in an inguinal lymph node of a 20-year-old man is likely to have spread from a testicular cancer while in a 75-year-old man, prostate cancer is more likely. An axillary lymph node with cancer in a 60-year-old woman is likely to have started in the nearby breast.

In choosing tests, it is better to start with ones that are not painful, do not cause serious complications, and are not too expensive. If these do not find the source of a cancer, then other tests are considered.

INVESTIGATIONS IN A CASE OF CARCINOMA OF UNKNOWN PRIMARY

1. Hematological studies
2. Urinalysis
3. Fecal occult blood test
4. Blood chemistry
5. Serum tumor markers
6. Pap smear
7. Biopsies, FNAC, core needle biopsy, bone marrow aspiration, excisional, incisional, and laparoscopic biopsy.
    All types of biopsies are examined under a microscope by a well-trained cytopathologist. In a few cases, the diagnosis of the primary lesion can be made by the histological evaluation. It can also classify

the cancers into broad categories to guide the treatment. If routine examination does not provide relevant information, further tests are necessary.

8. Immunohistochemistry
9. Electron microscopy
10. Cytogenetic assessment for diagnosis of translocation, inversion, deletion and addition.
11. Imaging studies-X-rays, CT scan, MRI, PET scan and Ultrasound.

Only after these examinations are complete, and the primary tumor site still remaining undetermined, the diagnosis of CUP is made.

CLASSIFICATION OF CUP

Carcinomas of unknown primary site require histologic evaluation and are categorized by pathology into:

a. squamous cell carcinomas
b. well and moderately differentiated adenocarcinomas
c. poorly differentiated carcinomas
d. undifferentiated neoplasms
e. carcinomas with neuroendocrine differentiation.

Immunohistochemistry should be routinely applied in poorly differentiated cases to exclude chemosensitive and potentially curable tumors (i.e. lymphomas and germ cell tumors).

In many cases, additional laboratory testing of a poorly differentiated malignant neoplasm will be done to classify it more precisely as a melanoma, lymphoma, sarcoma, small cell carcinoma, germ cell tumor, etc.

1. a. Evaluation for squamous cell CUP or poorly differentiated malignant neoplasm of CUP in cervical lymph nodes.

   Metastases to upper or middle cervical nodes usually come from cancers of the mouth, throat, sinuses, or larynx. Tests to find cancers of these sites are needed.

   The base of the tongue, the throat and the larynx are deep inside the neck and not easily seen. If the suspicion of cancer in the head and neck is very high, a very thorough examination of the oral cavity, oropharynx, larynx, esophagus, and the trachea and bronchi is performed with a fiberoptic pharyngo-laryngoscope. The examination is best done under general anesthesia and endoscopic biopsy of any suspicious area is done. Even if no abnormalities are seen, a few biopsies are routinely taken from the tonsils and other areas where cancers are often hard to see. Imaging tests such as CT and MRI scans of the sinuses and the neck area are also used to find small cancers that may have already spread to cervical nodes. Metastases to lower cervical nodes may also be from lung cancers, so a chest CT scan and bronchoscopy are often recommended to find lung cancers that may have been missed by a routine chest X-ray.

1. b. Evaluation for squamous cell CUP or a poorly differentiated malignant neoplasm of unknown primary in groin lymph nodes only.

   The likely sources of these metastases include cancers of the vulva, vagina, cervix, penis, skin of the legs, anus, rectum, or bladder. In women, a Pap test and examination of the vulva, vagina, and cervix are recommended. In men, the penis should be carefully examined. In both men and women, digital examination of the anorectal canal, and a proctoscopy examination must be conducted. Microscopic examination of urine, and pelvic CT scans may be useful.

2. a. Evaluation for adenocarcinoma of unknown primary or poorly differentiated malignant neoplasm of unknown primary in axillary lymph nodes only.

   In women, cancer that has spread to axillary nodes is most likely to have started in the breast. A thorough physical examination of the breast and diagnostic mammography are always done. An MRI of the breasts can be very useful. Tests to determine whether estrogen receptors (ER) and progesterone receptors (PR) are present are useful in planning treatment, and should be performed on the lymph node specimen. In men, a small cancer of the breast may rarely be responsible for axillary metastases.

2. b. Evaluation of adenocarcinoma of unknown primary or poorly differentiated malignant neoplasm of unknown primary in other locations.

   The main goal is to identify patients with types of cancer that respond well to specific treatments. Immunohistochemical tests for thyroglobulin can identify many thyroid cancers, which are often effectively treated with radioactive iodine injections. Other immunohistochemical tests can help identify breast cancers containing estrogen receptors (ER) and progesterone receptors (PR), and these cancers can be treated with hormonal therapy. Hormonal therapy is also used for prostate cancers, which can be identified by serum tests and immunohistochemical tests for prostate-specific antigen (PSA). A type of poorly differentiated malignant neoplasm called small cell carcinoma can develop in the lungs and, less often, in several other organs. Some small cell cancers respond to certain chemotherapy combinations. It is important to look for lymphomas since some can be cured by chemotherapy. It is also important to look for carcinoid tumors because these also have a fairly good outlook.

3. Evaluation of women with pelvic carcinomatosis of unknown primary: In this condition the spread of cancer on the surface of several pelvic organs is observed. The most likely source of a cancer that has spread in this way is the ovaries. Serum tests and immunohisto-chemical tests for CA 125 as well as CT scans of the abdomen and

pelvis are recommended to help determine whether the primary tumor is likely to be in the ovaries or some other organ. CA 125 is positive in most of the ovarian cancers. This is important because different chemotherapy drugs are used, and ovarian cancers have a better response to chemotherapy than many other cancers. Sometimes primary peritoneal carcinomatosis can arise in the peritoneum, which looks like and behaves like an ovarian cancer. Interestingly this condition is treated like ovarian cancer and responds well to treatment.

4. Evaluation of poorly differentiated malignant neoplasm of unknown primary in the retroperitoneum or mediastinum.
Germ cell tumors are one of the types of cancer that can start in these locations. CT scans of the chest and abdomen are used to try to exclude other types of cancers. Serum tests and immunohistochemical tests for alpha fetoprotein (AFP) and human chorionic gonadotrophin (HCG) are often positive in germ cell tumors. Cytogenetic studies may find chromosomal changes that support a diagnosis of germ cell tumor. It is important to identify germ cell tumors because they often respond well to certain combinations of chemotherapy drugs.

5. Evaluation for melanoma of unknown primary in neck, axilla, or groin lymph nodes only.
A thorough skin examination should be done to look for the primary melanoma. Some primary melanomas that have already metastasized may be quite small or may resemble ordinary moles to the untrained examiner. Rarely, primary melanomas regress and disappear on their own without treatment after metastasizing, leaving behind only an area of slightly lighter colored skin. Some patients may not recall that a primary melanoma had been previously removed. So it is important to specifically ask about any skin surgery and to look carefully for any small scars on the skin. The treatment of metastatic melanoma depends on whether or not it has spread only to lymph nodes or whether internal organs are also involved. Chest X-rays, CT scans of the head and abdomen, and blood tests that might suggest the site of the primary tumor. Liver metastasis has to be searched in any case of melanoma of unknown primary.

In a review reported by Hainsworth and Greco, approximately 60 percent of patients were found to have well-differentiated or moderately well-differentiated adenocarcinoma after light microscopy findings, 5 percent were found to have squamous carcinoma, and 35 percent of the patients were determined to have poorly differentiated neoplasm.

GENERAL PRINCIPLES OF TREATMENT OF UNKNOWN PRIMARY

It is most frustrating to the clinician to treat a patient with an unknown primary malignant tumor that already has proven metastatic lymph node or visceral secondaries. The patient too goes through agonizing days wondering what he can be offered by the clinician after the biopsy and expensive tests.

Surgery

It must be clearly understood that surgery has only a limited role in the treatment of CUP, as the primary is unknown. Most of the tumors come under Stage III or IV. At the same time it is seen that the removal of glandular and visceral metastatic sites can offer long term survival. The cervical, axillary and inguinal nodes can eventually enlarge and may cause skin necrosis and ulceration, which will increase the morbidity and the mortality. In case of peritoneal carcinomatosis, the patient must undergo laparotomy and surgical cytoreduction of the tumor mass. This will increase the survival time. The surgeon must be judicious in selecting cases that could withstand surgery and evaluate each case in the merit of the patient's willingness for surgery and the clinical status.

Radiation Therapy

Radiation therapy can be used with the goal of curing some cancers that have not spread too far from their sites of origin. Even when a cancer has spread too far to be cured by radiation therapy, radiation can still be used to palliate or relieve such symptoms as pain, bleeding, difficulty in swallowing, intestinal obstruction, compression of blood vessels or nerves by tumors. Radiation relieves the problems caused by metastases to bones. The radiotherapist has to plan the treatment of carcinoma of unknown primary once the oncologist feels that this modality of treatment would help the patient. If the neck area is treated with external beam radiation, the thyroid gland may be damaged, and drugs to replace thyroid hormone may be needed. External or internal radiation therapy to the head and neck area often causes damage to salivary glands, resulting in dry mouth, sore throat, hoarseness, difficulty in swallowing, partial or complete loss of taste and temporary tiredness. Radiation of the abdomen can also cause nausea, diarrhea, vomiting, and temporary or permanent damage to the intestines. Chest radiation may cause lung scarring that can eventually lead to shortness of breath. Chemotherapy may make some of the side effects of radiation worse.

Chemotherapy

Chemotherapy is used as *primary* (main) therapy with the intention of curing or at least inducing a remission in poorly differentiated carcinomas and some cancers such as germ cell tumors and lymphomas. Chemo-therapy drugs kill cancer cells but also damage some normal cells. Therefore, careful attention must be given to avoiding or minimizing side effects, which depend on the type of drugs, the amount taken, and the length of treatment. Temporary side effects might include nausea and vomiting, loss of appetite, loss of hair, and mouth sores. Because chemotherapy can damage the blood-producing cells of the bone marrow, patients may have low blood cell counts. This can result in an increased chance of infection, bleeding or bruising after minor cuts or injuries due to a shortage of blood platelets, and fatigue due to low red blood cell counts. Most side effects disappear once the treatment is stopped. There are remedies for many of the temporary side effects of chemotherapy. For example, *antiemetic* drugs to prevent or reduce nausea and vomiting can be given.

1. Treatment for squamous cell carcinoma of unknown primary or poorly differentiated malignant neoplasm of unknown primary in cervical lymph nodes only.

   If no primary tumor is found in spite of detailed investigations, the patient may be treated with surgery and/or with radiation therapy. Surgical treatment consists of a neck dissection. A modified radical neck dissection is preferred to simple node dissection for cervical node involvement. The common side effects of any neck dissection are numbness of the ear caused by injury to the greater auricular nerve, weakness in raising the arm above the head caused by injury to the spinal accessory nerve, and weakness of the lower lip caused by injury to the facial nerve. After a modified radical neck dissection, the weakness of the arm and lower lip usually disappear after a few months. However, if either nerve is removed as part of a radical neck dissection or because of involvement with the tumor, then the weakness is permanent. Radiation therapy might be used instead of surgery. One potential advantage is that the area treated would include the nodes with metastatic cancer and several of the areas of the neck likely to contain a primary tumor. Some patients are treated with both surgery and radiation therapy. This is considered when large and/or multiple tumors are present. Radiation may be given before or after surgery. When tumors are very large or present on both sides of the neck, chemotherapy and radiation therapy are often used together. The prognosis of these patients depends on the size, number and location of the nodes containing metastatic cancer. When the nodes are small and few, the 5-year survival rate is about 80 percent. When there is spread to both sides of the neck, about 70 percent of patients survive at least for 5 years. The spread of cancer to nodes in the lower part of the neck or nodes above the clavicle carries a less favorable outlook with a 5-year survival rate of about 5 percent.

2. The treatment of adenocarcinoma of unknown primary or poorly differentiated malignant neoplasm of unknown primary in axillary (underarm) lymph nodes only.

Because most axillary node metastases in women are from breast cancers, the recommended treatment is the same as for women diagnosed with stage II breast cancer. An axillary node dissection is done, and the breast on the same side is treated either with modified radical mastectomy or with radiation therapy. Depending on the patient's age and whether the cancer cells contain estrogen and progesterone receptor adjuvant treatment will include hormonal therapy with tamoxifen, chemotherapy, or both hormonal and chemotherapy. Although axillary lymph node metastases in men may represent spread from a breast cancer, spread from a lung cancer is much more likely. Treatment in men consists of the same chemotherapy combinations given for adenocarcinoma or poorly differentiated carcinoma of unknown primary in other locations. An axillary lymph node dissection may be recommended, while a few will rather observe how the enlarged lymph nodes respond to chemotherapy.

3. The treatment of squamous cell carcinoma of unknown primary or poorly differentiated neoplasm of unknown primary in groin lymph nodes only.

   The main goal of treatment in this situation is to prevent the cancer in the node from continuing to spread locally and causing problems such as skin ulceration and secondary infection. This is accomplished by simply removing the large node by excisional biopsy or by a superficial groin node dissection. The deeper nodes are not removed. The 2-year survival rate after these operations is about 50 percent. If the cancer spreads further and causes symptoms, palliative surgery, radiation or chemotherapy can be considered.

4. The treatment of women with pelvic carcinomatosis of unknown primary (spread of carcinoma of unknown primary on the surface of several pelvic organs).

   Unless tests have found a primary cancer outside the ovaries (in which case the diagnosis of carcinoma of unknown primary would no longer apply), these women are assumed to have an ovarian cancer that has spread within the pelvis. The treatment involves surgical removal of the uterus, both ovaries, both Fallopian tubes, and as much of the cancer as possible. After surgery, six to eight months of chemotherapy is recommended. The 3-year survival rate is in the range of 10-25 percent.

5. The treatment of poorly differentiated malignant neoplasm of unknown primary in the retroperitoneum or mediastinum.

   Once lymphoma has been excluded by appropriate laboratory testing of the tumor sample, the most likely diagnosis, particularly in men is a germ cell tumor. Even those cancers in one of these locations that do not have laboratory results typical of germ cell tumors often respond to chemotherapy combinations developed for treating testicular germ cell tumors. Depending on the exact location and amount of the cancer present, 5-year survival rates vary from 15-35 percent.

6. The treatment of poorly differentiated malignant neoplasm of unknown primary or adenocarcinoma of unknown primary in other locations. This group represents the majority of people with carcinoma of unknown primary. Usually the cancer is in the bones, lung, liver, breast, prostate or thyroid, and lymphoma. Amongst them lymphoma often responds well to specific treatments. Once laboratory testing of the biopsy specimen has excluded the lymphoma, many of the remaining patients are treated with chemotherapy for the purpose of palliation. The standard chemotherapy regimen consists of either cisplatin or carboplatin combined with etoposide. In some recent reports, other drugs like 5-FU, mitomycin and doxorubicin are added to this combination. The side effects of cisplatin are severe nausea and vomiting and, over time, numbness of hands and feet. The other side effects are hair loss and low blood counts. Sometimes the chemotherapy can be quite helpful. A significant minority (about 15%) of patients treated with aggressive chemotherapy will survive for a few years after diagnosis. For patients healthy enough to withstand aggressive chemotherapy, this treatment offers a chance for survival several years after diagnosis and, an average, extends survival by 3 to 11 months. Patients in poor health who would not be able to tolerate the side effects of aggressive chemotherapy are sometimes treated with lower doses or with drugs that cause fewer side effects. But the benefit of this approach is not clearly proven. Another option is to focus on relieving symptoms as they occur. Some poorly differentiated small cell cancers of unknown origin can respond dramatically to chemotherapy combinations originally developed to treat small cell lung cancer. The benefit is not longstanding usually, and 2-year survival rates are about 20 percent.

7. The treatment of melanoma of unknown origin in neck, axilla or inguinal lymph nodes only.

Once a carcinoma of unknown primary has been diagnosed as melanoma, it is no longer a true carcinoma of unknown primary. This situation is mentioned, nonetheless, because tests to identify some melanomas may take several days. Until they are complete, these patients are considered to have carcinoma of unknown primary. The recommended treatment of melanoma of unknown primary is simply removing lymph nodes of the affected area. If spread to additional nodes becomes apparent at a later time, but no unresectable metastases to internal organs are present, the nodes are also removed. It is seen that interferon alfa can slow the return of melanoma. The main side effects of this drug are fatigue and 'flu' like symptoms.

FOLLOW-UP AFTER TREATMENT OF CARCINOMA OF UNKNOWN PRIMARY

Frequent follow-up exams are needed for several years after the treatment for carcinoma of unknown primary is finished. Check ups include a careful physical examination, X-rays when necessary and laboratory tests. A relapse of carcinoma of unknown primary usually occurs while in treatment or shortly after a patient has finished chemotherapy. It is unusual for carcinoma of unknown primary to return if there are no signs of the disease five years after therapy is finished.

NEWER OPTIONS

Research into the causes, diagnosis, and treatment of cancer is being done at many cancer research centers. Scientists are making progress in understanding how changes in a person's DNA can cause normal cells to develop into cancer. A greater understanding of the genes involved in genetic abnormalities which can occur in cancer is providing insight into why these cells become abnormal. Some of this information is already being used to develop tests to classify carcinoma of unknown primary more precisely and predict prognosis and response to treatment. Because many patients with cancer face a serious prognosis, the need for advances in treatment is obvious. Clinical trials of new treatments are essential if progress is to occur. Some of these trials are testing new chemotherapy drugs, new drug combinations, and new ways to administer these drugs. Other trials are studying new approaches to treatment, such as biological therapy, immunotherapy, and gene therapy. The continued progress toward understanding the molecular basis of all cancers, will help in the study of carcinoma of unknown primary —a very diverse category of many types of cancers.

Needless to say that the presence of a metastatic node with an unknown primary gives anxious moments both to the oncology team and the patient and his dear ones. Some of the patients are too ill to be subjected to any diagnostic modalities. But now we know there is a cohort of patients who can be helped by radiation and chemotherapy. It is the duty of the treating physician to identify these subsets and treat them with modern therapeutic protocol.

FURTHER READING

1. Casciato DA, Lowitz BB (Eds). Metastases of unknown origin. In: Manual of Clinical Oncology (3rd ed). New York: Little, Brown and Company 1995;331-43.
2. Fisher DS, Knobf MT, Durivage HJ. The Cancer Chemotherapy Handbook (5th ed). St. Louis: Mosby-Year Book, Inc 1997;41:218-329.
3. Greco FA, Hainsworth JD. Cancer of unknown primary site. In: DeVita VT, Heilman S, Rosenberg SA (Eds). Cancer: Principles and Practice of Oncology (5th ed). Philadelphia, Pa: Lippincott-Raven Publishers 1997;2423-42.

4. Greco FA, Vaughn WK, Hainsworth JD. Advanced poorly differentiated cancer of unknown primary site: Recognition of a treatable syndrome. Ann Intern Med 1986;104:547-53.
5. Jame Abraham, Carmen J Allegra. Carcinoma of unknown primary. Bethesda Handbook of Clinical Oncology: Lippincott-Williams and Williams, 2001;387-96.
6. Steckel RJ, Kagan RA. Metastatic tumors of unknown origin: diagnostic and therapeutic implications. In: Murphy GP, Lawrence W, Lenhard RE Jr (Eds). American Cancer Society Textbook of Clinical Oncology. Atlanta: The American Cancer Society 1996;714-18.

Paraneoplastic Syndromes

10

Antony Thomas, K Pavithran

The term 'paraneoplasia' has been coined to denote the remote effects of malignancy that cannot be attributed either to direct invasion or metastatic lesions and may be the first sign of malignancy in 15 percent of patients. These may often be considered to be due to aberrant hormonal or metabolic effects, which are not produced by the tissue of tumor origin. Clubbing associated with bronchogenic carcinoma is recognized as a paraneoplastic syndrome. Clubbing is not due to direct invasion or metastasis but due to proliferation of connective tissue. Insulin produced by a tumor of endocrine cells of pancreas is not considered paraneoplastic while insulin produced by an unrelated neoplasm like fibrosarcoma is designated as paraneoplastic. Over the life span of the patient with cancer, the chance of developing paraneoplastic syndrome is around 50-60 percent.

FACTORS INVOLVED IN PARANEOPLASTIC SYNDROMES

1. The mediators involved in paraneoplastic syndromes are tropic (ectopic) hormones resembling those normally produced, e.g. Adreno-corticotropic hormone (ACTH) and ACTH-like substances in small cell carcinoma of the lung, pancreatic carcinoma and neural tumors, melano-cyte stimulating hormone (MSH) in colon carcinoma, antidiuretic hormone (ADH) in small cell carcinoma of the lung, certain intracranial tumors and parathormone-like substance associated with small cell carcinoma of the lung, breast carcinoma and renal cell carcinoma.
2. Immunologically active substances, e.g. myeloma proteins in multiple myeloma and physiologically active substances, like serotonin, bradykinin, and histamine are released in bronchial carcinoid, pancreatic carcinoma and gastric carcinoma.

3. Erythropoietin is released in renal cell carcinoma, cerebellar hemangioma and hepatocellular carcinoma.

4 In advanced cancers and in pancreatic and lung carcinomas there is hypercoagulability, which produces venous thrombosis (Trousseau's phenomenon) and non-bacterial thrombotic endocarditis.

5 It is also noted that there is depressed function of the tumor cells in a degree to which their capacity to divide is inhibited. The control mechanism is also lost. A good example is that the renal tissue produces erythropoietin only when there is tissue anoxia while in renal cell tumors, erythropoietin may be produced without regard to the control mechanism of anoxia.

A plausible theory is that the tumor which has the identical embryological analog of origin, may begin to secrete products of other tissues derived from the same analog, e.g. both anterior pituitary and lung are developed from the same branchial cleft. This results in lung cancers being associated with ACTH, ADH, and MSH production. Parathormone production in carcinoma of the lung may represent depression of synthesis of products of another branchial cleft tissue.

Synthesis of an abnormal hormone by inefficient tumor cells may result in large amounts of a product which block receptor sites and interferes with control by active hormone, e.g. in certain renal cell cancers, ineffective erythropoietin which coats marrow receptors may be produced which instead of polycythemia associated with renal tumors, anemia could develop.

PATHOGENESIS OF SYSTEMIC REACTIONS

1. Since cancer cells are not contact-inhibited, they invade basement membranes and secrete their specialized products into tissue spaces instead of secretory cavities such as gland ducts, lumens of gut and bronchus. These products, being foreign to the interior of the tissues, may excite antigenic reactions in the other tissues in the host, with resulting autoimmune phenomena such as fever, hemolysis, arthropathy, and vasculitis.

2. The endothelium of tumors is discontinuous with that of the normal capillaries. Much intratumor circulation is sinusoidal, blood circulating directly between the unendothelialized walls of tumor cells. Circulating red cells are damaged by contact with surfaces other than vascular endothelium, hence, hemolysis of the Starr valve type occurs in tumors.

3. Normal cells from these organs like skin, gut, breast and endometrium, die in response to the cell cycle in large numbers on to surfaces of these organs and are handled by specialized mechanisms. The body has a very limited capacity to handle other cells that die *in situ*. Tumor cells die frequently (high spontaneous death) in forbidden

places, releasing polypeptides and other products that are inflammatory and antigenic.

4. It was mentioned earlier about the different types of hormones produced in different types of tumors, that some of them represent the earliest symptoms of an unknown primary tumor while some others produce profound systemic changes.

ECTOPIC HORMONE PRODUCTION

Many tumors affect different metabolic functions of the host by the elaboration of circulating products that act at great distances from the tumor. The metabolic consequences of the neoplastic state can be clarified and at least partially understood on the basis of the pathophysiology of the neoplastic cell and tissues. It must be noted that one sixth of patients in late stage of cancer will have serious systemic effects due to different types of hormones secreted by the malignant tissue. It is seen that both primary tumor and secondary deposits are areas from where ectopic hormone is produced. Of the four classes of hormone-steroids, monoamines, amino acids and peptides/proteins, only the last one is secreted ectopically, as it requires less complicated derangements in cell metabolism. A few common paraneoplastic syndromes due to ectopic hormone production are given in the Table 10.1.

PARANEOPLASTIC NEUROLOGICAL SYNDROMES

Associated with malignancy, the physicians are recognizing a syndrome where different parts of the central nervous system both central and

Table 10.1: Ectopic hormones in paraneoplastic syndrome	
Hormones	*Common tumors*
Adrenocorticotrophin (ACTH)-(Cushing's syndrome)	Small cell lung carcinoma, Thymoma, Pancreatic islet cell tumor, Thyroid medullary carcinoma, Pheochromocytoma, Prostatic carcinoma.
Corticotrophin releasing hormone (CRH)	Small cell lung carcinoma, Carcinoid.
Vasopressin, Oxytocin, Neurophysin-(Syndrome of inappropriate antidiuretic hormone secretion- SIADH)	Small cell lung carcinoma, Carcinoid.
Chorionic gonadotropin	Lung carcinoma, Gastric carcinoma, Ovarian carcinoma, hepatoma, Hepatoblastoma.
Parathyroid hormone related protein (PTH-rp) (Hypercalcemia)	Renal carcinoma, Squamous carcinoma of lung, Hepatoma, Pancreatic islet cell tumors.
Insulin like factors (Hypoglycemia)	Mesenchymal tumors-fibrosarcoma, hepatoma.

peripheral, develop altered functions at different levels. This could occur even before the tumor clinically manifests. In some cases, these CNS symptoms can develop during the treatment and in some it may exhibit many years after the onset of the disease. The lesions are not due to the primary tumor or the metastasis. It is probably due to the deleterious effect of antigens, antibodies, and cytotoxic substances reaching the brain cells, spinal cord and peripheral nerves through blood stream. Common paraneoplastic neurologic syndromes are given in the order from brain to muscle in terms of the involved site (Table 10.2).

PARANEOPLASTIC DERMATOSIS

Paraneoplastic dermatosis can only be the presenting feature in a malignant disease. This can resemble any of the other skin diseases, and the early detection and initiation of therapy is important. The common paraneoplastic dermatoses are given in Table 10.3.

CLUBBING AND HYPERTROPHIC OSTEOARTHROPATHY

Selective bulbous enlargement of the distal segment of the fingers and toes due to proliferation of connective tissue is termed clubbing. The term

Table 10.2: Paraneoplastic neurologic manifestations		
Syndrome/ Clinical features	*Pathology*	*Common tumors*
Cancer associated retinopathy (progressive visual loss)	Associated with CAR-Antibodies	Small cell lung carcinoma
Encephalopathy, Sensory neuropathy	Associated with organ specific autoantibody-Anti-Hu	Small cell lung carcinoma
Cerebellar degeneration	Associated Purkinje cell antibody-Anti-Yo	Ovarian carcinoma, Small cell lung carcinoma
Acute demyelinating neuritis	Similar to Guillain-Barre syndrome	Hodgkin's disease
Lambert-Eaton myasthenic syndrome	Associated with LEMS-autoantibody (diminished acetyl choline activity at motor nerve terminals)	Small cell lung carcinoma, Breast, Prostate and Stomach tumors
Myasthenia gravis	MG-antibody mediated reduction in acetyl choline receptors at postsynaptic junction	Thymoma
Polymyositis-dermatomyositis	Myofiber necrosis, phagocytosis, and inflammation, high CPK	Breast tumors, Lung tumors, Lymphoma
Necrotizing myopathy	Myonecrosis with minimal inflammation	Bronchial carcinoma, Small cell lung carcinoma

Table 10.3: Paraneoplastic dermatosis	
Clinical features	*The common tumors*
Bazen syndrome; cutaneous eruption, nail dystrophy, paronychia, psoariasiform plaques on digits (acrokeratoses)	Squamous cell carcinoma of pyriform sinus, oral cavity, upper respiratory tract and gastrointestinal tract
Erythema gyratum refers to distinct skin eruptions with irregular urticarial bands of erythema	Lung, breast, cervical and gastric malignancies
Acanthosis nigricans; symmetric hyperpigmentation and thickening of flexural areas like axilla, inguinal region, side of neck, perineum, inframammary area etc.	Adenocarcinoma especially of stomach
Leser-Trelat sign; sudden appearance of multiple seborrheic keratosis along with pruritus	Gastric adenocarcinoma, hematopoietic, breast and lung neoplasms
Sweet's syndrome; acute febrile neutrophilic dermatoses with erythematous to voilaceous papules or plaques on arms, head and neck	Associated with acute myelogenous or myelomonocytic leukemia
Paraneoplastic pemphigus; polymorphous vesicobullous skin lesions that resemble pemphigus vulgaris, pemphigus foliaceous or erythema multiforme	Lymphoma, thymoma
Cryoglobulinemia; acral cyanosis, purpura, urticarial, Raynaud's phenomena, superficial ulceration or gangrene	Myeloma, lymphocytic leukemia, lymphoma, hairy cell leukemia, mycosis fungoidosis
Amyloidosis of heart, tongue, gastrointestinal tract, nerves and skin	In a variety of conditions (Primary amyloidosis in multiple myeloma)

hypertrophic osteoarthropathy is used when there is periosteal new bone formation in association with connective tissue proliferation. Clubbing may be hereditary, idiopathic or acquired in a variety of disorders, both neoplastic and non-neoplastic. Clubbing seen in association with bronchogenic carcinoma and mesothelioma are considered paraneoplastic. However clubbing can also be seen in conditions like cyanotic heart disease, infective endocarditis, metastatic lung carcinoma, bronchiectasis, lung abscess, cystic fibrosis, pulmonary tuberculosis, and gastrointestinal disorders like hepatic cirrhosis, ulcerative colitis and Crohn's disease.

HEMATOLOGICAL AND VASCULAR NEOPLASTIC SYNDROMES

One-sixth of malignant tumors produce life-threatening hematological problems like aplastic anemia, leucopenia, thrombocytopenia and purpura-like syndromes. It is not uncommon to see disseminated intravascular coagulopathy in certain types of tumors. Hypercoagulability is yet another feature of pancreatic and lung tumors and in women with carcinoma of the uterus and ovaries. Trousseau's syndrome was first described in 1865 when a close relationship was noticed between superficial thrombophlebitis of the leg veins and different types of cancers. This thrombophlebitis occurs spontaneously and is recurrent and migratory. Over a period of days, the thrombophlebitis resolves often to recur in the same or nearby vessels. Fever, tenderness and edema of the skin around the involved veins are seen. It is also seen that multiple areas are involved at the same time. Both superficial and deep veins of the legs are commonly involved, so too other veins like superior vena cava, inferior vena cava, portal and iliac veins. The underlying pathophysiology in this condition is variable but it is assumed that it is due to disseminated intravascular coagulation with associated depletion of fibrinogen and thrombocytopenia. In some patients direct tumor involvement of the veins is also noticed. Anticoagulant therapy is of limited use.

"Stimulation" of bone marrow elements in response to products secreted by tumor "hormones" is associated with increase in formed elements of blood. Enhanced erythropoietin secretion seen in renal cell cancer, hepatoma and cerebellar hemangioma are associated with erythrocytosis. Frank leukemoid reactions, thrombocytosis and eosinophilia are also seen. Vascular syndromes like Raynaud's phenomenon—unilateral as well as bilateral are seen in association with breast, mediastinal, esophageal and gastric malignancies. These do not respond to usual treatment modes with nifedipine or cervical sympathectomy. Various vasculitis syndromes are seen particularly in association with lymphoid malignancies and some of them may be due to direct vascular invasion.

IMMUNOSUPPRESSION

The mechanism for paraneoplastic immunosuppression is not clear. Defects in both T and B lymphocyte function and abnormalities in macrophages are noted. Immunosuppression is seen in association with primary lymphoid malignancies, various advanced cancers and also with chemotherapy and radiotherapy. Let's not forget that one approach to cancer treatment involves an attempt to stimulate an effective immune response against malignant cell population by using monoclonal antibodies against tumor cells or by use of cytokines.

TREATMENT OF PARANEOPLASTIC SYNDROMES

Proper treatment of the original tumor creates long-term control. Since most paraneoplastic syndromes are seen in the advanced stages of malignancy, the cure of tumor and syndrome is not likely. Yet for a lung cancer which is not amenable to surgical cure or chemoradiation, palliation may be worth trying with radiation or resection to control the PTH-rp hypercalcemia.

The treatment of the pathophysiologic mechanisms like inhibition of hormone production, may occasionally help:

1. Actinomycin D is used to inhibit biosynthesis of parathormone-like hormone by renal cancer.
2. The inhibition of adrenal response to ACTH from lung or thymus tumor causing Cushing's, diabetes, and bone fracture is possible with the use of metapyrone or aminoglutethimide. In case of bone fracture, surgical intervention like plating, intramedullary nail or cementation can be done. There should be calcium and vitamin D supplement in such cases.

THE PALLIATION IN PARANEOPLASTIC SYNDROMES

In many instances this is very important for the comfort of the patient and is operationally all that can be done. Some of the syndromes and therapies, which may be helpful, include:

1. The treatment of hypercalcemia is important and in certain situations, life saving. In mild cases, where the serum calcium is between 10 and 12 mg percent, adequate hydration with steroids and frusemide 40 mg i.v. would be helpful. If the serum calcium is more than 12 mg percent, pramidronate/zolendronate/calcitonin with adequate hydration should be carried out without delay.

2. In the case of syndrome of inappropriate antidiuretic hormone secretion, the severity of hyponatremia can be variable and may be as low as 100 mEq/L. This could be both relative due to dilution of sodium and absolute due to loss of sodium in the urine and sweat. Proper correction of sodium and chloride should be done by assessing the plasma electrolytes, at least once in 24 hours. Proper correction of hyponatremia should be done by normal saline.

3. Venous thrombosis, either superficial or deep is treated with anticoagulants. NSAID can relieve the pain. In severe cases, Pethidine may be given. The leg is kept elevated and the area is dressed with warm magnesium sulphate glycerin dressings. The thrombophlebitis resolves in 4 to 6 weeks time only to reappear after a few weeks.

FURTHER READING

1. Abeloff MD. Clinical Oncology (2nd ed). New York: Churchill Livingstone, 1999.
2. Andres R, Mayordomo JI, Ramon Y, Cajal S, Tres A. Paraneoplastic syndrome. Tumor 2002;88(1):65-67.
3. Bearz A, Giometto B, Freschi A, et al. Occult small cell lung cancer associated with paraneoplastic neurologic syndrome — Case report. Tumor 2001;87(6):447-50.
4. Esbrit P, Hurtado J. Treatment of malignant hypercalcemia. Expert Opin Pharmacother 2002;3(5):521-27.
5. Kristenson B, Ejlertsen B, et al. Prednisolone in the treatment in severe malignant hypercalcemia in metastatic breast cancer: A randomized study. J Intern Med 1992;232:237-45.
6. Marmur R, Kagen L. Cancer-associated neuromusculoskeletal syndromes: Recognizing the rheumatic-neoplastic connection. Postgrad Med 2002;111(4):95-98.
7. Oei ME, Kraft GH, Sarnat HB. Intravascular lymphomatosis. Muscle Nerve Study 2002;25(5):742-46.

Oncologic Emergencies

11

Jame Abraham, M Nageswara Rao

This condition is a very serious and sometimes life-threatening complication in bulky tumors or those tumors undergoing cancer therapy. The administration of anti-tumor agents can lead to cell death with subsequent release of intracellular contents. Tumor Lysis Syndrome (TLS) occurs when cellular disruption results in life-threatening lactic acidosis, with concomitant hyperuricemia, hyperkalemia, hyperphosphatemia and hypocalcemia. The patient can also present with renal failure.

Tumor lysis syndrome can be precipitated before the initiation of therapy or up to 5 days after the start of chemotherapy, especially with tumors that have a high level of growth with rapid turnover of cells and high sensitivity to chemotherapy. Burkitt's lymphoma and T cell acute lymphoblastic leukemia are most frequently associated with this complication. It has been seen also in association with solid tumors like hepatoblastoma and stage IV neuroblastoma.

SIGNS AND SYMPTOMS OF TUMOR LYSIS SYNDROME

TLS usually occurs when a patient with bulky tumors is treated with cytotoxic agents. It is more common in rapidly proliferating tumors. TLS most often occurs during the treatment of leukemia or high-grade lymphomas but may rarely occur during the treatment of solid tumors.

Cardiac arrhythmias may result from the severe hyperkalemia or hypocalcemia that accompanies TLS. Hypocalcemia can result in tetany, anorexia, vomiting, seizures, spasms, and altered mental status while hyperphosphatemia, and hyperuricemia can result in acute renal failure. Lethargy, nausea, and vomiting manifest at uric acid levels of 10-15 mg percent before the onset of renal failure.

TREATMENT OF TUMOR LYSIS SYNDROME

The pretreatment identification of individuals at risk, along with 24-48 hours of pre-hydration, use of pre-therapy allopurinol and vigilant metabolic monitoring (q 3-4 hour labs) after institution of therapy, are the hallmarks of TLS prevention and management. Elevated LDH, uric acid, or creatinine at presentation identifies a particularly high-risk patient.

Corrective measures should be directed toward any metabolic abnormalities that occur after starting cytotoxic therapy and particular care should be given to appropriate monitoring (e.g. continuous or serial EKGs) and early interventions during correction of hyperkalemia, ICU admission for severe hemodynamic instability, and hemodialysis when faced with worsening or severely compromised renal function.

The correction of metabolic abnormalities during TLS is similar to general ICU patient management with specific interventions for correction of hypocalcemia, hyperkalemia, hyperphosphatemia, hyperuricemia and renal failure.

PREVENTION

The pretreatment identification of individuals at risk, along with 24 to 48 hours of prehydration, use of pretherapy allopurinol, and vigilant metabolic monitoring, along with 3-4 hours laboratory tests after institution of therapy are the hallmarks of TLS prevention and management. Elevated lactate dehydrogenase (LDH), uric acid or creatinine at presentation identifies a particularly high-risk patient.

HYPERURICEMIA

Hyperuricemic acute renal failure may be avoided by: (1) pre-chemotherapy identification of patients at risk for developing TLS, (2) 24 to 48 hours of prehydration and (3) administration of allopurinol at doses of 600-900 mg qd starting several days before chemotherapy, with tapering doses to maintain uric acid levels of < 7 mg percent. Hyperuricemic acute renal failure is usually refractory to conservative therapy and may require hemodialysis as supportive therapy. The new drug uricase could well change this paradigm in the near future.

HYPERPHOSPHATEMIA

If mild to moderate, restrict dietary phosphate to 0.6 to 0.9 g/day or add aluminum hydroxide, 300 to 600 mg p.o. t.i.d before meals. If severe, volume expansion with 1,000 to 3,000 cc 0.9 percent sodium chloride injection i.v. over 1 to 2 hours is required.

HYPOCALCEMIA

If symptomatic and persisting after correction of hyperphosphatemia, 10cc of 10 percent calcium chloride i.v. is given slowly over 10 minutes, or diluted in 100 cc of 5 percent dextrose saline in water and infused over 20 minutes. Calcium gluconate, 10 percent solution, 20 cc i.v. over to 15 minutes can also be given. Serum calcium should be carefully monitored. Calcium chloride contains about 3 times more elemental calcium than an equal volume of calcium gluconate. Therefore, when hyperkalemia is accompanied by hemodynamic compromise, calcium chloride is preferred to calcium gluconate.

HYPERKALEMIA

Confirm that the elevation is genuine.
1. If mild, restrict food with potassium.
2. If moderate, administer calcium gluconate, 10 percent solution, 10 to 30 cc i.v. over 2 to 5 minutes (onset 0 to 5 minutes,1 hour duration).
3. Provide regular insulin, 10 U i.v. push with 10 cc of 50 percent glucose i.v. over 5 minutes.
4. Give kayexalate orally, 15 to 50 g in 50 to 100 cc of 20 percent sorbitol solution, repeated every 3 to 4 hours up to 5 times per day. Each modality has an approximate duration of 1 to 3 hours.
5. If emergent with onset of cardiac toxicity, paralysis, or levels greater than 6.5 to 7 mEq/L prepare for hemodialysis.

The majority of patients with acute renal failure can be managed conservatively, but peritoneal or hemodialysis must be considered if conservative management fails. The decision to initiate dialysis is usually not based on a single laboratory abnormality, but on the constellation of findings and the likelihood of further clinical deterioration. Each of the associated findings is much more worrisome in the setting of oliguria or anuria such as uncontrolled hyperkalemia (generally serum potassium >7 mEq/L) and worsening hyperuricemia (serum uric acid >10 mg%). Mere elevation of elevated uric acid in the absence of other abnormalities usually does not require dialysis but can be treated conservatively.

FURTHER READING

1. Chan FK, Koberle LM, et al. Differential diagnosis, causes, and management of hypercalcemia. Curr Probl Surg 1997;34:445-523.
2. Esbrit P, Hurtado J. Treatment of malignant hypercalcemia. Expert Opin Pharmacother 2002;3(5):521-27.
3. Gucalp R, Gill I, et al. Treatment of cancer associated hypercalcemia double blind comparison of rapid and slow intravenous infusion regimens of pamidronate disodium and saline alone. Arch Intern Med 1994;154:1935-44.
4. Kristenson B, Eilertsen B, et al. Prednisolone in the treatment in severe malignant hypercalcemia in metastatic breast cancer: A randomized study. J Intern Med 1992;232:237-45.
5. Percival RC, Yates AJ, et al. Role of glucocorticoids in management of malignant hypercalcemia. Br Med J 1984;289:87.

6. Raisz LG, Trummel CL, Wener JA, et al. Effect of glucocorticoids on bone resorption in tissue culture. Endocrinology 1972;90:961-67.
7. Ralston SH, Gallacher SJ, et al. Comparison of three intravenous bisphosphonates in cancer associated hypercalcemia. Lancet 1989;2:1180-82.

SUPERIOR VENA CAVA SYNDROME (SVCS)

Superior vena cava is a prominent vein in the superior mediastinum, formed by the confluence of two innominate veins. It is situated in a narrow space in the upper part of the chest anterior to the fourth thoracic vertebra, lateral to the trachea and the arch of the aorta and posterior to the sternal end of the first rib. In case a malignant mass, either a primary tumor or a metastasis, finds a place in this area, it is bound to compress this great vein. This could occur in either a non-Hodgkin's lymphoma, especially diffuse large cell, lymphoblastic lymphoma or extension of growth in a lung cancer, especially right-sided bronchogenic carcinoma. It could also develop in case of metastases from tumors of the lung, breast, testicle, etc. The malignant mass close to the SVC gradually becomes bigger and suddenly compresses the vein either by edema or bleeding within it. This is known as superior vena cava syndrome (SVCS). It can also develop as thrombosis resulting from a central venous access devise in total parenteral nutrition. The syndrome is not uncommon (SVCS) in cancer patients and can cause life-threatening cerebral edema by raised intracranial pressure or laryngeal edema by tracheal compression.

ETIOLOGY

It is most often due to extrinsic compression of the SVC by (intrathoracic) primary tumors like:
1. Non-Hodgkin's lymphoma, especially diffuse large cell or lymphoblastic lymphoma in the anterior mediastinum, soft tissue sarcoma, malignant melanoma.
2. Metastatic disease to the mediastinum, from primary tumors such as breast, testicular and gastrointestinal (GI) cancers.
3. Infective thrombosis from central venous access, central line thrombus and other iatrogenic causes, idiopathic fibrosing mediastinitis.

SYMPTOMS AND SIGNS

This condition can develop gradually or suddenly. The most important sign is a life-threatening edema due to the stasis of blood in both the internal jugular veins. There is marked rise in intracranial pressure. It is also noticed that the patient develops a sudden onset of stridor suggesting an airway obstruction.

The symptoms can be divided into 2 parts:
1. Due to venous congestion

2. Due to trachea compression
    i. In the first case the patient can develop distension of the neck or chest wall superficial veins, edema of the upper extremities, facial and periorbital edema, mental status changes, and lethargy, with altered sensorium.
    ii. The airway compression symptoms include dyspnea, orthopnea, facial cyanosis, cough with stridor, chest pain, dysphagia, hoarseness and restlessness.

DIAGNOSIS OF SVC

The diagnosis is one of exclusion after a careful clinical examination.

A chest radiograph may show widening of the superior mediastinum. A contrast-enhanced CT or MRI will show evidence of a space occupying lesion such as lymphadenopathy or a malignant mass in the superior mediastinum. Doppler examination of the neck veins or subclavian veins would differentiate between an infective thrombus from external compression.

TREATMENT OF SVC

Before actually planning therapy, biopsy of the lymph node and bone marrow must be carried out. Major thoracic surgical procedures must be avoided as the patient finds it difficult to lie in the normal supine position. The diagnosis can be reached by thoracentesis, bronchoscopy, or by sputum cytology. Mediastinoscopy may be required in some cases. If SVCS is a presenting symptom (i.e. no history of cancer), and if time allows (i.e. no respiratory distress or changing neurologic status), obtain tissues to establish a diagnosis before treatment.

The patients who require treatment are divided into non-emergent and emergent groups.

1. Non-emergent therapy includes elevation of the head of the bed, use of oxygen mask for supplementation of oxygen, and bed rest.
2. Hydrocortisone, 100 to 500 mg i.v., followed by lower doses of hydrocortisone every 6 to 8 hours.
3. Chemotherapy (lymphoma or germ cell tumor) once a positive diagnosis is reached.
4. Antibiotic therapy if the etiology is suggestive of infection.

Anticoagulant or thrombolytic therapy in case of catheter-associated thrombosis after withdrawing the catheter used for central venous access. Emergent therapy includes the following: radiation, surgery and intra-luminal stenting.

1. Emergent radiation therapy is required when respiratory compromise (e.g. stridor) or central nervous system (CNS) symptoms are present.
2. Chemotherapy and radiation therapy are recommended for limited-disease seen in small-cell lung cancer.

3. Surgery includes removal of the obstructing mass with video assisted thoracotomy or venous by-pass (especially in the setting of refractory disease or malignant causes).
4. Intraluminal, self-retaining stenting is provided from one of the neck veins through the superior vena cava to the right auricle.

FURTHER READING

1. Irabor DO. A giant retrosternal goiter with severe tracheal compression and superior vena cava syndrome: An operative experience. Med J 2003;41(1):63-68.
2. Lorenzo-Solar M, Lado-Abeal J, Cameselle-Teijeiro J, et al. Superior vena cava syndrome and insular thyroid carcinoma: The stent as a palliative therapeutic alternative. Med Internal 2003;(6):301-03.
3. Nguyen M, Tsou E. Superior vena cava syndrome in pregnancy. A case report. J Reprod Med 2003;48(4):299-301.
4. Saydam G, Sahin F, Bozkurt D, et al. Vena cava superior syndrome due to sternal plasmacytoma in the course systemic myeloma. Haematologia (Budap) 2002;32(4):529-33.
5. Sharoni E, Erez E, Birk E, Katz J, Dagan O. Superior vena cava syndrome following neonatal cardiac surgery. Pediatr Crit Care Med 2001;2(1):40-43.

SPINAL CORD COMPRESSION (SCC)

The classical presentation of malignant lesion of the spine especially metastatic deposits in the spinal axis is pain with local tenderness over the spinous process of the involved vertebra (most important and persistent symptom) followed by motor, sensory and bladder/bowel disturbances. The progression is usually rapid. Occasionally acute onset of neurological deficits is seen resulting in either partial (paraparesis) or complete weakness (paraplegia).

This condition is a serious oncologic emergency. Delay may cause permanent motor and sensory paralysis with loss of bladder and bowel functions. The majority of the cord compression is metastatic tumor or collapsed bone fragments. Most of them are epidural and rarely intradural and intramedullary.

ETIOLOGY

Metastatic tumors of breast, lung, prostate, renal and GI systems are the common lesions that cause SCC. It can also develop in cases of lymphoma, multiple myeloma and germ cell tumors. In a few cases SCC is the first sign of cancer and the first symptom may be retention of urine.

SYMPTOMS (TABLE 11.1)

1. Radiculitis
2. Slowly developing motor and sensory paralysis

Table 11.1: Pathophysiology of spinal cord compression

Pathological fracture of the vertebra due to: Vertebral bone metastases and primary tumors of vertebra (multiple myeloma, giant cell tumor) Secondary deposits from breast, prostate, lung, kidney etc.	Direct mechanical pressure over the spinal cord.	Partial weakness ↓ If immediate intervention is not taken up ↓
Epidural metastatic deposits	Vascular impedance of spinal/radicular arteries	(ischemic insult) Total weakness

3. Slowly developing bladder and bowel dysfunction
4. Autonomic dysfunction.

DIAGNOSIS

Careful clinical examination and evaluation of sensory and motor weakness are essential in evaluating the site of sudden compression. Light touch and pinprick examination from neck to toe is done to determine the level of sensory loss. Rectal examination is necessary for evaluation of sphincter tone.

DIAGNOSTIC IMAGING

1. Radiograph of spine to locate lesion in the vertebra or fracture or compression.
2. CT scan with intrathecal radiolucent agent.
3. Contrast MRI is done for the whole spinal axis to determine the level and also the higher and lower levels of cord of compression. It is a highly specific and sensitive examination for sudden cord compression. The usual level of compression is in the midthoracic level with lesser frequency at lumbar and cervical spine. It would require 60 minutes to complete the MRI imaging and a few patients have difficulty in lying supine.

(Implanted devices such as pacemaker and hip stabilization with metal pins are contraindications for MRI).

TREATMENT

As soon as the initial diagnosis is made, the patient must be given dexamethasone 10 mg i.v followed by dexamethasone 4 mg i.v every 6 hours for 7 days. Radiotherapy consultation is immediately sought for a case of acute cord compression. The therapy can be used to treat radio-sensitive tumors with stable vertebral bodies. Tumors of the breast, prostate and lymphoma, multiple myeloma and neuroblastoma are common radiosensitive tumors. Radiotherapy can also be used in multiple areas of compression to prevent slowly evolving spinal cord compression. Once the radiotherapy is started, the corticosteroid can be slowly tapered.

Surgery must be contemplated in patients with progressive lesions in spite of radiotherapy. It is also indicated in any lesion which causes mechanical instability or compression.

FURTHER READING

1. Brigden ML. Hematologic and oncologic emergencies. Doing the most good in the least time. Postgrad Med 2001;109(3):143-46, 151-54, 157-58.
2. Gupta R, Gupta S. Oncologic emergencies: superior vena cava syndrome. Cleve Clin J Med 2002;69(10):744.
3. Johnston PG, Spence RA. Oncologic emergencies. Oxford: Oxford University Press, 2002.
4. Krimsky WS, Behrens RJ, Kerkvliet GJ. Oncologic emergencies for the internist. Cleve Clin J Med 2002;69(3):209-10, 213-14, 216-17.
5. Tan SJ. Recognition and treatment of oncologic emergencies. J Infus Nurs 2002;25(3):182-88.

Section II

System or Organ Specific Cancer

- *Breast Cancer*
- *Non-small and Small Cell Lung Cancer*
- *Esophageal Cancer*
- *Gastric Cancer*
- *Colorectal Cancer*
- *Anal Cancer*
- *Primary Cancers of the Liver*
- *Biliary Tract Cancer*
- *Pancreatic Cancer*
- *Vulvar and Vaginal Cancers*
- *Cervical Cancer*
- *Gestational Trophoblastic Disease*
- *Endometrial Cancer*
- *Ovarian Cancer*
- *Renal Tumors*

- *Urothelial Tumors*
- *Bladder Cancer*
- *Cancer of the Prostate*
- *Testicular Carcinoma*
- *Penile Cancer*
- *Brain Tumors*
- *Spinal Cord Tumors*
- *Non-Hodgkin's Lymphoma*
- *Hodgkin's Lymphoma*
- *Multiple Myeloma—Plasma Cell Neoplasm*
- *Acute Leukemias*
- *Chronic Leukemias*
- *Myelodysplastic Syndromes*
- *Carcinoma Thyroid*
- *Adrenal and Retroperitonal Tumors*
- *Pediatric Solid Tumors*
- *Tumors of the Salivary Gland*
- *Head and Neck Tumors (Tumors of Oral Cavity, Lip, Tongue, etc.)*
- *Cancer of Head and Neck (Ear, Nose and Throat)*
- *Skin Tumors*
- *Musculoskeletal Tumors*
  - *Soft Tissue Sarcoma*
  - *Gastrointestinal Stromal Tumors*
  - *Osteosarcoma*
  - *Ewing's Family of Tumors*
  - *Metastatic Bone Tumors*

Breast Cancer

12

C Balachandran
Narayanan Kutty Warrier
K Pavithran

Breast cancer is the most common malignancy in women in the developed countries and the second commonest malignancy in women in India, second only to carcinoma cervix. Even in India, the incidence of breast cancer varies from Registry to Registry and has shown interesting difference between urban and rural populations. Its incidence has been steadily increasing over the past few decades and has become the commonest malignancy in women in metropolitan cities like Delhi and Mumbai. In Kerala breast cancer has taken the lead over carcinoma cervix to become the number one malignancy in women. The incidence of breast cancer is low in India compared to that in the West. The incidence is 28 cases per 1,00,000 women in India against 111 cases per 1,00,000 in the West.

Over the past few years, breast cancer morbidity appears to be declining in the West. This is because of early detection of breast cancer by way of increased awareness among the public and effective screening program. In India, the majority of breast cancer is diagnosed in the advanced stage and hence morbidity remains high. So our major challenge in the coming years will be implementing an effective, less costly screening program and making the public aware of the early detection methods of breast cancer such as breast self-examination.

EPIDEMIOLOGY

Breast cancer is relatively uncommon in men; the male to female ratio is approximately 1:100. Though this is a disease of middle-aged women, more and more women of less than 40 years are diagnosed to have breast cancer now-a-days. The incidence of breast cancer is greater in women of higher socio-economic background apparently due to differences in lifestyle.

The left breast is involved more frequently than the right and the most common sites are the upper outer quadrant and areolar regions.

ETIOLOGY AND RISK FACTORS

The etiology of the vast majority of breast cancer cases is unknown. However, a number of risk factors of the disease have been established. These risk factors include:
- Female gender
- Increasing age
- Early menarche
- Late menopause
- Nulliparity
- The first live birth after the age of 30
- History of radiation exposure
- BRCA-1, BRCA-2, p53 or PTEN mutations.

Except for female gender and increasing age, these risk factors are associated with only a minority of breast cancers.

GENETIC FACTORS

Hereditary forms of breast cancer constitute only 5 to 7 percent of breast cancers. Mutations in two tumor suppressor genes BRCA-1 and BRCA-2 have been identified in breast cancer patients.

BRCA-1 gene is located in chromosome 17 and mutations in this gene are inherited in an autosomal dominant fashion. BRCA-1 mutations are associated with an increased risk for ovarian and prostate cancers in addition to breast cancer. Mutations in BRCA-1 are associated with a 56 to 85 percent life-time risk of developing breast cancer with marked predisposition to the early onset of breast cancer.

BRCA-2 gene is located in chromosome 13 and mutations are associated with increased incidence of breast cancer in both women and men. Increased incidence is also noticed in ovarian and pancreatic cancer and melanoma. The incidence of BRCA gene mutations in the general population is estimated to be 1 in 500. But it is more prevalent in certain populations like Ashkenazi Jews, with the incidence as high as 1 in 40.

Breast cancer associated with BRCA-1 mutation is hormone receptor negative, high grade aggressive tumor. Li-Fraumeni syndrome, Cowden's syndrome, Muir syndrome and ataxia telangiectasia are the other familial syndromes associated with breast cancer.

FAMILIAL FACTORS

The overall relative risk of breast cancer is increased to 1.5 to 3-fold if a first degree relative (mother, sister or daughter) is affected by breast cancer. The risk is increased to 5-fold if the first degree relative has bilateral disease. The relative risk is higher when the first degree relative is affected by the disease before attaining menopause.

HORMONAL FACTORS

Menarche at an early age and establishment of regular ovulatory cycles (< 12 years) have been associated with two-fold increase in breast cancer. Women whose first full-term pregnancy occurs after the age of 30 have 2 to 5-fold increase in breast cancer risk in comparison with women who have a first full-term pregnancy before the age of 18. Nulliparous women are also at greater risk of developing breast cancer compared to multiparous women with a relative risk of 1.4. Studies of the effects of lactation on breast cancer are inconclusive.

Exogenous administration of estrogen as part of hormone replacement therapy causes a small increase in the risk of developing breast cancer; whereas there is no convincing evidence that use of oral contraceptives will increase the risk of developing this cancer.

PROLIFERATIVE BREAST DISEASE

Proliferative disease without atypia results in a small increase in risk— 1.5 to 2-fold; whereas atypical hyperplasia is associated with a greater risk of breast cancer, 4 to 5-fold.

RADIATION EXPOSURE

An increased risk of breast cancer was noticed in women who received mantle irradiation for Hodgkin's lymphoma before the age of 15. Environmental radiation exposure such as nuclear explosion also increases the risk.

LIFESTYLE AND DIETARY FACTORS

Diets that are high in fat have been associated with increased risk for breast cancer. Moderate alcohol intake also appears to increase breast cancer risk. Sedentary habits and obesity may enhance the breast cancer rate.

PATHOLOGY

In common usage, the term 'cancer of the breast' deals with the malignancy of the epithelial elements in the breast forming its ducts and tubules. The most commonly affected parts are the terminal ductules—which explains the tubular and ductal components existing within the same lesion. Malignant myoepithelioma/myoepithelial carcinoma is a rare tumor purely composed of myoepithelial cells.

Malignancies from other supporting connective tissues of the breast are also reported. They are sarcomas (fibrosarcoma, rhabdomyosarcoma, angiosarcoma, etc.) and lymphoma.

The main classification of breast cancers is based on their nature (noninvasive/invasive) and site of origin (duct/lobule). Ductal carcinoma constitutes nearly 85-90 percent of all breast carcinomas.

NONINVASIVE DUCTAL CARCINOMA: DUCTAL CARCINOMA IN SITU (DCIS)

DCIS is the preinvasive stage of ductal carcinoma. It is characterized by the proliferation of malignant breast epithelial cells, confined to the duct system. It does not invade the basement membrane or surrounding tissue. Earlier about 5-6 percent of DCIS was reported in nonsymptomatic autopsies. These tumors can be picked up by mammography due to the presence of microcalcification and screening mammography has raised the yield to 15-20 percent of all diagnosed breast cancers. These tumors are considered pervasive and have the potential to turn into infiltrating ductal carcinoma.

VARIANTS OF NONINVASIVE DUCTAL CARCINOMA

Different histological types of DCIS such as solid, comedo, cribriform, papillary, clinging, micropapillary and cystic hypersecretory are described. Comedo and papillary variants are more common and are associated with multicentricity. Comedo carcinoma has the greatest potential to become invasive and has the greatest expression of DNA aneuploidy and cerb-2 oncogene. Even though DCIS was classified by architectural pattern previously, it has now become apparent that nuclear grade, the size of lesion and the presence or absence of comedo type necrosis are of greater prognostic importance.

INVASIVE (INFILTRATING) DUCTAL CARCINOMA

As the name implies, the tumor does not respect the basement membrane and invades it and the surrounding tissues. It is usually referred to as infiltrating ductal carcinoma (IDC). The lesion is microscopically further classified into classic/not-otherwise specific (NOS) type and special types. Classic/NOS type is the commonest form, accounting for approximately 88 percent of all breast cancers. Grading of tumor depends upon the extent of tubular formation, nuclear pleomorphism and mitotic count (Nottingham modification of the Bloom-Richardson system). On microscopic evaluation each of them is given 1, 2 or 3 points. The total score is translated to grade (Grade I: 3-5, II: 6-7, III: 8-9).

Immunohistochemically the tumor cells show reactivity for low-molecular weight keratin (particularly 8, 18 and 19) and EMA. The majority are positive for lactalbumin and CEA.

SPECIFIC TYPES OF INFILTRATING DUCT CARCINOMA

a. Medullary carcinoma (6%) is usually seen in patients below 50 years of age. Macroscopically it is a soft, well-circumscribed tumor with uniform consistency and may appear to be encapsulated due to the presence of a pseudocapsule. Microscopically the tumor shows prominent lymphoplasmacytic infiltration. Axillary lymph node metastasis is common but they are usually few in number and limited to lower axillary groups. The variety is associated with good prognosis.

b. Tubular carcinoma is an uncommon variety of cancer. It is usually a small, hard nodule and on section shows radial appearance. Microscopically tubular arrangement is noticed with open central space lined by a single layer of epithelium. Prognosis is good. In a small group of cases, it shows a shift to more aggressive infiltrating duct carcinoma belonging to NOS.

c. Mucoid (mucinous) carcinoma usually presents as a small rounded tumor. It consists of a cluster of tumor cells arranged in a pool of mucinous material.

d. Papillary carcinoma is seen forming papillary structures. It exists in two forms, i.e. invasive and noninvasive. Noninvasive papillary carcinoma; also known as cystic papillary carcinoma, exhibits papillomatous structures within a cystic lesion with a fibrous capsule around it.

e. Cribriform carcinoma comprises the tumor cells that are arranged in a cribriform pattern. It has a good prognosis.

f. Clear cell carcinoma is associated with poor prognosis. The cells have distinctive staining features.

g. Juvenile/Secretory carcinoma is a rare tumor usually seen in children. Microscopically tumor cells with vacuolated cytoplasm are seen forming a lumina filled by an eosinophilic secretion. It has a good prognosis.

h. Inflammatory carcinoma is characterized by the occurrence of tumor emboli in dermal lymphatics leading to an appearance of inflammation. It is associated with poor prognosis.

i. Metaplastic carcinoma is a generic term for breast carcinoma of the ductal type in which the predominant component of neoplasm has an appearance other than that of epithelium and gland. It includes matrix (bone/cartilage) producing carcinomas, spindle cell carcinomas, etc.

Other rarer types of infiltrating duct carcinoma include those with neuroendocrine cells, apocrine cells and squamous cells.

PAGET'S DISEASE OF THE NIPPLE

This is a condition usually affecting the elderly. Clinically it presents as an itching vascular eruption of the nipple with induration. Biopsy demonstrates Paget's cells—large cells with pale cytoplasm and atypical nuclei in the epidermis. It is associated with underlying ductal carcinoma/ DCIS. Ultrastructurally the Paget's cells exhibit glandular differentiation.

LOBULAR CARCINOMA

Lobular carcinoma arising out of the lobular elements of the breast is also classified either as noninvasive (lobular carcinoma *in situ*) or as invasive.

LOBULAR CARCINOMA IN SITU

In this variety, the cancer arises from the distal ductules and acini and does not transgress the basement membrane of the lobule. Microscopically the tumor exhibits uniform proliferation of cells within the lobule, occluding any interstitial space. There is expansion of at least half of the acini of the tubular unit. It does not exhibit microcalcification and may not be picked up by mammography. The tumors are frequently multifocal (70%) and bilateral (30%) and over a period of time, one third of them develop into an invasive lobular/ductal carcinoma.

INVASIVE LOBULAR CARCINOMA (ILC)

It forms around 5 percent of breast cancers among which 20 percent can develop bilaterally. These tumors are poorly circumscribed and hard in consistency. Most of the time, it is difficult to palpate a discrete mass. In most cases, the cells are small, uniform and arranged in Indian file pattern. They surround a normal or cancerous acini and give a "bull's eye" appearance. As these tumors can develop in both the breasts, the clinician must evaluate the opposite breast with mammography and biopsy during the first visit. Five main subtypes of lobular carcinoma identified are classical, solid, alveolar, pleomorphic and mixed. Though lobular carcinomas are generally thought to be of better prognosis than infiltrating ductal carcinomas, the outcome of the pleomorphic variety is poor. Most cases of signet ring cell carcinomas are considered as variants of ILC.

CLINICAL FEATURES

A properly conducted clinical examination of the breast can detect up to 50 percent of the cancers not detected by mammography alone. Examination of breast in premenopausal women should be carried out one week after the onset of the last menstruation when breast engorgement and nodular texture of breast tissue are usually decreased.

The clinical features are grouped into local effects, lymph node involvement, distant metastases and systemic effects.

Local effects are: a breast lump, skin thickening, dimpling of the skin, peau d' orange and nipple discharge.

Axillary and supraclavicular glands require careful clinical evaluation.

The features of meatstases: pleural and pericardial effusion, hepatomegaly, ascites and other intraperitoneal masses.

Among CNS involvement, special attention must be paid to the presence of brain metastasis,spinal cord compression and meningitis carcinomata.

Among the systemic effects, loss of appetite, bone pains, headache and paresthesia of the extremities are not uncommon.

DIAGNOSIS ANY MASS IN THE BREAST SHOULD BE CONSIDERED FOR A BIOPSY EVEN IF MAMMOGRAMS ARE NEGATIVE

Virtually all breast cancers are diagnosed by Fine-Needle Aspiration Cytology (FNAC), Core Needle Biopsy, Incisional or Excisional Biopsy. Detected either on a mammogram or palpation. A palpable mass in a woman's breast represents a potentially serious lesion and requires triple assessment namely proper clinical examination, mammography and fine-needle aspiration biopsy regardless of the age of the women. The initial objective is to distinguish simple cysts from solid lesions, which can be accomplished with needle aspiration or a USG. A positive result on cytologic examination after aspiration is sufficiently accurate to justify one stage diagnosis and treatment, with confirmation by examination of a frozen section obtained during the procedure. An inconclusive or a negative cytology warrants a biopsy of the lesion. All solid masses should be subjected to FNAC or excision biopsy.

MAMMOGRAPHY (FIGURE 12.1)

Mammography is the radiological examination of the soft tissue of the breast. It has a major role in assessing clinically palpable and non-palpable breast lesions. Any abnormality found on mammography should be taken into account with the patient's symptoms and the results of other investigations, e.g. FNAC, core biopsy, etc. before planning definitive treatment. In the hands of an experienced radiologist, breast mass as small as 2-3 mm can be identified in 85 to 95 percent of cases. Mammography should be avoided in adolescence, pregnancy and lactation unless there is other evidence of malignancy. All women with breast cancer should have a mammogram in order to reveal the extent of the disease, to determine if there is multifocal disease or identify a lesion in the opposite breast. Scintimammography, is a newer device in which intravenous radioactive element, Technetium-99m (^{99m}Tc) is used to identify abnormal masses in the breast, and if any, can be imaged with a Digital Gamma

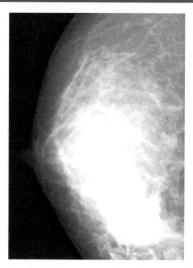

Figure 12.1: Mammogram showing a carcinoma

camera. This technique helps in differentiating benign and malignant lesions and to determine the presence of multicentric tumors in the breast.

ULTRASONOGRAPHY

Ultrasonography is a useful non-invasive imaging tool for investigating palpable lumps in the breast. It is complementary to mammography and will be able to pick out benign lesions more accurately.

MRI

It is not used routinely but is a sensitive tool for detecting occult breast cancer foci. MRI is useful in selective situations like detecting a subtle primary in the breast in patients presenting with carcinoma of unknown primary. It also helps in studying the local extent of the tumor and its multicentricity. MRI is very useful in distinguishing local recurrence from scar tissue in a previously irradiated breast.

STAGING AND EVALUATION (TABLES 12.1 AND 12.2)

The most widely used staging is the American Joint Committee on Cancer (AJCC) classification, which is based on the tumor size (T), the status of regional lymph nodes (N) and the presence of distant metastasis (M). Clinical staging is determined after physical examination and appropriate radiologic studies have been performed. Pathologic staging is determined following surgery for operable breast cancer. Pathologic tumor size may differ from clinical tumor size. In addition, axillary nodal metastases that were not clinically evident may be detected after pathologic examinations.

Table 12.1: The American Joint Committee on Cancer (AJCC) classification

T0	No evidence of primary tumor
T1	Tumor less than 2 cm in diameter
T2	Tumor between 2-5 cm in diameter
T3	Tumor greater than 5 cm in diameter
T4	Tumor fixation to chest wall or skin
T4a	Involvement of chest wall (ribs/serratus anterior/intercostal muscle)
T4b	Skin (satellite nodules/peau de orange/ulceration)
T4c	Both a + b
T4d	Inflammatory carcinoma
N0	No axillary nodes
N1	Palpable, mobile, ipsilateral axillary nodes
N2	Fixed ipsilateral axillary nodes
N3	Internal mammary nodes
M0	No metastasis
M1	Contralateral axillary nodes/supraclavicular nodes/contralateral breast tumor
M2	Distant metastasis

Table 12.2: Staging of cancer; TNM classification-1997

Stage				
0		Tis	N0	M0
I	2.2%	T1	N0	M0
IIA	11.8%	T0	N1	M0
		T1	N1	M0
		T2	N0	M0
IIB	21.9%	T2	N1	M0
		T3	N0	M0
IIIA	21.3%	T0	T2	M0
		T1	T2	M0
		T2	N2	M0
		T3	N1	M0
		T3	N2	M0
IIIB	28.7%	T4	Any N	M0
		Any T	N3	M0
IV	14.0%	Any T	Any N	M1

Adapted from AJCE Manual, 1997- Cancer Breast

SUMMARY OF MAJOR CHANGES IN THE AJCC CANCER STAGING MANUAL, SIXTH EDITION (TABLE 12.3)

Micrometastases are distinguished from isolated tumor cells on the basis of size. They are also more likely to show histologic evidence of malignant activity, but this is not an absolute requirement.

Table 12.3: Suggested new staging for cancer breast

TNM staging system for Breast Cancer

Primary Tumor (T)

Tx Primary tumor cannot be assessed

T0 No evidence of primary tumor

Tis Carcinoma *in situ*

Tis (DCIS) Ductal carcinoma *in situ*

Tis (LCIS) Lobular carcinoma *in situ*

Tis (Paget) Paget's disease of the nipple with no tumor

Note: Paget's disease associated with a tumor is classified according to the size of the tumor

T1 Tumor – 2 cm in greatest dimension

T1mic microinvasion – 0.1 cm in greatest dimension

T1a tumor – 0.1 cm but not – 0.5 cm in greatest dimension

T1b tumor – 0.5 cm but not – 1 cm in greatest dimension

T1c tumor – 1 cm but not – 2 cm in greatest dimension

T2 tumor – 2 cm but not –5 cm in greatest dimension

T3 tumor – 5 cm in greatest dimension

T4 tumor of any size with direct extension to:

Chest wall, or skin, only as described below

T4a extension to chest wall, not including pectoralis muscle

T4b edema (including Peau d' orange) or ulceration of the skin of the breast, or satellite skin nodules confined to the same breast

T4c both T4a and T4b

T4d Inflammatory carcinoma

Regional lymph nodes (N)

NX Regional lymph nodes cannot be assessed (e.g. previously removed)

N0 No regional lymph node metastasis

N1 Metastasis in movable ipsilateral axillary lymph node(s)

N2 Metastases in ipsilateral axillary lymph nodes fixed or matted, or clinically apparent in ipsilateral internal mammary nodes in the absence of clinically evident axillary lymph node metastasis

N2a Metastasis in ipsilateral axillary lymph nodes fixed to one another (matted) or to other structures

N2b Metastasis only in clinically apparent* ipsilateral internal mammary nodes and in the absence of clinically evident axillary lymph node metastasis

N3 Metastasis in ipsilateral infraclavicular lymph node(s), or in clinically apparent* ipsilateral internal mammary lymph node(s) and in the presence of clinically evident axillary lymph node metastasis; or metastasis in ipsilateral supraclavicular lymph

contd...

Table 12.3: contd...

node(s) with or without axillary or internal mammary lymph node involvement

N3a Metastasis in ipsilateral infraclavicular lymph node(s) and axillary lymph node(s)

N3b Metastasis in ipsilateral internal mammary lymph node(s) and axillary lymph node(s)

N3C Metastasis in ipsilateral supraclavicular lymph node(s)

Regional lymph nodes (pN)

pNX Regional lymph nodes cannot be assessed (e.g., previously removed or not removed for pathologic study)

pNO No regional lymph node metastasis histologically, no additional for isolated tumor cells.

pN0(i) No regional lymph node metastasis histologically, negative IHC

pN0(I) No regional lymph node metastasis histologically, positive IHC, no IHC cluster –0.2 mm

pNO (mol) No regional lymph node metastasis histologically, negative molecular findings (RT-PCR)

pNO (mol-) No regional lymph node metastasis histologically, positive molecular findings (RT-PCR)

pN1mi Micrometastasis (more than 0.2 mm, less than 2.0 mm)

pN1 Metastasis in one to three axillary lymph nodes and/or in internal mammary nodes with microscopic disease detected by sentinel lymph node dissection but not clinically apparent

pN1a Metastasis in one to three axillary lymph nodes

pN1b Metastasis in internal mammary nodes with microscopic disease detected by sentinel lymph node dissection but not clinically apparent

pN1c Metastasis in one to three axillary lymph nodes and in internal mammary lymph nodes with microscopic disease detected by sentinel lymph node dissection but not clinically apparent.

pN2 Metastasis in four to none axillary lymph nodes, or in clinically apparent* internal mammary lymph nodes in the absence of axillary lymph node metastasis

pN2a Metastasis in four to none axillary lymph nodes (at least one tumor deposit less than 2.0 mm)

pN2b Metastasis in clinically apparent* internal mammary lymph nodes in the absence of axillary lymph node metastasis

*T1 includes T1 mic.

Identifiers have been added to indicate the use of sentinel lymph node dissection and immunohistochemical or molecular techniques.

Major classifications of lymph node status are designated according to the number of involved axillary lymph nodes as determined by routine hematoxylin and eosin staining (preferred method) or by immunohisto-chemical staining.

The classification of metastasis to the infraclavicular lymph nodes has been added as N3.

Metastasis to the internal mammary nodes, based on the method of detection and the presence or absence of axillary nodal involvement, has been reclassified. Microscopic involvement of the internal mammary nodes is detected by sentinel lymph node dissection but not by imaging studies (excluding lymphscintigraphy) or clinical examination is classified as N1. Macroscopic involvement of the internal mammary nodes as detected by imaging studies (excluding lymphscintigraphy) or by clinical examination is classified as N2 if it occurs in the absence of metastases to the axillary lymph nodes or as N3 if it occurs in the presence of metastases to the axillary lymph nodes.

Metastasis to the supraclavicular lymph nodes has been reclassified as N3 rather than M1 of breast cancer staging.

Recent years have seen an explosion of studies analyzing IHC and genetic markers as prognostic indicators for breast cancer. While some of these markers show great promise for the future, lack of standardization measurement techniques for many of them (for example, Ki-67, cathepsin D, HER-2/Neu and p53) limit their current usefulness. As these technical problems are worked out, however, it is likely that some of these markers will provide powerful supplemental information to the existing staging system for breast cancer.

Since the immunohistochemical methods are not widely available in India and most of our cases are locally advanced, we have to follow the AJCC1997 (Fifth Manual) staging for routine management. The new system can be adopted on case to case basis in future.

Limitation of TNM Staging: Clinical staging system generally underestimates the extent of the disease and the inclusion of pathologic information improves staging accuracy. However, the tumor size or the presence of lymph node metastasis alone need not correlate the prognosis and treatment decisions. The biological aggressiveness of the tumor, sometimes will be out of proportion to the size of the tumor. Hence, it is proposed to include biological determinants of the tumor also in the staging in future.

BIOLOGICAL DETERMINANTS OF BREAST CANCER

Though not routinely included in the TNM staging, determination of these factors is very important in deciding prognosis, treatment selection and predicting the response to treatment.

Steroid receptors: Estrogen and progesterone are well-established endocrine steroid regulators that regulate mammary epithelial growth, differentiation and survival. Both estrogen and progesterone act through their nuclear receptors (ER and PR respectively) to modulate transcription of target genes. Determination of cellular concentration of ER and PR in the tumor is correctly used to predict which patients have a good prognosis and which may also benefit from antihormonal therapy. ER/PR estimation is done using radioimmunoassay. Immunohistochemical technique on tumor tissue—either on fresh tissue or on paraffin block—ER/PR positive tumors respond favorably to antihormone treatment and carries good prognosis. About 60 percent of breast cancers are ER positive.

HER-2/Neu (Cerb B₂): There are several growth factors needed for the normal secretory function of mammary epithelial cells. Epidermal growth factor (EGF) is one such family of growth factors needed for the regulation of proliferation and differentiation of the mammary gland. Overexpression of these growth factors is associated with aggressive proliferation and carcinogenesis. HER-2/Neu is a member of EGF receptor family. Overexpression of this growth factor receptor is seen inup to 25 percent human breast cancer cases. Estimation of this receptor should be done by using immunohistochemistry and its presence should be confirmed by fluorescent *in situ* hybridization (FISH). HER-2/Neu positivity indicates poor prognosis and predicts poor response to endocrine therapy. Such patients will respond better to Adriamycin. Trastuzumab (Herceptin) is a monoclonal antibody approved for the treatment of metastatic breast cancer, which overexposes HER-2/Neu.

Indices of Proliferation: Mitotic index, Ki-67 and S-phase fraction are some of the prognostic factors used to predict the prognosis and survival in breast cancer. This is done by flow cytometry which can be done on tumor tissue.

Bone marrow microinvasion is predicted to be a poor prognostic factor and its presence directly correlates with 4-year survival. BM microinvasion is detected by monoclonal antibodies against cytokeratin.

Certain specific antigens, especially CA-15-3 are found to be reliably elevated in advanced disease, Stages III and IV. It is more useful in monitoring the response to therapy and for follow-up of treated cases.

The other molecular markers such as tumor suppressor genes (p53) proteolytic enzymes that may be associated with invasion and metastasis (Cathepsin-D) and metastasis suppressor gene (nm 23) are under evaluation.

Routine work-up after the diagnosis includes full blood count. Liver function tests include serum alkaline phosphatase, chest X-ray and an abdominal USG to rule out liver metastasis. Bilateral mammogram is a mandatory investigation to rule out multifocal or synchronous lesions. A routine review of the pathology is needed to study invasive component, grade of tumor, tumor involvement of the margins and tumor prognostic factors like ER/PR status, and HER-2/Neu status.

Bone scan should be reserved for advanced cases like III or IV and with bone symptoms or raised serum alkaline phosphatase levels. CT-scan of chest, abdomen or brain may also be taken in selected cases if suspicion of metastasis is high due to symptoms.

PROGNOSTIC FACTORS OTHER THAN MOLECULAR MARKERS

Lymph node status: The number of positive axillary lymph nodes is an important independent prognostic factor. Survival decreases drastically when the number of positive lymph nodes in the axilla goes up and relapse rates are very high when the number of involved lymph nodes is more than four. The axillary lymph nodes should be dissected according to their relation with axillary artery (level I and II dissection) and at least 10 lymph nodes should be removed to rule out lymph node involvement.

Tumor size: The maximal size of the invasive component measured on microscopic sections. Patients with tumor size more than 1 cm have high probability of systemic relapses.

Tumor grade: Tumor grade is subjected to considerable variability and lacks reproducibility. Lymphatic and vascular invasion and tumor necrosis are other important prognostic factors.

TREATMENT

The understanding that breast cancer is no longer a regional disease but a generalized disease had led to the shift of treatment from drastic radical surgical procedures to the reliance on multidisciplinary treatment.

Over a century, the treatment of breast cancer was based on Halstead's theory, which taught that breast cancer spreads by direct permeation to regional nodes. These nodes act as filters from where disease spreads further up, once they are overloaded with tumor cells.

This concept was the basis of radical mastectomy, wide removal of a breast bearing tumor with en bloc dissection of the regional nodes.

But the occurrence of distant metastasis in "totally excised cancers" led to the detection of micrometastasis. It is now held that breast cancer is a systemic disease and micrometastasis occurs even at the time of detection of the disease. So a regional treatment alone does not solve this vexed problem of breast cancer. Patients may present with distant metastatic disease in the absence of metastasis in the axillary nodes at initial presentation.

At present, the management of breast cancer is multidisciplinary involving the surgeon, pathologists, radiotherapists, medical oncologists, psychologists and social workers. The success of the treatment depends on the coordinated approach of these specialists. The various options of treatment are as follows:

LOCOREGIONAL TREATMENT

Breast conserving therapy (lumpectomy, breast irradiation and surgical staging of the axilla).

Modified radical mastectomy (removal of the entire breast with level I-II axillary dissection) with or without breast reconstruction.

Adjuvant radiation after mastectomy—regional radiation
Adjuvant systemic therapy
Cytotoxic chemotherapy
Endocrine manipulations.

TREATMENT OF EARLY STAGE BREAST CANCER

Locoregional treatment.

BREAST CONSERVATIVE SURGERY

The last 3 decades of the 20th century has seen a shift from radical treatment to breast conservation. Different surgical techniques for the removal of the breast lump employed are:

Lumpectomy—when the lump is removed with little surrounding tissue.

Segmentectomy or quadrantectomy—where a segment or quadrant of breast harboring the tumor is excised.

However, with simple conservative surgical excision alone, patients are found to have high incidence of local recurrence. Hence adjuvant radiation to the remaining breast is added and it has now been proved that in suitable cases for breast conservation, limited resection with irradiation gives similar or even better prognosis when compared to radical surgical procedure.

FACTORS INFLUENCING BREAST CONSERVATION

Patient's preference: The patient should be given the option to decide the type of surgery she would like to be done on her. If she chooses a less radical surgery, she should be provided with the option of breast conservation. Needless to say, the surgeon must counsel her about the outcome of different types of surgery that are presently practiced.

Tumor size: The tumor size is an important parameter in selecting cases for breast conservation. Though many surgeons prefer tumors less than 3 cm for conservative surgery, the National Surgical Adjuvant Breast and Bowel Project (NSABP) recommends less radical procedure only if the tumor size is below 4 cm in diameter.

Fixity to muscle and/or skin is considered to be a factor against conservative resection.

Multicentricity: Multicentricity is a total contraindication for conservation. Some tumors especially lobular carcinomas are known to have multicentric origin in the same breast and a partial resection will lead to incomplete therapy. It is further advised to do a mammographic evaluation to pick up any multicentric tumor before giving the option of conservation to the patient.

Central location of tumor: Subareolar tumors are a relative contraindication to breast preservation. These tumors are more diffuse and are difficult to include in any segmental form of resection. Undesirable psychological effects of removal of the nipple have to be accepted in surgery for tumors of central location.

Poor tumor differentiation is another relative contraindication. Many poorly differentiated tumors are somewhat ill-defined and more rapidly growing. Hence breast conservation is hardly suitable in these cases.

The treatment of axillary nodes with breast cancer is again an area of controversy. For breast cancer, presence or absence of lymph node is not a criterion for deciding about surgical treatment. All localized breast cancer, stages I and II should be considered for lumpectomy. Even many stage III patients can be considered for lumpectomy, after neoadjuvant chemotherapy.

Local recurrence after surgery is a difficult problem faced after mastectomy or conservative resection.

FACTORS LEADING TO RECURRENCE

Positive axillary nodes: The presence of positive axillary nodes predisposes patients to develop local recurrence after partial or total mastectomy. Therefore, it has been suggested that all patients with spread to local lymph nodes should be subjected to postoperative field radiation.

Tumor size: The larger the size of the tumor, the greater is the possibility of local recurrence.

Highest tumor grade: Lymphatic and/or vascular invasion, younger age and presence of malignant tissue at the resected margin of the tumor are factors that add to increased recurrence.

To prevent local recurrence: Irradiation of postoperative field is found to reduce the incidence of local recurrence in breast conservation surgery from 30 percent to figures below 10 percent. In complete mastectomy, all node positive cases should undergo adjuvant radiotherapy to chest wall and axilla to reduce the incidence of local recurrence.

The treatment of local recurrence poses difficult problems for the oncology team. Small focal areas can be surgically removed and adjuvant irradiation may help in delaying the spread of the disease. Addition of chemotherapy and hormonal manipulation will be required to prevent further spread of the residual tumors.

RADICAL MASTECTOMY

Over the years, the mainstay of treatment has remained the radical removal of the tumor with breast and regional nodes. William Halstead (1852-1922) promoted this form of treatment and it consists of the removal of:

The whole breast with a large portion of skin, the center of which overlies the tumor, but always includes the nipple. When there is extensive skin involvement, more skin may need to be sacrificed.

The fat and fascia from the lower border of the clavicle to and including, the upper quarter of the rectus sheath and from the sternum to the anterior border of the latissimus dorsi.

The sternal portion of the pectoralis major and its fascial sheath.

The pectoralis minor and its fascial sheath.

The costocoracoid membrane.

All the fat, fascia and lymph nodes of axilla.

The fascia over, and a few of the superficial muscle fibers of, the anterior part of the external oblique, serratus anterior, the subscapularis, the expanded portion of the latissimus dorsi and the upper part of the rectus abdominus.

Axilla is cleared up to axillary vein. Special care is taken to protect axillary and cephalic veins, nerves to serratus anterior and latissimus dorsi. Primary approximation or split skin grafting with vacuum drainage achieves skin closure.

Modification to classical Halstead's operation, with more extensive clearance like Urban's operation where internal mammary chain of lymph nodes is also removed did not receive the acceptance of many surgeons. But scaled down procedures like Patey's (pectoralis minor muscle is sacrificed along with axillary contents sparing pectoralis major muscle) or Maddens' (where both pectoral muscles are spared) found greater acceptance due to reduced mortality, better chest wall appearance and better limb function with comparable results.

Simple mastectomy with radiation was practised by McWhirter who in the early 1950s, suggested that it was illogical to clear the axilla when internal mammary nodes were not cleared.

RADIOTHERAPY

The indications are:

Any patient undergoing lumpectomy or breast conserving treatment.

Tumors bigger than 5 cm (T3 lesions).

More than 4 axillary lymph nodes.

N2 nodes (nodes with extracapsular extension).

Chest wall invasion or skin invasion (T4 lesions).

It is usually given to patients after chemotherapy or patients after lumpectomy if they are not scheduled for chemotherapy.

Usually, radiotherapy is given in fractionated doses after completing a course of chemotherapy, 4500 to 5000 cGy (plus or minus 1000 to 1500 cGy) is applied to the tumor site to increase the tumoricidal activity. Postmastectomy radiation treatment to the chest wall and supraclavicular lymph nodes decrease the risk of locoregional recurrence in patients with four or more positive lymph nodes. The role of radiotherapy in patients with 1 to 3 lymph nodes is not generally accepted by radiotherapists.

Adjuvant Radiotherapy: is given in two situations: one as part of breast conservation treatment and the other following mastectomy. Radiotherapy is a standard option for breast conserving treatment. Postoperative external beam radiation is given to the entire breast with doses of 45 Gy to 50 Gy in 1.8 Gy to 2.0 Gy fractions over 5 week period. A further radiation boost is commonly given to the tumor bed to reduce local recurrence.

Postoperative chest wall and regional lymph node adjuvant radiation is given to selected patients considered high risk for locoregional spread following mastectomy. Patients in this category are those with 4 or more positive axillary nodes, grossly evident extracapsular nodal extension, large primary tumor (> 5 cm) and very close or positive deep margins of resection of primary tumor. For patients with positive nodes, radiation therapy to the supraclavicular fossa and/or internal mammary chain may be considered on individualized basis.

BREAST RECONSTRUCTION

Breast reconstruction has captured the imagination of surgeons and patients as an answer to the alteration in body image. Many patients accept total mastectomy in the hope of undergoing breast reconstruction. Reconstruction can be taken up along with mastectomy or can be done as a delayed procedure after completion of treatment like irradiation and chemotherapy. Immediate reconstruction, though having a positive advantage in the psychological well being of the patient has a disadvantage in masking early recurrence.

Reconstruction was earlier attempted with tissue implants like solstice material, which created problems due to skin necrosis, prosthesis displacements and extrusion. Presently, the emphasis is on tissue transfer through pedicle flaps from anterior abdominal wall, rectus muscle-based skin flaps or from back-latissimus dorsi based skin flap. Also, microvascular surgical advancement has contributed to free myocutaneous flaps. The nipple is reconstructed with skin from groin or thigh.

However, the patient and her partner must be counseled that the reconstructed breast only acts as a body image leveler and will not actually substitute an actual breast in its function.

SENTINEL LYMPH NODE MAPPING

The lymph node involvement in the axilla is an important predictor of prognosis and influences the treatment selection like addition of radiation or chemotherapy. Earlier treatment of breast cancer was radical mastectomy and even in cases where axillary nodes were not palpable, complete axillary clearance was carried out. The axillary dissection led to increased morbidity due to immediate postoperative complications like serum formation, damage to nerves to the serratus anterior and the latissimus dorsi muscles, and the later complications like lymphedema of the arm, restricted arm movement, etc. Many times, in early breast cancer the incidence of axillary involvement is much less and the extensive removal of the axillary lymph node is unnecessary. However, identifying lymph node involvement reliably prior to surgery is difficult clinically and requires a technique called sentinel lymph node mapping. This can avoid an unnecessary axillary dissection. The sentinel lymph node is defined as the first node in the lymphatic basin that receives primary lymphatic flow. Sentinel lymph node mapping allows the surgeon to accurately identify the sentinel node that stands at the entrance to the lymphatic system. Once the sentinel node is identified, it can be removed and tested for signs of metastatic cancer. If the sentinel node is cancer-free, other lymph nodes further along the chain will also be cancer-free. This is important for a woman undergoing breast cancer surgery because it can mean that those additional nodes can then be left in place, avoiding lymphedema and other complications. The procedure involves injecting a radioactive tracer Tc99 radio-colloid and a blue dye around the tumor site. These two substances travel from the tumor and drain into the sentinel or main lymph node. A hand-held radioactive detector, similar to a Geiger counter, is scanned after 20 to 24 hrs around the underarm area and a beeping sound pinpoints the location of the radioactive-filled node. After making a small incision, the surgeon can see the blue-dyed sentinel node. This node is subjected to frozen section, depending on the result of which, decision to clear or spare the axilla is made. The sentinel node detection has come to stay and in 50 percent of cases, axillary dissection is avoided in negative node biopsy.

ADJUVANT SYSTEMIC THERAPY

The treatment of breast cancer is multimodality which includes treatment of local disease with surgery or radiation therapy and the treatment of systemic disease with cytotoxic chemotherapy or hormonal therapy. For selecting the treatment and predicting survival and prognosis, invasive breast cancer can be broadly divided into three groups, early, locally advanced and metastatic breast cancers. Early breast cancer includes Stage I, II and IIIA. But In the case of locally advanced breast cancer, the size of the tumor is more than 5 cm and the tumor can be of any size with direct invasion of the skin of the breast or chest wall (T4) or it can be tumor of any size with fixed or matted axillary nodes. By virtue of the presence of supraclavicular nodes and metastasis to distant organs, this group of Stage 1V is known as metastatic breast cancer.

More than 50 percent of our patient population belongs to locally advanced category. In situ carcinomas are less than 2 percent.

TREATMENT OPTIONS

The various treatment options available for the treatment of breast cancers are:

Benefits of Adjuvant Chemotherapy

The benefit for chemotherapy after the local treatment has shown significant reduction in the mortality irrespective of lymph node status or ER status. This is proved in a large metaanalysis after analyzing the data collected from 47 trials: chemotherapy reduced recurrence by approximately 25 percent and death by 15 percent. However, the benefit of chemotherapy did vary substantially according to the patient's age and menopausal status. Currently chemotherapy is indicated in all patients with axillary lymph node metastasis or if the tumor size is more than 1 cm. Chemotherapy is more beneficial in younger women less than 69 years of age. The benefit of chemotherapy in terms of reduction in recurrence and mortality is less in women of more than 70 years. In younger patients, the chemotherapy acts in a number of ways in breast cancer. It has got direct tumoricidal effect on tumor cells. In addition, it induces menopause; thereby it has got an endocrine effect also in tumor cells. That is why chemotherapy is more effective in younger women. But newer studies have shown benefit from chemotherapy irrespective of age.

The decision regarding advising adjuvant systemic chemotherapy in node negative early breast cancer is difficult. An international consensus panel proposed a 3 tiered risk classification for patients with negative axillary lymph nodes at St.Gallen's meeting (Table 12.4).

Previously age 35 years or older and certain uncommon histologies (like tubular, medullary or mucinous) were also included in the low risk category. But biological factors like tumor proliferative fractions (S-phase) and HER-2/neu overexpression may be more useful in deciding the risk and thereby adjuvant system therapy.

Chemotherapy is indicated in all patients except for a small group– axillary node negative, ER/PR +ve and HER-2/neu negative and mostly belonging to the low risk early breast cancer (i.e. tumor <1 cm, low grade). This small group requires only surgery and hormonal therapy.

Table 12.4: Risk categories			
	Tumor size	*ER/PR status*	*Tumor grade*
Low risk (all factors should be present)	<1cm	Positive	Grade 1 time
Intermediate risk (risk classified between low risk and high risk)	1 – 2 cm	Positive	Grade 1 to 2
High risk (if at least one factor is present)	>2cm	Negative	Grade 2 to 3

CHEMOTHERAPY DRUGS (TABLE 12.5)

Several chemotherapy drugs are effective in breast cancer. These drugs are listed below:

Conventional drugs	*Newer drugs*
Cyclophosphamide	Paclitaxel
5-Fluorouracil	Docetaxel
Methotrexate	Vinorelbine
Doxorubicin	Gemcitabine

A combination of two or three drugs is used to avoid drug resistance and for better response. Several such combinations (regimens) are available. For axillary lymph node negative breast cancer, appropriate regimens include cyclophosphamide, methotrexate and 5-fluorouracil (CMF), fluorouracil, doxorubicin and cyclophosphamide (FAC/CAF) or doxorubicin and cyclophosphamide (AC).

In women with node positive disease, FAC/CAF or cyclophosphamide and Adriamycin (AC) at a higher dose or AC followed by paclitaxel are all considered to be appropriate options. Adriamycin containing regimen will be more appropriate for those who over express HER-2/Neu.

It is important to use these drugs in the recommended dose (dose intensity) to derive the adequate response. Compromising the dose to reduce toxicity will jeopardize the expected response and thereby survival.

AC chemotherapy followed by paclitaxel-sequential chemotherapy will be superior to other regimens for women with 4 or more positive axillary lymph nodes.

The duration of chemotherapy is also an important factor affecting the response and overall survival. Chemotherapy should be continued for at least 4 to 6 months and is given as 21 day cycle. Four to Six such cycles are given conventionally.

Table 12.5: Dosage of commonly used chemotherapeutic agents		
CMF	Cyclophosphamide	600 mg/m^2 Day 1 and 8
	Methotrexate	40 m/m^2 Day 1 and 8
	5-Fluorouracil	600 mg/m^2 Day 1 and 8
	Repeat cycles every 4 weeks × 6 cycles	
AC	Adriamycin	60 mg/m^2 Day 1
	Cyclophosphamide	600 mg/m^2 Day 1
	Repeat cycles every 3 weeks × 6 cycles	
FAC	5-Fluorouracil	600 mg/m^2 Day 1
	Adriamycin	60 mg/m^2 Day 1
	Cyclophosphamide	600 mg/m^2 Day 1
	Repeat cycles every 3 weeks × 6 cycles	
AT	Adriamycin	60 mg/m^2 Day 1
	Docetaxel	75 mg/m^2 Day 1
	Repeat cycles every 3 weeks × 6 cycles	

HORMONE THERAPY

More than 60 percent breast cancers are hormone dependent. Steroid hormones like estrogen and progesterone are essential for growth differentiation and survival of these cells. Hence hormones play an active role in the treatment of these cancers. The main sources of these hormones in the body are ovaries in premenopausal and adrenal gland in postmenopausal women. Estrogen is a highly potent mammary mitogen, therefore most forms of endocrine therapy for breast cancer are directed towards inhibiting, ablating or interfering with estrogen activity.

The major drugs available are:

Tamoxifen

Aromatase inhibitor

Progestins

LHRH agonists

Tamoxifen It is a nonsteroidal antiestrogen that is structurally related to diethylstilbesterol (DES). Tamoxifen inhibits estrogen mediated protein synthesis and also has direct tumor inhibiting activity.

Tamoxifen reduces the recurrence by 47 percent and mortality by 26 percent. Again, there is an additional benefit that it reduces the incidence of contralateral breast cancer by 50 percent. The benefit of tamoxifen is irrespective of age, menopausal status or axillary lymph node involvement. It is indicated only in estrogen receptor positive tumors. Tamoxifen is given in a dose of 20 mg daily and should be continued for at least 5 years. It should be started only after the completion of chemotherapy. Major side effects of tamoxifen are endometrial cancer, deep venous thrombosis, ovarian cysts, hot flushes and vaginal discharge. It has some positive effects also like reduction in coronary artery disease and prevention of osteoporosis in postmenopausal women.

Aromatase Inhibitors: After menopause major sources of estrogen are adrenal and adipose tissues. The enzyme aromatase converts androstenedinone to estrone which is subsequently converted to estradiol. Aromatase inhibitors block this enzyme, thereby reducing estradiol production. The aromatase inhibitors available are letrozole, anastrozole and exemestane. Currently these agents are recommended as second line drug when the disease progresses under tamoxifen and also as primary therapy in HER-2/Neu overexpressed tumors.

OVARIAN ABLATION

In premenopausal ER +ve patients, medical, surgical or radiation ablation of ovaries further add to the effects of chemotherapy and tamoxifen. Luteinizing hormone-releasing hormone analogues like gosorelin are available to suppress ovarian function. Major advantage of medical ablation is the reversibility of ovarian suppression.

LOCALLY ADVANCED BREAST CANCER

Locally advanced breast cancer includes the following:

Large tumor size of more than 5 cm irrespective of their lymph node involvement.

Tumor of any size with direct skin involvement regardless of lymph node involvement.

Tumors of any size but with matted/fixed axillary lymph node involvement.

Inflammatory breast cancer.

Large tumors in relation to the size of the breast. Though technically operable, they require radical mastectomy close to their size.

NEOADJUVANT THERAPY

Patients with locally advanced breast cancer do have distant metastasis. More than 80 percent of the patients treated only with local therapy such as surgery or radiotherapy died of distant metastasis within 10 years of diagnosis and their local recurrence often exceeds 50 percent. Therefore it is clear that the major problem in locally advanced breast cancer is the development of micrometastases, months or years before the diagnosis is made. Tackling the micrometastasis first along with locoregional control of the disease by giving chemotherapy initially prior to surgery is not new and is called neoadjuvant chemotherapy. This method has several advantages. It permits *in vivo* chemosensitivity testing, and can downstage locally advanced disease and render it operable and may allow breast conservation surgery to be performed. But this method has got a disadvantage—accurate pathological staging is not possible with this method. Clinically complete pathological disappearance of the tumor was observed in 10 to 25 percent of these patients. Most of the tumors require three to four cycles of chemotherapy for downstaging the disease. Patients should be followed carefully while receiving neoadjuvant chemotherapy to determine treatment response. If operable after 2 or 3 cycles of chemo-therapy, patients should be taken up for surgery and the rest of chemo-therapy should be completed after surgery.

Multidisciplinary, multimodality approach is the best treatment option for locally advanced breast cancer. The treatment approach is primary chemotherapy followed by surgery or radiation therapy and additional adjuvant systemic therapy. Traditionally the surgical procedure of choice for patients with locally advanced breast cancer has been mastectomy. But recently, it was found that breast conservative surgery in patients, which responds to neoadjuvant chemotherapy also gives equal results compared to mastectomy. Hence patients who respond to initial chemotherapy should be evaluated carefully and the option of breast conservation should be offered. Preoperative chemotherapy regimens, reported to result in high response rates are the same as that used in the adjuvant settings (postoperative chemotherapy).

About 10-20 percent patients with locally advanced breast cancer will not achieve either complete response or partial response. Such patients carry very poor prognosis. These patients will not be benefited by surgery and are candidates for palliation.

PROGNOSTIC FACTORS IN LOCALLY ADVANCED BREAST CANCER

The initial size of the primary tumor or the extent of lymph node metastases represents the most important prognostic factor. However, the response to primary chemotherapy and the extent of residual disease of the primary chemotherapy remain the most influencing factor for outcome.

METASTATIC BREAST CANCER

Metastatic breast cancer is beyond the scope of complete cure. The median survival for women with metastatic breast cancer is in the range of 2 to 3 years. But this is highly variable, a minority of patients live even a decade longer with treatment.

Patients with metastatic breast cancer can be divided into two groups: those with Stage IV disease at presentation and those who develop metastases after primary treatment. The majority of women diagnosed with breast cancer today will never experience a systemic recurrence. Patients with delayed metastatic disease can be divided into two groups, i.e. low risk and intermediate/high risk, based on biological aggressiveness of the tumor.

Many patients have metastatic involvement that is confined to bone or soft tissue, while others have predominantly visceral disease. Metastasis in some of the sites like bone will not pose any danger to life immediately.

Favorable prognosis: Patients include those who develop metastatic diseases after a long disease-free interval following treatment of the primary or those with estrogen or progesterone receptor positive tumors, those without extensive visceral organ involvement.

Unfavorable patients include those with rapidly progressive disease or visceral involvement or hormone refractory disease or HER-2/Neu positivity.

The primary goal of treatment in these patients is improvement or maintenance of good quality of life and prolongation of survival.

The patients with favorable prognosis having positive hormone receptor may be treated with a trial of hormone therapy. Tamoxifen is the first line hormonal agent in premenopausal women who have not been treated with hormone previously. Ovarian ablations followed by aromatic inhibitor is the second line hormone therapy for those who progress under tamoxifen. In postmenopausal women also tamoxifen is the first line hormonal therapy. Aromatic inhibitors have also been tried with equal efficacy. In patients with HER-2/Neu positive tumors aromatase inhibitors may have better response over tamoxifen. If the tumor initially responds to the first line hormone therapy and then progresses, a second hormonal manipulation is warranted.

Patients with unfavorable prognosis, metastatic breast cancer or hormone refractory favorable prognosis patients are candidates for systemic chemotherapy. Combination chemotherapy is preferred to single agent. Doxorubicin/epirubicin and docetaxel containing regimens are more popular. Chemotherapy should be continued for 4 to 6 months or until the disease becomes stable and can be resumed if the patient experiences progression of disease after stopping the treatment. Other agents that are used in the salvage chemotherapy are capecitabine, vinorelbine and gemcitabine.

Trastuzumab: About 25 percent of breast cancer patients overexpress HER-2/Neu receptors. These tumors are more aggressive and predict poor response to endocrine therapy. They have high risk of recurrence, higher frequency of visceral disease at first recurrence. Trastuzumab is a monoclonal antibody to the HER-2/Neu protein and has been approved for use in metastatic breast cancer. It can be used as a single agent or in combination with chemotherapy for better response. However, the duration of the therapy with trastuzumab has not yet been decided. Dosage is 4 mg/kg IV over 90 minutes first dose, then 2 mg/kg IV over 30 minutes every week if the initial infusion was well tolerated. Trastuzumab is generally well tolerated. Rarely it may produce cardiac toxicity, especially if it is combined with other cardiotoxic drugs like doxorubicin and paclitaxel.

BISPHOSPHONATES

Bisphosphonates are potent inhibitors of osteoclastic bone resorption. They are indicated in the treatment of malignancy related hypercalcemia and metastatic bone disease. These agents reduce the skeletal related events such as bone pain, pathologic fracture and new bone metastasis. Commonly used bisphosphonates are pamidonate, ibandronate and zolendronic acid. Oral bisphosphonates are not very effective. Pamidronate (90 mg) is given in 500 ml of normal saline over 3 hours and zolendronate (4 mg) in 100 ml normal saline over 15 minutes; the frequency is once in 4 weeks. Bisphosphonates can be continued as long as the patient has benefit. Toxicities are generally tolerable like conjunctivitis, and hypersensitivity reactions. Now-a-days bisphosphonates are used routinely with hormone therapy or chemotherapy as an adjunctive treatment in breast cancer patients with bone metastasis.

MALE BREAST CANCER

Male breast cancer remains an uncommon disease. Male breast cancer has biological differences compared with female breast cancer, including a high prevalence in certain parts of Africa, a higher incidence of estrogen receptor positivity and more aggressive clinical behavior. The mean age of presentation is approximately 10 years later than the corresponding mean age for breast cancer in women. It responds to hormonal manipulation and chemotherapy, but optimal treatment regimens in males are unknown.

HORMONE REPLACEMENT THERAPY AFTER TREATMENT OF BREAST CANCER

Reports from certain centers have shown that breast cancer survivors treated with low-dose HRT did not show adverse impact upon survival. So if necessary it may be used, but further study of this issue is ongoing.

PREGNANCY AFTER BREAST CANCER

The issue of pregnancy following the diagnosis and treatment of breast cancer is important because the incidence of breast cancer is increasing in women of childbearing age. The survival of women with breast carcinoma who subsequently become pregnant is not reported to be decreased in any of the published series. Women should be advised to avoid pregnancy till 5 years of completion of chemotherapy.

FOLLOW-UP FOR PATIENTS WITH OPERABLE BREAST CANCER

History and physical examination are a must after every 3 months for the first year, every 6 months for the next 2 years and then annually. Annual mammograms and monthly self-breast examination are needed. Annual Pap smear and pelvic examination are required in women who are on tamoxifen.

FUTURE

The use of cytotoxic drugs against breast cancer is limited by a number of factors, including toxicity, tumor resistance and lack of targeted cell death. New strategies are based on increasing and improved knowledge of the molecular events responsible for disordered cellular growth. They include antibodies to block receptors, small molecules that inhibit receptor tyrosine kinase (RTK) mediated cell signaling, agents directed at suppressing the growth of blood vessels that feed cancer growth, vaccines to stimulate immune recognition of cancer cells, cell cycle inhibitors, and gene therapy to turn off signaling pathways or provide a missing tumor suppressor.

FURTHER READING

1 Bonadonna A, Brusamolima B, Valagussa P, et al. Combination chemotherapy as an adjuvant treatment in operable breast cancer. N Engl J Med 1976:294(8): 405-13.

2 Charles V, Mann RCG, Russel Norman S. Williams Bailey and Love Short Practice. of Surgery (22nd ed). ELBS With Chapman & Hall, London.

3. Early Breast cancer trialants collaborative group. Systemic treatment of early breast cancer by hormonal, cytotoxic or immune therapy. Lancet 1992; 339:1-15.

4. Hortobagyi GN. Treatment of breast cancer. N Engl J Med 1998;339,974-84.

5. Hartman LC, Schaid DJ, Woods JE, et al. Efficacy of bilateral prophylatic mastectomy. N Engl J Med 1999;340:77-84.

6. Karge D, Weaver D, Askikagi, et al. The sentinel node biopsy in breast cancer. N Engl J Med 1998;339:941-46.

7. Seymour I, Schwartz MD. Principle of Surgery (6th ed). McGraw-Hill Book Company, New York.

APPENDIX 1

International comparison; India and five continents—AAR (ICMR and IARC).

BREAST CANCER (FEMALE)

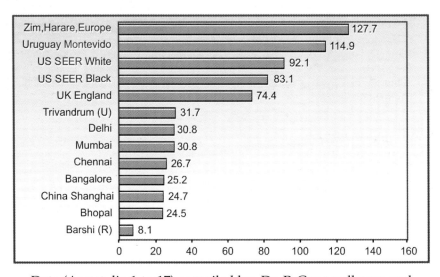

Data (Appendix 1 to 17) compiled by Dr. P. Ganagadharan and published with his kind permission.
Rate per 1000,000
(SEER-Surveillance, Epidemiology and End Result Reporting)

Non-small and Small Cell Lung Cancer

13

TK Jayakumar
K Pavithran
Shirley George

NON-SMALL CELL LUNG CANCER

Lung cancer is among the most commonly occurring malignancies in the world and it is one of the few that continues to show an increasing incidence. Non-small cell lung cancer (NSCLC) is a heterogeneous aggregate of at least 3 distinct histologies of lung cancer including squamous cell carcinoma, adenocarcinoma and large cell carcinoma. These histologies are often classified together because when localized, all have the potential for cure with surgical resection.

EPIDEMIOLOGY

The incidence of lung cancer in India is 9.7 per 100,000 among men and 4.45 among females. The lung is the leading site of cancer among males in Bhopal, Delhi and Mumbai and the second and third leading sites in Chennai and Bangalore respectively. In females also, except in Bangalore, all the urban registries have shown lung to be one of the ten leading sites. Its epidemiology differs in several respects from that in Western countries. The male-female ratio is around 4:5 in the urban registries. Almost a third of all patients and 90 percent of the women had never smoked. Squamous cell carcinoma was more frequent in the 1980s, however, the trend is changing in India also. A study done in 1999 showed predominance of adenocarcinoma.

ETIOLOGY

a. By far the biggest causal factor in lung cancer is smoking. eighty percent of lung cancer deaths among men and 75 percent of lung cancer deaths among women are attributable to smoking.

b. Passive smokers are at increased risk (30%) to develop cancer when living with a smoker. Environmental tobacco smoke (ETS) has also been strongly linked to an increased risk of lung cancer as the smoldering end of a lighted cigarette can emanate the carcinogenic compounds within the smoke to the atmosphere. Similarly stopping of smoking does not provide immunity against development of lung cancer. It depends on the number of cigarettes the person has smoked and the years of smoking.

c. Exposure to carcinogens like nickel, beryllium, chloromethyl ether chromium, polycyclic aromatic hydrocarbons, arsenic compounds, mustard gas and silica dust has increased the risk of developing lung cancer. There is also a strong link between asbestos and mesothelioma.

d. Dietary factors: Two recent evaluations have shown that, those people in the high risk group who were administered beta carotene and retinol had an adverse effect on lung cancer (NSCLC) with higher mortality.

e. Genetic mutations in cancer of the lung: In NSCLC, the most frequently identified abnormalities are 3p deletions (80%), deregulation of tumor suppressor gene p53 (seen in > 50%), aberrant expression of the epidermal growth factor receptor (EGFR) and one of its ligands, and the presence of K-ras abnormalities in adenocarcinoma. No single genetic factor is sufficiently predictive to be of diagnostic use. The lung tumors arise via a multistep carcinogenesis. Carcinogenic agents affect DNA by several molecular mechanisms. Generally they form molecular intermediaries that bind to DNA causing abnormalities in DNA synthesis. It has been demonstrated that in lung cancer, large areas or 'fields' of genetic mutations are found throughout the lung, even when no histological abnormality is seen.

f. NSCLC is more common in the scarred and chronically diseased lung. In developing countries, tuberculosis of the lung is not uncommon and has a role as an etiological factor in cancer of the lung. Chronic lung infections such as bronchiectasis, lung abscess and chronic tuberculosis should be actively treated.

PATHOLOGY OF LUNG CANCER

Cancer of the lung mainly affects the bronchi and hence bronchial carcinoma is synonymous with carcinoma of the lung. In NSCLC, squamous cell is the most frequently diagnosed cancer both in men and women, but this trend is changing the world over.

WHO CLASSIFICATION OF NSCLC

1. Squamous cell carcinoma—papillary, clear cell, basaloid
2. Adenocarcinoma—acinar, papillary, bronchoalveolar carcinoma, solid adenocarcinoma with mucin formation

3. Large cell carcinoma
4. Adenosquamous

Squamous cell carcinoma arises most frequently in the proximal segmental bronchi and is associated with squamous metaplasia. These tumors tend to be slow-growing, and it is estimated that a period of 3 or 4 years is required from the development of *in situ* carcinoma to a clinically apparent tumor. Adenocarcinoma most often is peripheral in origin and, arises from alveolar surface epithelium or bronchial mucosal glands; they can also present as peripheral tumors arising in areas of previous scars. The bronchoalveolar carcinoma, a subset of adenocarcinoma is different from the classical type of adenocarcinoma. They are more commonly seen in women, can occur in nonsmokers and are seen in both lung fields. There is lesser tendency for extrathoracic metastases and better survival than NSCLC in the particular stage.

CLINICAL MANIFESTATIONS

Carcinoma lung occurs in a wide range of age spectrum. It is rare before the age of 30 and the peak incidence is the sixth or the seventh decade.

Symptoms will depend upon the following factors:
a. Anatomical location of the tumor.
b. Involvement of adjacent structures.
c. Extent and location of metastatic spread.
d. Metabolic byproducts of the tumor (paraneoplastic syndromes).
e. About 5 to 6 percent of the patients may be asymptomatic and the lesion may be accidentally detected in routine radiography.

BRONCHOPULMONARY SYMPTOMS

This is due to the tumor producing block, ulceration or irritation. Central tumor with intraluminal component will be more symptomatic.

The following are the usual symptoms:
a. *Cough:* Persistent cough lasts for three to six months duration, usually an irritant type which can be productive once there is associated infection or tumor necrosis.
b. *Hemoptysis:* It can be mild to massive and even a single episode warrants full investigation.
c. *Fever:* Though tumor itself can produce fever, commonly it is due to secondary pneumonitis.
d. Obstructive symptoms like stridor and wheezing will depend upon the location of the tumor. Typically the wheezing is a late onset and can be unilateral.
e. *Dyspnea:* Central tumors cause breathlessness because of the block to airways. Peripheral tumors can impair respiration because of the compression and collapse produced by pleural effusion or because of the loss of lung reserve due to mass effect and pneumonitis.

SYMPTOMS DUE TO ADJACENT STRUCTURE INVOLVEMENT AND CHEST WALL INVASION

a. *Chest pain:* This can be of two types—pleuritic or neuralgic. Pleuritic pain can be due to direct tumor invasion of the pleura or can be due to pleurisy. Neuralgic pain of direct involvement of brachial plexus or intercostal nerves can be the first symptom. This may be ignored by many as myalgia or nonspecific chest pain.

b. Hoarseness of voice can be the first symptom and may indicate inoperability. This is commonly due to the left recurrent laryngeal nerve involvement.

c. Dysphagia is rare. It can be due to compression of esophagus by primary tumor or lymph nodes or due to direct infiltration as well.

d. Pericardial effusion, tamponade or arrhythmia can occur due to direct infiltration of pericardium and heart. It is rarely a presenting symptom but it is a feature of advanced malignancy (15 to 30%).

e. Superior vena caval syndrome also may indicate advanced disease.

SYMPTOMS DUE TO METASTATIC DISEASE

Metastatic spread can occur to supraclavicular nodes, brain, adrenals, kidneys, liver and bone. Any symptom pertaining to these in a patient with lung cancer requires further evaluation.

EXTRAPULMONARY NONMETASTATIC SYMPTOMS (PARANEOPLASTIC SYNDROMES)

This can precede the other manifestations of lung cancer. This can be categorized as:

a. *Metabolic:* Cushing's syndrome, hypercalcemia, excessive ADH, carcinoid syndrome, gynecomastia.

b. *Neuromuscular:* Peripheral neuropathy, cortical cerebellar degeneration, Eaton-Lambert syndrome, myopathy etc.

c. *Dermatological:* Acanthosis nigricans, dermatomyositis.

d. *Skeletal:* Clubbing, pulmonary hypertrophic osteoarthropathy.

e. *Vascular:* Migratory thrombophlebitis, nonbacterial verrucal endocarditis.

f. *Hematological:* Anemia.

Common ones are discussed.

Cushing's syndrome: This syndrome is more common in squamous cell carcinoma and carcinoid syndrome and differ from classical Cushing's syndrome. This group of patients tend to be males in the older age group.

SIADH: Immunoreactive Arginine-Vasopressin and atrial natriuretic peptide (ANP) can be secreted by carcinoma of the bronchus. It is seen with especially small cell carcinoma and patients can present with water intoxication.

Hypercalcemia can be due to parathormone or PTH related protein (PTHrP) and it is seen more in squamous cell carcinoma.

Neuromyopathy: It is the commonest extrathoracic manifestation of lung cancer (15%). Eaton-Lambert myasthenic syndrome mainly affects pelvic girdle and thigh muscles. Response to Neostigmine is poor.

PROGNOSTIC FACTORS

1. Patients with poor performance status will be poor candidates for surgery or chemotherapy.
2. The higher the stage, the poorer the prognosis.
3. Women have better prognosis than men.
4. Weight loss and the presence of paraneoplastic syndrome have poorer prognosis.
5. Squamous cell and bronchoalveolar cell carcinomas have better prognosis than large cell or adenocarcinoma.

DIAGNOSIS

Detailed history and clinical examination can give a clue to the diagnosis. *X-ray chest* will show some abnormality in at least 98 percent of patients with lung cancer. The usual radiographic features include hilar prominence, mediastinal widening, single or multiple mass lesions of varying sizes, air entrapment, evidence of collapse, consolidation, thick-walled cavity, pneumonitic changes, pleural effusion and vertebral or rib erosion. Squamous cell carcinoma is usually central. A peripheral thick-walled cavity also can be squamous cell carcinoma. Adenocarcinoma is peripheral and cavitation is unusual.

CT SCAN THORAX AND UPPER ABDOMEN

This is a routine investigation in lung cancer. CT should include the thorax from apex to upper abdomen, i.e. include liver and adrenals.

CT will help to see:
a. The exact location and extent of tumor.
b. Involvement of ribs or vertebrae.
c. Chest wall involvement may not be that specific to assess in all cases.
d. Mediastinal lymph node enlargement: This is the most important use of CT thorax in carcinoma lung.
e. Involvement of mediastinal structures like pericardium, great vessels etc. They are not 100 percent predictive.

CT also helps to rule out synchronous and metachronous lesions.

MRI

This investigation is not used for routine diagnostic or staging procedures. The area, where MRI is superior, is in assessing chest wall invasion and differentiating between benign and malignant lymph node enlargement.

ULTRASONOGRAPHY (USG)

USG abdomen is useful in evaluating intra-abdominal metastasis and pleural effusion. Endoscopic ultrasonogram using an esophageal probe is the most sensitive method to assess circumferential spread of the tumor. Endoscopic ultrasonogram has been proved to be the most effective method to detect paraesophageal lymph node involvement as well as the subcarinal or inferior pulmonary ligament nodes.

SPUTUM CYTOLOGY

Different series show 40-90 percent positivity. More chance of positivity exists in central rather than peripheral lesions.

INVASIVE PROCEDURES

Bronchoscopy

This is a routine investigation in the preoperative workup of lung cancer. This helps in getting a tissue diagnosis, staging of lung cancer as well as to assess resectability. Biopsy from a visible lesion gives the maximum positivity. Bronchial washing cytology is more useful in central lesions whereas transbronchial FNAC can be of some help in peribronchial or hilar growth.

Percutaneous Transthoracic Needle Aspiration

The indications for this procedure include clinically nonresectable tumor, medically unfit patient or the patient refusing resection. A negative FNAC will not exclude the possibility of a malignancy.

Video-assisted Thoracoscopic Surgery (VATS)

VATS is becoming popular not only in the diagnosis of the tumors but also in staging. By this modality, biopsy can be taken, and the extent and resectability can be assessed. Different types of resection like wedge resection of a peripheral tumor or lobectomy can be undertaken. This, being a minimally invasive surgery, is cosmetically better and reduces the pain, the hospital stay and morbidity.

Mediastinoscopy

There is a role for mediastinoscopy especially in those having CT-proved mediastinal lymphadenopathy. This helps in precise staging and also in assessing operability.

Metastatic work up includes bone scan and CT scan abdomen.

Screening for Cancer Lung

Early detection of cancer of the lung by chest radiograph has not shown any significant reduction in mortality with this dreaded disease. But in many centers, the cancer-prone individuals particularly the smokers must undergo yearly chest radiograph study.

At the same time, the lack of evidence of early detection of lung cancer by screening cannot be recommended as a public health project.

The public health authorities must use all methods: press, television and roadside posters telling the citizens that smoking is the prime etiological factor in cancer lung. They also must form 'Citroen Protection Groups' to spread this idea: no smoking, no lung cancer.

The staging is undertaken with this information:

Occult carcinoma	T × N0 M0
Stage 0	Tis N0 M0
Stage IA	T1 N0 M0
Stage IB	T2 N0 M0
Stage IIA	T1 N1 M0
Stage IIA	T2 N1 M0
	T3 N0 M0
Stage IIIA	T1 N2 M0
	T2 N2 M0
	T3 N1 M0
	T3 N2 M0
Stage IIIB	Any T N3 M0
	T4 any N M0
Stage IV	Any T any N M1

PRINCIPLES OF TREATMENT

Therapeutic decision-making depends on the TNM stage of non-small cell carcinoma (Table 13.1). A joint consultation with different disciplines can be done to plan therapy. The questions to be answered are:
  a. Is there a role for surgery and if so, whether it is going to be curative, palliative or pain relieving?
  b. What is the role of chemotherapy/radiotherapy?
  c. What is going to be the outcome?

Surgery

Surgery should be considered in TNM stages I, II and IIIA. The contraindications for surgery in these stages are:
  a. Associated other systemic illnesses like recent MI, uncontrolled congestive cardiac failure and arrhythmias.
  b. Inadequate lung reserve: Pulmonary function tests are used to assess the reserve. If FEV1 and FVC are more than 60 percent of predicted

Table 13.1: Staging

The TNM staging

Note: The staging is mostly done for NSCLC.

Tx: Imaging modality or bronchoscopy does not identify tumor. Tumor cells are present in the bronchopulmonary secretion.

T0: No evidence of primary tumor.

Tis: Carcinoma *in situ*, which means the cancer, is contained within the bronchial epithelium.

T1: Tumor 3 cm or less in its greatest dimension. Surrounded by normal lung or visceral pleura without bronchoscopic evidence of invasion more proximal than lobar bronchus.

T2: Tumor with any of the following features of size or extent: more than 3 cm in its greatest dimension, involves main bronchus 2 cm or more distal to the carina, invades visceral pleura, associated with atelectasis or obstructive pneumonitis that extends to the hilar region but does not involve the entire lung.

T3: Tumor of any size that directly invades any of the following—chest wall (including superior sulcus tumors), mediastinal pleura, parietal pericardium, diaphragm; or tumor in the main bronchus less than 2 cm distal to the carina, but without involvement of the carina or associated atelectasis or obstructive pneumonitis of the entire lung.

T4: Tumor of any size that invades any of the following—mediastinum, heart, great vessels, trachea, esophagus, vertebral body, carina; or separate tumor nodules in the same lobe, or tumor with malignant effusion.

Nodal involvement (N)

N0: No evidence of regional lymph node metastasis.

N1: Metastasis to ipsilateral peribronchial or ipsilateral hilar nodes, and intrapulmonary nodes including involvement by direct extension of the primary tumor.

N2: Metastasis to ipsilateral mediastinal and subcarinal lymph nodes.

N3: Metastases to contralateral mediastinal, contralateral hilar, ipsilateral or contralateral scalene or supraclavicular lymph node(s).

Distant metastasis

M0: No known or identifiable distant metastasis

M1: Distant metastasis to bone, brain, liver, adrenal glands, etc.

value, resection including pneumonectomy can be planned. If it is less than 30 percent of predicted value, surgery is contraindicated. If the PFT values are marginal radionuclide ventilation, perfusion scans will help to predict postoperative lung function and if it is acceptable they can be taken up for resection.

Lung resection can be done through thoracotomy or by video-assisted thoracoscopy. Final decision of resectability and the extent of resection is made at the operating table. Contraindications for resection at the table include fixity to vital structures like great vessels, trachea, etc. non-resectable lymph nodes, N3 disease and pleural deposits. The basic principle to be observed is that residual macroscopic or microscopic tumor should be avoided. The resection can be wedge resection, segmentectomy, lobectomy or pneumonectomy. Wedge resection can be done for small peripheral lesions. Segmentectomy is done for T1 disease confined to a segment. Both these limited resections have the advantage of preserving more pulmonary parenchyma but have the disadvantage of compromising on local clearance. Different studies showed that survival rates of limited resection are comparable with lobectomy but with a higher local recurrence rate. Pneumonectomy is done when lobectomy will not be sufficient to clear all the tumor tissues (e.g. T1/T2 disease involving more than one lobe across the fissure). Mediastinal lymph node dissection or sampling of different stations also should be done for proper staging. The common postoperative problems include bleeding, ventilatory failure, persistent air leak, infection of residual space and bronchial stump blow out.

Multimodality treatment of NSCLC (surgery, radiotherapy and chemotherapy) in different stages.

Stage I—Surgery is the treatment of choice. This therapy is curative in 60-70 percent of patients with pathologic stage I disease. If inoperable due to poor pulmonary functional reserve, the patient is treated with radiotherapy. Primary radiation therapy should consist of approximately 60 Gy delivered with megavoltage equipment. A boost to the conedown field of the primary tumor is frequently used to further enhance local control.

Stage II—If the pulmonary function tests (PFTs) are favorable, the tumor can be resected (either lobectomy, pneumonectomy, segmental, wedge, or sleeve resection as appropriate) with curative intent. About 40-50 percent of these patients are cured. If inoperable, radiotherapy with concurrent chemotherapy shall be the treatment of choice.

Stage III A—If the performance status is within normal, resection can be done, followed by combination chemotherapy.

Stage III B—These patients with regionally advanced disease are not amenable to surgical resection with curative intent. They should be given induction chemotherapy followed by radiotherapy.

Stage IV—Chemotherapy improves survival and palliates symptoms, thereby improving quality of life in patients with stage IV NSCLC in both the first-line and second-line setting. Patients with performance status 0-2 can be considered for combination chemotherapy. Others are only given supportive treatment. No one regimen has been demonstrated to be superior in the first-line therapy for patients with advanced NSCLC. A cisplatin-based or carboplatin-based combination regimen that includes one of the new agents (gemcitabine, paclitaxel, docetaxel, vinorelbine) remains the appropriate drugs for first-line therapy in patients with stage IV NSCLC. Patients with a good PS who are experiencing disease progression after receiving platinum-based chemotherapy should be offered second-line chemotherapy. Radiotherapy is given for residual disease or for metastatic sites.

DOSES AND SCHEDULE OF CHEMOTHERAPEUTIC AGENTS

Paclitaxel/Carboplatin
Paclitaxel 175 mg/m^2 IV over 3 hours on Day 1
Cisplatin 75 mg/m^2 Day 1.
Gemcitabine/Cisplatin
Gemcitabine 1.2 g/m^2 Day 1 and 8
Cisplatin 75 mg/m^2 Day 1.
Docetaxel 75 mg/m^2 Day 1
Cisplatin 75 mg/m^2 Day 1.
Vinorelbine 25 mg/m^2 Day 1 and Day 8
Cisplatin 75 mg/m^2 Day 1.
Carboplatin can be used instead of cisplatin in all of the above regimens at AUC 6, IV over 60 minutes.
Cisplatin 75 mg/m^2 Day 1
Etoposide 100 mg/m^2 Day 1-3.

All treatment cycles are repeated every 21 days for 6 cycles depending upon the response.

ADVANCED STAGE III OR IV WITH MALIGNANT EFFUSION

It must be realized that the survival of patients at these stages is extremely poor. The median survival rate is only a matter of weeks (16 to 18 weeks). Pleurodesis can be done to counteract recurrent pleural effusions due to malignant pleural seeding. These substances are of no value if the effusion is caused by tumor of lymph nodes which blocks lymph drainage of pleura and lung.

Pancoast Tumor

This syndrome, initially described by Pancoast, is characterized by rib erosion, shoulder pain radiating down the arm and Horner's syndrome. On radiographic study of the chest, a small homogeneous mass will be seen at the apex of the lung with erosion of the first rib and infiltration of the 7th cervical vertebra. These tumors are also called superior sulcus tumors and are better evaluated using MRI scans than CT scans. Most of these tumors are adenocarcinoma. Ipsilateral supraclavicular nodal involvement has a better prognosis than ipsilateral mediastinal nodal involvement and both of them suggest poor prognosis. Untreated patients have a survival rate of 10 to 11 months. Preoperative radiation with lobectomy and resection of the first rib has been advocated with better survival rates. In fact the survival rate is twice that obtained by wedge resection (65% vs 30%).

Pulmonary Metastases

The lungs are frequent sites for metastatic tumors. If the radiographic abnormalities are multiple and there is a history of previous malignancy, the diagnosis is not difficult. If there is a solitary lesion, it may be difficult to exclude a benign nodule or a primary carcinoma of the lung. The typical cannon ball appearance on chest radiography is often seen with primary lung tumors. Metastatic disease may assume a variety of radiographic appearances from finely nodular disease to an infiltrate, poorly defined opacity.

In selected cases surgical excision of pulmonary metastases may be feasible and worthwhile. A 5-year survival of 35-55 percent has been reported following the surgical excision of carcinomatous and sarcomatous deposits. The selection for such surgery must be rigorous. In addition to ensuring the patient's fitness, selection should ensure that the primary tumor has been reliably controlled, usually by excision. Extrathoracic metastases have been excluded using the most sensitive investigations appropriate, and the extent of intrathoracic metastases has been documented by CT scans of the whole of both lungs. The disease-free interval and the number of metastases do not appear to influence the effectiveness of pulmonary resection. The excision of each metastasis is performed by the most conservative resection feasible—usually removing only the deposit with a thin surrounding rim of normal lung. If metastases are large or impinge on hilar structures, segmentectomy or lobectomy may be necessary. Pneumonectomy is rarely justified for the removal of metastatic disease (Figs 13.1 and 13.2).

The prospect of surgery in lung metastasis is grim and most patients relapse within 1 year. The role of adjuvant chemotherapy remains controversial.

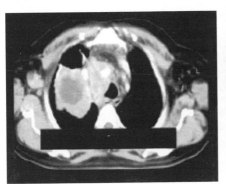 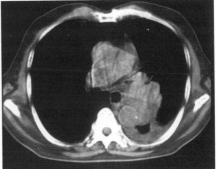

Figure 13.1: CT scan of a case of melanoma in a 50-year-old male with pulmonary metastases. Mediastinal adenopathy and involvement of the first rib-Pancoast tumor

Figure 13.2: CT scan of a case of 46-year-old male patient with carcinoma of the left lung with pleural effusion

Malignant Pleural Effusion

Malignant pleural effusion is one of those most commonly referred conditions to the thoracic surgeon. Malignant bronchial obstruction will lead to consolidation of the lung and may result in a benign effusion. Once these have been shown to be serous and cytologically negative, they have little impact on the management of the underlying condition. Malignant effusions, however, may result from visceral pleural invasion by a peripheral carcinoma of the lung or by metastatic involvement of the pleura by adenocarcinoma derived from the lung, breast or other sites. On certain occasions the primary may not be identified.

The diagnosis is usually made by aspiration cytology or needle biopsy of the pleura. Should these techniques fail, open pleural biopsy through a limited thoracotomy or by video-assisted thoracoscope (VATS) is indicated. Repeated attempts at pleural aspiration may lead to empyema, a troublesome complication that seriously hampers the patient's remaining life. The treatment consists of pleurodesis and combination chemotherapy depending upon the etiology.

FURTHER READING

1. American Society of Clinical Oncology. Clinical practice guidelines for the treatment of unresectable non-small cell lung cancer. J Clin Oncol 1997;15:2996-3018.
2. Donnadieu N, Paesmans M, Sculier J-P. Chemotherapy of non-small cell lung cancer according to disease extent: A meta-analysis of the literature. Lung Cancer 1991;7:243-52.
3. Jain NK, Madan A, Sharma TN, Agnihotri SP, Saxena A, Mandhana RG. Bronchogenic carcinoma: A study of 109 cases. J Assoc Physicians India 1989;37:379-82.
4. Jindal SK, Malik SK, Malik AK, Singh A, Sodni JS. Bronchial Carcinoma (A review of 150 cases). Indian J Chest Dis Allied Sci 1979;21:59-64.
5. Leef JL 3rd, Klein JS. The solitary pulmonary nodule. Radiol Clin North Am 2002;40:123-43.
6. Marino P, Pampallona S, Preatoni A, et al. Chemotherapy vs supportive care in advanced non-small cell lung cancer: Results of a meta-analysis of the literature. Chest 1994;106:861-65.
7. Ross JA, Rosen GD. The molecular biology of lung cancer. Curr Opin Pulm Med 2002;8:265-69.
8. Socinski MA. Chemotherapy for stage IV non-small cell lung cancer. In: Detterbeck FC, Rivera MP, Socinski MA, et al (Eds). Diagnosis and treatment of lung cancer: An evidence-based guide for the practicing clinician. Philadelphia, PA: WB Saunders 2001;307-25.
9. Souquet PJ, Chauvin F, Boissel JP, et al. Polychemotherapy in advanced non-small cell lung cancer: A meta-analysis. Lancet 1993;11:1866-72.
10. The Non-Small Cell Lung Cancer Collaborative Group. Chemotherapy in non-small cell lung cancer: A meta-analysis using updated data on individual patients from 52 randomized clinical trials. BMJ 1995;311:899-909.
11. Vigano A, Binera E, Jhangri GS, et al. Clinical survival predictors in patients with advanced cancer. Arch Intern Med 2000;160:861-68.

SMALL CELL LUNG CANCER

The small cell lung cancer (SCLC) is a distinct variety of lung cancer and accounts for 10-20 percent of all lung cancers. It is considered to be a systemic disease with different histologic patterns. This type of cancer is characterized by rapid growth and greater tendency to be widely disseminated at the time of diagnosis. Without treatment, small cell carcinoma has the most aggressive clinical course in any type of pulmonary tumor. The median survival from the time of initial diagnosis is only 2 to 4 months. At the same time, this kind of tumor is much more responsive to treatment than NSCLC. The overall survival at 5 years is 5 percent to 10 percent.

ETIOLOGY

The etiology is similar to NSCLC.
   a. By far the biggest causal factor in lung cancer is smoking. More than 95 percent of patients with small cell lung cancer are current or past cigarette smokers. Among tobacco related cancers, SCLC is higher than other histologic types of lung cancer. This is true as regards both men and women. In fact, the number of SCLC is on the increase in young women due to increased tobacco consumption. The risk of exposure of nonsmokers in public places is similar to that noted in NSCLC.
   b. Miners working in uranium mines and those exposed to radon gas have a higher chance of developing SCLC.

GENETIC MUTATION IN INITIATION OF SCLC

Unlike other epithelial tumors, the tumor suppressor genes play a vital role in the initiation of these tumors. More than 90 percent of p53 and Rb are inactivated in SCLC and both these genes have a critical role in the G1/S cell-cycle check-points. More than 90 percent show deletions on the short arm of chromosome 3, suggesting the presence of additional important tumor suppressor genes in SCLC.

SCLC shows overexpression of many dominant oncogenes like the oncogene Myc, a family of nuclear phosphoproteins that regulate transcription, KIT, growth factor receptor with tyrosine kinase activity and telomerase, which is believed to block sequences by preventing telomeric shortening.

PATHOLOGY

An accurate pathologic diagnosis is essential for treatment planning. Tumor blocks have to be obtained either by VATS or CT-guided wide bore needle. Ordinary needle aspirations or bronchoscopy can lead to mistaken diagnoses of SCLC. SCLC cells are thought to arise from

Kulchitsky's cells. These cells often stain with silver and have demonstrable neurosecretory granules.

THREE CLASSES OF CELLS ARE IDENTIFIED IN SCLC

Small cell carcinoma (commonest, comprising more than 90 percent of all SCLC).

Mixed cellular pattern of large and small cells.

Combined small and non-small cell carcinoma.

It is essential to determine whether the pathologist is dealing with an SCLC or an NSCLC since the prognosis in the former is dismal.

CLINICAL FEATURES

As mentioned before, both NSCLC and SCLC share the same pulmonary symptoms.

1. Most of the SCLC begins as a central endobronchial tumor with cough, dyspnea, hemoptysis and chest pain. Fever with post-obstructive pneumonitis can be present. Chest radiography shows hilar prominence due to lymphadenopathy. About 15 to 19 percent of patients have early signs of superior vena caval syndrome of prominent neck veins, edema of face and upper limbs. If situated in the periphery pleural pain, fever and dyspnea occur.

2. Due to either direct or metastatic local involvement the following symptoms may be observed: hoarseness (involvement of recurrent laryngeal nerve), tracheal obstruction, dysphagia (esophageal obstruction), superior vena cava obstruction, malignant pleural effusion, pericardial effusion, phrenic nerve and sympathetic nerve palsy (Horner's syndrome).

3. Approximately two thirds of patients have distant metastases at the time of first presentation. Metastasis spread can reach virtually any extrathoracic organ of the body commonly head and neck region, brain, liver, bones and adrenal glands. Headache, seizures, visual disturbances, jaundice, asymptomatic elevations of liver enzymes etc. can occur. Bone marrow involvement with resultant anemia, leucopenia, thrombocytopenia, etc. may be experienced.

4. Extrapulmonary manifestations of lung carcinoma or the well-known paraneoplastic syndrome may be recognized before lung cancer itself produces symptoms. They are often related to the secretion of polypeptide hormone from the neuroendocrine cells.

Hyponatremia (SIADH, secretion of excess atrial natriuretic peptide), Cushing's syndrome due to ectopic adreno-corticotropic hormone (ACTH), Eaton-Lambert myasthenia like syndrome, etc. can be associated with SCLC.

Neurological symptoms such as cerebellar ataxia, subacute sensory neuropathy, with proximal and distal myopathy and unexplained severe neuralgic type of pain too can be seen in these patients.

Loss of weight, loss of appetite, anemia and unexplained fever are some of the evidences of extrathoracic metastases.

STAGING

The TNM staging system is not used typically for patients with small cell lung cancer because the patients usually do not undergo evaluation for surgical resection after the diagnosis is established. The staging classification for these patients is a simple, two-stage—Veterans Administration Lung Study Group system—that categorizes patients as having limited or extensive stage disease.

1. Limited stage disease is confined to one hemithorax and nodes. It can be brought within a radiotherapy field.
2. In extensive stage there is evidence of distant metastases.

Contralateral hilar, mediastinal, or supraclavicular nodes are usually included in limited-stage disease.

Ipsilateral malignant pleural effusion is considered extensive disease.

Necessary components of an adequate staging and pretreatment evaluation include:

1. Complete history and physical examination.
2. Chest radiography, CT of chest and upper abdomen, tissue biopsy, hemogram, renal and liver function tests, LDH, bone marrow examination, bone scan and CT scan of the brain.

It has been already mentioned that 65 percent of the patients on the initial phase of the diagnosis have distant metastases and 10-15 percent of patients present with evidence of paraneoplastic syndrome. Hence it is essential that accurate staging of the disease is mandatory before starting any form of therapy. Those patients who may benefit from combined-modality treatment (combination chemotherapy with concurrent thoracic radiation) must be identified and aggressive multimodality therapy must begin.

The most important factors that suggest favorable prognosis are limited stage disease, good performance status, normal lactic dehydrogenase and female gender. Patients with involvement of the central nervous system or liver at the time of diagnosis have a significantly worse outcome.

TREATMENT IN LIMITED-STAGE DISEASE

Combined chemotherapy with concurrent thoracic irradiation is generally recommended. Toxicities of therapy, including dysphagia, esophagitis, pneumonitis, myelosuppression and fatigue may be observed more frequently in patients receiving concurrent treatments. Some stage I patients may be candidates for surgical resection combined with multiagent chemotherapy on re-evaluation after the initial chemotherapy treatment.

STAGE-DEPENDENT TREATMENT OF SCLC

Stage	*Treatment*
Limited-stage disease	Combination chemotherapy
	Thoracic radiation recommended
	Prophylactic cranial irradiation may be
	considered in complete responders
Extensive-stage disease	Combination chemotherapy

RADIOTHERAPY

Thoracic radiation provides a marginal survival advantage and reduced local recurrence rate when added to chemotherapy in limited-stage disease.

Most regimens incorporating radiation therapy use a total dose of 45 to 50 Gy. The optimal timing of radiotherapy is unclear, but administration either concurrent or interdigitating with chemotherapy is favored over sequential regimens.

Radiation therapy is also used in local control of disease (CNS and other isolated metastatic sites not responding to systemic chemotherapy).

CHEMOTHERAPY

Different protocols are used in different centers with each one of them having strong advocates for its use. Instead of using a single agent, survival with multiagent therapy has made combination chemotherapy the standard approach in initial treatment in patients with SCLC. Combination chemotherapy produces results that are clearly superior to single-agent treatment and moderately intensive doses of drugs are superior to doses that produce only minimal or mild hematologic toxic effects. Because of the frequent presence of metastatic disease, chemotherapy is the cornerstone of treatment in SCLC. Optimal regimens yield 80 percent to 90 percent response rates, 50 to 60 percent complete response rates, and 2-year survival rates of 15 to 40 percent. Several combinations have been used successfully. The most commonly used regimen currently is etoposide and cisplatin (EP) because of its favorable toxicity profile and reports of activity in tumors initially treated with cyclophosphamide-containing regimens. A recent study that compared cisplatin and etoposide to a combination of cisplatin and irinotecan showed improvement in response rates (65% vs 52%) and 2 year survival (19.5% vs 5.2%) in the cisplatin and irinotecan group compared to cisplatin and etoposide arm.

The optimal duration of chemotherapy is four to six cycles. Longer duration of treatment has not been shown to be of any benefit. High-dose chemotherapy with autologous stem cell reinfusion has not been demonstrated to be superior in phase III trails to conventional therapy and is currently used only in clinical trials. Other chemotherapeutic regimens are mentioned below.

DIFFERENT PROTOCOLS IN THE TREATMENT OF SCLC

The drugs are used in combination and the commonly used combination of drugs is etoposide and cisplatin cyclophosphamide, doxorubicin and vincristine (CAV) cyclophosphamide, doxorubicin, vincristine and etoposide (CAVE) cisplatin and irinotecan

In regimen,

a. Etoposide 100 mg/m^2 IV day 1-3 and cisplatin 100 mg/m^2 IV day 1 Repeated every 3 weeks, for 6 cycles.

b. Cyclophosphamide 1,000 mg/m^2 IV day 1 doxorubicin 45 mg/m^2 IV day 2 and vincristine 1.4 mg/m^2 IV day 3 (maximum dose of 2 mg). Each cycle is repeated every 3 weeks and continued for 6 cycles.

c. Cyclophosphamide 1,000 mg/m^2 IV day 1, doxorubicin 50 mg/m^2 IV day 2, vincristine 1.4 mg/m^2 IV day 3 and etoposide 60 mg/m^2 IV day 4. Each cycle is repeated every 4 weeks and continued for 6 cycles.

d. Irinotecan 60 mg/m^2 day 1, 8 and 15; cisplatin 60 mg/m^2 day 1.

Each cycle is repeated every 4 weeks and continued for 6 cycles.

The clinician must be alert to different types of toxicities, some of them mild and some others severe while using these drugs. Before every cycle, blood and platelet count, LFT and urea and creatinine must be evaluated. In case of low white cell count, whole blood transfusion must be given. Platelet transfusion also must be given if the platelet count is less than 50,000/cmm. The patient must be adequately hydrated by oral route or intravenous route before each cycle.

PROPHYLACTIC CRANIAL IRRADIATION (PCI)

It has been noted that 50 to 60 percent of survivors develop cerebral metastasis. Prophylactic cranial irradiation (PCI) typically in doses of 24 to 36 Gy given in 8 to 15 fractions has been used to prevent the development of brain metastases. Although PCI reduces the frequency of brain metastases, no significant survival advantage was observed in earlier randomized studies. Despite concerns about impaired intellectual function in patients successfully treated for small cell lung cancer, prospective studies have not confirmed these initial observations. A recent study group reported that PCI improved both overall survival and disease-free interval with better survival among patients with SCLC. Patients with SCLC achieving a complete remission should be treated with prophylactic cranial irradiation.

EXTENSIVE-STAGE DISEASE

Combination chemotherapy without thoracic irradiation is the cornerstone of therapy. Combination chemotherapy identical to those used in limited-stage disease is used with overall response rates of 60 to 80 percent, complete response rates of 15 to 20 percent, and median survival of 7 to 11 months. Two-year survival is uncommon with current therapy. Because of the poor performance status commonly encountered in this stage and the low cure rate with standard treatment, single-agent chemotherapy with oral VP-16 is used in selected cases.

RECURRENT DISEASE OR PROGRESSIVE DISEASE ON INITIAL THERAPY

Recurrent disease or a progressive disease has an extremely poor prognosis, with a median survival of 2 to 3 months. Treatment options in this group are limited. The relative effectiveness of different drug combination programs appears similar and there are a large number of potential combinations. Some clinicians have administered two of these or other regimens in alternating sequences, but there is no proof that this strategy yields substantial survival improvement. Optimal duration of chemotherapy is not clearly defined. At the same time, there is no obvious improvement in survival when the duration of drug administration exceeds six months.

Thoracic irradiation should be considered in those patients whose recurrence is confined to the thorax and who have not received irradiation previously. Patients who have not received a platinum, containing regimen may benefit from combinations containing cisplatin, taxol and topotecan. Single agents have also been shown to have some activity in this setting.

Long-time survivors of SCLC are at a high risk of developing second primary tumor of NSCLC in addition to recurrent SCLC. The patients who are able to quit smoking seem to do better than the patients who continue to smoke. These patients should be considered for chemoprevention strategies.

FURTHER READING

1. Arriagada R, Auperin A, et al. On behalf of the PCIO Collaborative group: Prophylactic cranial irradiation overview (PCIO) in patients with small cell lung cancer (SCLC) in complete remission (CR). Proc Am Soc Clin Oncol 1998;17:1758, 1777.
2. Auperin A, Arriagada R, Pignon JP, et al. Prophylactic cranial irradiation for patients with small-cell lung cancer in complete remission. Prophylactic Cranial Irradiation Overview Collaborative Group. N Engl J Med 1999;341:476-84.
3. Hirsch FR, Matthews MJ, Aisner S, et al. Histopathologic classification of small cell lung cancer: Changing concepts and terminology. Cancer 1988;62:973-77.
4. Noda K, Nishiwaki Y, Kawahara M, et al. Irinotecan plus cisplatin compared with etoposide plus cisplatin for extensive small-cell lung cancer. N Engl J Med 2002;346:85-91.
5. Rawson NS, Peto J. An overview of prognostic factors in small cell lung cancer of the United Kingdom Coordinating Committee on Cancer Research. Br J Cancer 1990;61:597-604.
6. Urban T, Lebeau B, Chastang C, et al. Superior vena cava syndrome in small-cell lung cancer. Arch Int Med 1993;153:384-87.
7. Wurschmidt F, Bunemann H, Heilmann HP. Small cell lung cancer with and without superior vena cava syndrome: A multivariate analysis of prognostic factors in 408 cases. Int J Radiat Oncol Biol Phy 1995;33:77-82.

APPENDIX 2

International comparison; India and five continents—AAR (ICMR and IARC).

CANCER LUNG (MALE)

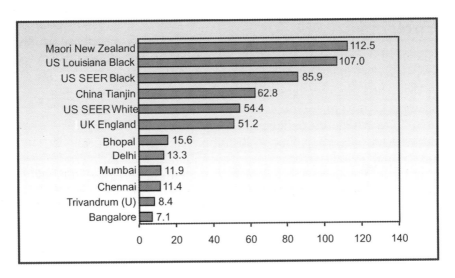

CANCER LUNG (FEMALE)

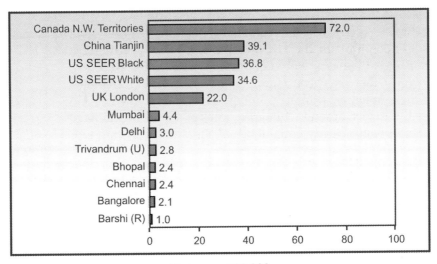

Rate per 100,000

Esophageal Cancer

14

Sanjay Joseph

PERSPECTIVE

Cancers of the alimentary tract are of special surgical interest since at earlier stages, surgical resection is eminently suited for their cure. Aggressiveness diminishes as it descends from the upper GI tract to the anorectal area. Most tumors are adeno-carcinomas which are radioresistant and hence radiotherapy can be used only for palliation in tumors of the esophageal and the anal regions which are mostly of squamous cell variety. Now there is a growing interest in combination of surgery with pre- or postoperative irradiation and chemotherapy in tumors of the alimentary tract. Multimodality treatment either in the pre- or postoperative stages has increased the cure rate and ensured a better 5-year survival rate.

ESOPHAGEAL CANCER

Esophageal cancer is the ninth most common cancer worldwide. In the developing areas of the world (Asia, Africa and Latin America), this type of cancer is not uncommon but is less common in the UK and the US. Historically, most esophageal cancers were squamous cell tumors. Recently, however, there has been a marked increase in adenocarcinoma of the esophagus, primarily among white men in the UK and the US. In fact, among white men, rates of adenocarcinoma of the esophagus nearly equal those of squamous cell variety.

EPIDEMIOLOGY

IN INDIA

The cancers seen in stomach and esophagus are more common than cancer of the lung in men and rarer than cancer of the breast and cervix in women. There is variation in the statewise distribution in the various population groups. Esophageal cancers are not uncommon in the southern regions of India such as Bangalore and Chennai. The occurrence of the esophageal tumor in different communities is listed in Table 14.1. The median age is 55 and rarely earlier than 30 years. Esophageal cancer occurs six times more commonly in men than in women. Use of alcohol, smoking *bidi* and cigarettes and using smoked salmon in food, (North Malabar area, Kerala, India) are the common etiological factors. Lye strictures are seen as an etiological factor (Table 14.1).

IN ASIA (OTHER THAN INDIA)

It is seen as clusters in certain provinces in China (e.g. Luxian), Japan, Iran, East Africa and South Africa. In fact, there is an area known as 'cancer belt' from Northern Iran to China. The highest incidence in the world is in Luxian in Henan province in China where cancer of the esophagus is the commonest single cause of death. It is also endemic among blacks in Transkei and Durban provinces in South Africa. A variety of causes like infection of food materials with fungus, poor nutrition, genetic mutation of p53 in early life, etc. are said to be the etiological factors. Smoking and chewing tobacco, drinking country made alcohol, etc. add to the list of carcinogens initiating this form of cancer. Food rich in vitamins, beta-carotene, vitamin E and selenium is known to reduce the incidence of esophageal cancer.

PREDISPOSING DISEASES

Cancer of the esophagus is seen more commonly than gastric cancer in India. This has been attributed to both dietary and nondietary factors. Dietary factors that have been reported as risk factors are high temperature of food; the consumption of very strong chillies, pickles and spices; and the consumption of Kalahari. Kalahari is used by the indigenous population of Assam and other North-Eastern states. It is a highly alkaline (pH 11–12) substance made from the skin of a particular variety of banana. It

Table 14.1: Carcinoma of the esophagus, National Cancer Registry Programme 1981-2001				
	Male		*Female*	
	CR	AAR	CR	AAR
Bangalore	8.6	9.1	6.0	8.3
Barshi	8.5	4.1	4.2	2.6
Bhopal	6.9	7.5	4.4	4.9
Chennai	8.1	8.8	5.0	6.1
Delhi	4.6	6.2	2.8	4.4
Mumbai	6.8	8.5	5.0	6.7

is used as an additive during the preparation of curry or "*dhal*". Consumption of Kalahari was associated with an eight-fold increased risk. Nondietary factors that were noted to have a significant association with esophageal cancer were betelnut and tobacco chewing and "*bidi*" smoking.

It is well known that Barrett's esophagus is an important risk factor in adenocarcinoma of the lower end of esophagus at least in 50 percent of esophageal malignancy. In Barrett's esophagus, the normal stratified squamous epithelium of the esophagus is replaced by metaplastic columnar epithelium that is premalignant. The progression is from epithelial metaplasia, low-grade dysplasia, to high-grade dysplasia, and ultimately to invasive cancer.

Tylosis, achalasia cardia, lye strictures, esophageal diverticuli, with webs, Plummer-Vinson syndrome, celiac disease, etc. are also suggested as predisposing factors.

Environmental factors such as radioactive chemicals and asbestosis and nitrosamines are also thought to be etiological factors.

Among dietary factors identified in areas of high incidence are low intake of proteins, fruits and vegetables, vitamins B and C and beta-carotene and essential minerals such as magnesium, molybdenum and zinc.

CLINICAL PRESENTATION

In almost all cases, dysphagia is the presenting symptom and more so in solids than liquids in its early days of malignancy. The dysphagia is relentlessly progressive. The loss of weight too is significant. Pain while swallowing—odynophagia—is felt in more than half the number of cases; retrosternal and epigastric pain is noted in 25 percent of cases. Later dysphagia becomes a distressing symptom where the patient finds it difficult to take liquid food and even swallow his own saliva. Hoarseness of voice (involvement of recurrent laryngeal nerve) and cough with every meal (tracheoesophageal fistula) are late symptoms. Horner's syndrome is not unusual in certain esophageal cancers. Hematemesis and regurgitation of undigested food, aspiration pneumonia, superior vena caval syndrome, cervical lymphadenopathy, etc. are late symptoms. Malignant hypercalcemia due to bone metastases and hemoptysis due to lung metastases are also seen in the later stages of esophageal cancer.

INVESTIGATIONS

1. CBC
2. Liver function tests
3. Fiberoptic endoscopy and biopsy
4. Endoscopic ultrasound
5. Cat scan of chest and upper abdomen
6. PET scan can be considered if the CT scan suggests involvement of celiac group of glands. CT scan of the chest and abdomen are done to

identify mediastinal and lung involvement and the involvement of liver, adrenals and peritoneal lymph glands. CT scan also helps in correct staging of the disease.

7. Laparoscopy can reveal small liver and peritoneal metastases particularly on their surfaces.

LOCATION OF THE ESOPHAGEAL TUMORS

Twenty percent of the tumors are seen in the upper one third, 38 percent in the middle one third and 42 percent in the lower one third.

FAMILIAL AND GENETIC FACTORS

There is no evidence of familial pattern in esophageal cancer. Ostroweski et al (1991) have found that there is p53 alteration in esophageal squamous cell cancer (ESC), while others have noticed that there is high incidence of p53 alteration in nontumor esophageal mucosal changes. Both the loss of heterozygosity and replication errors have been identified as genetic alterations in esophageal cancer. Allelic losses at frequencies of at least 30 percent were observed at loci on chromosomal arms 3p, 3q, 5q, 9p, 9q, 10p, 13q, 17p, 17q, 18q, 19q, and 21q, suggesting that several putative tumor-suppressor genes may be associated with the development and/ or progression of esophageal cancer.

MTS-1 (CDKN2) is a tumor-suppressor gene on chromosome 9p21-22. This region is frequently observed to have a loss of heterozygosity in patients with esophageal squamous cell carcinomas and adenocarcinomas. There is evidence of mutations of this gene in esophageal tumors. It has been shown that 67 percent of esophageal squamous cell carcinoma cell lines have deletions of both exons 1 and 2 of the MTS-1 gene, suggesting that it has a role in the pathogenesis of esophageal cancer (Shirely George).

PROGNOSTIC FACTORS

The poor prognosis of the esophageal tumors is recognized in all centers in spite of modern diagnostic technique. The delay of the patient to reach a center where endoscopic evaluation is available is pointed out as the main reason in the poor prognosis. The spread of the tumor along the submucosal lymphatics to different levels in the esophagus, and the spread to regional lymph nodes are poor prognostic factors. Similarly the spread of the tumor in discontinuity and the development of satellite nodules proximal to the tumor and spread to the celiac axis group of nodes from the intrathoracic esophagus are also suggested as the causes for the poor prognosis.

STAGING OF ESOPHAGEAL CANCER

ACJC and UICC have together developed a new system of staging based on TNM staging.

TNM definitions

Primary tumor (T)

TX Primary tumor cannot be assessed

T0 No evidence of primary tumor

Tis Carcinoma *in situ*

T1 Tumor invades lamina propria or submucosa

T2 Tumor invades muscularis propria

T3 Tumor invades adventitia

T4 Tumor invades adjacent structure

Regional lymph nodes (N)

   NX Regional lymph nodes cannot be assessed

   N0 No regional lymph node metastasis

   N1 Regional lymph node metastasis

Distant metastasis (M)

   MX Distant metastasis cannot be assessed

   M0 No distant metastasis

   M1 Distant metastasis

Lower thoracic esophagus

   M1a Metastasis in celiac lymph nodes

   M1b Other distant metastasis

   Midthoracic esophagus

   M1a Not applicable

   M1b Nonregional lymph nodes and/or other distant metastasis

Upper thoracic esophagus

   M1a Metastasis in cervical nodes

   M1b Other distant metastasis

AJCC Stage Groupings

Stage 0	Tis, N0, M0
Stage I	T1, N0, M0
Stage IIA	T2, N0, M0
	T3, N0, M0
Stage IIB	T1, N1, M0
	T2, N1, M0
Stage III	T3, N1, M0
	T4, Any N, M0
Stage IV	Any T, Any N, M1
Stage 1Va	Any T, Any N, M1a
Stage 1Vb	Any T, Any N, M1b

Note: For tumors of midthoracic esophagus, use only M1b, since these tumors with metastasis in nonregional lymph nodes have an equally poor prognosis as those with metastasis in other distant sites.

TREATMENT IN CANCER OF THE ESOPHAGUS

The treatment of the cancer of the esophagus is essentially the resection of the tumor, restoring continuity of the lumen either with stomach, small intestine or with colon, either inside or outside the chest. Surgical resection is considered the standard approach for patients with stages I and II and even early stage III carcinomas. Curative resection is feasible in only about 50 percent of patients because often the lesions are more extensive than what is judged by the routine clinical staging. A high rate of local recurrence following resection has been reported in some series, and the median survival of patients with resected tumors is approximately 11 months. Over the past 10 years, surgical mortality has declined substantially and is well below 10 percent at centers where the procedure is frequently performed. The type of surgical resection does not seem to alter the long-term outcome of these patients.

The ultimate goal is to cure the cancer and to remove dysphagia. The principle is wide resection of the esophagus with a clear margin of 5 cm and clearing of the local lymph nodes. The results are better with improved staging techniques, better choice of patients, and better anesthetic strategy. Age is not a contraindication for surgery.

SURGERY

There are different types of surgery for carcinoma of the esophagus. The type of resection depends on the location of the tumor, and the six common approaches are:

1. Left thoracoabdominal approach of Sweet
2. Laparotomy and right thoracic approach of Lewis
3. Transhiatal approach originally described by Grey Turner and later modified by Orringer
4. Endothoracic endoesophageal resection
5. Laryngoesophagectomy for cancer of cervical esophagus
6. Video-assisted thoracoscopic (VATS) esophagectomy is carried out with minimal thoracotomy incision at many centers. Thoracoscopic esophagectomy is done in a semiprone position (Cuschieri) which will avoid injury to the lung and major blood vessels.

The surgeon can choose the type of surgery he is familiar with, and the other determinants are the level of the tumor and the nodal involvement. The proponents of extensive esophagectomy with resection of contiguous tissue and regional lymph nodes have not constantly shown a superior survival rate.

Postoperative reflux esophagitis can be a distressing problem after esophagectomy. Conversion of the anastomosis by a Roux-en-Y reconstruction with a long ascending jejunal loop or interposition of colon or jejunum are some of the techniques used to reduce gastroesophageal reflux.

MORBIDITY AND MORTALITY

The most common complications are the pulmonary complications regardless of the types of approach. The other feared complication is the anastomotic leak in 5 to 10 percent of cases. They occur both in cervical and thoracotomy incisions and are associated with 2 layer anastomosis. They present themselves with fever, cough and breathlessness. The leak at the cervical anastomosis appears as a painful swelling at the site of the original incision. The neck incision is reopened and a good drainage is established and suitable antibiotic is started.

In case of intrathoracic leak, unless treated early, there is 40 to 50 percent mortality. The immediate duty is to remove all infected material from the pleural cavity. Re-exploration is necessary to rule out gastric necrosis. Wide drainage is established and all patients require appropriate antibiotics. One problem, which can develop after the leak, is a stricture, which requires several gentle dilatations.

RADIOTHERAPY

The survival of patients, with locoregional spread of carcinoma of the esophagus, who receive radiotherapy alone has not changed appreciably in the past 2 decades. five-year survival is approximately 5 percent and median survival is approximately 12 months. Radiotherapy alone, although clearly inferior to concurrent chemoradiotherapy, can still be considered for palliation in patients in whom chemotherapy is contraindicated. In this circumstance up to 60 Gy of radiotherapy (daily fraction-200 cGy) may be warranted to achieve optimal palliation. It must be understood that the curative dose of radiation should be at least 65 Gy if radiation alone is given.

The current standard nonsurgical treatment for esophageal cancer is concurrent chemoradiotherapy.

The value of preoperative chemoradiotherapy has yet to be fully defined in patients with potential resectable carcinoma of esophagus. A single institution, randomized study of 100 patients, assigned to receive either intensive preoperative chemotherapy with hyperfractionated radiotherapy or surgery alone has not demonstrated a statistically significant survival difference between the two groups (Urba et al 1997).

The randomized data did not favor the routine use of preoperative combined modality therapy, but rather strongly support further investigation of this approach in a larger randomized trial. Neither preoperative chemotherapy nor radiotherapy alone has improved survival over surgery alone. Similarly, recipients of postoperative radiotherapy alone did not show any survival advantage compared to those who did not receive postoperative radiation.

(Personal communications, Babu Zachariah MD, Radiotherapy in esophageal cancer, University of South Florida, USA).

MULTIMODALITY THERAPY

Over the years, multimodality therapy has emerged as a result of the failure of single modalities against esophageal carcinoma. The clinicians have realized that esophageal carcinoma is more a systemic disease than a locoregional one, and even if the locoregional disease is controlled, the patient ultimately succumbs within a year to distant metastases on the liver, lungs, bone and brain.

In discussing multimodality therapy of esophageal carcinoma, two factors require special consideration. They are the role of radiation for the local control and chemotherapy for systemic control. The role of radiation has already been discussed in the previous paragraph.

CHEMOTHERAPY

Systemic therapy is an important cornerstone of multimodality therapy because more than 75 percent of the patients harbor occult metastases at presentation. Sixteen different antitumor drugs have been investigated in depth in patients with metastatic disease, and the majority of these agents have been evaluated in patients with the squamous cell carcinoma histologic subtype. In case of adenocarcinoma, pilot studies suggest that adenocarcinoma would probably respond to chemotherapy with a frequency similar to that of squamous cell carcinoma.

Among the groups of drugs, Cisplatin (Platinol) is one of the most active agents, with a single-agent response rate that is consistently around 20 percent. Other drugs that have been tried with limited success are 5-fluorouracil (5-FU), mitomycin, bleomycin, paclitaxel, vinorelbine and gemcitabine. The most popular combination has been infusional fluorouracil and cisplatin. Fractionating the dose of cisplatin over several days can result in less nausea and vomiting than what occurs with a single total dose. This combination of Cis-platinum and 5-FU has been used with response rate of 20 percent to 50 percent combined with radiation.

PREOPERATIVE CHEMOTHERAPY (NEOADJUVANT)

Preoperative chemotherapy allows an assessment of *in vivo* chemosensitivity and can guide postoperative therapy. Major responses were achieved in 47 percent of the patients but with only one pathologically complete response. Resectability and survival were similar regardless of whether patients received preoperative chemotherapy.

The dose cycle suggested is:

Cisplatin, 100 mg/m^2 IV day 1 (Total dose cycle,100 mg/m^2)

5-FU 1000 mg/m^2 per day by continuous IV Infusion for 5 days.1–5 days total infusion 5,000 mg/m^2.

The duration of the treatment cycle is 28 days and 3 such cycles are given before surgery. This treatment cycle is repeated in the postoperative period if the earlier results show favorable clinical response. Despite the early positive response in preoperative chemotherapy, the Intergroup trial conducted in the United States did not show any increase in the survival rate in patients with surgically resectable cancer of the esophagus with either subgroups.

MULTIMODALITY THERAPY ALTERNATIVE TO SURGERY

Definitive chemoradiation for locoregional carcinoma of the esophagus is considered an alternative to surgery in a few centers in the UK, France and the USA.

Total number of cases—123 eligible patients (RTOG 85-01):

Chemotherapy with radiation therapy or radiation therapy alone:

Fluorouracil, 1,000 mg/m^2 per day by continuous IV infusion for 4 consecutive days, during 1, 5, 8 and 11 weeks (total dose/4-day cycle, 4,000 mg/m^2)

Cisplatin, 75 mg/m^2 IV daily, during weeks 1, 5, 8 and 11 (total dose/ cycle 100 mg/m^2)

Radiation therapy, 2 Gy/fraction for five fractions per week, weeks 1-5 (total dose/course, 50 Gy)

Radiation therapy, 2 Gy /fraction for five fractions per week, weeks 1-6.4 (total dose/course, 64 Gy).

This trial demonstrated a 4-month median survival advantage for patients receiving combined-modality therapy compared with those given radiation alone. Seventy-three additional patients were then registered directly to receive chemoradiation. Long-term follow-up indicated that the median survival was 14.1 months versus 9.3 months, in favor of the combined-modality arm. At 5 years, no patients who received radiation therapy alone was alive compared with 26 percent who received chemoradiation (p < 0.001).

A SUMMARY OF TREATMENT FOR ESOPHAGEAL CANCER STAGE BY STAGE

Stage I

Surgical resection—transthoracic or transhiatal

Stage IIa

Surgical resection:

If surgical margins are positive, postoperative radiation therapy is often used to improve locoregional control.

Postoperative chemotherapy with radiation therapy may be considered, but the benefit of this approach has not been tested in randomized trials.

Primary chemotherapy plus radiation (as per RTOG 85-01[2] or INT 0123[3]) is an alternative procedure.

Surgery may be considered after recovery from chemoradiation, but the benefit of this approach has not yet been proven in multi-institutional phase III trials.

Stage IIb
Surgical resection
The outcome is poor in patients with nodal involvement with esophagectomy alone. Primary chemotherapy plus radiation (as per RTOG 85-01[2] or INT 0123[3]) is also used in phase trials. Surgery may be considered after recovery from chemoradiation, but the benefit of this approach has not yet been proved in multi-institutional phase III trials. In patients selected for primary surgery, there is no clear survival advantage with pre- or postoperative radiation alone or chemotherapy alone.

Stages III and IV
Radiation therapy, 2 Gy/fraction (total dose/course, 50 Gy).
Cisplatin, 75 mg/m^2 IV day 1 of weeks 1, 5, 8, and 11 (total dose/cycle, 75 mg/m^2).
Fluorouracil, 1,000 mg/m^2/day by continuous IV infusion for 4 days, day 1 to 4 during weeks 1, 5, 8, and 11 (total dose/4-day course, 4,000 mg/m^2).
Radiation therapy, 1.8 Gy/fraction (total dose/course, 50.40 Gy).
Cisplatin, 75 mg/m^2 IV day 1 of weeks 1, 5, 9, and 13 (total dose/cycle, 75 mg/m^2).
Fluorouracil, 1,000 mg/m^2/day by continuous IV infusion for 4 days, days 1 to 4 during weeks 1, 5, 9 and 13 (total dose/4-day course, 4,000 mg/m^2).

PALLIATION

External beam radiation either alone or in combination chemotherapy offers palliation of dysphagia in approximately 80 percent of patients; approximately half have ongoing palliation until the time of death. Radiation therapy constitutes 2 Gy fractions, days 1-5, weeks 1-3, the total dose 30 Gy in 3 weeks time. If a patient requires rapid palliation, laser therapy or stenting is recommended. Brachytherapy also should be considered if external beam radiation therapy is unresponsive.

Current methods of endoscopic palliation include balloon dilatation or bougienage, thermocoagulation (laser), photodynamic therapy, intra-cavitary irradiation, and placement of expandable metal stents or hollow plastic tubes.

A wide variety of simple stents are available in Asian markets. Atkinson, Souttar, Celestin, Medinova (Indian) and Procter-Livingstone are some of the esophageal stents that can be used with simple bougienage. The intubation is made easier by the use of fiberoptic endoscopes. Another type that is gaining popularity is the covered and uncovered expansile metal stents. These expansile metal stents are placed under X-ray or endoscopic control. In cases of tracheoesophageal fistula, which is a sign of incurable stage IV disease, the expansile metal stent can be used to prevent regurgitation and tracheal exclusion.

Endoscopic laser treatment may be used to core a channel through the malignant tumor masses. It provides temporary palliation. Laser is also used to reopen a stent blocked by tumor overgrowth.

The placement of a gastrostomy or jejunostomy tube may improve the patient's nutritional status.

CURRENT OPTIONS, FUTURE DIRECTIONS

Significant advances have been made in the management of patients with carcinoma of the esophagus. Improvements in short-term outcome have resulted from advances in all disciplines. Combined-modality therapeutic approaches have taken the central stage in the management of carcinoma of the esophagus. The major limitations at present include the lack of more effective cytotoxic therapy and less toxic chemoradiotherapy. Substantial efforts are under way to improve combined modality therapy for carcinoma of the esophagus. Newer modalities such as immunotherapy and hyperthermia with chemoradiotherapy show promises and are tried in a few centers. Both these modalities are at the investigational stage and may require proper evaluation in different centers.

The aim of preoperative therapy must be to increase the rate of pathologically complete responses. Hyperfractionated radiation therapy, the search for new radiation enhancers and sequential therapy must also be investigated. Nevertheless, the combined modality therapy has provided short-term benefits for patients with locoregional carcinoma of the esophagus, and further research efforts will translate into long-term benefits for the patients. The search must continue for novel therapeutic agents, novel approaches and exploitation of the unique biologic features of precancerous and cancerous tissues. Analyses of molecular events underlying the development of esophageal cancer may yield new strategies for diagnosis, prevention and therapy.

FURTHER READING

1. Avoki T, Mori T, Du X, et al. Allelotype study of esophageal carcinoma. Gene Chromosome Cancer 1994;10:177-82.
2. Blot WJ, Devesa SS, Kneller RW, et al. Rising incidence of adenocarcinoma of the esophagus and gastric cardia. JAMA 1991;265:1287-89.
3. Fok M, Sham JS, et al. Postoperative radiotherapy for carcinoma of the esophagus: A prospective, randomized controlled study. Surgery 1993;113:138-47.
4. Huibregtse JM, Scheffner M, Howley PM. A cellular protein mediates association of p53 with the E6 oncoprotein of human papillomavirus types 16 or 18. EMBO J 1991;10:4129-35.

5. Itakura Y, Sasano H, Shiga C, et al. Epidermal growth factor receptor overexpression in esophageal carcinoma. An immunohistochemical study correlated with clinicopathologic findings and DNA amplification. Cancer 1994;74:795-804.

6. Jones DR, Davidson AG, Summers CL, et al. Potential application of p53 as an intermediate biomarker in Barrett's esophagus. Ann Thorac Surg 1994;57:598-603.

7. Liu Q, Yan YX, McClure M, et al. MTS-1 (CDKN2) tumor suppressor gene deletions are a frequent event in esophagus squamous cancer and pancreatic adenocarcinoma cell lines. Oncogene 1995;10:619-22.

8. Mori T, Avoki T, Matsubara T, et al. Frequent loss of heterozygosity in the region including BRCA1 on chromosome 17q in squamous cell carcinomas of the esophagus. Cancer Res 1994;54:1638-40.

9. Neshat K, Sanchez CA, Galipeau PC, et al. Barrett's esophagus: The biology of neoplastic progression. Gastroenterol Clin Biol 1994;18:D71-76.

10. Powell SM, Papadoupoulos N, Kinzler KW, et al. APC gene mutations in the mutation cluster region are rare in esophageal cancers. Gastroenterology 1994; 107:1759-63.

11. Rice TW, Goldblum JR, Falk GW, et al. p53 immunoreactivity in Barrett's metaplasia, dysplasia, and carcinoma. J Thorac Cardiovasc Surg 1994;108:1132-37.

12. Sarbia M, Porschen R, Borchard F, et al. p53 protein expression and prognosis in squamous cell carcinoma of the esophagus. Cancer 1994;74:2218-23.

13. Stemmermann G, Heffelfinger SC, Noffsinger A, et al. The molecular biology of esophageal and gastric cancer and their precursors: Oncogenes, tumor suppressor genes, and growth factors. Hum Pathol 1994;25:968-81.

14. Tarmin L, Yin J, Zhou X, et al. Frequent loss of heterozygosity on chromosome 9 in adenocarcinoma and squamous cell carcinoma of the esophagus. Cancer Res 1994;54:6094-96.

15. Vijeyasingam R, Darnton SJ, Jenner K, et al. Expression of p53 protein in oesophageal carcinoma. Br J Surg 1994;81:1623-26.

16. Zhou X, Tarmin L, Yin J, et al. The MTSI gene is frequently mutated in primary human esophageal tumors. Oncogene 1994;9:3737-41.

APPENDIX 3

International comparison; India and five continents—AAR (ICMR and IARC).

CANCER ESOPHAGUS (MALE)

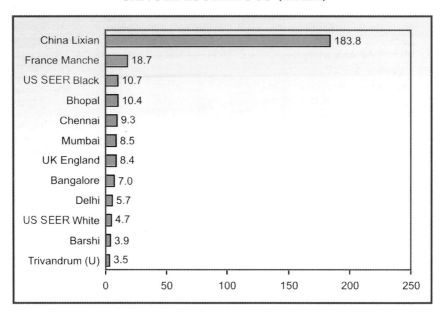

CANCER ESOPHAGUS (FEMALE)

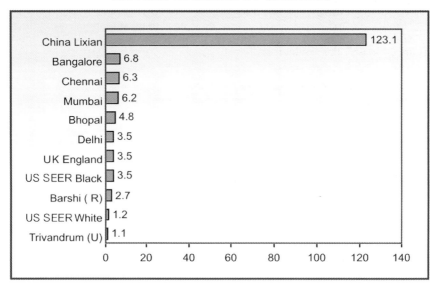

Rate per 100,000

Gastric Cancer

15

Sanjay Joseph, K Pavithran

Carcinoma stomach is described as one of the 'captains of men's death'. Gastric cancer has a wide geographic variation. Countries in Asia with a high incidence include Japan, China, and South Korea; those with a low incidence are India, Pakistan, and Thailand. Until recently stomach cancer was the second most common cancer worldwide. Now it has moved to the third place, behind breast cancer. It is the second most common cause of death from cancer (734000 deaths annually). Two thirds of the cases of stomach cancer occur in developing countries. Incidence rates in men are twice that in women, in both low-risk and high-risk areas.

EPIDEMIOLOGY

UNITED STATES AND UNITED KINGDOM

In the United States, there is an overall decrease in the number of gastric cancers, especially distal gastric cancers. The age-adjusted mortality per 100,000 has fallen from 28 in men (1935) to 9.7 (1967) and 8.3 (1986).

Even in the UK about 80 percent of the cases present in advanced stage. The male: female ratio is 1.4:1 for young adults but rises to 2:1 in the 6th and 7th decades. It has been reported that there is a worldwide increase in proximal gastric cancers and its annual increase at a rate of 4.3 percent is higher than the rate of lung cancer.

INDIA

The age-adjusted incidence rates (AAR) of stomach cancer in urban registries (3.0-13.1) is on the lower side among those reported worldwide (4.1-95.5). The least incidence in the world is reported from Barshi (AAR 1.2). It is a disease mainly of males. Stomach cancer occurs a decade earlier among South Indians compared with the North Indians.

In India, across the various registries there is a wide variation in the incidence of carcinoma stomach. The incidence rate of stomach cancer is 4 times commoner in Southern India compared to Northern India. An exception to the relatively low incidence of gastric cancer in Northern India is Kashmir where the AAR is reported to be 36.7. Among the 6 registries the highest incidence is reported from Chennai in both sexes (AAR 13.6 in males, 6.5 in females) and lowest from Barshi (AAR 1.2 in males and 0.8 in females). In Kerala, the southernmost region in India, the incidence is 5.1 and 3.8 per 100,000 for male and female respectively. Over the years, there has been an overall decrease from 7.8 per 100,000 in 1986 to 7.7 in 1995 in men and 5.3 to 3.6 in women. The AAR reported from Delhi is 3.9 in males and 2.5 in females. Incidence varies among different religious groups also. In Kashmir Muslims have a higher incidence compared to Hindus whereas a reverse trend is seen in Mumbai.

In most developed countries there has been a persistent and progressive decline of both incidence and mortality of gastric cancer in the last 50 years. This is principally because of changes in diet, food preparation and food preservation (increased use of refrigeration). In India also this trend is seen among most registries. In Chennai there was a slight increase in the early 80s but has flattened or shows a decline thereafter. However, this has not been found to be statistically significant. A declining trend is seen in Mumbai and Bangalore also.

ETIOLOGY AND PATHOGENESIS

Several etiological factors have been identified as being important in the initiation of carcinoma of the stomach.

AGE

Carcinoma of the stomach is clearly related to age and occurs predominantly between the 5th and the 7th decades in men and the 4th and 7th decades in women. At the same time, people of younger age groups are also known to develop cancer of the stomach particularly those in poor socioeconomic groups where the intake of food is less nutritious with lack of essential vitamins and minerals.

RACE

Among the different races the Japanese have the highest incidence, the next highest being in African Americans and the least in Buddhists and Jains in India.

BACTERIAL INFECTION

Helicobacter pylori (HP) have been accepted as being carcinogenic (3-5 fold increased risk of gastric cancer) in humans. *H. pylori* cause atrophic gastritis after an initial period of chronic inflammation, which may initiate intestinal metaplasia where apoptosis and adhesion of gastric epithelial cells are impaired. There is a strong link between *H. pylori* infection and gastric cancer in many countries such as Japan. Even though the prevalence of *H. pylori* infection is high (49.4% to 83.3%) in India, gastric cancer rates are low. The role of *H. pylori* in gastric cancer has been studied in 3 studies from India. Out of these only one study showed a positive association. Factors for this Asian enigma in the etiology of gastric cancer includes the genetic diversity of the infecting *H. pylori* strains and differences in the host genetic background in various ethnic groups, including gastric acid secretion and genetic polymorphisms in proinflammatory cytokines. Smokers with Cag A-positive *H. pylori* infection have a strongly increased risk of gastric cancer and this is particularly important in developing countries where both are widely prevalent. *H. pylori* may act as a cofactor in the pathogenesis of gastric carcinoma along with other risk factors.

OTHER FACTORS

Intestinal type of gastric carcinoma develops in a multistep pathway. In a case control study from Chennai, smokers had a two-fold increased risk of stomach cancer compared to non-smokers and the risk seen among current smokers was significantly higher than from that seen among ex-smokers. The risk among those who smoke '*bidi*' was thrice more than that seen among cigarette smokers. However, the habits of drinking alcohol and chewing quid (containing leaf of *piper betel*, small pieces of arecanut and a pinch of aqueous lime) did not emerge as risk factors. In another study, high consumption of rice, high consumption of chilli and consumption of high-temperature food were (seven-fold increased risk) found to be independent risk factors. Consumption of vegetables and fruits was found to reduce the risk. Salted tea prepared in Kashmir by brewing green tea leaves with sodium bicarbonate shows high methylating activity upon *in vitro* nitrosation. In addition other dietary items containing substantial amounts of N-nitroso compounds are sun-dried vegetables, dried fish and red chillies. Deficiencies of vitamins A, C, E, β-carotene, selenium and lack of fiber are a few etiological factors that are suggested in gastric cancer.

A few of the gastric cancers (10%) are familial. Germline E-cadherin mutations lead to an autosomal dominant predisposition to diffuse gastric carcinoma. Premalignant conditions include gastric polyps, Menetrier's disease, gastric ulcer, pernicious anemia (achlorhydria) and previous gastric surgery to reduce acid output.

In contrast to other gastrointestinal cancers, there is DNA aneuploidy and loss of heterozygosity. The latter two are seen more in the intestinal form and encode epidermal growth factor. Among the tumor suppressor genes p53 and APC are seen mutated in 40 to 60 percent of cases by allelic loss and base conversion mutations. There is loss of heterozygosity: in chromosomes 5q or APC gene (deleted in 34% of gastric cancers), 17p, and 18q (DCC gene). E-cadherin, a cell adhesion mediator, is also observed in diffuse type of undifferentiated cancers.

PATHOLOGY

Approximately 95 percent of all malignant gastric neoplasms are adeno-carcinomas, and in general, the term gastric cancer refers to adenocarci-noma of the stomach. Other malignant tumors are rare and include squamous cell carcinoma, adenoacanthoma, carcinoid tumors, and leiomyosarcoma. The stomach is the most common site for lymphoma of the gastrointestinal tract and with the relative decrease in the incidence of gastric carcinoma, lymphomas represent a larger proportion of gastric malignancies. In terms of location, any area of the stomach can be affected—anterior and posterior walls, lesser curvature, and greater curvature (in that order of frequency). Multiple tumors are found in about 6 percent of the cases. The non-neoplastic mucosa adjacent to the carcinoma is often thickened, due to production of epidermal growth factor by the tumor. It may result in false-negative endoscopic biopsies.

LAUREN'S CLASSIFICATION (INTESTINAL AND DIFFUSE TYPES)

Lauren has divided gastric cancer into two distinctive histologic types—'intestinal' gastric cancer (53 percent) and 'diffuse' gastric cancer (33%). The former is also known as the 'epidemic' form and the latter the "endemic" form.

In intestinal gastric cancer, there is gland formation and it is defined by its cellular architecture. The amount of mucin production is highly variable; when abundant, it is often accompanied by calcification. Some-times, metaplastic ossification is present either in the primary tumor or the metastasis. Scattered endocrine cells and paneth cells may be demons-trated.

They are also associated with precancerous lesions, gastric atrophy, and intestinal metaplasia. It is also associated with *H. pylori* infection, parti-cularly in young people. This type of cancer resembles cancer anywhere in the tubular gastrointestinal tract and accounts for the superficial and polypoid types. In fact, this type of cancer has been declining in incidence in recent years. It must be realized that there is an interplay of environ-mental factors leading to glandular atrophy, relative achlohydria and increase in gastric pH. This results in bacterial overgrowth of *H. pylori* and subsequent production of nitrites and nitrosamine compounds, which are carcinogens as far as the gastric mucosa is concerned.

The diffuse form is more common in younger patients and exhibits undifferentiated signet-ring histology. There is a predilection for sub-mucosal spread because of lack of cell cohesion. They infiltrate deeply into the submucosa without producing an ulcer or a malignant mass. The diffuse gastric cancer leads to linitis plastica. Contiguous spread to the peritoneum is common. These cancers occur in the proximal stomach where worldwide increase in incidence has been observed, stage for stage. The diffuse variety has a much worse prognosis.

EARLY GASTRIC CANCER

The great interest evinced by the oncologists in early gastric cancer produced a separate classification on the basis of endoscopic appearances. Early gastric cancer, by definition is a carcinoma confined to the mucosa or to the mucosa and submucosa (not extending into the muscularis externa), regardless of the status of the regional lymph nodes. The cancers in this group are divided into 3 subsets: (1) protruding, (2) superficial and (3) excavated.

SPREAD AND METASTASIS IN GASTRIC CANCER

Carcinomas of the stomach can spread by local extension. Deeper penetration will involve deeper layers of the stomach wall and later breach the serosa. Lateral spread along the lamina propria is within 3 cm but a large number of tumors are seen penetrating beyond this level to reach up to 6 cm intramurally. Once the serosa is penetrated, the tumor also extends to adjacent structures like omentum, spleen, kidney, liver, pancreas or bowel. Tumor spread is often through the intramural lymphatics in submucosal, intramuscular or subserosal layers. Local spread can also occur into the esophagus and the duodenum. Spread into the esophagus occurs primarily through lymphatic channels. Duodenal extension is principally through the muscular layer by direct infiltration and through subserosal lymphatics. If serosa is breached, 80 percent of cases have lymph node involvement with poor prognosis and curative resection is not possible. At the same time, if the serosa is not penetrated, in spite of lymph node involvement, curative resection is possible.

Once the serosa is breached by the tumor, shedding of malignant cells from its surface into the celomic cavity takes place, with wide dissemination. The Krukenberg tumors seen bilaterally on the ovaries and Blumer's shelf are examples of transcelomic spread.

LYMPHATIC SPREAD

At least 50 percent of patients have evidence of lymphatic disease at the time of resection and it occurs early. The spread is mainly due to emboli or permeation to different lymphatic sites. For the purpose of identifying the different sets of lymph nodes with tumor spread, the stomach is divided into upper 1/3, middle 1/3 and lower 1/3. The term N1 and N2 are given to those nodes. N1 are nodes within 3 cm and N2 nodes 3 cm away from the primary tumor. Japanese workers have allotted specific numbers to these nodes, 1 to 12, 1 being left cardiac and the 12 celiac axis group of nodes.

UPPER THIRD

N1 nodes: Left cardiac, right cardiac, lesser curvature and greater curvature.
N2 nodes: Supra- and infrapyloric, left gastric, common hepatic, nodes along splenic artery, splenic hilum and around the celiac axis artery.

MIDDLE THIRD

N1 nodes: Right gastric, nodes within lesser curvature, greater curvature supra- and infrapyloric regions.
N2 nodes: Along the splenic artery, splenic hilum, left cardiac, left gastric, common hepatic and celiac axis.

LOWER THIRD

N1 nodes: Lesser curvature and greater curvature, supra- and infrapyloric.
N2 nodes: Right cardiac, left gastric, common hepatic and celiac axis.

SYMPTOMS AND SIGNS

The most common presenting symptom is abdominal or epigastric pain that cannot be distinguished from benign dyspepsia. The symptoms are vague, nonspecific and mentioned as indigestion or dietary indiscretion. Definite symptoms occur only when the tumor is large enough to produce gastric outlet obstruction or causes disordered functions of the stomach by its penetration into the gastric wall. Over 70 percent have had symptoms for more than 6 months before attending the clinic for the first consultation.

There may be associated weight loss and general weakness.

The symptoms and signs can be classified into three different groups:
— upper abdominal symptoms and signs
— signs due to lymphatic spread
— paraneoplastic syndrome.

UPPER ABDOMINAL SYMPTOMS AND SIGNS

Dysphagia, early satiety, nausea with emesis, excessive belching, reflux, fatigue and anemia are the symptoms of gastric malignancy. Gastrointestinal bleeding can occur but it is a late symptom. On examination, intra-abdominal masses or subcutaneous nodules can be felt in the epigastrium. Other common sites of spread are the liver (49%), lung (14%) and bones (11%).

A firm, smooth, enlarged liver or irregular hepatic masses may indicate metastases. An epigastric mass may represent a large metastatic mass in the liver. Ascites is a late sign. Clinical findings also include anemia, weight loss, electrolyte abnormalities, and liver enzyme elevations. Occult blood is positive in 95 percent of cases.

The following lymph nodes are felt in different sites in the body:

1. The left supraclavicular lymph node is known as Virchow's node (Troisier's sign).
2. Irish's node is felt at the left anterior axillary lymph node resulting from proximal primary cancer spread to lower esophageal and then intrathoracic lymphatics.
3. Sister Mary Joseph's nodules or periumbilical lymph nodes, named after The Mayo Clinic operating room nurse, which form as the tumor spreads along the falciform ligament to subcutaneous sites.

PARANEOPLASTIC SYNDROMES IN GASTRIC CANCER

These symptoms can exhibit themselves at the early or late period of this disease. Skin syndromes include acanthosis nigricans, dermatomyositis, patchy erythemas, pemphigoid ulcers and acute onset of seborrheic keratosis (sign of Leser-Trelat). Among the CNS syndromes, dementia and cerebellar ataxia can be seen. Migrating thrombophlebitis, microangiopathic hemolytic anemia and rarely membranous nephropathy can develop in patients with gastric cancer.

INVESTIGATIONS

Upper GI barium series is an accurate (and the most common) method of detecting malignant gastric lesions, but approximately 10 percent of malignant gastric lesions may be missed unless a double-contrast technique is used. Malignant lesions generally have elevated irregular margins and rugal folds disappear at the crater instead of converging to it. There is also lack of clear delineation of the rugae. The upper GI contrast study usually underestimates the extent of the disease.

ENDOSCOPIC FINDINGS

The fiberoptic flexible forward-viewing endoscope allows direct visualization of the stomach and accurate biopsy of the lesion. The endoscopic view of the malignant ulcer has certain distinct characteristics. The diameter of the ulcer is more than 1 cm. The borders are elevated and heaped up and there is centrifugal radiation of the mucosal folds. The stomach wall is rigid and not distensible on air insufflation.

If 10 biopsies are taken, the diagnostic specificity reaches up to 100 percent. The whole stomach should be examined with care, because tumors in the region of the fundus, if any, can be missed. The working recommendation is six biopsies from the ulcer, deeper to the slough if any, and four from its inner edges. Medically refractory persistent peptic ulcer disease may prompt endoscopic evaluation.

CYTOLOGY

The cytological study of gastric aspirate for exfoliated cells has been reported in patients with Stage III and Stage IV disease, but the accuracy in cytological studies is variable in early mucosal lesions. Cytological study of brushings under endoscopic view has an accuracy of 91 percent.

CT scan, ultrasound of abdomen and magnetic resonance imaging are used widely to evaluate the presence of metastasis in gastric cancer.

ENDOSCOPIC ULTRASONOGRAPHY (EUS)

EUS has been used extensively to evaluate potentially curative gastric cancer. EUS uses a high-frequency (7.5 to 12 MHz) transducer at the end of an endoscope and allows accurate evaluation of the primary tumor (T), its size, site and depth of infiltration. It also assesses submucosal linear extension and the size of perigastric lymph nodes, if greater than 3 mm.

STAGING

The American Joint Committee on Cancer-2002 (AJCC) has designated staging by TNM classification (Table 15.1).

PROGNOSIS

Poor prognostic factors include the age of the patients (older people), the location (proximal tumors), the type (linitus plastica) and the weight loss (greater than 10%). Prognostic factors for patients who undergo resection include the type of resection (R), depth of invasion (T), the presence and the number of nodal metastases (N), and the ratio of involved and removed lymph nodes. Molecular markers associated with poor prognosis are expression of *PDGF-α*, *Her-2/neu*, *TGF-β* and *EGFR*. In addition, high *TS* and *ERCC1* expression have been linked to poor prognosis among patients receiving fluoropyrimidine and platinum-based chemotherapy.

PRETREATMENT EVALUATION

It is necessary to determine the operability, the extent of gastric resection and the type of lymphadenectomy to be carried out for curative intent.

The major steps include:
1. Proper history taking and physical evaluation
2. Review of histology
3. WBC and platelet count
4. Blood chemistries and liver function tests
5. Digital rectal exam—blood in stool or the presence of Blummer's shelf
6. Upper GI barium series
7. Esophagogastrodeuodenoscopy
8. Endoscopic ultrasonography

Table 15.1: Definition of TNM

Primary Tumor (T)

TX	Primary tumor cannot be assessed
T0	No evidence of primary tumor
Tis	Carcinoma *in situ*: Intraepithelial tumor without invasion of the lamina propria
T1	Tumor invades lamina propria or submucosa
T2	Tumor invades the muscularis propria or the subserosa
T3	Tumor penetrates the serosa (visceral peritoneum) without invasion of adjacent structures
T4	Tumor invades adjacent structures

Regional Lymph Nodes (N)
(There must be at least 15 nodes for proper staging)

NX	Regional lymph nodes cannot be assessed
N0	No regional lymph node metastasis
N1	Metastases in 1 to 6 regional lymph nodes
N2	Metastases in 7 to 15 regional lymph nodes
N3	Metastases in more than 15 regional lymph nodes

Distant Metastasis (M)

MX	Presence of distant metastasis cannot be assessed
M0	No distant metastasis
M1	Distant metastasis

Stage Grouping

Stage 0	Tis N0 M0
Stage IA	T1 N0 M0
Stage IB	T1 N1 M0
	T2 N0 M0
Stage II	T1 N2 M0
	T2 N1 M0
	T3 N0 M0
Stage IIIA	T2 N2 M0
	T3 N1 M0
	T4 N0 M0
Stage IIIB	T3 N2 M0
Stage IV	T4 N1-3 M0
	T1-3 N3 M0
	Any T Any N M1

9. CT lower chest and abdomen with barium contrast study
10. Diagnostic laparoscopy (to evaluate the stage of the disease and to provide a histological diagnosis) is a part of pretreatment assessment. The presence of serosal perforation, lymph node metastases, and the involvement of the adjacent structures of the stomach can be evaluated by this method.

TREATMENT

Carcinoma of the stomach is a type of cancer eminently suited for cure if identified early. Surgical resection is the only treatment that offers any prospect of cure.

ENDOSCOPIC TUMOR RESECTION

This treatment is specially suited if the tumor is limited to the mucosa, of a size not greater than 6 mm with no histologic ulceration nor lymphatic vessel invasion. A cancer-negative resection line should be identified by the EUS. The tumor can be treated with mucosectomy using a conventional endoscopic snare and pure coagulation current. A piecemeal technique can be used to achieve complete removal in a single session with no major complications.

SURGERY

Different types of surgery are offered in gastric cancer. Tumor size and location dictate the type of surgical procedure and the histomorphological type described by Lauren.

SUBTOTAL GASTRECTOMY

The extent of resection depends on the site and the preoperative diagnosis of histomorphological type described by Lauren. The curative resection is suited for patients with distal tumors with Stages I, II and III diseases with minimal lymph node involvement. The intestinal type requires a proximal margin of 5 cm, the diffuse type, 8 cm measured *in situ* in an unstretched stomach. With proximal gastric tumors, subtotal gastrectomy (proximal gastrectomy) may be performed, provided the fundus or cardioesophageal junction is not involved. It is important that the margins should be free of tumor that can only be correctly ascertained by frozen section evaluation at the time of surgery.

RADICAL TOTAL GASTRECTOMY

The surgeons, in the UK, the US and elsewhere are of the opinion that even in Stages I, II, and III diseases, involving the middle of the corpus and proximal one third of the stomach, total gastrectomy with identifiable node resection must be done with curative intent. The whole stomach, greater and lesser omentum and N1 nodes of the upper, middle and lower groups are removed en bloc. This type of gastrectomy is more appropriate if tumor is diffuse and within 6 cm from the cardia. Roux-en-Y procedure or jejunal-interposition or pouch-reconstruction can be performed for the reconstruction of the upper GI tract. Total gastrectomy has certain inevitable problems with increased morbidity and mortality.

If cardia is involved, the correct curative surgery is thoracoabdominal exploration with distal esophagectomy and total gastrectomy (R3) with Roux-en-Y jejunal anastomosis. Lesions at the cardia metastasize to all lymph nodes including mediastinal group and hence N1, N2 and mediastinal lymphadenectomy should be done.

Intraoperative frozen sections on both resection margins are carried out, so that the margins are free from tumor.

There is no universal acceptance to the levels of the lymphadenectomy, which has to be done with curative intent in gastric cancer. There are surgeons in the UK and the US who advocate limited lymphadenectomy in the early stages of the disease, while both the Japanese and European surgeons are proponents of extended lymphadenectomy in similar stages.

Both the Japanese and German workers claim that there is therapeutic benefit with D2 extended lymphadenectomy (second tiers or N2 nodes) in all resectable gastric cancers. In fact, a few Japanese surgeons advocate D3 and D4 (higher tiers) in Stage II and early Stage III diseases.

If the performance of R0-resection does not seem practicable according to the staging procedures (EUS and laparoscopy), the importance of preoperative chemotherapy must be considered so as to downgrade the locally advanced gastric cancer. This could increase the chance of curative resection. There is no marked difference in postoperative morbidity or mortality in extended N2 lymphadenectomy.

Reconstruction of the upper GI-tract can be performed by Billroth II antecolically (48%) and retrocolically (47%) or by Roux-en-Y procedure.

In case of synchronic tumor, total gastrectomy offers a better form of treatment.

PALLIATIVE SURGERY

Palliative distal gastrectomy
Palliative proximal gastrectomy
Palliative total gastrectomy
Gastroenterostomy
Intubation by stent at the cardia for infiltrating tumor at the cardia

Palliative surgery is considered in patients with obstruction, bleeding or pain. Pain can be distressing which may be intermittent or constant. Resection of the tumor may relieve the pain even though without increase of mean survival time.

The selection of patients most likely to benefit from this palliative effort requires further evaluation and should be tailored to suit each patient. By-pass (gastroenterostomy), resection with exclusion and intubation are done as the cases demand. One of the common operations in Indian hospitals as palliation of distal gastric tumor with obstruction is anterior gastrojejunostomy with jejunojejunal anastomosis. It is found that the posterior gastroenterostomy produces stomal obstruction due to overgrowth of the tumor mass.

RECURRENCE

Local and regional recurrences are not unusual problems with gastric resections. The risk is higher in patients with serosal breach, positive nodes and residual tumor at the margins. Re-exploration and resection of the stump cancer is undertaken with care, as such a procedure would increase morbidity and mortality. These results have led to the use of radiotherapy and chemotherapy to prevent recurrence almost immediately after resection. Gastric adenocarcinoma is regarded as radioresistant when compared to squamous carcinoma but with newer protocols, useful palliation has been achieved with mean survival up to 5 years in 50 percent of cases.

POSTOPERATIVE THERAPY

Adjuvant Chemotherapy

Many trials have been done using single agents and in combination using drugs like 5-FU, mitomycin C, cisplatin, methotrexate and adriamycin. Results of these trials have been disappointing and occasionally conflicting. Gastric cancer overviews to date, suggest a modest benefit. The meta-analysis showed a slight benefit to postoperative adjuvant therapy. These meta-analyses were fraught with limitations as they are reviews of the literature, rather than a pooled analysis of individual patient data. In the older trials, agents were used with limited activity and the number of patients was relatively small.

Adjuvant Intraperitoneal Therapy

Continuous hyperthermic intraperitoneal perfusion (CHPP) A significant proportion of postoperative relapses occurs in the peritoneal cavity. This has made intraperitoneal therapy an attractive venue of investigation. The continuous perfusion increases the dose intensity to the abdominal and pelvic surface, as there is increased tissue perfusion to the cancerous surface. This type of perfusion can be done with total removal of the peritoneal surface or without such a procedure. With increased tissue perfusion, there may be increased toxicity too.

A Tenchkoff infusion catheter is placed with suitable outflow drains fixed with purse string sutures so that the peritoneal cavity is made watertight. The peritoneal cavity is then primed with 1.5 percent dextrose peritoneal dialysis solution. Later 3 liters of chemotherapy solution is used to wash the abdomen and peritoneal cavity. The perfusate is heated to 41-46°C so that it develops a core perfusion temperature of 41-42°C and the perfusion is allowed to run through for 90 minutes. The CHP is repeated once in 7 days for 4 cycles after evaluating the Hb, total leucocyte count and platelet count. Some of the trials have shown no survival benefit whereas others have shown some improvement.

Postoperative Chemoradiation

Postoperative radiation therapy has been accepted to have a useful role in gastric cancer. The gastrointestinal cancer Intergroup 0116, in a randomized study using surgery followed by 5-FU, leucovorin and external beam irradiation versus surgery alone showed an improvement in overall survival and disease-free survival. The schedule used —(1) 5-FU 425 mg/m^2/day IV on days 1-5 of 28 day cycle and folinic acid 20 mg/m^2/day IV on days 1-5 of 28 day cycle, and (2) 5-FU 400 mg/m^2/day IV on days 1-4 and on the last 3 days of radiotherapy. Folinic acid 20 mg/m^2/day on the same schedule. External beam irradiation, 4500 cGy at 180 cGy per day 5 days per week. Based on the results of this trial postoperative chemoradiotherapy has been accepted as the standard of care for gastric cancer patients who have undergone gastric resection.

Chemoimmunotherapy

The incorporation of immunotherapy (levamisole and OK-432) in the postoperative setting has also been explored. Data from Japanese and Korean investigators suggest that immunotherapy may improve outcome for patients undergoing potentially curative resection. The number of patients in any given trial is small, however, and the power of the observation therefore relatively weak. Large-scale confirmatory trials are necessary before accepting immunochemotherapy as a standard of care.

Chemotherapy for Advanced Gastric Cancer

Chemotherapy Versus Best Supportive Care
Three randomized studies clearly demonstrated an advantage for combination chemotherapy over best supportive care in both survival and symptom palliation. The most widely used single agent chemotherapy was 5-fluorouracil (5-FU), with partial response rates up to 20 percent. Combination chemotherapy has become the standard therapy with the response rate range between 25 percent and 40 percent with median survival of 6 to 8 months. A variety of regimens such as FAM (5-FU, adriamycin, mitomycin-c), FAMTX (5-FU, adriamycin, methotrexate), FEP (5-FU, etoposide, cisplatin), FAP (5-FU, adriamycin, cisplatin), EAP (etoposide, adriamycin, cisplatin) and ECF (infusional 5-FU, epimbicin, and cisplatin) have been tried without definite superiority but with significant toxicities. Recently, studies with taxanes, irinotecan and oxaliplatin have shown important activity in gastric cancer. The combination of docetaxel 75 mg/

m^2 + cisplatin 75 mg/m^2 every 3 weeks yielded 58 percent response rate and paclitaxel 175 mg/m^2 + 5-FU 1.0 gm/m^2 every 3 weeks resulted in 63 percent response rate. S-1 (oral 5-FU prodrug) showed 40-50 percent response rate in the recent Phase II trials.

Currently, there is no uniformly accepted best regimen in advanced gastric cancer. It is hoped that Phase III trials with newer agents will further improve survival in patients with advanced gastric cancer.

FOLLOW-UP

It should include hospital visits once a month with liver function tests. A chest radiograph is also warranted at intervals of every 3 months for the first 2 years, then 6 months for 3 years, and then once every year. If total gastrectomy is not performed, yearly upper endoscopy is dictated by the fact that there is 1 percent to 2 percent incidence of second primary tumors. Vitamin B$_{12}$ deficiency develops in most total gastrectomy patients and 20 percent of subtotal gastrectomy patients, typically within 4 to 10 years. Vitamin B^{12} supplementation is administered at 1,000 mcg intramuscularly every month.

FURTHER READING

1. Abraham J, Allegra CJ. Bethesda Handbook of Clinical Oncology: Lippincott, Philadelphia, Baltimore 2001;71-80.
2. Barreda BF, Sanchez LJ. Endoscopic treatment of early gastric cancer and precancerous gastric lesions with mucosectomy. Rev Gastroenterol Peru 1998;18:214-26.
3. Fochs CS, Meyer RJ. Gastric carcinoma. N Eng J Med 1995;333:32-41.
4. Gonzalez CA, Sala N, Capella G. Genetic susceptibility and gastric cancer risk. Int J Cancer 2002;100:249-60.
5. Im JJ, Tao H, Carloni E, Leung WK, Graham DY, Sepulveda AR. Helicobacter pylori impairs DNA mismatch repair in gastric epithelial cells. Gastroenterology 2002;123:542-53.
6. Jemal A, Murry T, Samuels A, Ghafoor A, Ward E, Thun MJ. Cancer statistics, 2003. CA Cancer J Clin 2003;53:5-26.
7. Karpeh MS, Kelson DP, Tepper JE. Cancer of the stomach. In: Devita VT, Hellman S, Rosenberf SA (Eds), Cancer: Principles and Practice of Oncology. Philadelphia: Lippincott Williams & Wilkins 2001;1092-1125.
8. Lechner S, Muller-Ladner U, Schlottmann K, et al. Microsatellite instability in Japanese vs European American patients with gastric cancer. Carcinogenesis 2002;23:1281-88.
9. Lee JH, Abraham SC, Kim HS, Nam JH, Choi C, et al. Inverse relationship between APC gene mutation in gastric adenomas and development of adenocarcinoma. Am J Pathol 2002;161:611-18.
10. Lin CH, Hsu CW, Chiang YJ, et al. Esophageal and gastric Kaposi's sarcomas presenting as upper gastrointestinal bleeding. Med J 2002;25:329-33.
11. Ma ZQ, Tanizawa T, Nihei Z, et al. Barrett's esophagus is characterized by expression of gastric-type mucins (MUC5AC, MUC6) and TFF peptides (TFF1

and TFF2), but the risk of carcinoma development may be indicated by the intestinal-type mucin, MUC2. J Med Dent Sci 2000;47:39-47.

12. Pavithran K, Doval DC, Pandey KK. Gastric cancer in India. Gastric Cancer 2002;5:240-43.
13. Schöffski P. New drugs for treatment of gastric cancer. Ann Oncol 2002;13 Suppl 4:13-22.
14. Tokunaga Y, Kitaoka A, et al. Gastrointestinal tumor study group. A comparison of combination chemotherapy and combined modality therapy for locally advanced gastric cancer. Cancer 982;49:1771-77A.
15. Tsai JY, Safran H. Status of treatment for advanced gastric carcinoma. Current Oncol Rep 2003;5:210-18.
16. Waki T, Tamura G, Tsuchiya T, Sato K, et al. Follicular gastritis associated with Helicobacter pylori. Am J Pathol 2002;161:399-403.

APPENDIX 4

International comparison;India and five continents—AAR (ICMR and IARC).

CANCER STOMACH (MALE)

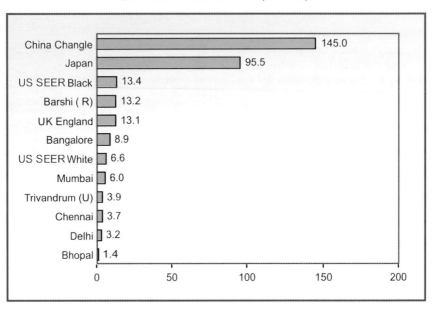

CANCER STOMACH (FEMALE)

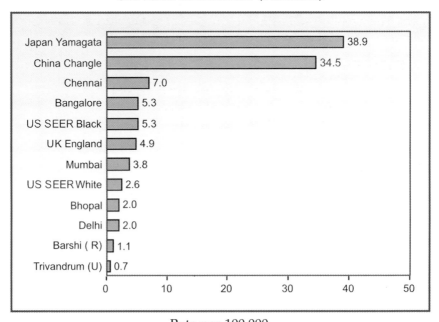

Rate per 100,000

Colorectal Cancer

16

S Sudhindran

The past decade has brought great progress in the under-standing of the environmental and genetic basis of colorectal neoplasia and in the ability to treat it successfully. Armed with new evidence and effective therapies there is the prospect of preventing or even curing most of the colorectal cancers.

EPIDEMIOLOGY

Colorectal cancer is the fourth commonest form of cancer worldwide, with about 400,000 new cases in men annually and 380,000 in women. It represents almost 10 percent of all incident cancers. It is estimated that 394,000 deaths occur from colorectal cancer worldwide annually.

Colorectal cancer, however, is not equally distributed throughout the world. While colorectal cancer represents 13 percent of all incident cancers in westernized countries like the USA, Western Europe, Australia and New Zealand, elsewhere it represents fewer than 8 percent of all incident cancers. The age-adjusted incidence in various cities of India varies from 0.8 to 3.3 in 100,000 persons.

RISK FACTORS

Ethnic and racial differences in the incidence of colorectal cancer as well as studies immigrants suggest that environ-mental factors (cultural, social, dietary and lifestyle practices) play a major part in the etiology of this cancer.

Dietary Factors

Analytical epidemiology has given us some clear ideas on how individuals can reduce their risk of colorectal cancer. Many studies have consistently shown that high-fiber, low-calorie, and low-animal-fat diets may significantly reduce the risk of colorectal cancer. High fiber from vegetables and fruits increa-ses the fecal bulk and reduces the transit time in the colon.

Deficiency of micronutrients like folate and vitamins E and D may increase the risk of this cancer.

Daily intake of 1.25-2.0 gm of calcium is associated with a reduced risk of recurrent adenomas in a randomized placebo-controlled trial.

PHYSICAL ACTIVITY

Epidemiological studies show strong evidence of inverse relationship between physical activity and colorectal cancer.

Hormone Replacement Therapy

There is mounting data to support a link between hormone replacement therapy and reduced incidence of colorectal cancer.

Age

More than 90 percent of cases occur in patients older than 50 years.

Gender

Colon cancer is higher in women (1.20:1.0), whereas rectal cancer is more common in men (1.27:1.0).

Colorectal Adenomas

70 percent of all colorectal carcinomas develop from sporadic adenomatous polyps. Flat adenomas accounting for 10 percent of all polyps have a higher rate of malignant change.

The factors determining the increased risk of malignant transformation within colonic polyps are:
- Size more than 1.5 cm
- Sessile or flat polyps
- Severe dysplasia
- Villous architecture
- Presence of squamous metaplasia
- Polyposis syndromes with multiple polyps

Family History

The immediate family member of a patient with colorectal cancer will have a 2-3 fold increased risk of disease.

Recognized family syndromes account for about 5 percent colorectal cancers and include familial adenomatous polyposis (FAP), hereditary non-polyposis colon cancer or Lynch syndrome (HNPCC), attenuated familial adenomatous polyposis or hereditary flat adenomas (AFAP/HFAS), Peutz-Jeghers syndrome and juvenile polyposis. The main clinical and molecular differences between these are shown in (Table 16.1).

Table 16.1: Comparison of familial adenomatous polyposis (FAP), Lynch forms of hereditary colorectal cancer (HPCC/Lynch); ulcerative colitis associated neoplasia (UCAN) and attenuated familial adenomatous polyposis/hereditary flat adenoma syndrome (AFAP/HFAS)

1. Familial adenomatous polyposis (FAP)
2. Lynch forms of hereditary colorectal cancer (HPCC/Lynch)
3. Ulcerative colitis associated neoplasia (UCAN)
4. Attenuated familial adenomatous polyposis/hereditary flat adenoma syndrome (AFAP/HFAS)

Mean age at diagnosis of colorectal cancer
1. FAP 32-39
2. HPCC/Lynch 42-49
3. UCAN 40-70
4. AFAP/HFAS 45-55

Distribution of cancer
1. FAP Random
2. HPCC/Lynch Mainly right colon
3. UCAN Mainly left colon
4. AFAP/HFAS Mainly right colon

No. of polyps
1. FAP>100
2. HPCC/Lynch 1 (i.e. tumor)
3. UCAN 1-100
4. AFAP/HFAS 1-100

Sex ratio (male: female)
1. FAP 1:1
2. HPCC/Lynch 1.5:1
3. UCAN 1:1
4. AFAP/HFAS 1:1

Endoscopic view of polyp
1. FAP Pedunculated
2. HPCC/Lynch Pedunculated (45%); flat (55%)
3. UCAN None
4. AFAP/HFAS Mainly flat

Lag time from early adenoma to occurrence of cancer
1. FAP 10-20 years
2. HPCC/Lynch 5 years
3. UCAN <8 years (?)
4. AFAP/HFAS 10 years

Distribution of polyps
1. FAP Distal colon or universal
2. HPCC/Lynch Mainly proximal to splenic flexure
3. UCAN None
4. AFAP/HFAS Mainly proximal to splenic flexure with rectal sparing

contd...

Table 16.1: contd...

Carcinoma histology
1. FAP More exophytic growth
2. HPCC/Lynch Inflammation, increased mucin
3. UCAN Mucosal ulceration and inflammation
4. AFAP/HFAS Non-exophytic but very variable

Gene (chromosome) mutation
1. FAP APC (5q 21) distal to 5'
2. HPCC/Lynch MHS2 (2p), MLH1 (3p21), PMS1 (2q31), PMS2 (7p22)
3. UCAN Multiple mutations, 17p (p53), 5q (APC), 9p p16)
4. AFAP/HFAS APC (5q 21) proximal to 5'

INFLAMMATORY BOWEL DISEASE

Ulcerative colitis increases the risk of colorectal cancer by 2 to 9 times and Crohn's colitis is associated with a two-fold increase in risk.

The factors affecting risk of colorectal cancer in patients with ulcerative colitis include long duration of disease (especially >10 years), extensive disease, dysplasia, presence of primary sclerosing cholangitis, family history of colorectal cancer and coexisting adenomatous polyp.

MOLECULAR BASIS OF COLORECTAL CANCERS

Colon carcinogenesis involves progression from hyperproliferative mucosa, to polyp formation with dysplastic involvement, to transformation to non-invasive lesions and subsequent tumor cells with invasive and metastatic capabilities. Colorectal cancer is a unique model of multistep carcinogenesis resulting from the accumulation of multiple genetic alterations. Molecular alterations in colorectal cancer can be classified into two broad categories: chromosomal instability (subdivided into aneuploidy and chromosomal alterations) and microsatellite instability. As a consequence of these two phenomena, other specific genetic events occur at increased frequency. These include inactivation of tumor suppressor genes by deletion or mutation, activation of proto-oncogenes by mutation and dysregulated expression of molecules such as E cadherin (the cell to cell adhesion molecule) and mucin related sialosyl -Tn antigen.

The p53 gene locus is the commonest site demonstrating loss of heterozygosity. p53 is a DNA binding protein transcription activator and can arrest the cell cycle in response to DNA damage; hence its title "guardian of the genome." The effect of normal p53 is antagonized by mutation or by action of the antiapoptotic gene Bcl-2. Most mutations in p53 cause the protein to become hyperstable and lead to uncontrolled growth.

In familial adenomatous polyposis there is a germline mutation in the tumor suppressor gene for adenomatous polyposis coli (APC) on chromosome 5. Patients with heredity non-polyposis colon cancer show germline mutations in DNA mismatch repair enzymes. Mutations are particularly demonstrable in DNA with multiple microsatellite (microsatellite instability).

OTHER ASSOCIATED TUMORS

Duodenal adenoma, cerebral and thyroid tumors, medulloblastoma and desmoids, endometrial, ovarian and gastric cancers, and glioblastoma are associated with colorectal cancers.

FAMILIAL ADENOMATOUS POLYPOSIS (FAP)

FAP accounts for less than 1 percent of all colorectal cancers and is characterized by the presence of 100 or more tubovillous adenomas in the colon, with intervening microadenoma on histological examination. The mean age of diagnosis of polyps is during teenage, and almost all the gene carriers have polyps by the age of 40. If these polyps are left untreated, malignant transformation is inevitable, with a mean age of colorectal cancer occurring during the patients' mid-30s, often with synchronous tumors. This condition is an autosomal dominant disorder, with the offspring of affected individuals at 50 percent risk of being gene carriers. The cloning of the causative gene APC on chromosome 5 in 1991 dramatically changed the management of familial adenomatous polyposis. If DNA is available from an affected individual, mutation detection is possible in about 70 percent of families. Non-gene carriers should be reassured and surveillance stopped. Gene carriers should be offered annual flexible sigmoidoscopy from the age of 12. Once several polyps have been identified, the timing and type of surgery available should be discussed. The two most common options are ileal-rectal anastomosis with annual surveillance of the remaining rectal tissue; and ileal-anal anastomosis with reconstruction of a rectal pouch using terminal small bowel (Table 16.1).

HNPCC OR THE LYNCH SYNDROMES

Named after Henry T. Lynch, they include Lynch I or the colonic syndrome, which is an autosomal dominant trait characterized by distinct clinical features including proximal colon involvement, mucinous or poorly differentiated histology, pseudodiploidy and the presence of synchronous or metachronous tumors. The Lynch II or extracolonic individuals are susceptible to endometrial, ovary, stomach, hepatobiliary, small intestine, and genitourinary malignancies. The name hereditary non-polyposis colon cancer is potentially misleading as many gene carriers will develop a small number of tubovillous adenomas, but not more than 100, as seen in familial adenomatous polyposis. The proportion of colorectal cancers due to hereditary non-polyposis colon cancer ranges from 1 percent to 20 percent; most observers, however, suggest about 2 percent.

The diagnosis of HNPCC is made on the family history as the appearance of the bowel, unlike in familial adenomatous polyposis, is not diagnostic. To improve the recognition of hereditary non-polyposis colon cancer, diagnostic criteria were devised in Amsterdam in 1991 and were subsequently modified to include non-colonic tumors.

MODIFIED AMSTERDAM CRITERIA

Three or more cases of colorectal cancer occur in a minimum of two generations.
- One affected individual must be a first degree relative of the other two (or more) cases.
- One case must be diagnosed before the age of 50.
- Colorectal cancer can be replaced by endometrial or small bowel adenocarcinoma.
- Familial adenomatous polyposis must be excluded.

SCREENING

Colorectal cancer is probably a good example of a disease that fulfils the WHO prerequisites for introduction of screening for a disease.

Colorectal cancer is a common cause for mortality from cancer, especially in the western world. There is a known premalignant condition (adenomatous polyp). There is a long lag time for the adenoma-carcinoma transformation sequence. There are sufficient facilities for the treatment of any lesions detected. Recent evidence suggests that removal of adenomas by flexible sigmoidoscopy decreases the mortality from distal colorectal cancer.

For a screening test to be widely applicable it must be sufficiently sensitive and specific, inexpensive and have high patient compliance.

TESTS FOR SCREENING

Digital Rectal Examination (DRE) and rigid sigmoidoscopy suffer from the limitations that they detect only rectal or rectosigmoid cancers and are unpleasant and invasive.

FECAL OCCULT BLOOD TESTING

These are the most extensively studied screening tests for colorectal cancer. They detect hematin from partially digested blood in the stool. The individuals are requested to undergo a "six-sample test" (2 samples each from 3 consecutive stools) and if 4 out of 6 are positive, the participants need colonoscopy. Studies have shown that such screening reduces mortality and that the cancers detected by screening tended to be at an early stage than those presenting symptomatically. But the disadvantages are the low sensitivity (30 to 50% cancers may be missed) and low patient compliance.

FLEXIBLE SIGMOIDOSCOPY

Flexible sigmoidoscopy examines the whole of the left colon and the rectum and thus detects 80 percent of the colorectal cancers. Once detected, the lesions can be removed or biopsied in the same sitting. It is much less uncomfortable and has much higher yield than rigid sigmoidoscopy. There are various studies now nearing completion but as yet, the effect of screening with flexible sigmoidoscopy on the incidence and mortality of colorectal cancer is uncertain.

COLONOSCOPY AND BARIUM ENEMA

These examine the whole colon and rectum. Both are invasive and require full bowel preparation. Colonoscopy is expensive and there is a small risk of perforation. While colonoscopy may be therapeutic, barium enema does not allow for removal or biopsy of the lesions seen.

Carcinoembryonic antigen (CEA) is a tumor marker which may be raised in many cancers including colorectal cancers. It is not useful for general colorectal cancer screening purposes. CEA has a low positive predictive value whereby approximately 60 percent of cancers are missed.

K-RAS DETECTION

The K-ras gene is mutated in 50 percent of colorectal cancers, and its detection in stool represents a potential powerful screening strategy. This is currently an active area of clinical investigation.

CT COLOGRAPHY OR VIRTUAL COLONOSCOPY

This is a new radiological technique which is minimally invasive and quick. Preliminary data suggest comparable sensitivity to colonoscopy or barium enema. But it requires full bowel preparation and is currently enormously expensive.

PATHOLOGY AND CLINICAL FEATURES

More than 90 percent of colorectal cancers are adenocarcinomas. Mucoid adenocarcinoma is a histological subtype associated with particularly poor prognosis. When the accumulation of mucoid material is intracellular, individual cells have a "signet ring" appearance. Survival with signet ring adenocarcinoma is unusual.

Approximately half of large bowel tumors are situated in the rectum. Of those developing in the colon, approximately half occur in the sigmoid colon and a quarter in the cecum and the ascending colon.

Primary symptoms include persistent rectal bleeding and change in bowel habits (increasing frequency or loose stools or both). Secondary symptoms include anemia and intestinal obstruction. The site of the carcinoma often dictates the symptoms. Carcinoma of the right colon is usually polypoidal, soft and friable and bleeds easily. Thus the patient presents with symptoms of anemia from occult bleeding. Sometimes the patient complains of abdominal pain and a mass may be palpable in the right iliac fossa. Left-sided cancers tend to be annular and therefore more likely to obstruct, particularly since the intraluminal contents are more solid on the left. Constipation is therefore a frequent initial symptom and is often accompanied by abdominal colic. Overt bleeding and passage of mucus per rectum are more common with left sided tumors.

Unusual presentations include deep venous thrombosis, *Streptococcus bovis* bacteremia and nephrotic range proteinuria.

DIAGNOSIS

As an initial evaluation, a double-contrast barium enema may be more cost-effective, but endoscopic studies provide histologic information, potential therapeutic intervention, and overall greater sensitivity and specificity. Colonoscopy should probably be done in all patients with colorectal cancer to rule out coexistent polyps or synchronous carcinomas.

Additional studies which may be helpful in staging the disease include blood counts, renal and liver function tests, chest films, CEA estimation and computed tomography. Elevation of alkaline phosphatase and CEA is associated with high incidence of liver metastasis. It may be useful to determine the preoperative CEA level, because if it is elevated prior to excision of tumor and returns to normal postoperatively, it can be of value in following patients for metastasis or recurrence. However, CEA elevations occur in a number of unrelated benign conditions like in cirrhosis, cigarette smokers, etc as well as in other malignancies including cancers of the breast and lung.

Preoperative computed scanning of the abdomen and pelvis is an important step in the evaluation of patients with colorectal cancers, especially those with rectal cancer. CT scan can detect nodal enlargement, assess the degree of lateral spread, spot liver metastasis, identify ureteric obstruction and occasionally determine whether transperitoneal seeding has occurred.

STAGING AND SURVIVAL OF COLORECTAL CANCER

The accepted method of staging patients with colorectal cancers is based on Duke's staging (Table 16.3). However there has been a gradual move from Duke's staging to TNM classification system as this has a more accurate independent description of the primary tumor and its spread. Both the staging systems are shown in (Table 16.2).

Independent factors which affect the survival include the number of positive lymph nodes, histopathologic differentiation, vascular or lymphatic invasion and incomplete resection margin.

MANAGEMENT

Surgery

The primary curative intervention requires en bloc extirpation of the involved bowel segment with adequate margins and inclusion of the

Table 16.2: TNM classification		
	Modified	*(%)*
Stage 0	Carcinoma in situ	
Stage I	Tumor invades submucosa, no nodal involvement, no metastasis (T1,N0,M0). Tumor invades muscularis propria, no nodal involvement, no metastasis (T2,N0,M0)	90-100
Stage II	Tumor invades subserosa, no nodal involvement, no metastasis (T3,N0,M0). Tumor invades other organs, no nodal involvement, no metastasis (T4,N0,M0)	75-85
Stage III	Involvement of up to 3 regional nodal, no metastasis (any T, N1,M0) Involvement of 4 or more nodes, no metastasis (any T, N2, M0)	30-40
Stage IV	Distant metastasis	<5

Table 16.3: Duke's pathological staging		
	Extension of invasion	*Node involvement*
Duke's A	Limited to mucosa	N0
Duke's B1	Tumor invades into muscularis propria	N0
Duke's B2	Tumor invades through muscularis propria	N0
Duke's C1	Tumor invades into muscularis propria	Lymph node involvement is present
Duke's C2	Tumor invades through muscularis propria	Highest lymph node involved
Duke's D	Distant metastases	not applicable

corresponding lymphatic drainage. As the lymphatic drainage parallels the regional circulation, the major vessels must be resected near their margins. The options depend on the location of the primary tumor.

Lesions of the right colon require right hemicolectomy, which includes 10-15 cm of terminal ileum, cecum, ascending and transverse colon. The ileocolic vessels, the right colic and the right branch of middle colic artery along with the mesentery are resected. For lesions of hepatic flexure dissection is extended to include the middle colic artery at its origin.

Lesions in the transverse colon are treated by transverse colectomy or extended right hemicolectomy. Carcinomas of the splenic flexure and proximal descending colon require resection of the transverse colon and descending colon to the first branch of the inferior mesenteric artery including the left colic vessels but preserving the sigmoid branch of inferior mesenteric artery.

Sigmoid carcinomas require a resection that includes the inferior mesenteric artery close to its origin. For rectal lesions, total mesorectal excision (TME) is mandatory to decrease local recurrence. Lesions in the middle and upper rectum (up to 5 to 6 cm from the anal verge) may be treated by resection and primary anastomosis using stapling devices (anterior resection). A proximal diverting colostomy or ileostomy is advocated to protect a less than perfect anastamosis after low anterior resection.

Low rectal lesions may require abdominoperineal excision, where after complete tumor extirpation and excision of anal canal, the sigmoid colon is brought out as a permanent colostomy.

ADJUVANT THERAPY

Despite apparently curative surgery more than half of operated patients develop recurrence and die of their disease. This is a result of occult viable tumor cells that have metastasized before surgery and which are undetectable by current radiological techniques. Adjuvant chemotherapy and radiotherapy have developed as a complementary tool to surgery and is aimed at eradicating these micrometastatic cancer cells before they become established.

Fluorouracil has remained the mainstay of chemotherapy for colorectal cancer. It is a prodrug that is converted intracellularly to metabolites that bind to the enzyme thymidylate synthase, inhibiting synthesis of thymidine, DNA and RNA. Addition of folinic acid increases the inhibition of thymidylate synthase and seems to confer superior clinical outcome in advanced disease. The side effects of fluorouracil based chemotherapy include nausea, vomiting, increased susceptibility to infection, oral mucositis, diarrhea, desquamation of the palms and soles, and, rarely, cardiac and neurological toxic effects.

A meta-analysis of data from randomized studies of adjuvant chemotherapy has shown reduction in failure of events by 35 percent and currently combination therapy with 5-FU and leucoviron is accepted as standard therapy for Duke's C colon cancer. Patients with high overall mortality have shown reduction by 22 percent compared with surgery alone. Patients with high risk features, e.g. T3 or N2 disease benefit from oxaliplatin, 5-FU and leucoviron-based therapy every 2 weeks for 12 cycles.

METASTATIC DISEASE

A combination of chemotherapy with oxaliplatin, irinotecan with 5-FU and leucoviron is the regimen of choice. Recent trials using antiangiogenesis agent bevacizumab, and epidermal growth factor cetuximab in combination with irinotecan and 5-FU containing regimen have shown good response.

ADJUVANT THERAPY IN RECTAL CANCER

Rectum is less accessible to the surgeon anatomically, so it is much more difficult to achieve wide excision of the tumor, and about 50 percent of recurrences are in the pelvis itself rather than at distant sites. Consequently locally directed radiotherapy is a useful adjuvant weapon, and this has been assessed for rectal cancer both before and after surgery.

The standard postoperative treatment for rectal cancer is adjuvant chemotherapy for patients with stage II rectal cancer (node negative disease with transmural invasion) and stage III rectal cancer (node positive disease). However the role of preoperative radiotherapy has been investigated in many trials and has been found to be better than postoperative treatment in terms of local recurrence. This has been substantiated in the Swedish trials (11% in the preoperative radiotherapy vs 27% in the group treated with surgery alone), the German trials (6% in the preoperative chemoradiotherapy group vs 13% postoperative chemoradiotherpy) and the Dutch trials (2.4% in the radiotherapy and surgery vs 3.2% in the surgery group). An improvement in the overall is seen only in the Swedish trials (48% in the surgery only group vs 58% in the combined treatment group).

ROLE OF PORTAL VENOUS INFUSIONAL THERAPY

Fluorouracil is an S phase specific drug, and its active metabolites have a half life of about 10 minutes, which limits its target when given as a bolus, to the small fraction of cells in the S phase at the time of administration. Infusional therapy may affect a greater proportion of cells. Furthermore, the most common site for micrometastases after resection of a colorectal tumor is the liver. In contrast with grossly identifiable metastases of the advanced disease, which derive their blood supply from the hepatic artery, these micrometastases are thought to be supplied by the portal vein. Therefore delivering chemotherapy via the portal vein should provide high concentrations of the drug at the most vulnerable site and lead to substantial first pass metabolism, which should attenuate any systemic toxicity. Results of trials are still awaited for a final decision on this modality of therapy.

OTHER APPROACHES TO ADJUVANT THERAPY

Nonsteroidal Anti-Inflammatory Drugs

Evidence strongly suggests a protective effect of non-steroidal anti-inflammatory drugs in colon cancer. Patients with familial adenomatous polyposis who took the non-steroidal anti-inflammatory drug, sulindac had reductions in the number and size of their polyps. Inhibition of the cyclo-oxygenase type 2 pathway by non-steroidal anti-inflammatory drugs may be the mechanism of action. The side effect from using non-steroidal anti-inflammatory drugs is the increased incidence of gastrointestinal bleeds. On the current evidence, non-steroidal anti-inflammatory drugs could be used as secondary prevention after surgical resection of colonic tumors.

IMMUNOTHERAPY

Several immunostimulatory approaches have been advocated to augment the innate immune response against tumors. These include:
- Vaccination with autologous cells derived from the patient's tumor to elicit a cell mediated immune response against the tumor. To increase the efficacy of this response, tumor cells are co-administered with an immunomodulatory adjuvant, such as BCG.
- Vaccination against tumor associated antigens such as the carcinoembryonic antigen.
- Monoclonal antibodies directed against tumor antigens like the 17-1A antigen which is a surface glycoprotein with a role in cell adhesion and present in over 90 percent of colorectal tumors.

GENE THERAPY

This is a new approach at a developmental stage for the treatment of colon cancer. Two gene therapy strategies are currently used, gene correction and enzyme-prodrug systems.

GENE CORRECTION

The logical approach to gene therapy is the correction of a single gene defect, which causes the disease phenotype. The p53 gene regulates the cell cycle and can cause growth arrest or apoptosis in response to DNA damage. Loss of p53 control leads to uncontrolled growth and is associated with more aggressive tumors. Restoration of wild-type p53 in p53 mutated tumors inhibits growth.

VIRUS DIRECTED ENZYME-PRODRUG TREATMENT

Enzyme-prodrug systems are used to localize the toxic drug effects to tumor cells. This involves gene transfer of an enzyme into tumor cells, which converts an inactive prodrug into a toxic metabolite, leading to cell death. An important feature of enzyme-prodrug systems is the "bystander effect," whereby surrounding cells are also killed by active metabolites. Gene transfer is achieved by viral vectors, such as retroviruses or adenoviruses.

THE MATRIX METALLOPROTEINASE

These are a group of enzymes involved in the physiological maintenance of the extracellular matrix. They degrade the extracellular matrix and promote the formation of new blood vessels and are involved in tissue remodeling processes, such as wound healing and angiogenesis. Matrix Metalloproteinase is overexpressed in various tumors, including colorectal cancers, and has been implicated in facilitating tumor invasion and metastasis. The Matrix Metalloproteinase inhibitor, marimastat, has shown reductions in levels of tumor markers in phase I studies, and its clinical efficacy is currently being tested.

FURTHER READING

1. American Joint Committee on Cancer. AJCC Cancer Staging Manual (5th ed). Philadelphia: Lippincott-Raven, 1997.
2. Bennett RC, Duthie HL. Br J Surg 1964;51:335-57.
3. Johnston PG, Fisher ER, et al. The role of thymidylate synthase expression in prognosis and outcome of adjuvant chemotherapy in patients with rectal cancer. J Clin Oncol 1994;12:2640-647.
4. Keighley MRB, and Williams NS. Surgery of the Anus, Rectum and Colon (2nd ed), WB Saunders, London.
5. Leichman CG, Fleming TR, Mussia FM, et al. Phase II study of fluorouracil and its modulation in advanced colorectal cancer: a Southwest Oncology Group Study. J Clin Oncol 1995;13:1303-11.
6. Miller R, Bartolo DCC, et al. Br J Surg 1988;75:40-43.
7. Mortel CG, Fleming TR, Macdonald JS, et al. Levamisole and fluorouracil for adjuvant therapy of resected colon carcinoma. N Engl J Med 1990; 322: 352-58.
8. Nigro ND. Dis Colon Rectum 1984;27:736-66.
9. OPCS 1983 HMSO, London.
10. Orda R, Bawbik JB, et al. Dis Colon Rectum 1976;19:626-31.
11. Pack GT, Miller TR, Trinidad SS. Dis Colon Rectum 1963;6:1-6.

12. Petrelli N, Herrera L, Rustum Y, et al. A prospective randomized trails of 5-fluorouracil versus 5-fluorouracil and high dose leucovorin versus 5-fuorouracil and methotrexate in previously untreated patients with advanced colorectal carcinoma. J Clin Oncol 1987;5:1559-65.
13. Stein RB, Hanauer SB. Medical therapy for inflammatory bowel diseases. Gastroenterol Clin North Am 1999;28:297-321.
14. Wolmark N, Fisher B, Rockette H, et al. Postoperative adjuvant chemotherapy or BCG for colon cancer: Results from NSABP protocol C01. J Natl Cancer Inst 1988;80:30-36.
15 Wolmark N, Rockette H, Mamounas E, et al. Clinical trail to assess the relative efficacy of fluorouracil and leucovorin, fluorouracil and levamisole, and fluorouracil, leucovorin, and levamisole in patients with Duke's B and C carcinoma of the colon: results from National Surgical Adjuvant Breast and Bowel project CD4. J Clin Oncol 1999;17:3553-59.

APPENDIX 5

International comparison; India and five continents—AAR (ICMR and IARC).

CANCER COLON (MALE)

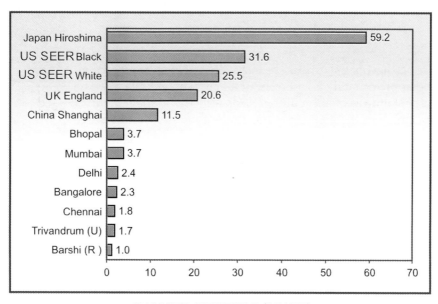

CANCER RECTUM (MALE)

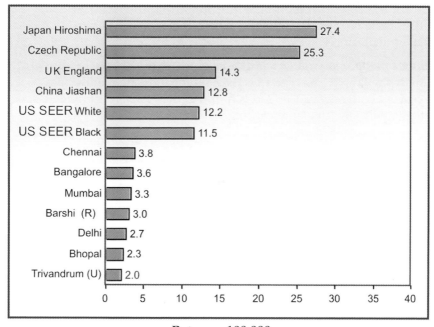

Rate per 100,000

Anal Cancer

17

S Sudhindran

Neoplasms of anal cancer are relatively uncommon, representing approximately 1-2 percent of all large bowel cancers. The understanding of the pathogenesis and the management of carcinoma of the anal canal has undergone profound change over the last 30 years. Anal cancer remains the only carcinoma of the gastrointestinal tract that is curable without the need for definitive surgery.

EPIDEMIOLOGY

Anal cancer was initially believed to develop in areas of chronic irritation as a result of benign conditions such as hemorrhoids, fissures and fistulae. However, a series of case-control studies have shown that there is little risk associated with the presence of hemorrhoids, fissures or fistulae. Epidemiological surveys suggest that the majority of anal cancers are due to infection with human papillomavirus (HPV). Table 17.1 lists the principal risk factors for the development of anal cancer.

Human papillomavirus: As is the case for cervical cancer, human papillomavirus type 16 is the subtype most frequently associated with anal cancer and is found in over 70 percent of patients with invasive anal cancer.

Sexual activity: Anal receptive intercourse, history of sexually transmitted disease and more than 10 sexual partners have all been found to significantly increase the risk of anal cancer. The association between sexual activity and anal cancer is strengthened by the strong links between this malignancy and prior history of cervical, vulval or vaginal cancer.

Immunosuppression: Chronic immunosuppression from medications is a risk factor for several types of squamous-cell carcinomas, including those of the anal canal. In recipients of renal allografts, persistent human papillomavirus infection has been associated with a 100-fold increase in the risk of anogenital cancer.

HIV Infection: HIV-positive patients are two to six times as likely as HIV-negative persons to have anal human papillomavirus infection and to subsequently develop high grade intraepithelial neoplasia and anal cancer.

Smoking: Several case-control studies have shown that a history of smoking increases the risk of anal cancer by a factor of 2 to 5. This fact is supported by the finding that lung cancer is twice as frequent in patients with a history of anal cancer as in the general population (Table 17.1).

PATHOLOGY

The anal canal is 3 to 4.5 cm long extending from anal verge to rectal mucosa. The anal verge corresponds to the introitus of the anal orifice which is covered by skin (epidermis) and not by mucosa.

Cancer of the anal canal may be divided into carcinoma of the anal canal (mucosa covered) and carcinoma of the anal margin (epidermis covered). Carcinomas of the anal canal occur at or above the dentate line, whereas carcinomas of the anal margin arise distal to the dentate line.

The columnar epithelium of the rectum is replaced by squamous epithelium in the anal canal at an area corresponding to the zone of fusion between the embryonic hindgut and proctodeum. This mucocutaneous junction is the visually identifiable dentate or pectinate line. Distal to this line, the anal canal is lined by stratified squamous epithelium. This zone can therefore give rise to morphologically dissimilar malignancies. Tumors arising within the transitional zone are now referred to as non-keratinising squamous cell carcinomas, whereas tumors developing in the more distal anal canal are termed keratinising squamous cell carcinomas (Table 17.3).

Lymphatic drainage of anal cancers is dependent upon the anatomic site of its origin. Above the dentate line, drainage flows to perirectal and paravertebral nodes in a manner similar to rectal adenocarcinoma, whereas below the dentate line lymphatics drain to the inguinal and femoral nodes. The inguinal, femoral, and iliac nodes are the most frequent sites of nodal metastases of anal canal cancer.

Table 17.1: Risk factors for anal cancer

Strong association
1. Human papilloma virus infection (anogenital warts)
2. History of receptive anal intercourse
3. History of sexually transmitted disease
4. More than 10 sexual partners
5. History of cervical, vulvar or vaginal cancer
6. Immunosuppression after solid organ transplantation

Moderate association
1. HIV infection
2. Long term use of corticosteroids
3. Cigarette smoking

SYMPTOMS

Anal cancers often remain asymptomatic for long periods. Pain, bleeding and increasing difficulty in defecation are the leading symptoms. Unfortunately these are often indistinguishable from those associated with lesions such as hemorrhoids, fissures or pruritus ani. Consequently the disease may be discovered late in its course. There are situations when the patient presents with acute or subacute intestinal obstruction.

An incision biopsy is required to establish the histological diagnosis and local staging.

STAGING AND PROGNOSTIC FACTORS

Staging work up should include digital rectal examination, anoscopy, proctoscopy and assessment of inguinal nodes. An examination under anesthesia may not only allow a biopsy for diagnosis but in addition permits assessment of local infiltration.

Work up to exclude metastatic disease include liver function tests, chest radiograph and ultrasound scan of liver. Computed tomography (CT) of abdomen and pelvis and endoanal ultrasound may allow more accurate locoregional assessment of the disease.

Endoanal ultrasound is useful to evaluate changes in the mucosa, submucosa and the internal and external sphincter. It can determine the depth of penetration of carcinoma into the sphincter complex. It is also used to assess the response of these tumors to chemoradiation therapy.

The UICC (Union Internationale Contre Cancer) and AJCC (American Joint Committee on Cancer) have proposed a practical staging system for anal cancer. Cancer of the anal margin is staged identically to squamous cell cancer of skin. The staging system for both types of tumors is outlined in Tables 17.2 and 17.3.

There are three major prognostic factors:

Size: The size of the tumor is the most important prognostic factor. Mobile lesions that are no more than 2 cm in diameter can be cured in approximately 80 percent of cases, whereas tumors of 5 cm or more can be cured in less than 50 percent of cases. The probability of nodal involvement is also directly related to the size of the tumor.

Site: Anal canal carcinomas fare worse than those of perianal skin.

Differentiation: Well-differentiated tumors are more favorable than are poorly differentiated tumors.

TREATMENT

A major determinant of appropriate treatment is the location of the primary tumor.

Table 17.2: AJCC classification of anal canal tumors

Primary tumor (T)

TX	Primary tumor cannot be assessed
T0	No evidence of primary tumor
Tis	Carcinoma *in situ*
T1	Tumor <2 cm in greatest dimension
T2	Tumor >2 cm but <5 cm in greatest dimension
T3	Tumor >5 cm in greatest dimension
T4	Tumor of any size that invades adjacent organs [e.g. vagina, bladder, urethra; involvement of sphincter muscle(s) alone is not classified as T4]

Regional lymph nodes (N)

Nx	Regional lymph nodes cannot be assessed
N0	No regional lymph node metastasis
N1	Metastasis in perirectal lymph node(s)
N2	Metastasis in unilateral internal iliac and/or inguinal lymph node(s)
N3	Metastasis in perirectal and inguinal lymph node(s) and/or bilateral internal iliac and/or inguinal lymph nodes

Distant metastasis (M)

MX	Distant metastasis cannot be assessed
M0	No distant metastasis
M1	Distant metastasis

Stage groupings

Stage 0	Tis	N0	M0
Stage I	T1	N0	M0
Stage II	T2	N0	M0
	T3	N0	M0
Stage IIIA	T1-3	N1	M0
	T4	N0	M0
Stage IIIB	T4	N1	M0
	Any T	N2-3	M0
Stage IV	Any T	Any N	M1

CANCER OF ANAL CANAL

Surgery

Traditionally the treatment of cancers of the anal canal has been surgical, often involving an abdominoperineal resection (APR), thus necessitating a permanent colostomy. The overall survival ranged from 40 to 70 percent following surgery.

Primary Radiotherapy

Use of primary radiotherapy was associated with local eradication of tumor and cure in 70 to 90 percent of selected patients. Radiation was given either as external-beam radiation or as brachytherapy (implantation

Table 17.3: WHO classification of carcinoma of the anus

1. Carcinoma of the anal canal (mucosa covered)
   - Squamous cell carcinoma (cloacogenic)
     - Large cell keratinising (from distal anal canal)
     - Large cell non-keratinising (from transitional zone)
     - Basaloid
   - Adenocarcinoma
     - Rectal type
     - Anal glands
     - Within anorectal fistula
2. Carcinoma of anal margin (epidermis covered)
   - Squamous cell carcinoma
   - Giant condylomata
   - Basal cell carcinoma
   - Bowen's disease
   - Paget's disease
   - Others

of radioactive seeds in tumor). However results were similar or inferior to that of surgery in patients with nodal involvement or tumors larger than 5 cm. Moreover approximately 10 percent of patients later required a colostomy for adverse effects of radiation such as anal ulcers, stenosis and necrosis.

Combined Modality Treatment (CMT)

The concomitant administration of fluoropyrimidines potentiates the therapeutic effect of radiation on a variety of gastrointestinal cancers. Thus preoperative administration of fluorouracil and mitomycin combined with an intermediate dose of radiation therapy (30 Gy) to patients with anal cancer was found to leave no residual tumor thus obviating the need for a permanent colostomy but still achieving cure in 70 percent of patients.

The value of substituting platinum compounds like cisplatin for mitomycin in combination-therapy regimens is being investigated currently.

Three randomised trials showed that CMT resulted in a reduction in local recurrence and a lower probability of a subsequent colostomy because of persistent disease. Overall survival, however, was not significantly altered. The presence of nodal involvement or tumor ulceration is a poor prognostic factor.

CURRENT STRATEGY

Chemotherapy

The primary treatment of anal canal cancer is with concomitant chemotherapy (fluorouracil and mitomycin) and radiation therapy (CMT).

Local Recurrence

For patients with persistent or locally recurrent carcinoma of the anal canal after CMT, an abdominoperineal resection remains the treatment of choice. Among patients who do not have a complete clinical or pathological response to combination therapy, approximately 50 percent can be cured after undergoing a salvage surgical resection.

Treatment for Anal Margin Cancer

Cancers arising in the anal margin are considered as skin cancers and best treated by local excision. Malignant melanomas may occur in this region and will have to be treated accordingly

FURTHER READING

1. American Joint Committee on Cancer. AJCC Cancer Staging Manual (5th ed). Philadelphia: Lippincott Raven, 1997;91-95.
2. Carcinoma of the Anal Canal. Ryan DP, Compton CC, Mayer RJ. N Engl J Med 2000;342:792-800.
3. Hrmanek P, Sobin LH (Eds). TNM Classification of Malignant Tumors (4th ed). Berlin: Springer-Verlag 1987;50-52.
4. Peiffert D, Seitz JF, Rougier P, et al. Preliminary results of a Phase ll study of high dose radiation therapy and neoadjuvant concomitant 5-fluorouracil with CDDP chemotherapy for patients with anal canal cancer: A French co-operative study. Ann Oncol 1997;8(6):575-81.
5. Peley G, Farkas E, Sinkovics I, Kovacs T, et al. Inguinal sentinel lymph node biopsy for staging anal cancer. Scand J Surg 2002;91(4):336-38.
6. Tanum G, Tveit K, et al. Chemotherapy and radiation therapy for anal carcinoma: survival and late morbidity. Cancer 1991;67:2462-66.

Primary Cancers of the Liver

18

S Sudhindran

HEPATOCELLULAR CARCINOMA

Most primary liver cancers arise from the parenchymal liver cells or hepatocytes, and are called hepatocellular carcinoma (HCC). Tumors arising from the intrahepatic bile ducts are called cholangiocarcinomas.

HCC is one of the commonest cancers in the world, particularly in Asia. It is unusual among human cancers in that the causative agent is by and large readily identifiable. There is now strong evidence that the prevalence of HCC is rising all over the world, corresponding with that of the viral hepatitis. In addition, it is expected to be seen more frequently over the next few years, largely as a result of Hepatitis C virus (HCV) epidemic.

The incidence of primary cancers of the liver shows striking geographic variation. In India, it is 3.8 per 100,000 (National Cancer Registry Programme, Indian Council of Medical Research 2001). In China, South East Asian countries and sub-Saharan regions in Africa, it ranges from 20 to 150 per 100,000. In the US, the UK and Scandinavia, it is 5 per 100,000.

ETIOLOGY

The Presence of Hepatic Cirrhosis

Cirrhosis is present in over 90 percent of patients with HCC. Patients with a more advanced stage of underlying liver disease have higher risk of occurrence of HCC. It is unclear whether cirrhosis *per se* is important in the development of HCC. It could be that tumorogenesis and cirrhosis occur concurrently but cirrhosis takes a shorter time period than HCC.

Viral Cirrhosis

The prevalence of HCC worldwide parallels that of viral hepatitis and the majority of cases are associated with

Hepatitis B virus (HBV) or Hepatitis C virus (HCV). Cirrhotic patients with either infection have approximately 3-10 percent annual risk of HCC development. In HBV, those with ongoing viral replication have a higher incidence of HCC.

Non-Viral Cirrhosis

Patients with cirrhosis due to genetic hemochromatosis have a very high risk of HCC development (7–9% per year). The risk falls with venesection but not to baseline levels (1–3% per year).

Alcoholic cirrhosis carries an increased risk of development of HCC. The available data suggest that abstinence from alcohol does not protect against HCC development and that tumor development is seen in 1–4 percent of male cirrhotics per year. For unclear reasons, the rate of HCC development in women seems significantly lower.

In contrast to the above, patients with cirrhosis of autoimmune hepatitis, primary biliary cirrhosis and Wilson's disease have a very low risk of HCC development. Patients with other metabolic diseases including hereditary tyrosinemase, α-1 antitrypsin deficiency, porphyria cutanea tarda, glycogen storage disease 1 and 3, citrullinemia, and aciduria are also at a slightly increased risk of developing HCC.

Non-cirrhotic HCC

Approximately 7 percent of hepatocellular cancers, excluding the fibrolamellar variant, arise without cirrhosis. Non-cirrhotic HCCs occur in young patients (fibrolamellar variant) and in the elderly (apparent *de novo* HCC). Fibrolamellar HCC has an equal sex incidence and an average age at diagnosis of 30 years. Non-cirrhotic HCC does occur in patients with viral liver disease, particularly HBV where direct viral integration into host DNA may play a role. Non-cirrhotic HCC can develop in a patient with HCV or the rarely occurring hemachromatosis.

Sex

The incidence is 3 to 5 time more in males compared to females of all ages.

Age

The average age of HCC development is 66 years, which probably reflects the long term nature of most underlying liver diseases producing tumor development. This tumor is rare among those below the age of 45 years in areas with low levels of HBV infection. In high HBV prevalence areas, HCC has a bimodal age distribution with peaks at ages 45 and 65.

Race

Within regions, the incidence varies by race: Asians more than blacks and blacks more than whites.

Environmental Factors

The role of Afflotoxin B, a product of fungus Aspergillosis as a carcinogenic agent that can infect unrefrigerated food material is under scrutiny by public health officials. It has been suggested as an incriminating factor in primary tumors of the liver.

Chemicals

Other risk factors include ingestion of nitrites and nitrate-treated foods, androgenic steroids, exposure to pesticides and insecticides, and exposure to industrial solvents (dioxane, chloroform, carbon tetrachloride, vinyl chloride, polychorinated biphenyls and trichloroethylene).

Histology

The majority of primary liver cancers are adenocarcinoma and arise from the epithelial cells. The primary tumors include:
- HCCs: HCC usually appear either as diffuse or massive form, but a few appear as nodular variety and often multiple, presenting in both the lobes. In general, the malignant cells are larger than normal hepatocytes, have a polygonal shape and appear finely granular with eosinophilic cytoplasm. Distinctive histologic patterns include trabecular, compact, acinar, and clear cell variety.
- Fibrolamellar variant of HCC: This variant has a more favorable prognosis. It tends to occur in young subjects unassociated with cirrhosis, and is often solitary. The histology is distinctive: eosinophilic, polygonal cells separated by lamellar fibrosis
- Cholangiocarcinoma
- Mixed cholangiocarcinoma and HCC
- Undifferentiated cancers

One interesting feature of HCC is the involvement of hepatic veins. This is commonly seen in large and massive tumors. The hepatic vein invasion is also seen in 20 percent small primary tumors, less than 2 cm in diameter, but ranges from 70 to 90 percent with tumors more than 5 cm in diameter. Thrombosis of the hepatic vein, vena cava and portal veins can occur in association with HCC.

Fewer than 3 percent of primary liver tumors arise from mesenchymal cells; these include sarcoma, angiosarcoma, epithelioid tumors and hemangioendothelioma. Hepatoblastoma is a very rare cancer that occurs in children with an incidence of one per 100,000.

NATURAL HISTORY AND PROGNOSIS OF HCC

HCCs develop as small nodules. The majority of them grow in an asymptomatic phase, which may be years in length. Estimated median doubling time of HCC is six months.

The major factors influencing overall survival are severity of underlying liver dysfunction and tumor size at initial detection. Overall survival with tumors of less than 5 cm is 80–100 percent at one year and 17–20 percent at three years with no therapy. This suggests that if earlier diagnosis can be made, the opportunity for intervention may be greater.

SCREENING TESTS FOR HCC

α- Fetoprotein (AFP), a normal serum protein synthesised by fetal liver cells and yolk sac cells, is the most widely studied screening test used as a tumor marker for HCC. The normal range for AFP is 10–20 ng/ml and a level >400 ng/ml is usually regarded as diagnostic of HCC. However up to 20 percent of HCCs do not produce AFP, even when very large. A rising AFP over time, even if the level does not reach 400 ng/ml, is virtually diagnostic of HCC.

Desgamma-carboxy prothrombin has been used as an alternative tumor marker for HCC. It has not gained wide acceptance.

Ultrasound can detect large HCCs with high sensitivity and specificity. Ultrasound detects 85-95 percent of lesions 3-5 cm in diameter.

Combining AFP and ultrasound improves detection rates.

CLINICAL FEATURES

Abdominal pain is the most common symptom, other symptoms being increasing abdominal girth, weight loss, anorexia, vomiting and jaundice. In fact, patients can present with symptoms of chronic liver disease or with symptoms of an advanced liver tumor.

The most common physical signs are hepatomegaly and stigmata of cirrhosis, but may include abdominal bruit (reflecting increased vascularity), ascites, splenomegaly, Budd-Chiari syndrome, Virchow's node, and cutaneous metastasis. HCC may be associated with a variety of paraneoplastic features including hypoglycemia, erythrocytosis, hypercalcemia, hypercholesterolemia, dysfibrinogenemia, carcinoid syndrome, increased thyroxine-binding globulin, sexual changes, and porphyria cutanea tarda.

INVESTIGATIONS

Common chemistry abnormalities include elevations in alkaline phosphatase, liver transaminases, bilirubin and $\mu_1$globulin. Very high serum bilirubin levels suggest intrahepatic or extrahepatic obstruction. AFP is elevated in about two-thirds of patients with HCC in western countries. The des-¡-carboxy prothrombin protein induced by vitamin K abnormality is elevated in more than 90 percent of patients with HCC, but is not specific for this disease. Hepatitis A, B, C, and D serology should be measured.

ABDOMINAL ULTRASOUND

As explained above, it is useful for screening high-risk populations. It has very high sensitivity and specificity for large tumors. It can detect 85-95 percent tumors more than 3 cm in diameter. Detection of tumors less than 2 cm is uncommon.

COMPUTED TOMOGRAPHY, TRI-PHASIC SPIRAL CT EVALUATION

CT scan delineates the extent of hepatic involvement, invasion or thrombosis of the portal and hepatic veins, regional lymph node involvement, splenomegaly and ascites.

The tri-phasic spiral CT involves:

1. An initial *non-contrast* CT scan to show gross liver abnormalities such as hemochromatosis, glycogen storage disease, confluent fibrosis, etc.
2. The *hepatic arterial phase* which is a second CT scan obtained 20-30 seconds after contrast injection to view primary liver tumors that receive their blood supply from the hepatic arterial system.
3. *Portal venous phase* (a third sequence acquired approximately 60-70 seconds after contrast injection) to confirm tumors with a rich arterial supply which will quickly fade during this phase and to help characterize other liver abnormalities.

CT PORTOGRAPHY

Contrast injected in superior mesenteric artery enters portal vein and permits good contrast between normal and tumor tissue.

ETHIODOL (LIPIODOL) CT SCANNING

If, after initial imaging, confusion remains as to whether a lesion represents HCC or another hypervascular lesion (focal nodule hyperplasia, metastatic disease from carcinoid, islet cell tumors, etc.), a lipiodol CT scan can be used. This technique involves an initial study of the liver's arterial supply, followed by a small injection of lipiodol (a thick, oily substance that is an iodized ethyl ester of the fatty acid of poppy seed oil) into the hepatic artery. HCC nodules hold the lipiodol much longer than other cells, enabling radiologists to view these nodules during a follow-up CT scan performed 7 to 28 days after the lipiodol injection. This technique has an accuracy of approximately 90 percent.

HEPATIC ANGIOGRAPHY

Hepatic angiography reveals multiple, tortuous tumor vessels, and a characteristic early venous tumor blush providing important details about the vascular anatomy in planning hepatic intra-arterial therapy.

MRI WITH INTRAVENOUS GADOLINIUM

To complement the CT scan, radiologists may use the T1 and T2 MRI weighting of different lesions. This helps differentiate between regenerative or dysplastic nodules and frank HCC. T2-weighted spin-echo sequence can detect small hepatic tumors.

DIAGNOSTIC WORK UP FOR A LIVER MASS

Algorithm of a diagnostic work up in a liver mass is given in Figure 18.1. AJCC stage grouping is given in Table 18.1

LIVER BIOPSY

In the few cases where real diagnostic doubt persists, percutaneous fine needle aspiration or biopsy may be indicated. There is an associated risk of seeding of HCC, which does not appear to be related to tumor size. If surgical therapy is possible biopsy should be avoided.

If surgery is planned, a laparoscopic biopsy or an open biopsy at laparotomy is usually preferred to decrease the risk of tumor seeding.

When a patient presents with a liver mass, there is a requirement to make a diagnosis and to stage the disease. If the patient is known to have

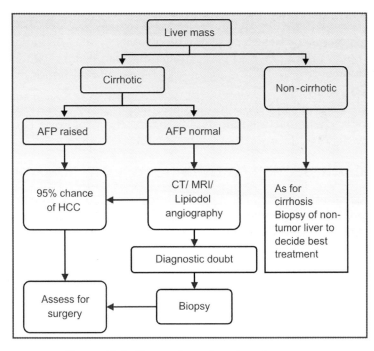

Figure 18.1: Diagnostic work up for a liver mass

Table 18.1: AJCC stage grouping	
Stage I	T1, N0, M0 T1: Solitary tumor ≤ 2 cm, no vascular invasion
Stage II	T2, N0, M0 T2: Solitary tumor ≤ 2 cm, with vascular invasion: multiple tumors (one lobe only), none > 2 cm, no vascular invasion; solitary tumor >2 cm, no vascular invasion
Stage III A	T3, N0, M0 T3: Solitary tumor >2 cm, with vascular invasion; multiple tumors (one lobe only) with no tumor >2 cm with vascular invasion; multiple tumors (one lobe only) with any tumor >2 cm vascular invasion
Stage III B	T1-3, N1, M0 N1: Regional lymph node involvement including nodes in hepatoduodenal ligament, hepatic and periportal nodes, and nodes along inferior vena cava, portal vein, and hepatic artery
Stage IV A	T4, any N, M0 T4: Multiple tumors in more than one lobe; tumor(s) involving a major branch or portal or hepatic vein
Stage IV B	Any T, any N, M1: Distant metastases

pre-existing cirrhosis and the mass is greater than 2 cm in diameter, there is a greater than 95 percent chance that the lesion is an HCC. If AFP is raised, this confirms the diagnosis and further investigation is only required to establish the most appropriate therapy. If AFP is normal, further radiological imaging is required to allow a confident diagnosis to be made and to assess treatment without the need for biopsy. In a few cases, when real diagnostic doubt exists, a percutaneous biopsy may be indicated.

In a patient not known to be cirrhotic, the plan of investigation is as before. However once HCC is diagnosed, biopsy of non-tumor liver may be done to assess the best treatment.

In this staging, no evaluation is undertaken of the underlying liver pathology, particularly cirrhosis and hence the prognosis cannot be properly evaluated.

SURGICAL RESECTION OR LIVER TRANSPLANTATION FOR HCC

Both techniques are primarily suited to small unifocal disease, but only a small proportion of patients with HCC will be suitable for either of these potentially curative treatments. The decision as to which therapy is appropriate will depend on the availability of resources and individual tumor characteristics.

SURGICAL RESECTION

Resection is only suitable for patients with excellent liver function (Child Pugh class A cirrhosis) because of the high risk of hepatic decompensation after surgery. Child Pugh's class A cirrhosis is defined as bilirubin less than 2.0 mg/dl, serum albumin more than 3.5 g/dL, no ascites, no neurologic dysfunction, and excellent nutritional status. Perioperative mortality depends on the extent of the resection and the severity of preoperative liver dysfunction. Even in experienced centers mortality remains between 5 and 20 percent, the majority of which is due to liver failure. In addition, the residual liver after resection continues to have a malignant potential. Consequently, recurrence rates of 50–60 percent after five years of follow up are usual following surgical resection.

Fibrolamellar HCC has a very different biology and arises in non-cirrhotic liver. Surgical resection for this tumor is therefore less likely to produce liver failure. Because it arises without pre-existing liver disease, fibrolamellar hepatoma usually presents with late symptoms, and therefore even though resection may be undertaken, there is often vascular or diaphragmatic involvement. Survival rates following resection vary from 15 to 65 percent.

Other HCCs in non-cirrhotic liver too present at an advanced stage but five-year survival after resection tends to be longer than that of tumors arising in cirrhosis (approximately 25%).

LIVER TRANSPLANTATION

Transplantation probably offers the best chance of cure for patients with small tumors and cirrhosis, and is therefore the treatment of choice, even in Child Pugh class A cirrhosis. It is well-established that patients with single lesions of 5 cm diameter or up to three lesions of less than 3 cm in the absence of vascular invasion have an almost zero recurrence rate for HCC and the prognosis after transplantation is the same as for a similar underlying liver disease without HCC. In contrast, unfavorable factors that suggest a poor outcome after transplantation include tumors larger than 5 cm, multiple tumors, involvement of more than one lobe, vascular invasion and diffuse tumor infiltration.

In selected patients, 5-year survival rates after transplantation for stages I, II and III disease are 75, 60, and 40 percent respectively, whereas fewer than 10 percent of stage IV patients who have received a transplant are alive at 5 years. The recurrence rate appears to be lower than that expected with surgical resection alone for patients with stage II and III tumors.

Disadvantages of transplantation include the expenses, the availability at only a few selected centers, the limited supply of donor livers, and the potential for tumor progression before a suitable donor liver is available.

NON-SURGICAL THERAPIES

A number of non-surgical therapies are in clinical use for HCC.

Percutaneous ethanol injection or PEI is well-described to produce tumor necrosis and many series show that morbidity and mortality are low. Although PEI has not been subjected to randomised controlled trials there is a considerable evidence in the literature on its use in HCC. In large series, complete response rates of 75 percent in tumors less than 3 cm in diameter have been reported, with five year survival rates of 35-75 percent.

Treatment of larger and multiple lesions is possible, often requiring repeated sessions and a general anesthetic, but recurrence occurs in more than 50 percent at one year. Treatment is technically very difficult in lesions affecting the posterior segments of the liver. Complications are uncommon, but seeding in the needle tract occurs in 3 percent and serious bile duct injury in 1 percent. Most centers still regard surgery as the best proven therapy, providing a chance of cure, but PEI probably represents the best therapy for patients with small inoperable HCCs.

Experimental studies have been undertaken using agents other than ethanol as a tumor damaging agent (cisplatinum, cold acetic acid) but to date none has shown convincing advantages.

RADIOFREQUENCY ABLATION

It is a relatively new technique where high frequency ultrasound probes are placed into a liver mass, usually under ultrasound control. It generates heat at the probe tip which can destroy tissue. A single probe can destroy lesions of up to 3 cm and a multiple tipped probe has been used to target lesions of up to 6 cm in diameter. There are few data on long term outcome in HCCs.

EMBOLIZATION/CHEMOEMBOLIZATION

Chemoembolization has been widely used as primary therapy for inoperable HCC. This is done using lipiodol and doxorubicin. There is good evidence that it is effective at reducing tumor size and treating pain or bleeding from HCC. No increase in survival has been shown, however. There is evidence from non-controlled series that small HCCs are more likely to respond to chemoembolization. Side effects of chemoembolization are those of the chemotherapeutic agent used (usually doxorubicin) in addition to the complications of arterial embolization such as pain, fever, hepatic decompensation, and rarely infarction of organs other than the liver. Serious complications occur in 3–5 percent of treated patients. A small number of studies have combined ethanol injection with chemo-embolization. There is as yet no evidence available to support this.

CRYOSURGERY

In situ destruction of tumor by application of subzero temperatures by specially designed probes that contain circulating liquid nitrogen can be performed in patients with multifocal lesions and limited hepatic reserve. Complications include cracking of the liver, bile leakage, hemorrhage, infection, myoglobinuria, and renal failure.

HORMONAL MANIPULATION WITH TAMOXIFEN

It has been the subject of randomised clinical trials. Initial data suggesting a positive effect on survival in patients with inoperable HCC has not been confirmed in larger randomised studies. Other agents with hormonal targets, stilbesterol, and flutamide have been used in HCC but there is no evidence of effectiveness.

CHEMOTHERAPY

Given intravenously, it has a very limited role in the treatment of HCC. The best single agent is doxorubicin with response rates of 10-15 percent. More aggressive combination chemotherapy regimens show no improvement in response rates and may even produce a reduction in survival of treated patients.

OCTREOTIDE

A somatostatin analogue, given intravenously as a form of therapy for HCC, it has shown inconsistent results so far.

PREVENTION OF HCC

Hepatitis B Vaccine

Given the dismal prognosis for most patients with HCC, strategies focusing on primary prevention offer the promise of reducing mortality. It is hoped that more widespread use of the hepatitis B vaccine will decrease the incidence of patients with chronic hepatitis B, although the cost of such vaccination in developing nations may be prohibitive. Transmission of the hepatitis B virus at birth through the vaginal canal is a major source of viral infection, and infants and children exposed to hepatitis B virus have a greater chance of becoming chronic carriers than do newly infected adult patients. These observations form the rationale for a large intervention study, sponsored by the World Health Organization that is currently under way in Asia involving vaccination of newborns. However, it will take many years of follow-up to ascertain whether this strategy indeed reduces the incidence of HCC.

Interferon α

The use of interferon-α in patients with chronic hepatitis C reduces the onset of liver damage and progression to cirrhosis in about 10 to 30 percent of the patients. There is a scientific rationale for this therapy as interferon-α has a broad range of antitumor activity and is known to be the effective therapy for some hematological malignancies. Initial data from both Japan and Europe showed a lower risk of HCC in cohorts of patients with hepatitis C cirrhosis who were given interferon therapy compared with those who were not treated.

RETINOIDS

Retinoids and compounds involved in the vitamin A metabolic pathway are known to be differentiation inducing agents with hypoproliferative effects. A single study using retinol showed a 20 percent reduction in second tumor development in patients who had been treated with PEI.

ADAPTIVE IMMUNOTHERAPY

This method using primed peripheral lymphocytes has also been used in the context of prevention of second tumor development after initial tumor resection or ablation. One study showed a significant increase in tumor free survival.

CONTROL OF AFLATOXIN IN FOOD

Refrigerated storage of food grains and transportation of grains in refrigerated vehicles should help reduce the risk of ingesting aflatoxin.

OTHER PRIMARY LIVER TUMORS

Hepatoblastoma is the most common primary malignant tumor of the liver in children affecting those below 3 years of age. The presenting symptoms are abdominal distension and ill-defined upper abdominal pain. Sexual precocity due to ectopic sex hormone production is also noticed in a few cases. Alpha fetoprotein is increased in >75 percent. Other tumor markers have no relevance in hepatoblastoma.

CT scan identifies a solitary enhancing mass in 80 percent and speckled calcification is seen in 50 percent in angiography.

Surgical resection is possible in 50 percent of cases and 30-70 percent of those resected cases are cured. Hepatoblastoma is more chemosensitive than HCC. Active agents include doxorubicin, vincristine, cyclophosphamide, and 5-FU. It seems that preoperative chemotherapy may increase resectability rate. Postoperative adjuvant chemotherapy may improve survival.

Angiosarcoma is a highly aggressive primary liver tumor (median survival is <6 months). 50 percent of cases have distant metastases at the time of presentation. 85 percent patients are male and peak incidence in the 6th and 7th decades. Surgical resection is the treatment of choice. The tumor is insensitive to chemotherapy and radiation therapy.

Hemangioendothelioma: Workers associated with the manufacture of vinyl chloride are more prone to develop this type of tumor. It is commonly seen in middle aged men and the median age is 50. Tumor is generally of low grade but can metastasize in 30 percent. Surgical resection is the treatment of choice. Liver transplantation has also been done in many cases.

FURTHER READING

1. Ahmed A, Keeffe EB. Treatment strategies for chronic hepatitis C: Update since the 1997 National Institutes of Health consensus development conference. J Gastroenterol Hepatol 1999;14(suppl):S12-18.
2. Bottelli R, Tibballs J, Hochhauser D, et al. Ultrasound screening for hepatocellular carcinoma (HCC) in cirrhosis: The evidence for an established clinical practice. Clin Radiol 1998;53:713-16.
3. Carr BI, Flickinger JC, Lotze MT. Hepatobiliary cancers. In: De Vita VT Jr, Hellman S, Roseberg SA (Eds). Cancer: Principles and Practice of Oncology (5th ed). Lippincott-Raven, 1997;1087-1114.
4. Finch MD, Crosbie JL, Currie E, et al. An 8 year experience of hepatic resection: indications and outcome. Br J Surg 1998;85:315-19.
5. McGinn CJ, Ten Haken RK, Ensminger WD, et al. Treatment of intrahepatic cancers with radiation doses based on a normal tissue complication probability model. J Clin Oncol 1998;16:2246-52.
6. Mor E, Kaspa RT, Sheiner P, et al. Treatment of hepatocellular carcinoma associated with cirrhosis in the era of liver transplantation. Ann Intern Med 1998;129:643-53.
7. Schafer DF, Sorrel MF. Hepatocellular carcinoma. Lancet 1999;353:1253-57.
8. Soni P, Dusheiko GM, Harrison TJ. Genetic diversity of hepatitis C virus: Implications for pathogenesis, treatment, and prevention. Lancet 1995;345:562-66.
9. Venook AP. Treatment of hepatocellular carcinoma: Too many options? J Clin Oncol 1994;12:1323-34.
10. Yoshida H, Shiratori Y, Moriyama M. Interferon therapy reduces the risk for hepatocellular carcinoma: National surveillance program of cirrhotic and noncirrhotic patients with chronic hepatitis C in Japan. Ann Intern Med 1999;131:174-81.

APPENDIX 6

International comparison; India and five continents—AAR (ICMR and IARC)

CANCER LIVER (MALE)

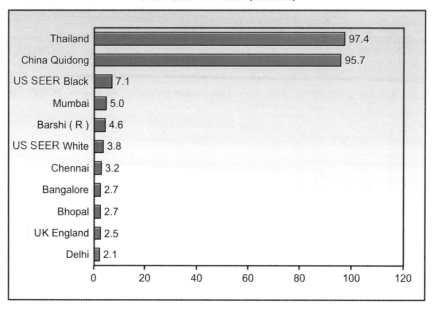

CANCER LIVER (FEMALE)

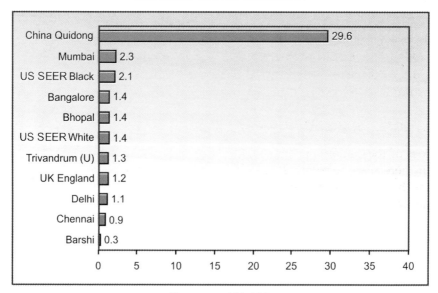

Rate per 100,000

Biliary Tract Cancer

19

Shirley George, S Sudhindran

BILIARY TRACT CANCER

Carcinomas of the biliary tract include those cancers arising either in the gallbladder or the bile ducts. The term cholangio-carcinoma was initially used to designate tumors of the intrahepatic bile ducts, but more recently refers to the entire spectrum of tumors arising in the intrahepatic, perihilar, and distal bile ducts. The prognosis from these tumors is very poor.

The clinical features, staging, and surgical treatment are different for carcinoma of the gallbladder and the bile duct, and these are described separately.

CARCINOMA OF THE GALLBLADDER

EPIDEMIOLOGY AND ETIOLOGY

Almost all gallbladder tumors are associated with a long history of calculus disease of the gallbladder. The chronic irritation of the gallbladder walls by the calculus produces metaplastic changes in the columnar epithelium of the walls which eventually becomes malignant.

Other risk factors include calcified gallbladder wall, gall-bladder polyps, typhoid carriers, chemical carcinogens like nitrosamines and obesity.

CLINICAL FEATURES

Most of the patients have a long history of calculus disease but there may be recent alteration in the type of pain which may become continuous and localized to the right upper quadrant. There may be a recent history of jaundice with asso-ciated anorexia, nausea and vomiting. Weight loss and fever are not uncommon symptoms. A frequent finding on physical examination is a tender firm mass associated with the liver. Hepatomegaly and ascites are noticed in a few cases in the later stages of the disease.

IMAGING STUDIES

Ultrasound is very sensitive in detecting gallbladder stones. In gallbladder cancer, ultrasound typically shows a thick irregular solid intramural mass associated with the gallbladder not varying its position with that of the patient. It may also demonstrate tumor extension into the liver. Computed tomography (CT) scan is useful in identifying adenopathy and spread of disease into adjacent structures. Endoscopic Retrograde Cholangiopancreatography (ERCP), Magnetic Resonance Cholangiopancreatography (MRCP) or Percutaneous Transhepatic Cholangiography (PTC) are all valuable in identifying the site of biliary obstruction.

PATHOLOGIC FEATURES AND STAGING

About 85 percent of gallbladder cancers are mucus-secreting adenocarcinoma. A squamous component is seen in 10 percent of cases and certain tumors are entirely squamous. The rest are composed of squamous or mixed tumors (Table 19.1).

The lymphatic drainage is rich and the spread is along the common bile duct to the lymph nodes in porta hepatis. In addition, direct extension into the adjacent organs especially liver is commonly seen.

SURGICAL TREATMENT

Curative surgical resection is possible only in Stage 1 disease. It is seen that in 1 to 2 percent of cholecystectomy specimens, incidental cancer is seen and the best prognosis is seen in such patients. In fact, these patients have undergone cholecystectomy for calculus disease. For T1 tumors, cholecystectomy alone is adequate, and 5-year survival is approximately 85 percent. If the tumor invades to or through the serosa (T2, T3), resection of the gallbladder and gallbladder bed and porta hepatic lymphadenectomy are recommended; the median survival after 'curative' resection

Table 19.1: AJCC stage grouping for gallbladder cancer		
Stage I	T1, N0, M0	T1a: invades lamina propria T1b: invades the muscle layer
Stage II	T2, N0, M0	T2: invades perimuscular connective tissue
Stage III	T3, N0, M0	T3 : perforates the serosa and/or directly invades one adjacent organ (< 2 cm into liver)
	T1-3, N1, M0	N1: metastases in cystic duct, percholedochal, and/or hilar lymph nodes
Stage IVA	T4, N0-1, M0	T4: tumor extends > 2 cm into the liver and/or into ≥ 2 adjacent organs
Stage IVB	Any T, N2, M0	N2: metastases in peripancreatic (head only), periduodenal, periportal, celiac, and/or superior mesenteric lymph nodes
	Any T, any N, M1	M1: distant metastases

is approximately 17 months, and 5-year survival is approximately 33 percent. The presence of nodal involvement reduces the 5-year survival to less than 15 percent. In patients who undergo a palliative procedure only, the median survival is 6 months. In patients who have more advanced local or metastatic disease and cannot undergo surgical resection, the median survival is 3 months.

CHOLANGIOCARCINOMA OR CARCINOMA OF THE BILE DUCTS

Cholangiocarcinoma includes tumors involving intrahepatic, perihilar (Klatskin tumors) and extrahepatic bile ducts.

RISK FACTORS

1. Primary sclerosing cholangitis with or without ulcerative colitis is the commonest known predisposing factor in western countries (lifetime risk of 5-15%). Smoking augments this risk.
2. In South East Asia where the prevalence of cholangiocarcinoma is high, liver fluke (*Opisthorchis viverrini* and clonorchis sinensis) has a strong association.
3. Chronic typhoid carriers have a six fold increased risk.
4. Intraductal gallstones
5. Bile duct adenoma and biliary papillomatosis
6. Caroli's disease has a lifetime risk of 7 percent
7. Choledochal cysts (5% will transform into cholangiocarcinoma)
8. Thorotrast (a radiological agent currently not in use)

CLASSIFICATION

Anatomic:
- Intrahepatic: 20–25%
- Perihilar: 50–60%. Those involving the bifurcation are called "Klatskin" tumors.
- Extrahepatic: 20-25%

Bismuth classification:
The extent of duct involvement by perihilar tumors is classified as suggested by Bismuth and is a valuable guide to the extent of surgery required.

Type I- tumors below the confluence of hepatic ducts

Type II- tumors at the confluence of hepatic ducts

Type III- tumors at the confluence and extending into either right (3a) or left (3b) hepatic duct

Type IV-tumors involving confluence as well as *both* right and left hepatic ducts *or* multicentric tumors

HISTOLOGY AND STAGING

Most cholangiocarcinomas (95%) are adenocarcinomas. Adenocarcinomas are graded from 1-4 according to the percentage of tumor that is composed of glandular tissue (Table 19.2).

DIAGNOSIS

Clinical features
- Perihilar and extrahepatic tumors typically present with *biliary obstruction*: jaundice, pale stool, dark urine and pruritus.
- Intrahepatic tumors and perihilar tumors obstructing one hepatic duct usually present after the disease is advanced, as jaundice may occur late in such cases. They often present with malaise, weight loss and fatigue.
- Right hypochondriac pain, fever with rigors and jaundice (Charcot's triad) suggest cholangitis. This is particularly common after attempts at drainage of the obstructed biliary ducts.
- Some cases are detected incidentally as a result of deranged liver function tests or ultrasound scans performed for other indications.

BLOOD TESTS

- Liver function tests often show an obstructive picture i.e. elevated bilirubin, alkaline phosphatase and gamma glutamyl transpeptidase. Although aminotransferases are frequently normal they may be raised due to cholangitis.
- Prolonged obstructive jaundice causes deficient absorption of fat soluble vitamins including vitamin K and prolongs the prothrombin

Table 19.2: Staging		
AJCC stage grouping for cancers of the bile ducts		
Stage I	T1, N0, M0	T1a: invades subepithelial connective tissue T1b: invades the fibromuscular layer
Stage II	T2, N0, M0	T2 : invades perimuscular connective tissue
Stage III	T1-2, N1-2, M0	N1 : metastasis to cystic duct, percholedochal, and/or perihilar nodes N2 : metastasis in peripancreatic area (head only), periduodenal, periportal, celiac, superior mesenteric, and/or posterior pancreaticoduodenal nodes
Stage IVA	T3, Any N, M0	T3 : tumor invades adjacent structures
Stage IVB	Any T, N, M1	M1 : distant metastases including parapancreatic in body and tail of pancreas

time. This typically returns to normal after administration of vitamin K.

- Although there are no tumor markers specific for cholangiocarcinoma, it may be useful in conjunction with other diagnostic modalities when doubt persists. CA 19.9 is elevated in up to 85 percent patients with cholangiocarcinoma. However, CA 19.9 elevation can occur in patients with obstructive jaundice without malignancy. Carcinoembryogenic antigen (CEA) is raised in 30 percent and CA-125 in 40-50 percent of patients with cholangiocarcinoma.

IMAGING TECHNIQUES

Ultrasonography remains the first line investigation for biliary obstruction. Cholangiocarcinoma should be suspected when intrahepatic, but not when extrahepatic ducts are dilated. Colour duplex scans can detect invasion of hepatic artery or portal vein by the tumor.

Computed tomography with contrast enhancement can visualize intrahepatic mass lesions, liver metastases as well as regional lymphadenopathy. Additionally, it can provide information on the involvement of hepatic artery and portal vein.

Magnetic resonance imaging (MRI) offers good quality assessment of the extent of the tumor, hepatic parenchymal abnormalities and liver metastasis. In conjunction with MR cholangiography (MRCP) and MR angiography (MRA), it can evaluate the extent of bile ductular and vascular involvement by the tumor and is currently the best possible initial investigation for cholangiocarcinoma.

Cholangiography can be acquired in many ways and is essential for diagnosis as well as for assessing resectability. MRCP is noninvasive. Endoscopic Retrograde Cholangiopancreatography (ERCP) and Percutaneous Transhepatic Cholangiography (PTC) are invasive but permit bile sampling and brush biopsies for cytological diagnosis which are positive in about 40 percent cases. They also allow stent insertion for palliative purposes in irresectable tumors or for biliary decompression prior to surgery in selected cases. PTC is usually favored over ERCP for more proximal tumors.

Angiography is useful in evaluating the involvement of the main stem of the hepatic artery, portal vein or hepatic veins. But contrast spiral CT or MRA can provide equally accurate information and has replaced invasive angiography in most centers.

Newer techniques under evaluation include endoscopic ultrasound, positron emission tomography, intraductal ultrasound and flexible cholangioscopy.

TREATMENT

Surgery

Surgery is the only curative treatment and is possible in approximately 20 percent of proximal cancers and in up to two-thirds of distal tumors. The appearance of jaundice early in the disease makes the clinicians more alert to these types of tumors. Lymph node involvement is present in 50 percent of all patients at presentation and is associated with poor prognosis. The 5-year survival for proximal bile duct cancers is 10-20 percent and for distal bile duct lesions 20-30 percent.

Criteria that exclude a patient from attempts at resection include the following:
1. Encasement of the main hepatic artery or portal vein.
2. Bilateral tumor extension into secondary hepatic ducts.
3. Ductal involvement of one side with contralateral vascular involvement.
4. Peritoneal and distant metastasis.

The aim of surgical resection is tumor free margin of more than 5 mm.

For Klatskin tumors the Bismuth classification is a guide to the extent of surgery required:
- types I and II: en bloc resection of the extrahepatic bile ducts and gallbladder, regional lymphadenectomy, and Roux-en-Y hepaticojejunostomy;
- type III: as above plus right or left hepatectomy;
- type IV: as above plus extended right or left hepatectomy.

Distal cholangiocarcinomas are managed by pancreatoduodenectomy as with ampullary or pancreatic head cancers.

The intrahepatic variant of cholangiocarcinoma is treated by resection of the involved segments or lobe of the liver.

Liver transplantation is currently contraindicated except within clinical trials as it is usually associated with rapid recurrence of tumor and death.

PALLIATIVE TREATMENT

Endoscopic or percutaneously placed metal or plastic stents are used for palliation of symptoms relating to biliary obstruction (pain and distressing pruritus). Metal stents have a larger diameter and are less prone to occlusion or migration. Metal stents are advantageous in patients surviving more than six months whereas plastic stents are acceptable for patients surviving six months or less.

RADIOTHERAPY

Radiotherapy did not improve survival or the quality of life in patients with resected perihilar cholangiocarcinoma. There is no evidence for radiotherapy improving survival or the quality of life in advanced disease. Radiation still may have potential palliative value for painful localized metastases and uncontrolled bleeding.

CHEMOTHERAPY

There is currently no evidence to support postoperative adjuvant therapy outside a trial setting. Early conclusions from ongoing studies suggest that cholangiocarcinomas are relatively chemosensitive, with most studies being 5-fluorouracil (5-FU) based. Gemcitabine in combination with cisplatin shows 30–50 percent partial response rates. Quality of life is significantly improved in responders.

Survival benefit of non-surgical oncological intervention compared with best supportive care is still lacking. However there are many newer promising agents with optimistic efficacy and tolerability.

FURTHER READING

1. Barish MA, Kent Yucel E, Ferrucci JT. Magnetic resonance cholangio-pancreatography. N Engl J Med 1998;341:258-64.
2. de Groen PC, Gores GJ, LaRusso NF, et al. Biliary tract cancers. N Engl J Med 1999;341:1368-78.
3. Faivre J, Forman D, Esteve J, et al. Survival of patients with primary liver cancer, pancreatic cancer and biliary tract cancer in Europe: EUROCARE Working Group. Eur J Cancer 1998;34:2184-90.
4. Hejna M, Pruckmayer M, Raderer M. The role of chemotherapy and radiation in the management of biliary cancer: A review of literature. Eur J Cancer 1998;34:977-86.
5. Saini S. Imaging of the hepatobiliary tract. N Engl J Med 1997;336:1889-94.
6. Whittington R, Neuberg D, Tester W, et al. Protracted intravenous fluorouracil infusion with radiation therapy in the management of localized pancreaticobiliary carcinoma: A phase I Eastern Cooperative Oncology Group Trial. J Clin Oncol 1995;13:227-32.

APPENDIX 7

International comparison; India and five continents—AAR (ICMR and IARC.)

CANCER GALLBLADDER (MALE)

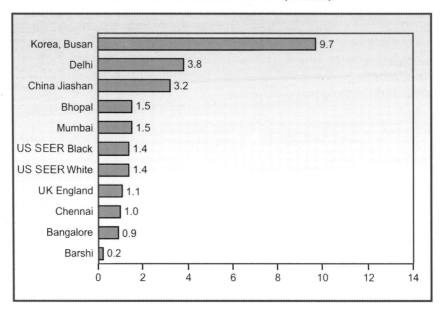

CANCER GALLBLADDER (FEMALE)

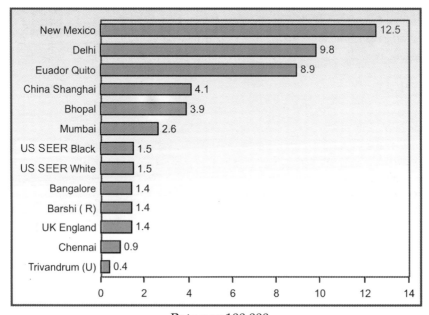

Rate per 100,000

Pancreatic Cancer

20

AR Rama Subbu, K Pavithran

Pancreatic cancer is relatively common (age-adjusted incidence rate 10 per 100,000 population) in Western countries. It is the 13th commonest cancer and the 8th leading cause of cancer death in the world. The incidence rises steadily with age and the disease is slightly more common in men than in women. While the incidence was steadily increasing earlier, it has leveled off in the last decade in the Western world. Pancreatic carcinoma is a disease with a poor prognosis and less than 20 percent of patients survive one year after the diagnosis. The overall five-year survival is only 3 percent. Despite this dismal picture, significant progress has been made in recent years in the early diagnosis and better management of this disease.

IN INDIA

Age-adjusted incidence rate for pancreatic cancer in India is the lowest in the world. The mean incidence for 8 population based cancer registries is 1.8 for men and 1.1 for women (per 100,000 population). Men are 1.5 to 2 times more affected than women. It is uncommon below the fifth decade of life.

PATHOLOGY

Approximately 95 percent of pancreatic malignancies arise from exocrine pancreas and are classified as adenocarcinomas. eighty-five percent are ductal carcinoma and the rest are acinar carcinoma, cystadenocarcinoma, anaplastic carcinoma, sarcoma and squamous cell carcinoma. Approximately 65 percent of pancreatic carcinomas arise in the proximal pancreas and are part of a larger group of tumors known as periampullary malignancies, which include cancers of the ampulla of Vater, distal bile duct and duodenum. These tumors manifest early with obstructive type of jaundice due to the obstruction of the common bile duct. Cancers of the body and the tail of the pancreas are usually diagnosed at a more advanced stage because of their lack of specific symptoms.

Cystic neoplasms of the pancreas also arise from the exocrine pancreas and are classified as benign serous cystadenomas, potentially malignant mucinous cystadenomas, or malignant cystadenocarcinoma. These neoplasms are much less common than ductal adenocarcinomas and tend to occur in women and are found throughout the gland. Endocrine or islet cell tumors such as gastrinoma and insulinoma form less than 1 percent. These tumors can be malignant or benign and many islet cell neoplasms are functional with excessive hormonal production resulting in clinical manifestations. Nonfunctional islet cell tumors are also seen and do not produce any recognizable hormonal manifestations, and are detected because they cause obstruction or are discovered as accidental findings.

RISK FACTORS

Environmental and Dietary

Up to 30 percent of pancreatic cancer is associated with cigarette smoking and the intake of food containing nitrosamines. The mechanism of causing pancreatic cancer by smoking is unknown but smoking 10 cigarettes per day increases the risk in both men and women. Among the dietary factors, increased intake of fat and meat as well as decreased consumption of vegetables is suggested as risk factors in the development of this type of cancer. The type of diet used by the Japanese with increased fat has caused fourfold increase in pancreatic cancer from 1960 onwards. In certain countries, nitrosamine is used as a meat preservative, which may be a carcinogen in pancreatic cancer.

Those patients with long-standing diabetes (NIDDM) have two-fold increase in the development of pancreatic cancer. Chronic pancreatitis both due to consumption of tubers particularly tapioca and drinking country brewed alcohol is associated with 5 percent of pancreatic cancer. In certain hilly terrains of Kerala in the southern part of India, fibrocalculus pancreatitis is not uncommon in the middle-aged men and they have five-fold increased incidence of pancreatic cancer. Increased serum gastrin levels associated with peptic ulcer surgery too are incriminated as causative factors.

Genetic

Approximately 5 percent to 8 percent of pancreatic cancer cases are associated with a familial predisposition. Several hereditary disorders predispose persons to pancreatic cancer. These include multiple endocrine neoplasia type 1, hereditary pancreatitis, hereditary nonpolyposis colon cancer, Lynch syndrome II, Von Hippel-Lindau and ataxia-telangiectasia. K-ras mutations are associated with most of the pancreatic cancer.

Occupational

Workers in chemical industry involved in the production of petrochemical products, benzidine and b-Naphthylamine are more prone to pancreatic cancer and they require yearly examination specific for early detection of pancreatic malignancy.

Clinical Presentation

The early symptoms of pancreatic carcinoma include anorexia, weight loss, abdominal discomfort and nausea. Unfortunately, these symptoms are so nonspecific that they often contribute to a delay in diagnosis by both the patient and the physician. Specific symptoms like jaundice and backpain develop after the invasion or obstruction of an adjacent structure. The jaundice is progressive and often associated with significant pruritus. Invasion of the tumor into the splanchnic plexus, retroperitoneum and the obstruction of the pancreatic duct cause severe backpain, often worse in the supine position and relieved by sitting forward. This most often indicates an unresectable pancreatic cancer. Duodenal obstruction with nausea and vomiting is also a late manifestation of the carcinoma of pancreas. Glucose intolerance is present in the majority of patients with pancreatic cancer. An occasional patient may present with acute pancreatitis or troublesome diarrhea.

Prognosis

Pancreatic cancer is a dismal disease. Patient survival depends on the extent of disease and performance status at diagnosis. Resectable tumors amount to 10 percent. Small-sized tumors with absence of lymph node metastases, and histological differentiation have better prognosis when compared to large tumors, positive lymph node metastases and poor histological differentiation. Three-year survival of node negative tumors is between 20 to 30 percent while it is only 2 to 3 percent in node positive tumors in the same period. In patients who successfully undergo a potentially curative surgical resection, long-term survival is seen in about 20 percent. Tumors with extension to celiac plexus and splanchnic nerves, encasement of superior mesenteric artery and superior mesenteric vein and portal vein have poor prognosis and most of these tumors are unresectable.

INVESTIGATIONS

Screening Test

There are no good screening tests for pancreatic cancer. CA 19-9, a sialated Lewis antigen, is elevated in 70 percent to 90 percent of patients with pancreatic cancer. However, because of low specificity, it is not useful as a screening test. The CA19-9 may have greater utility in monitoring recurrent or advanced disease.

Imaging Techniques

Chest radiographs and abdominal computed tomography (CT) preferably the spiral CT, abdominal and endoscopic ultrasound and endoscopic retrograde cholecystopancreatography (ERCP) are the common modalities of investigations used in staging the disease.

A minimally invasive tool, upper GI endoscopic ultrasound is used widely in different centers in the diagnosis of pancreatic carcinoma. The usefulness of this test is in detecting small cancers, the width of the common bile duct, mucosal changes in the ampulla, lymph node metastasis and vascular involvement. However, endoscopic ultrasound is operator dependent and the results should be carefully evaluated by examination with computed tomography. In case of a mass in the pancreas, CT-aided percutaneous needle aspiration of the mass is undertaken for histological diagnosis. This type of fine needle aspiration of pancreatic masses is safe and generally reliable. The reader must note that a negative result cannot exclude malignancy because small and curable tumors can be missed by the needle aspiration technique. Seeding of the tumors along the needle tract can develop thus making a potentially curable tumor an incurable one. The percutaneous biopsy is also undertaken in case of a tumor of the body of the pancreas, which is considered unresectable based on CT scan findings, for correct histological evaluation. Similarly the technique is useful for patients with carcinoma of the head of the pancreas, who are not surgical candidates and can be palliated nonoperatively.

If the patient presents himself with jaundice, he should promptly undergo evaluation with endoscopic ultrasound and computed tomography (CT). Both tests confirm the obstructive nature of jaundice by demonstrating dilated intrahepatic ducts. Computed tomography defines the level of obstruction, demonstrates the presence of a pancreatic mass and identifies the liver metastasis and local vascular invasion. Currently the use of intravenous and oral contrast-orientated spiral CT offers the best form of imaging of the pancreas. Magnetic resonance imaging has no apparent advantage over CT.

The next step in evaluation of the jaundiced patient is cholangiography, either by the endoscopic or percutaneous routes. Usually the endoscopic approach is preferred because ampullary and duodenal carcinomas can be visualized and biopsies performed. In addition, a pancreaticogram may be obtained, which may be important if the differential diagnosis includes chronic pancreatitis. In patients in whom neoadjuvant therapy is considered, ERCP is indicated for the placement of an endoscopic stent to relieve jaundice while the patient is prepared for surgery. Endoscopic pancreatic stenting too is done to relieve pain with obstruction to the flow of pancreatic juice.

Liver metastasis and peritoneal seedlings are the common sites of metastases in pancreatic carcinoma. Liver metastases larger than 2 cm can be detected by CT but approximately 30 percent of these metastases are smaller and may be detected on diagnostic laparoscopy.

Staging classification is reviewed in Table 20.1

DIFFERENTIAL DIAGNOSIS

Anicteric patients with suspicious lesions in pancreas are usually initially investigated for their pain by gastroscopy or ultrasonography. Unless good views are obtained by the latter, computed tomography is required for the diagnosis.

Chronic pancreatitis with or without pancreatic lithiasis may have a similar presentation, but there is usually a history of alcoholic misuse or intake of tapioca in younger days. However, the two conditions may be radiologically indistinguishable and fine needle aspiration cytology or histological assessment is needed. For prognosis, it is important to disting-

Table 20.1: AJCC/UICC staging classification (2002)	
Primary tumor	
TX	Primary tumor cannot be assessed
T0	No evidence of primary tumor
Tis	*In situ* carcinoma
T1	Tumor limited to the pancreas < 2 cm
T2	Tumor limited to the pancreas > 2 cm
T3	Tumor extends beyond the pancreas but without involvement of the celiac axis or the superior mesenteric artery
T4	Tumor involves the celiac axis or the superior mesenteric artery
Regional lymph nodes	
NX	Regional lymph nodes cannot be assessed
N0	No regional lymph node metastasis
N1	Regional lymph node metastasis
pN1a	Metastasis in a single regional lymph node
pN1b	Metastasis in multiple regional lymph nodes
	Distant metastasis
MX	Distant metastasis cannot be assessed
M0	No distant metastasis
M1	Distant metastasis
Stage grouping	
Stage 0	Tis N0 M0
Stage I	T1-2 N0 M0
Stage II	T3 N0 M0
Stage III	T1-3 N1 M0
Stage IVA	T4 Any N M0
Stage IVB	Any T Any N M1

uish malignant periampullary lesions from tumors of the head of the pancreas.

TREATMENT

The patients with carcinoma of the pancreas can be divided into three groups:
1. Resectable—curative resection is possible with postoperative chemoradiation (10%).
2. Locally advanced—treated with radiation and chemotherapy (25%).
3. Metastatic—only chemotherapy is applicable (65%).

Surgery remains the only potentially curative modality. However, it is of value only if the primary tumor is no more than few centimeters in diameter, there is no lymph node or hepatic metastases and if it is free of vascular encasement. The portal vein-superior mesenteric vein confluence should be patent. Patients may have isolated involvement of the superior mesenteric vein, portal vein, or hepatic artery, which can be resected, and vascular anastomosis established. Unfortunately only a few patients, less than 10 percent meet these criteria.

If the jaundice is of short duration, stenting of biliary duct may not be necessary; if it is more than 2 weeks old, an endoscopic biliary stent must be done to drain the held up bile. A coagulation profile should be done and suitable corrections must be made if necessary.

Suitable patients undergo Whipple's procedure or modified Whipple's (pylorus preserving) surgery. The head of the pancreas, the distal bile duct, the gallbladder, the duodenum and the distal stomach are excised. Reconstruction involves anastomosis of the pancreatic duct, the common hepatic duct, and the distal stomach to a loop of jejunum. Whipple's procedure is a formidable operation, and patients must be fit in order to undergo this surgery. A modification allows preservation of the distal stomach and pylorus, which may have long-term nutritional benefits. There are a few options for the treatment of pancreatic remnant. They include pancreaticojejunostomy, pancreatic-gastrostomy, pancreatic ductal occlusion, isolated Roux-en-Y anastomosis and duct to mucosal anastomosis.

The patients who have undergone resection for carcinoma of ampulla of Vater have better prognosis than those who underwent resection for tumors in the head of the pancreas. The 5-year survival under competent hands in case of former is 40 percent while in case of the latter it is only 20 percent during this period. The overall survival is 20 weeks and 5-year survival of either of the tumors is less than 3 percent.

ADJUVANT THERAPY FOLLOWING RESECTION

Even after complete resection, there is more than 70% risk of locoregional recurrence. This has led to many studies, however, the results of randomized trials have been inconclusive. The recently published European Study Group for Pancreatic Cancer 1 Trial showed that estimated five-year survival rate was 10 percent among patients assigned to receive chemoradiotherapy and 20 percent among patients who did not receive chemoradiotherapy. Chemotherapy consisted of an intravenous bolus of leucovorin (20 mg/m^2), followed by an intravenous bolus of fluorouracil (425 mg/m^2) on each of 5 consecutive days every 28 days for six cycles. This study showed that adjuvant chemotherapy has a significant survival benefit in patients with resected pancreatic cancer, whereas adjuvant chemoradiotherapy has a deleterious effect on survival.

Distal pancreatectomy may be suitable for carcinoma of the body or tail; but in most cases, the tumor is unresectable. The tumors are large, lymph node is usually positive and there may be extension to retropancreatic area. Total pancreatectomy and extended vascular resections are rarely advocated.

LOCALLY ADVANCED DISEASE

Another set of patients with pancreatic cancer has locoregional involvement at the time of the first presentation and the tumor is found to be unresectable. They form a quarter of the patients. The present-day approach in this group is a planned chemoradiation protocol and it has shown to prolong survival significantly. The performance status of the patient must be good so that he could withstand the after effects of radiation and chemotherapy. The commonly used regimen is 4,500 to 5,400 cGy in 20 fractionated doses of 200 cGy with 5-FU, 500 mg/m^2/day daily on the first and last 3 days of radiation. The treatment scheme is identical to those used for adjuvant treatment of resectable disease as described earlier. Median survival is approximately for 10 months with treatment. A chemotherapy protocol used in many centers consists of gemcitabine, 1,000 mg/m^2/week iv for 3 weeks (days 1, 8 and 15) followed by 1 week without gemcitabine (total dose/cycle, 3,000 mg/m^2).

Treatment cycles are repeated every 28 days 5-Fluorouracil, 600 mg/m^2/day by iv bolus injection at the end of every cycle.

For those patients with poor performance status, supportive care is recommended. The goal of treatment for locally advanced disease is to prolong survival.

METASTATIC DISEASE

Approximately half of new diagnoses of pancreatic cancer have metastasis, with common sites including the liver and lungs. Needless to say the treatment is purely palliative. It also depends on the performance status of the patient.

5-FU has been the most extensively evaluated agent for metastatic pancreatic cancer. However, gemcitabine has recently become the treatment of choice for first line therapy for metastatic pancreatic cancer. The drug gemcitabine is given on day 1 and day 8 (1200 mg/m^2) with cisplatin every 3 weeks for 4-6 cycles depending on the response. The response rate is about 20 percent. More recently, "clinical benefit response" is taken as a marker of efficacy. Clinical benefit response is measured by analgesic consumption, pain intensity, performance status and weight change, so that more emphasis is given to quality of life, even if there is no objective response.

The goal of treatment for metastatic disease remains to decrease symptoms. Gemcitabine has even been advocated for palliation for patients with poor performance status.

PALLIATIVE TREATMENT

Stenting the malignant stricture at the lower end of the common bile duct can be done by ERCP technique. This procedure has superseded operative palliation of jaundice. If stenting is difficult with an ERCP procedure, percutaneous stenting can be attempted. In certain centers, cholecysto-jejunostomy is done to relieve the jaundice and very troublesome pruritus. Some 15-20 percent of patients develop duodenal obstruction, which can be relieved by laparoscopic gastrojejunostomy. Palliation of pain and of other symptoms is best managed by a hospice with a multidisciplinary palliative care team. Celiac plexus block or transthoracic splanchnicectomy is of immense help to the patient.

FURTHER READING

1. Buchler M, Freiss H, Kelmpa I. Role of ostreotide in the prevention of postoperative complications following pancreatic resection. Am J Surg 1992;163:125-31.
2. Chari ST, Mohan V, Pitchumoni CS, Viswanathan M, Madanagopalan N, Lowenfels AB. Risk of pancreatic carcinoma in tropical calcifying pancreatitis: An epidemiologic study. Pancreas 1994;9:62-66.
3. Delcore R, Thomas JH, Hermerck AS. Pancreaticoduodenectomy for malignant pancreatic and periampullary neoplasms in elderly. Am J Surg 1992;162:532-36.
4. Dhir V, Mohandas KM. Epidemiology of digestive tract cancers in India IV. Gallbladder and Pancreas. Indian J Gastroenterol 1999;18:24-28.
5. Freboug T, Bercoff E, Mouchon N, et al. Evaluation of CA19-9 antigen level in the early detection of pancreatic cancer 1988;62:2287-90.
6. Freeny DC, Marks WM, Ryan JA, Traverso LW. Pancreatic ductal adenocarcinoma: Diagnosis and staging with dynamic CT. Radiology 1988;166:125-33.
7. Jemal A, Murry T, Samuels A, Ghafoor A, Ward E, Thun MJ. Cancer Statistics, 2003. CA Cancer J Clin 2003;53:5-26.
8. Kalra MK, Maher MM, Sahani DV, Digmurthy S, Saini S. Current status of imaging in pancreatic diseases. J Comput Assist Tomogr 2002;26:661-75.
9. Kaufman AR, Sivak MV. Endoscopic ultrasonography in the differential diagnosis of pancreatic disease. Gastrointest Endosc 1989;35:214-19.

10. Klinkenbijl JH, Jeekel J, Sahmoud T, et al. Adjuvant radiotherapy and 5-fluorouracil after curative resection for the cancer of the pancreas and periampullary region. Phase III trial of the EORTC gastrointestinal tract cancer cooperative group. Ann Surg 1999;230:776.

11. Kuvshinoff BW, Bryer MP. Treatment of resectable and locally advanced pancreatic cancer. Cancer Control 2000;7:428-36.

12. Lillemoe KD, Cameron JL, Kaufman HS, et al. Chemical sphlancinisectomy in patients with unresectable pancreatic cancer. Ann Surg 1993;217:447-57.

13. Lillemoe KD, Sauter P, Pitt HA, et al. Current status of surgical palliation of periampullary carcinoma. Surg Gynecol Obstet 1993;176:1-10.

14. Parsous L, Palmer LH. How accurate is fine needle biopsy in malignant neoplasm of the pancreas. Acta Cytol 1989;33:145-52.

15. Potts JRIII, Broughan TA, Hermann RE. Palliative operations of pancreatic carcinoma. Am J Surg 1990;159:73-79.

16. Rosemurgy AS, Serafini FM. New directions in systemic therapy of pancreatic cancer. Cancer Control 2000;7:437-44.

17. Shemesh E, Czerniak A, Nass S, Klien E. Role of endoscopic retrograde cholangiopancreotography in differentiating pancreatic cancer coexisting with chronic pancreatitis. Cancer 1990;65:893-96.

18. Spencer MD, Sarr MG, Nagorney DM. Radical pancreatectomy for pancreatic cancer in elderly. Is it safe and justified? Ann Surg 1990;212:140-47.

19. Trede M, Scwall G, Saeger H. Survival after pancreaticoduodenectomy: 118 consecutive resections without an operative mortality. Ann Surg 1990;211:447-58.

20. Warshaw AL, Compton CC, Lenandrowski K, et al. Cystic tumors of the pancreas: New clinical radiologic and pathologic observations in 67 patients. Ann Surg 1990;212:432-45.

21. Watanapa P, Williamson RCN. Surgical palliation for pancreatic cancer: Developments during the past 2 decades. Br J Surg 1991;79:8-20.

Vulvar and Vaginal Cancers

21

Abraham Peedicayil

Gynecologic malignancies account for about 15 percent of all cancers in women. In developing countries, cervical cancer is the most common cancer affecting women. In contrast, breast cancer is the most frequently seen cancer in women of developed countries. In this chapter, the various gynecologic cancers will be dealt with from external to internal structures, i.e. vulva, vagina, cervix, uterus, fallopian tubes and ovaries. Preinvasive and invasive diseases will be considered at each site. In addition, gestational trophoblastic tumors will also be discussed at the end. In many countries, breast cancers are not managed by gynecologists and this topic will be dealt with in a separate chapter.

THE VULVA

Non-neoplastic disorders of the vulvar skin were previously described as vulvar dystrophies. In 1987, the International Society for the Study of Vulvar Diseases (ISSVD) adopted a new classification system that should be accepted by gynecologists, dermatologists and pathologists. Non-neoplastic conditions were clearly separated from those that showed atypia and included squamous cell hyperplasia, lichen sclerosis and other dermatoses such as seborrheic dermatitis, psoriasis, tinea corporis, lichen simplex and lichen planus. Neoplastic conditions were squamous displasia, Paget's disease and melanoma *in situ*.

Malignant tumors of the vulva account for 1 percent of cancers in women and for 3 to 5 percent of all female genital malignancies. The frequency of various histological types is given in Table 21.1.

The average age at diagnosis is 65 years. However, with increasing awareness among women as well as physicians, the diagnosis is being made earlier and in younger women.

Table 21.1: Frequency of types of vulvar cancer	
Histologic type	*Percentage of all cases*
Squamous cell carcinoma	86
Melanoma	6
Adenocarcinoma	4
Basal cell carcinoma	2
Sarcoma	1.5
Paget's disease with invasion	0.5

Thus there has been a move away from radical surgery to more conservative treatments that minimize anatomic deformity and psychosexual problems without compromising the cure rate.

VULVAR INTRAEPITHELIAL NEOPLASIA (VIN)

This can occur at any age but is usually seen in women above the age of 45 years. In premenopausal women the lesions tend to be multifocal (multiple vulvar lesions) and multicentric (also involving vagina and cervix) and human papilloma virus (HPV types 16, 18, 31, 33, 35 and 51) is positive. In postmenopausal women, lesions are usually unifocal, keratinizing and HPV negative.

VIN is characterized by a loss of epithelial cell maturation with associated nuclear hyperchromatism and pleomorphism, cellular crowding and abnormal mitosis. If the full thickness of the epithelium is involved, it would be VIN III and lesser grades would be VIN II and VIN I. Although spontaneous remission in young women has been reported, in women above 40 years VIN invariably progresses to invasive cancer.

Patients usually present with pruritus but the condition is often diagnosed after a routine gynecological examination. VIN is associated with immunosuppression and hence should be carefully looked for in patients with HIV infection, or long-term corticosteroid therapy and in women who have had organ transplantation.

DIAGNOSIS

The diagnosis is made by inspecting the vulva in bright light. Lesions on the vulvar skin appear, as hyperkeratotic whitish plaques while those on the mucosa are usually macular and reddish. Some lesions may be hyperpigmented and multiple lesions may be discrete or coalescent. A hand-held magnifying lens is very helpful and suspicious areas should be examined again after application of 5 percent acetic acid for 5 minutes. Toluidine blue and Lugol's iodine are alternatives but have higher false positive and false negative rates. If a clinical diagnosis is made, colposcopic examination of the entire vulva and perianal region should follow. The diagnosis is confirmed by biopsy taken with a 3 mm Keye's punch or a wedge biopsy under local anesthesia. In all cases, the vagina and the cervix have to be evaluated as multicentric involvement is common. In about 10 percent of cases, VIN is associated with underlying invasive cancer, especially if the lesion is pigmented.

TREATMENT

The treatment is surgical and can be excisional or destructive. The advantage of excisional treatment is that adequate tissue can be obtained for histopathological evaluation and invasive disease is often found this way. In the older women, wide local excision for discrete single lesions and simple vulvectomy for diffuse and multifocal lesions are the treatments of choice. In the women below 40 years, lesions must be observed for at least 6 months to ensure that they do not regress spontaneously. Persistent lesions can be excised by the "skinning vulvectomy" followed by skin grafting which gives a good cosmetic result and does not cause sexual dysfunction.

Instead of excising it, the lesion can be destroyed by laser, cautery or cryosurgery. The disadvantages are that such treatments do not provide tissue for examination and that if extensive and deep, a necrotic ulcer may result and healing may take several weeks. The treated area may be painful for most of this time. In patients with extensive and multifocal lesions, laser vaporization under general anesthesia is the treatment of choice, however, great care should be taken to exclude invasive cancer prior to the treatment. Recurrence rates are quite high especially if the margins are involved but seem to be lowest for the laser. Topical 5-FU has been tried but not recommended as failure and slow painful healing limit its use.

BENIGN TUMORS OF THE VULVA

Non-neoplastic conditions of the vulva may be cystic or solid. The cystic lesions include epidermal inclusion cysts, Bartholin cysts, cysts arising from vestiges of the urogenital sinus, Gartner's duct, canal of Nuck and paramesonephric embryonic remnants. Solid conditions include fibroepithelial polyp, nevi, hemangiomas, hernias, scar endometriosis, breast tissue and Fox-Fordyce disease.

Benign neoplasms include hidradenomas, syringomas, condyloma acuminata, schwanoma, fibroma, lipoma, leiomyoma and nodular fasciitis. Most vulvar ulcers are infectious (syphilis, chancroid, herpes genitalis, hidradenitis suppurativa) or inflammatory (lichen sclerosis, lichen simplex, lichen planus, pemphigus vulgaris, pemphigoid, Behçet's syndrome, Crohn's disease) or neoplastic (squamous cell carcinoma, adenocarcinoma and malignant mesodermal tumor).

Pigmented lesions are common and usually innocuous. Most frequent is the lentigo. Nevi may be junctional, compound or mature. Raised lesions of any hue need to be excised. Acanthosis nigricans is a progressive diffuse dermatosis resembling condyloma acuminata or seborrheic keratosis. On microscopic examination it shows hyperkeratosis, acanthosis, papillomatosis and pigmentation.

The above benign conditions will enter the differential diagnosis and often only a biopsy will determine the final diagnosis.

SQUAMOUS CELL CARCINOMA OF THE VULVA

Most women with vulvar carcinoma present with a vulvar mass or pruritus (50%). Other presentations in descending order of frequency are pain or burning sensation, bleeding, ulceration, dysuria, discharge, groin mass and swelling of legs. Sometimes, the diagnosis is made in patients while they are being evaluated for VIN or lichen sclerosis. Since fear and embarrassment make women postpone seeing a physician, the majority of women would have had the symptoms for over six months.

The inguinal regions, the mons pubis, the perineum and anal region should be inspected and palpated for cutaneous lesions and subcutaneous nodules. Palpation for groin nodes is essential and the extent of the tumor needs to be determined by noting the proximity to the urethra, vagina, labiocrural folds and anus. Rectal examination should be routine and the integrity of the pelvic floor and the adequacy of the venous and arterial systems in the lower limbs should be assessed.

Physician delay in diagnosis is common because lesions are treated for condyloma acuminata, vulvar dystrophy and Bartholin's abscess. A greater willingness to perform outpatient biopsy would clinch the diagnosis at the appropriate time. Fine needle aspiration cytology (FNAC) of inguinal nodes is done only if a positive result would alter management.

Most patients with vulvar cancer have a dominant lesion that distracts the clinician from less apparent multifocal lesions. The majority of lesions arise from the labia majora (50%), labia minora (25%), perineum (15%) and clitoris/mons (10%). It tends to be indolent, often arising in a background of chronic vulvar disease. Local extension to adjacent structures such as the anorectal junction, anal sphincter, pubic bone, skin of the leg and bladder neck, urethra and perineal body is common.

Superficial and deep lymphatics from the perineum and labia course towards the mons pubis and thence to the superficial and deep inguinal lymph nodes. Decussation of vulvar lymphatic channels occurs in the mons pubis and posterior fourchette. Spread could occur to the contralateral side and also directly to the deep inguinal lymph nodes without first involving the superficial nodes.

The FIGO staging for vulvar cancer is surgical as shown in Table 21.2. Prognosis as reflected in the staging is influenced mainly by the extent of

Table 21.2: Staging of vulvar carcinoma	
Ia	Tumor confined to vulva/perineum, 2cm or less in largest diameter and depth of invasion 1 mm or less
Ib	Tumor confined to vulva/perineum, 2 cm or less in largest diameter and depth of invasion more than 1 mm
II	Tumor confined to vulva/perineum, more than 2 cm in largest diameter
III	Tumor of any size with spread to lower urethra, vagina or anus and / or ipsilateral groin node metastasis
IVa	Tumor of any size infiltrating upper urethra, bladder mucosa, rectal mucosa, pelvic bone and/or bilateral groin node metastasis
IVb	Tumor of any size with pelvic lymph node or other distant metastasis

of local spread and regional node metastasis. Clinical assessment of nodal spread is unreliable as up to 10 percent of cases thought to be Stage I and 25 percent of cases believed to be Stage II, are actually Stage III. Node status is undoubtedly the most important prognostic factor that overrides all others in Stage I through Stage III vulvar cancer. Pelvic node involvement is rare without ipsilateral inguinal node metastasis. In patients with clinically nonsuspicious inguinal nodes, only 5 percent of pelvic nodes are histologically positive. In case, the groin has nodal metastases, 33 percent of cases have positive pelvic nodes. In fact, there are two groups of patients; in one only less than 3 groin nodes are positive (33%) and in the other more than 3 groin glands have metastases (60%). In the second group, pelvic nodes too are positive for metases in 33 percent of cases.

Large lesions, central location, infiltrative lesions, lymph-vascular space invasion, poor differentiation, depth of invasion and a confluent pattern of invasion are poor prognostic factors. The 5-year survival for Stage I is 90percent, Stage II 80 percent, Stage III 50 percent and for Stage IV it is only 15 percent.

TREATMENT

The treatment consists of managing the local lesion as well as the regional lymph nodes. Traditional radical vulvectomy with bilateral groin node dissection even for early invasive vulvar cancer has given place to individualized and conservative treatment. Radical surgery is well tolerated and can be done in stages if the patient has other medical problems.

When the primary tumor is less than 2 cm with only microinvasion (< 1 mm) and without lymphovascular space invasion, only deep wide excision is sufficient.

If the tumor is less than 2 cm and lateralised but depth of invasion is more than 1 mm, and groin nodes are negative, the treatment is radical local excision/hemivulvectomy and ipsilateral superficial and deep inguinal node dissection. If the primary tumor is not lateralised, i.e. it is less than 2 cm from the clitoris, urethra or posterior fourchette, then the treatment is radical local excision with bilateral groin dissection. If the cancer is advanced, then radical vulvectomy is done with bilateral groin dissection. Treatment in these cases will have to be individualized with consideration of chemoradiation prior to surgery. Adjunctive treatment consists of contralateral groin dissection if even one ipsilateral inguinal node is positive and radiation therapy for groin and pelvic nodes if three or more groin nodes are positive. For microinvasion, a margin of 1 cm is needed and for lesions with a greater depth of invasion, a margin of at least 2 cm is required. The dissection should extend to the deep fascia or the aponeurosis of the pubic symphysis.

Complications of radical vulvectomy and groin node dissection are wound breakdown, chronic leg edema, lymphocyst, genital prolapse, stress incontinence, thrombophlebitis and hernia. Death is rare but may occur from pulmonary embolism, myocardial infarction and stroke. Patients who undergo surgery should be given prophylactic anticoagulants. Conservative surgery and the use of the three-incision technique as well as omitting pelvic node dissection when radical vulvectomy is done have made the treatment much safer.

Radiation therapy is effective against these cancers but is limited by the reaction of the normal tissues in this region. Radiation therapy to pelvic nodes or even preoperatively for large primary tumors is again becoming popular. Palliative radiation therapy without surgery is also used for very advanced cancers. Chemoradiation consists of daily 5-FU for 5 days prior to radiation as well as 4 weeks later. Radiation sensitizers such as metronidazole have been used with high dose radiation.

VARIANTS

Verrucous carcinoma is a variant of squamous cell carcinoma. It is a rare, indolent, locally invasive growth. It is often associated with HPV and lichen sclerosis. It is clinically and histologically similar to the giant condyloma. The treatment recommended is wide local excision as radiation is not very effective.

Adenosquamous carcinoma is believed to arise from the skin appendages and is composed of glandular cells and squamous cells. It is associated with a higher incidence of lymph node metastasis and carries a poorer prognosis, stage for stage, than squamous cancers but the two types of cancers are managed in the same way.

BASAL CELL CARCINOMA

This is an invasive malignancy, arising from the skin or hair follicles, accounting for 2 percent of vulval cancers. It occurs almost invariably in the white races. Patients are usually in the late 50s and present with pruritus or a nodule. It may ulcerate to form a "rodent ulcer" or have an eczematoid appearance. It is usually located on the labium majus and is less than 2 cm in diameter. Suspected nodes should be evaluated by FNAC or excision biopsy. Regional node metastasis is extremely rare and associated with lesions 4 cm or more. Such cases should have groin node dissection.

ADENOCARCINOMAS

These form only 1 percent of vulvar cancers and arise from Bartholin's gland, Skene's glands, skin adnexal glands, endometriosis, ectopic breast and cloacal tissue. Secondary adenocarcinoma of the vulva is also possible with the primary malignancy in the rectum or upper genital tract.

Bartholin's gland carcinomas are usually more advanced at diagnosis than the typical squamous cancer of the vulva. Management consists of radical local excision with bilateral groin dissection. Adenoid cystic carcinoma occurs at an average age of 42 years. It is characterized by an indolent course, late recurrence and tendency for perineural and local invasion. Radical excision and ipsilateral groin node dissection are recommended.

Paget's disease is an intraepithelial adenocarcinoma. Patients usually present with pruritus several years before the diagnosis is made. The lesion is well demarcated with irregular borders with red and white areas representing ulceration and hyperkeratosis. Some lesions are velvety and uniformly erythematous. Lesions often extend to the anus and occasionally to the vagina, thigh or urethral meatus. Less than 20 percent of cases have an underlying invasive adenocarcinoma. Patients are prone to develop extragenital adenocarcinomas and need to be followed up for this reason. Histologically, the large, clear Paget's cells form a characteristic pattern. In the absence of invasion, the treatment of choice is simple excision with a 1cm margin. If very extensive, skinning vulvectomy, with skin grafting or skin flaps, is appropriate. Local recurrence is related to inadequate excision of lesions, hence, intraoperative margin checks are recommended. When invasion is present, bilateral groin dissection should be done.

Merckel cell carcinoma is a neuroendocrine small cell tumor arising from touch sensitive cells. These tumors are aggressive and the treatment consists of radical local excision with margin checks, bilateral groin dissection and chemotherapy.

MALIGNANT MESODERMAL TUMORS

Vulvar sarcomas make up less than 2 percent of vulvar malignancies. More than a dozen histological types have been reported but the majority are leiomyosarcomas and malignant fibrous histiocytomas. Tumors tend to recur locally and have a protracted course. Other tumors include dermatofibrosarcoma, epithelioid sarcoma, histiocytosis X and rhabdomyosarcoma.

MALIGNANT MELANOMA

Although rare, this is the second most common malignancy of the vulva. It is seen in the perimenopausal age group and usually arises in the labia minora and clitoris. It can arise from a nevus or *de novo*. Most lesions are elevated, pigmented, with an irregular border and often ulcerated and surrounded by an inflammatory margin. The amelanotic variety may resemble a furuncle or epidermoid carcinoma. There are various staging methods depending on the thickness of the invasive portion (Breslow), depth of invasion (Clark), metastasis, and local extension. For melanomas less than one mm thick and without lymphovascular space invasion, local excision with a 1 cm margin is sufficient. Thicker lesions require a 2 to 3 cm margin and bilateral groin node dissection. Routine pelvic lymph node dissection is not warranted but if the groin nodes are involved, pelvic dissection should be performed. Involvement of the vagina requires total vaginectomy along with hysterectomy while extension to the urethra and rectum would require exenteration. Adjuvant interferon therapy seems to be useful. Inoperable or recurrent melanomas may benefit from chemotherapy, radiation therapy and immunotherapy.

VAGINAL CANCER

Primary cancers of the vagina account for only 1 to 2 percent of all gynecological cancers. The cell type varies with the age of the patient: rhabdomyosarcoma and endodermal sinus tumors occur in infancy, botyroid tumors and diethylstilbestrol related adenocarcinomas occur in adolescence, leiomyosarcomas occur in the later reproductive years and the squamous cancers and melanoma are common in the seventh decade. Primary cancers are less common than secondary deposits in the vagina.

VAGINAL INTRAEPITHELIAL NEOPLASIA (VAIN)

This condition is associated with HPV, radiation and immunosuppression. Almost 60 percent of patients with VAIN have cervical intraepithelial neoplasia (CIN) or vulvar intraepithelial neoplasia (VIN). Most cases of VAIN are diagnosed in women who have had hysterectomy for CIN or invasive cervical cancer. The Pap smear is the single most important test that alerts the clinician to the presence of VAIN. Annual vaginal cytology is recommended for patients who have had hysterectomy for CIN or cervical cancer. Abnormal smears are evaluated by colposcopy or Lugol's iodine. Almost all the abnormal areas are in the upper third of the vagina and these should undergo tissue biopsy. Bimanual rectal/vaginal palpation is essential to rule out an invasive cancer at the vault.

Limited lesions are excised and the defect is closed. Larger lesions are excised but the defect is not closed in order to prevent vaginal shortening. Hemostasis is achieved in these cases by packing the vagina for 24 hours.

Radiation therapy can be used but is not recommended as it can shorten the vagina and produce ovarian failure in premenopausal patients. Topical 5 percent fluorouracil (5-FU) weekly for 10 weeks can be used for multifocal disease. The vagina should be well estrogenized and the perineum protected with petrolatum or zinc oxide paste during this treatment. Patients who have been treated for VAIN have to be followed up after a week to monitor healing, to detect development of synechiae and evaluate vaginal capacity. Thereafter, they are seen every 6 months with vaginal cytology.

BENIGN LESIONS OF THE VAGINA

Vaginal cysts can be epidermoid inclusion cysts and, cysts arising from paramesonephric or mesonephric remnants. Benign vaginal ulcers could be infectious (herpetic), autoimmune (Behçet's syndrome), traumatic (pessaries) or dermatoses (pemphigoid). Benign polyps are rare but could resemble malignant conditions. Leiomyomas usually occur on the anterior vaginal wall of perimenopausal women.

SQUAMOUS CARCINOMA

The most common site is the upper third of the vagina but extension to the cervix might obscure the actual site of origin. Similarly, growths in the lower third may be confused with vulvar cancers. The tumor is usually exophytic and spreads locally extending to the underlying muscularis and the adjacent bladder or rectum. Lymphatics from the upper vagina drain to the pelvic nodes while those from the lower vagina drain to the inguinal nodes. About 20 percent of the cancers are detected by routine Pap smear or speculum examination. A large proportion of patients has had hysterectomy and many give a history of previous cervical or vulval cancer. The full extent of the tumor and its relationship to the cervix, urethra, vestibule and vulva must be appreciated before treatment planning. Biopsy is taken in the outpatient clinic and the diagnostic work up includes cystourethroscopy, proctosigmoidoscopy, endocervical curettage, endometrial curettage, chest radiograph, CT scan abdomen, renal and liver function tests. Serum carcinoembryonic antigen (CEA) and squamous cell carcinoma antigen (SCA) or CA125 may be useful in post-treatment surveillance (Figs 21.1a and b, Plate 1).

The prognosis is mainly a function of the stage of the disease as given in Table 21.3. Clinical staging is done although staging laparotomy has been suggested for medically fit patients.

TREATMENT

In planning treatment, the factors to be considered are stage, size of lesion, location, presence of uterus and whether the patient has been previously

Plate 1

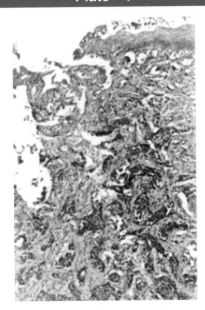

Figure 21.1a: Squamous cell carcinoma cervix: Low power view of wall of cervix showing surface ulceration

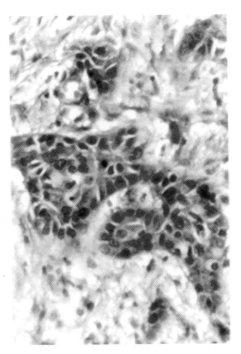

Figure 21.1b: Squamous cell carcinoma cervix: High power view with infiltrating nests of mitotically active squamous cells

Table 21.3: FIGO staging for carcinoma of the vagina

I Limited to the vagina

II Extension to the subvaginal tissue but not to the pelvic wall

III Extension to the pelvic side wall

IV Extension to bladder/rectal mucosa or beyond the true pelvis

irradiated. Combined external beam and internal radiation therapy is the treatment of choice. For early lesions, surgery provides equally good results but many of these patients are frail and elderly. Radical hysterectomy and upper vaginectomy should be considered for lesions in the fornices where the parametrium/paracolpos is not involved and coital function needs to be preserved. External beam radiation with 4000 to 5000 cGy to the pelvis followed by 3000 cGy of interstitial therapy is definitive treatment. When the distal vagina is involved, the inguinal nodes should also be treated.

Radiation sensitizers, neoadjuvant chemotherapy and chemoradiation may be used in very advanced cases. Whole pelvis radiation followed by radical surgery has also been advocated.

The prognosis for early stages is relatively good but only about 15 percent of patients present in Stage I which carries a 5-year survival rate of 75 to 80 percent. In advanced cases, 50 percent of patients have local treatment failure and 20 percent have major treatment complications. The 5-year survival in this group is less than 30 percent.

ADENOCARCINOMA

These are usually secondary deposits from endometrium, ovary, cervix, kidney, breast, colon or pancreas. Primary tumors arise from residual glands of mullerian origin. The treatment is the same as that for squamous cancers but the prognosis is believed to be worse.

Clear cell adenocarcinomas are also thought to arise from Müllerian remnants. These tumors are associated with maternal DES exposure but occur without that as well. The average age of women with this tumor is 20 years. The tumor cells appear clear, as the cytoplasmic glycogen is lost during processing. Older patients have the tubocystic or 'hobnail pattern' with a better prognosis than the papillary or solid patterns seen in younger patients. Early stages are managed by radical surgery (partial or total vaginectomy with pelvic lymphadenectomy) with ovarian preservation and split-thickness skin grafting of the raw areas. In patients with Stage I disease where laparoscopic or retroperitoneal lymphadenectomy has shown that nodes were free of tumor, local excision and interstitial radiotherapy would allow future pregnancies.

EFFECTS OF DIETHYLSTILBESTROL

The DES exposed females' risk of developing clear cell adenocarcinoma is 1 in 1000. The most common effects are vaginal adenosis, structural changes and infertility. Squamous dysplasia (VAIN and CIN) can also occur in these patients. Loop and laser therapy can be used in these women. The majority of structural changes induced by DES (cervical collar, cocks-comb, transverse septa) tend to disappear as the individual matures and has sexual activity and childbirth.

FURTHER READING

VAGINAL TUMORS

1. Granberg S, Wikland M, Norstrdam. Vaginal bleeding in postmenopausal women. Ultrasound Obstet Gynecol 1991;1(1):63-65.
2. Kim H, Jung SE, Lee EH, Kang SW. Case report: Magnetic resonance imaging of vaginal malignant melanoma. J Comput Assist Tumor 2003;27(3):357-60.
3. Long-term morbidity in children treated with fractionated high-dose-rate. J Pediatr Hematol Oncol 2003;25(6):448-52.
4. Massad LS, Collins YC. Strength of correlation between colposcopic impression and biopsy histology. Gynecol Oncol 2003;89(3):424-28.
5. Menell JH, Chi DS, Hann LE, Hricak H. The use of MRI in the diagnosis and management of a bulky cervical carcinoma. Gynecol Oncol 2003;89(3):517-21.
6. Sesti F, La Marca L, Pietropolli A, Piccione E. Multiple leiomyomas of the vagina in a premenopausal woman. Arch Gynecol Obstet 2003.
7. Solomon LA, Zurawin RK, Edwards CL. Vaginoscopic resection for rhabdomyo-sarcoma of the vagina: A case report and review of the literature. J Pediatr Adolesc Gynecol 2003;16(3):139-42.
8. Varras M, Polyzos D, Akrivis CH. Effects of tamoxifen on the human female genital tract: Review of the literature. Eur J Gynaecol Oncol 2003;24(3-4):258-68.

VULVAR TUMORS

1. Aboul-Nasr Al. Malignant tumors of the female external genital organs. J Egypt Med Ass 1961;44:809-19.
2. Barton DP, Shepherd JH, et al. Identification of inguinal lymph node metastases from vulval carcinoma by magnetic resonance imaging: An initial report. Clin Radiol 2003;58(5):409-14.
3. Crowley LV. Malignant tumors of the vulva. J Maine M Ass 1958;49(5):171-73.
4. DiSaia PJ, Creasman WT. Clinical Gynecologic Oncology (5th ed). St. Louis: Mosby, 1997.
5. Gualco M, Bonin S, Foglia G, et al. Morphologic and biologic studies on ten cases of verrucous carcinoma of the vulva supporting the theory of a discrete clinico-pathologic entity. Int J Gynecol Cancer 2003;13(3):317-24.
6. Handa Y, Yamanaka N, Inagaki H, Tomita Y. Large ulcerated perianal hidradenoma papilliferum in a young female. Dermatol Surg 2003;29(7):790-92.
7. Huang YH, Chuang YH, et al. Vulvar syringoma: A clinicopathologic and immunohistologic study of 18 patients and results of treatment. J Am Acad Dermatol 2003;48(5):735-39.

8. Jackson KS, Das N, Naik R, et al. Contralateral groin node metastasis following ipsilateral groin node dissection in cancer: A case report. Gynecol Oncol 2003;89(3):529-31.

9. Milde-Langosch K, Riethdorf SJ. Role of cell-cycle regulatory proteins in gynecological cancer. Cell Physiol 2003;196(2):224-44.

10. Miranda JJ, Shahabi S, Salih S, et al. Vulvar syringoma: Report of a case and review of the literature. J Biol Med 2002;75(4):207-10.

11. Moore RG, DePasquale SE, Steinhoff MM, et al. Sentinel node identification and the ability to detect metastatic tumor to inguinal lymph nodes in squamous cell cancer of the vulva. Gynecol Oncol 2003;89(3):475-79.

12. Neto AG, Deavers MT, et al. Metastatic tumors of the vulva: A clinicopathologic study of 66 cases. Am J Surg Pathol 2003;27(6):799-804.

13. Rose PG. Local relapse in patients treated for squamous cell vulvar carcinoma: Incidence and prognostic value. Obstet Gynecol 2003;101(5 Pt 1):1022.

14. Shihara M, Hasegawa G, Mori M. Histochemical observations of oxidative enzymes in malignant tumors of female genital organs. Am J Obset Gynecol 1964;90:183-94.

15. Vlastos AT, Malpica A, Follen M. Lymphangioma circumscriptum of the vulva: A review of the literature. Obstet Gynecol 2003;101:946-54.

Cervical Cancer

22

Abraham Peedicayil

Cancer of the uterine cervix is one of the leading causes of cancer death among women worldwide. The estimated new cancer cervix cases per year worldwide is 500,000 of which 79 percent occur in the developing countries. Cancer cervix occupies either the top rank or second among cancers in women in the developing countries. Cancer of the cervix is the number one cancer in females in Bangalore, Barshi, Bhopal and Chennai. Chennai has the highest age-adjusted incidence rate (AAR) of 30.7 per 100,000. Average AAR across various registries in India is 25.2 per 100,000 (range 17.2-30.7). Incidence rates begin to rise in the early twenties in all registries and reach a peak in the 50-54 age group and only slowly thereafter. An overall decline in the incidence rate was observed in all registries. Over 90 percent of cases of cancer of the cervix are squamous cell carcinomas. Adenocarcinomas constituted 2-4 percent of all cervical cancers. In spite of mass screening programs for cervical cancer, 80 percent of patients with invasive cancer are symptomatic at diagnosis. The reported five-year relative survival in the registries is as follows: Bangalore: 40.4 percent; Chennai: 60.0 percent; Mumbai: 50.7 percent.

CERVICAL INTRAEPITHELIAL NEOPLASIA (CIN)

This is an intraepithelial neoplasia that encompasses a continuum of morphologic changes arising in the basal layer of the stratified squamous epithelium of the transformation zone and extending to the entire thickness of the epithelium. The progression is divided into CIN I, CIN II and CIN III which are histological diagnoses.

Patients are in the reproductive or perimenopausal age group. These women may complain of discharge per vaginum or intermenstrual bleeding but the diagnosis is most often made on screening asymptomatic women.

The causes of CIN are multifactorial but sexual activity is a necessary cause. Almost all lesions have HPV DNA and it is the persistence of this infection that results in carcinogenesis. Almost 60 percent of CIN I and 50 percent of CIN II lesions regress spontaneously. The remainder either persists or progresses through intermediate stages to invasive cancer. The majority of CIN III lesions progress to invasive cancer over 10 to 20 years. The majority of high-grade lesions are associated with HPV 16, 18, 31 and 33.

DIAGNOSIS

Cervical cytology or the Pap smear has been the mainstay of screening. The most effective method of obtaining a specimen is to use a cytobrush for the endocervical canal and scraping the ectocervix with an Ayre's spatula. The false-negative rate of the Pap smear is 15 to 25 percent, thus repetitive screening is necessary for optimal results. Cytological screening has been established in most developed countries resulting in marked decreases in incidence of invasive cervical cancer. In developing countries that have the maximum number of cervical cancers, national screening programs are nonexistent due to absence of laboratory infrastructure and lack of personnel and resources. In these countries opportunistic screening of women attending tertiary care centers is all that is being done. The World Health Organization has advocated that women have at least one cervical smear in their lifetime and has encouraged countries to look toward less expensive screening programs such as Visual Inspection with Acetic acid (VIA). Cheaper tests to detect oncogenic HPV DNA may be another strategy that might replace or complement cytology.

In the Bethesda Reporting System, Low-grade Squamous Intraepithelial Lesions (LSIL) include HPV infections and combined HPV and mild dysplasia. High-grade Squamous Intraepithelial Lesions (HSIL) include moderate and severe dysplasia. Squamous cells that are atypical but not dysplastic are termed atypical squamous cells of uncertain significance (ASCUS). Similarly, glandular cells that are atypical are classified as atypical glandular cells of uncertain significance (AGCUS). The proportion of abnormal Pap smears that show ASCUS and AGCUS is less than 5 percent and 1 percent respectively. Patients with ASCUS should be treated for vaginitis or given estrogen therapy before repeating the Pap smear while those with AGCUS should have colposcopy and endocervical and endometrial curettage.

Patients with HSIL, persistent LSIL and those with an abnormal looking cervix should be evaluated with colposcopy. The cervix is treated with 3 to 5 percent acetic acid that removes the mucus and dehydrates abnormal cells and makes them appear thickened and white. Colposcopically directed biopsy of abnormal areas is done along with endocervical curettage.

Special techniques are also applicable to cytology smears including immunohistochemistry, *in situ* hybridization and DNA cytometry. The new tests for cervical cancer screening include liquid based/thin layer preparations of cells to improve quality and adequacy of Pap smear, computer-assisted screening (Auto Pap, Auto Cyto Screen, etc) to improve interpretation of smear and new generation human papilloma virus testing methods like hybrid capture II.

TREATMENT

The principles in the management of CIN are to:
1. find out the lesion,
2. rule out concurrent invasive cancer,
3. prevent progression of the dysplasia to cancer,
4. use the most cost-effective and safe treatment and
5. preserve reproductive integrity.

A cervical lesion should never be ablated without being completely evaluated by Pap smear, colposcopy and biopsy and excluding invasive cancer. The entire squamocolumnar junction should be evaluated by colposcopy or, if not visible, by histopathology of LLETZ (large loop excision of transformation zone)/cone biopsy specimens. A keratinizing lesion should be excised rather than ablated and cervical dysplasia should not be treated during pregnancy.

If only CIN is present and the LLETZ or conization has cleared the entire lesion, the treatment is complete. If the margin is involved, the lesion may still have been cleared by the fulguration but these women will have to be followed up closely. If there is evidence of residual dysplasia, then repeat conization is mandatory. However, if the patient is perimenopausal, unlikely to be regular with follow-up or declines conservative management, simple hysterectomy is a good option (Table 22.1).

LLETZ or LEEP is a simple, inexpensive, safe test and provides tissue for histopathology. A shiny tungsten wire is used with an insulated stem. Electricity cuts tissue by an arcing phenomenon that produces a steam envelope around the wire. Wire loops come in various sizes and one appropriate for the patient is selected. The procedure is done in the outpatient clinic under local anesthesia. It would help if the speculum was insulated and a smoke extractor was available. The area to be excised is examined and stained with Lugol's iodine. The loop is positioned 3 mm from the cervix and the current is activated. A blend of cutting and coagulating current is set at about 40 watts. The loop is then passed through the tissue vertically or horizontally at a slow and even pace. If the technique is correct, there should be hardly any bleeding. The specimen is removed and additional passes of the loop are made if needed. A smaller loop can be used to remove more of the canal in a 'top hat' fashion. The raw bed is cauterized with a ball electrode and hemostasis ensured with Monsel's solution or packing. Secondary bleeding is reported in 3 to 4 percent of patients and cervical stenosis in 1 percent. Patients may have a brownish watery discharge for about 10 days and should be advised not

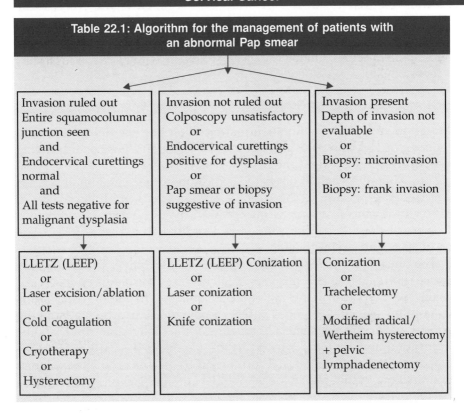

Table 22.1: Algorithm for the management of patients with an abnormal Pap smear

Invasion ruled out Entire squamocolumnar junction seen and Endocervical curettings normal and All tests negative for malignant dysplasia	Invasion not ruled out Colposcopy unsatisfactory or Endocervical curettings positive for dysplasia or Pap smear or biopsy suggestive of invasion	Invasion present Depth of invasion not evaluable or Biopsy: microinvasion or Biopsy: frank invasion
LLETZ (LEEP) or Laser excision/ablation or Cold coagulation or Cryotherapy or Hysterectomy	LLETZ (LEEP) Conization or Laser conization or Knife conization	Conization or Trachelectomy or Modified radical/ Wertheim hysterectomy + pelvic lymphadenectomy

to have coitus for 2 weeks. They are then followed up at 6 monthly intervals with Pap smear/endocervical curettage/colposcopy.

BENIGN TUMORS OF THE CERVIX

These may present with bleeding and/or discharge and be associated with abnormal Pap smears. They may mimic or mask cervical or endometrial cancer. The most common lesion would be an endocervical polyp, which should be removed for pathological examination. Microglandular hyperplasia is associated with pregnancy and oral contraceptives. No treatment is required for this condition. Condyloma acuminatum and squamous papilloma also present as polypoidal lesions in cervix. Cervical hemangiomas or hamartomas and benign mixed mesodermal tumors are rare.

MICROINVASIVE SQUAMOUS CELL CARCINOMA

Invasive squamous cell carcinomas in which depth of stromal invasion is 5 mm or less have been segregated from others and designated as microinvasive carcinoma/superficially invasive carcinoma. This corresponds to stage 1A in FIGO system. The natural history is akin to high-grade

CIN. Accordingly, the treatment can be generally conservative, although it needs to be individualized. The majority of tumors are located in the anterior lip of cervix and microinvasion originates practically always from a focus of CIN.

SQUAMOUS CELL CARCINOMA

Most patients present with abnormal bleeding per vaginum: too heavy, too long or too many. Postmenopausal bleeding and postcoital bleeding should also alert a patient and her physician to the possibility of a cervical cancer. Although vaginal discharge is a common presentation, it is often overlooked especially in the younger patient as a symptom of cervical cancer. In advanced cases there may be pelvic pain and urinary symptoms. In spite of mass screening programs, less than 20 percent of cases are early stage and asymptomatic.

The cancer may be exophytic, ulcerative or infiltrative. The cervix may appear normal if the lesion is very small or if it is within the endocervical canal. A watery, purulent, malodorous and blood-stained discharge is usually present. In advanced cases, the diagnosis can be made as the patient walks into the clinic. Other signs of the malignancy are friability, induration and fixity. Extension to the vagina is best appreciated by palpation and the parametrial infiltration by per rectal or rectovaginal examination. In thin patients, the inguinal and iliac lymph nodes may be palpable. If the uterus is enlarged, the possibility of pyometra should be considered. Treatment of symptoms without proper examination or, reliance on the Pap smear when an obvious lesion is present are causes for delayed diagnosis. Biopsy should be taken from viable tissue at the heart of the cancer. LLETZ and cone biopsy are contraindicated in patients with overt cancer.

PATHOLOGY

Squamous cancers arise at the active squamocolumnar junction from a pre-existing dysplastic lesion. Once the basement membrane is breached the malignant process is irreversible. Progression of the tumor is by local infiltration and lymphatic invasion. Vascular spread can occur from lymphovascular anastomosis and direct invasion of venous channels. If the tumor penetrates through the posterior cervix or corpus, intraperitoneal dissemination occurs.

PROGNOSIS

Prognosis is worse if the patient is old, the stage is advanced, the tumor is undifferentiated, the tumor is composed of small cells and without keratin, there is lymph-vascular space invasion, the tumor volume is large, and if the patient is immunocompromised. The risk of nodal metastases accounts for the prognostic importance of many of the above variables. Survival is almost halved if there is nodal metastasis. The site, size and number of nodes involved influence the outcome.

Cervical cancer staging is clinical since surgery will add to cost, morbidity and complications from radiation therapy (Tables 22.2 and 22.3). Investigations that can be done for staging include biopsy, endocervical curettage, cystoscopy, chest radiograph, ultrasonography and intravenous pyelogram (IVP). CT scan and MRI scan should be obtained only if they would have a bearing on the treatment decisions (Figs 22.1 to 22.3).

One of these tests should be done in cases of poorly differentiated tumors, large IB2/IIA lesions and endocervical barrel-shaped lesions. In advanced cases, anemia, renal failure, electrolyte barrel-shaped lesions. In advanced cases, anemia, renal failure, electrolyte disturbances and hepatic as well as skeletal involvement should be excluded.

Table 22.2: FIGO staging of carcinoma cervix	
0	Carcinoma in situ
IA	Invasive cancer identified microscopically and confined to the cervix
IA1	Stromal invasion less than 3mm deep and 7mm wide
IA2	Stromal invasion 3-5mm deep and less than 7mm wide
IB	Clinical lesions confined to the cervix or preclinical lesions greater than IA
IB1	Lesions 4cm or less in size
IB2	Lesions >4cm in size
II	Cancer that extends beyond cervix but not to the pelvic side wall or the lower third of vagina
IIA	No obvious parametrial involvement, involvement of up to the upper two thirds of the vagina
IIB	Medial part of parametrium involved
III	Cancer has extended to pelvic sidewall or lower third of vagina; cases with hydroureter or non-functioning kidney should be included
IIIA	Involvement of lower third of vagina
IIIB	Extension to pelvic side wall / hydronephrosis / non-functioning kidney
IV	Cancer has extended to mucosa of bladder / rectum or beyond the true pelvis
IVA	Spread to bladder/rectum
IVB	Spread to distant organs

Table 22.3: Frequency of lymph node metastases in cervical carcinoma		
Clinical stage	*Percent with pelvic nodes*	*Percent with aortic nodes*
IA	1	0
IB	5	3
IIA	10	5
IIB	25	20
III/ IV	50	30

Cervical cancer is not a disease localized to the pelvis. Even in early stages of the disease, aortic and common iliac lymph nodes may have metastases as shown in Figures 22.1 to 22.3. The chance that pelvic and aortic lymph nodes are involved increases, if there is lymphovascular space involvement, increased tumor volume or if the tumor is poorly differentiated. If the aortic nodes are greatly enlarged, they need to be removed. However, microscopic disease can be treated by extended field radiation which should be given for all patients at high risk for aortic lymph node metastases.

TREATMENT

All stages of cancer of the cervix can be treated effectively with radiation therapy. However, surgery is preferred for early stages as well as in young women. Surgery is not the primary modality of treatment for stage II b and above.

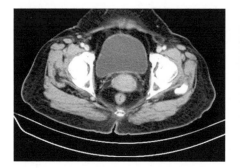 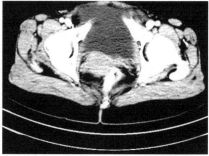

Figure 22.1: CT scan showing an enhancing mass lesion confined to the cervix. Carcinoma of the cervix: Stage I

Figure 22.2: CT scan showing a cervical mass lesion infiltrating the right parametrium: Carcinoma Stage II B

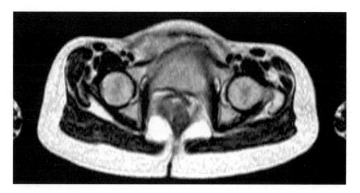

Figure 22.3: T2W axial MRI scan through the pelvis of the same patient (Fig. 22.2) confirms right parametrial infiltration

Surgery by Stages

Some patients may present with vesicovaginal or rectovaginal fistula. Urinary diversion or a colostomy may be done before the radiation. Patients presenting with bilateral ureteric obstruction and uremia should have a percutaneous nephrostomy prior to radiation/chemotherapy. Patients with pyometra should have this drained prior to radiation. Patients who have torrential bleeding from the tumor should have their vagina packed. Bleeding is usually controlled with the initiation of external beam therapy. Treatment may need to be modified in special situations such as pregnancy, prolapse, co-existing pelvic disease like fibroids, ovarian cysts, cervical stump cancer and vaginal stenosis.

The majority of recurrences occur in the first two years. Patients are reviewed every three months during this time and then every six months. After 5 years, they need to be seen less frequently as recurrence after this period is very rare. The likelihood of salvage after recurrence is determined to a great extent by the extent of the disease at the initial diagnosis. The most important recurrences to identify are the ones that can be cured namely, the central ones involving the cervix, vagina, parametrium, bladder or rectum.

Patients with a small central persisting lesion or recurrence could have radical hysterectomy. However, complications of surgery in this situation may be seen in 50 percent of cases. Hence salvage radical hysterectomy should be reserved for patients with small Stage I or II cancer. Up to 50 percent of patients with central failure after radiation therapy and no metastatic disease can be cured by exenteration. Lymph node metastasis or inability to obtain tumor free margins is a contraindication to exenteration. Even with advances in reconstructive techniques, this surgery is quite formidable and the patient requires expert postoperative medical and psychological support.

Metastases at distant sites such as bone, brain or lung are treated by palliative radiation. If the lesion is isolated, it may be resected. Patients who have disease that is not amenable to surgery or radiation therapy present a very difficult problem. Chemotherapy is often not tolerated and has a response of 20-30 percent.

VERRUCOUS CARCINOMA

This is characteristically an indolent, warty, locally invasive fungating growth that rarely metastasizes. Radiation therapy is not very effective and in fact may make it more aggressive. Stages I and II can be treated by radical hysterectomy without pelvic lymphadenectomy. Recurrent verrucous carcinoma can spread to the nodes and has a poorer prognosis.

ADENOCARCINOMA

Adenocarcinoma *in situ* is usually diagnosed in the evaluation of an abnormal Pap smear. A cone biopsy has to be done to exclude invasion and unless the patient desires to preserve her fertility, simple hysterectomy is done. Although adenocarcinomas have been believed to have a worse prognosis than squamous cancers, the same definition of microinvasion can be used. Frankly invasive cancers account for 5 to 20 percent of all cervical cancers. They may be associated with CIN and a common etiological agent like HPV. In the early stages, the gross examination, Pap smear, and colposcopy may be negative as the lesion is situated higher in the cervical canal than squamous lesions. Two thirds of cervical adenocarcinomas are progesterone receptor positive. The management of adenocarcinomas is similar to that of squamous carcinomas except for the fact that a combination of hysterectomy and radiation seems to be better than just one modality. The rationale for this is that patients with adenocarcinoma have a 30 percent chance of residual cancer after intracavitary radiation while those with squamous cancers have only a 10 percent risk of residual tumor. In early cases radiation therapy followed by simple hysterectomy is done while for very advanced cases, chemoradiation is given. Adenocarcinomas can be mucinous, endometrioid, papillary or clear cell types. Although these patterns are predominantly Müllerian in origin, rarely they may arise from mesonephric remnants.

MIXED CARCINOMAS

Adenosquamous carcinomas have intimately mixed malignant glandular and squamous parts. They form up to 25 percent of cervical adenocarcinomas and may have a poorer prognosis than pure squamous cancers.

Adenoid cystic carcinoma resembles the homonymous tumors of the salivary gland and the upper respiratory tract. Overall survival may be poorer than in squamous cancers.

Adenoid basal carcinoma behaves more like the basal cell carcinoma of the skin, slow growing and locally invasive.

Glassy cell carcinoma is a poorly differentiated variant of the mixed carcinoma. It occurs in the younger age group (mean age 41 years) and has often been associated with pregnancy. Prognosis is poor.

NEUROENDOCRINE CARCINOMA

A small number of cervical carcinomas exhibit various degrees of neuroendocrine differentiation. They are called carcinoid tumor/Apudoma/small cell carcinoma/carcinoma with neuroendocrine differentiation. They also show association with HPV. Most cervical small cell carcinomas are not associated with endocrine activity but carcinoid syndrome and the production of ACTH, insulin and parathormone have been reported. In contrast to the classical carcinoid tumors of appendix, small intestine and lung, a large majority of cervical neoplasms are histologically and clinically aggressive. These tumors have a very poor prognosis.

MISCELLANEOUS TUMORS OF THE CERVIX

Botryoid rhabdomyosarcoma, leiomyosarcoma, stromal sarcoma, mixed mesodermal sarcoma, Müllerian adenosarcoma and liposarcoma can occur. Radical hysterectomy is sometimes applicable with or without adjuvant radiation and chemotherapy. Lymphomas, granulocytic sarcomas, melanomas and metastatic tumors are rare. In metastasis, the most common sites of primaries are ovary, large bowel, stomach, breast and kidney.

RADIATION THERAPY IN CERVICAL CANCER (STAGE IA, IB, IIA)

In the majority of cases radiotherapy is the treatment of choice. The aim is to deliver, a lethal dose of radiation to the primary tumor in the cervix, parametrium and the lymph nodes in the lateral pelvic walls. The primary malignant tumor is irradiated from a source of radioactive material, radium, carefully placed in the cervical canal. The use of intracavitary radium has now been replaced by cesium 137 since this isotope is less expensive and can be artificially produced. It has the advantage of giving high dose of radiation directly to the tumor, but a low dose to normal tissues around the cervix like the bladder and the rectum. As the intensity of radiation diminishes by the distance from the source, the therapeutic level of radiation reaching the pelvic wall is inadequate. Hence deep X-ray therapy to the pelvic wall too is added for an optimum biological effect against the cervical lesion.

Modern machines like Curitron/Selectron and Microselectron are being used in many advanced radiotherapy centers. In Microselectron, the isotope used is Iridium 192. It is a high radioactivity source and a lethal dose is delivered to the lesion in a few minutes time. The total dose can thus be reduced to 30 or 40 percent to have the required biological effect. Once the required dose of radiation is given, the sources and the applicators will be removed. Certain anatomical points are identified in relation to the cervix and the pelvic wall so that maximum dose is delivered to the standard pelvic points. They are point A, point B and point P. Point A is located 2 cm cranial and 2 cm lateral to the cervical os. Anatomically it correlates with the medial parametrium/lateral cervix, the point where the ureter and uterine artery cross. Point B is located 5 cm lateral to the center of the pelvis at the same level as point A. Anatomically it correlates to the obturator lymph node or lateral parametrium.

Point P is located at the most lateral point of the bony pelvic side wall. Radiation to this area represents the minimal dose to the external iliac lymph node.

Typical doses of external radiation are 40 to 50 Gy followed by 40 to 50 Gy to point A with brachytherapy for a total dose of 80 to 90 Gy to point A. Depending on the extent of the disease, a parametrial boost may be applied to point B or P for a total dose of 60 Gy with external beam radiation.

Surgery and radiation are equivalent treatment options for stages IB and IIA with identical 5-year overall survival (OS) and disease-free survival (DFS). Expected cure rate is 75 percent to 80 percent (85-90 in small-volume disease).

The choice of surgery versus radiation depends on many factors including tumor size, younger women wishing to preserve their ovaries, other comorbid conditions, and the availability of local expertise.

For bulky (4 cm or greater) stage IB2 disease, the pelvic control, which is 57 percent, and survival, which is 40 percent, are lower than for non-bulky tumors (smaller than 4 cm; total pelvic control and survival rates are 93% and 82%, respectively) if treated with radiation alone. Adjuvant hysterectomy could potentially improve these statistics. Based on current data, both radiation alone and radiation combined with hysterectomy are acceptable local therapy options for bulky IB2 disease. However, recently published data from the GOG study, support addition of (weekly) cisplatin (40 mg/m^2 for up to six doses) to radiotherapy followed by hysterectomy, because it reduces recurrence and death rate in this patient population. The use of adjuvant hysterectomy remains controversial in disease of smaller than 4 cm IB2 disease.

Postradiation surgery may be a consideration in patients with residual tumor confined to the cervix or in patients with suboptimal brachytherapy due to vaginal anatomy (Table 22.4).

POSTOPERATIVE PELVIC IRRADIATION

Postoperative pelvic irradiation (with or without chemotherapy) after radical hysterectomy and bilateral pelvic lymph node dissection is applied to patients with negative pelvic nodes who are at risk of pelvic metastasis (primary tumor greater than 4 cm, outer third cervical stromal invasion, lymph-vascular space invasion, close vaginal margins). This provides reduction in recurrence rate and improved survival.

It is also recommended for patients with positive pelvic nodes, as this was shown to reduce pelvic metastasis rates by 25 percent. However, radiation therapy alone did not improve survival compared with surgery.

Radiation doses used are 45 to 50 Gy by external pelvic radiation, with boosts given to specific sites (as needed) either with external beam, intra-cavitary, or interstitial radiation.

The advantage of radiation is that it can be applied to all patients while the disadvantages are 0-1 percent operative mortality in the case of intracavitary application, 2-6 percent serious bladder/bowel damage,

Table 22.4: Surgery by stages

Stage I A1:	If the woman is young and desires to preserve fertility, conization of the cervix would be sufficient as long as there is no lymphovascular space involvement and the cone margins are free. For the older woman who has completed her family, simple hysterectomy would be the better option.
Stage I A2:	If the woman has no children and wants to retain her fertility then, radical vaginal trachelectomy with curettage is done. Given the increased risk of lymphatic spread, a modified radical hysterectomy with pelvic lymphadenectomy is the best option for women who have at least one child.
Stage I B1, I B2 and II A:	Radical hysterectomy with pelvic lymphadenectomy is the best option. For debilitated women who are at high risk for surgery, radiation therapy is the alternative. In patients with very bulky tumors, neoadjuvant chemotherapy with cisplatin and vincristine is given prior to surgery. In patients with bulky tumors receiving radiation, concomitant chemotherapy should be given (chemoradiation).
Stage IIB to IVA:	Radiation is by far the best treatment. External beam radiotherapy is followed by intracavitary radiation. Computerized treatment planning, after-loading techniques and megavoltage machines are some of the technological advances that have made radiation therapy safe, precise and effective. Patients with large aortic and common iliac nodes should have these removed prior to radiation. The radiation therapy field should be extended to one nodal group above the highest level of known metastases. Radiation sensitizers such as cisplatin (50 mg weekly) or 5-fluorouracil are used routinely along with external-beam pelvic irradiation. Concurrent chemoradiotherapy has been found to increase overall survival. Patients with persistent disease following radiation should have adjuvant hysterectomy.
Stage IVB:	There is no standard chemotherapy treatment for patients with stage IVB cervical cancer that provides significant palliation. Chemotherapeutic agents that are useful in this setting are cisplatin, ifosfamide or paclitaxel and its combinations.

destruction of ovary function, vaginal stenosis, and sexual dysfunction, especially common in postmenopausal women.

SPECIAL CONSIDERATION

Patients with suspected or confirmed para-aortic nodal disease should receive extended-field radiation encompassing pelvic and para-aortic areas. Current data confirm survival advantage (in stage IB, larger than 4 cm, IIA, IIB) with addition of external beam para-aortic radiation over external beam pelvic irradiation alone. Some patients with small-volume disease in para-aortic lymph nodes and controllable pelvic disease can potentially be cured. However, in gross para-aortic disease, the role of radiation is limited, as tolerance of surrounding organs (bowel, kidney, spinal cord) precludes delivery of adequately high radiation doses.

Toxicity from para-aortic lymph node radiation is somewhat greater than that in pelvic radiation alone, but is seen mostly in patients with prior abdominopelvic surgery.

Different surgical techniques alter the rate of complications (e.g., extra-peritoneal lymph node sampling led to fewer complications than seen in transperitoneal approach).

STAGE IIB, III, IVA

The role of surgery as a curative treatment decreases when tumor spreads beyond the cervix and vaginal fornices. Patients presenting with tumors at these stages are treated with radiation therapy plus chemotherapy, where brachytherapy is given for central pelvic disease and external beam radiation is provided for lateral parametrial and pelvic nodal diseases. Chemotherapy used is weekly cisplatin chemotherapy combined with radiation.

For patients without para-aortic lymph node involvement, external beam pelvic radiation of 45 to 50 Gy is followed by brachytherapy with 40 to 50 Gy to point A for a total dose of 80 to 90 Gy (applies to stages IB2-IVA). Patients with para-aortic lymph nodes involved will benefit from extended-field radiation covering para-aortic area.

FURTHER READING

1. Elkas J. Farias-Eisner R. Cancer of the uterine cervix. Curr Opin Obstet Gynecol 1998;10:47-50.
2. Hoskins WJ, Perez CA, Young RC. Principles and Practice of Gynecologic Oncology (2nd ed) Philadelphia: Lippincott-Raven, 1997.
3. Keys H, Bundy B. Cisplatin, radiation, and adjuvant hysterectomy compared with radiation and adjuvant hysterectomy for bulky stage IB crevical cancer. N Engl J Med 1999;340:1154-61.
4. Morris M, Eifel PJ, Lu J. Pelvic radiation with concurrent chemotherapy compared with pelvic and para-aortic radiation for high risk cervical cancer. N Engl J Med 1999;340:1137-43.
5. Orr JW. Cervical cancer. Surg Oncol Clin North Am 1998;7:299-317.
6. Rose P, Bundy B, Watkins E. Concurrent cisplatin-based radiotherapy and chemotherapy for locally advanced cervical cancer. N Engl J Med 1999;340:1144-53.
7. Sabbatini P, Aghajanian C, Spriggs D. Chemotherapy in gynecological cancer. Curr Opin Oncol 1998;10:429-33.
8. Shanta V, Krishnamurthi S, Gajalakshmi CK, et al. Epidemiology of cancer of the cervix: global and national perspective. J Indian Med Assoc 2000;98:49-52.

APPENDIX 8

International comparison; India and five continents—AAR (ICMR and IARC).

CANCER CERVIX

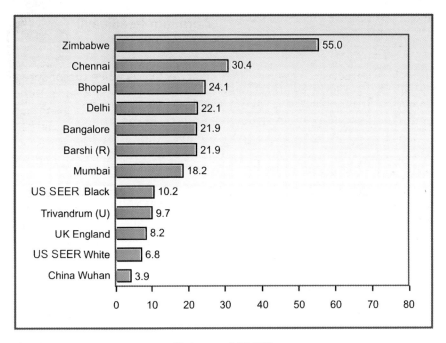

Rate per 100,000

Gestational Trophoblastic Disease

23

Abraham Peedicayil

Tumors of the placental trophoblast are collectively called Gestational Trophoblastic Neoplasia (GTN). GTNs are rare but highly curable tumors arising from the products of conception in the uterus. GTN is a clinical spectrum extending from the benign hydatidiform mole at one end to the highly malignant choriocarcinoma at the other end. The other distinct forms are invasive mole (chorioadenoma destruens) and placental site trophoblastic tumor. GTN is more frequent in South-East Asia, India and Africa, and rare in European and North American populations. In the United States, the frequency of GTN was 1.08 per 1000 pregnancies compared to 9.93 in Indonesia and 6.67 per 1000 pregnancies in China. The prevalence rate is much higher in the state of Kerala, India, than in other parts of the world (12 per 1000 deliveries). High incidence of GTN in some populations has been attributed to nutritional and socioeconomic factors.

HYDATIDIFORM MOLE

This term is derived from the Latin word *'hydatis'*-'watery vesicle' or 'moles' which means a shapeless mass. It is also called a molar pregnancy. Previously the rate of occurrence of molar pregnancies was described as a ratio of the number of viable deliveries. However, it is best to state it as a proportion of the total number of pregnancies. Hospital-based statistics are prone to referral bias and hence, importance should be given only to population-based data.

The risk for molar pregnancy increases if maternal age is less than 20 or more than 40 years. If a woman has had one molar pregnancy, the risk of another one in a subsequent gestation is 0.5 to 2.5 percent. After two molar pregnancies the risk of a third one is 30 percent. Other reported risk factors are a low protein and low folate diet, professional occupation, artificial insemination, consanguinity and nulliparity. A molar pregnancy is caused by the fertilization of an anucleate ovum by one or more sperms. This may be enhanced by factors that affect the quality of the gametes.

A complete mole is characterized by gross vesicular swelling of all the placental villi. The embryo is invariably absent on gross and microscopic examination. The partial mole is invariably associated with an embryo or fetus, cord and membranes. The hydropic swelling of the villi is focal and less pronounced. The differences between these two forms of molar pregnancy are presented in Table 23.1.

The complete mole is composed of chromosomes that are of paternal origin. The 46 XX complete mole results from reduplication of a single haploid (23 X) sperm within the ovum, while the 46 XY mole originates from two separate sperms, one with 23 X and the other with 23 Y chromosomes. The triploid partial moles contain two sets of paternal and one set of maternal chromosomes. Partial moles that are associated with a live born infant may have one set of paternal and two sets of maternal chromosomes.

Patients present with amenorrhea and bleeding per vaginum. They may also have hyperemesis or give a history of passing vesicles. On physical examination, the uterus is usually larger than 12 weeks of gestation and inappropriate for gestational age. There may be bilateral theca-lutein cysts of the ovaries. The diagnosis is confirmed by ultrasound examination that reveals a honeycomb or snowstorm appearance inside the uterus. The fetus will be absent in a complete mole whereas in a partial mole or a twin gestation with a complete mole there would be a fetus. The latter two can be differentiated by placental biopsy that will show triploidy in a partial mole. The main differential diagnosis would be a "missed abortion" or intrauterine fetal demise and an ovarian neoplasm. The serum β–hCG levels are usually above 100,000 mIU/ml.

Table 23.1: Clinicopathologic characteristics of complete and partial moles		
Feature	*Complete mole*	*Partial mole*
Synonym	Classic, true	Incomplete
Villi	All are hydropic	Crinkled, focally hydropic
Trophoblast	Cyto and syncytial hyperplasia	Focal mild syncytial hyperplasia
Embryo survival to term	Dies very early, may survive to term	Usually dies by 9 weeks
Capillaries	No fetal blood cells	Fetal blood cells present
Gestational age	8-12 weeks	10-24 weeks
Serum hCG	> 50,000 mIU/ml	< 50,000 mIU/ml
Uterine size	Small for dates 33% Large for dates 33%	Small for dates 65% Large for dates 10%
Karyotype	95% are 46 XX	90% Triploid
Malignant potential	15-25%	5-10%

Patients may have anemia from chronic blood loss, early onset pre-eclampsia, hyperthyroidism, high output cardiac failure, torrential hemorrhage and trophoblastic embolization. A dramatic life-threatening complication is acute pulmonary insufficiency that usually occurs a few hours after evacuation of the uterus. This may be due to pulmonary edema as a result of cardiac dysfunction or excessive fluid administration. The condition can be aggravated by hyperthyroidism and trophoblastic embolization to the pulmonary vasculature.

A molar pregnancy should be terminated by suction evacuation. If there is active bleeding, an oxytocin drip is begun while waiting for the operation theater to be prepared. Hysterotomy, oxytocin induction and prostaglandin therapy are reserved for the patient with a mole and a fetus. Suction evacuation is carried out under general anesthesia and at least two pints of blood cross-matched must be made available. A central line is helpful in fluid management. Following suction evacuation, sharp curettage is performed to ensure that the uterine cavity is in fact empty. Rh antigen is present on trophoblasts, hence Rh negative patients who are not sensitized should be given Rh immunoglobulin. Prophylactic chemotherapy to cover the evacuation or primary hysterectomy is not recommended.

INVASIVE MOLE AND CHORIOCARCINOMA

Clinically, these are clubbed together as persistent trophoblastic disease (PTD). In 5 to 10 percent of all molar pregnancies, trophoblastic tissue invades the myometrium. This diagnosis can be made with certainty only at hysterectomy. The tumor can penetrate the full thickness of the uterine wall and cause serious hemorrhage into the broad ligament or peritoneal cavity. It may be associated with trophoblastic embolization to the vagina or lungs.

In 3 to 5 percent of cases, choriocarcinoma develops. This is a highly malignant tumor that spreads through blood vessels. Metastases usually occur, in decreasing order of frequency, to lung, vagina, cervix, vulva, brain, liver, kidney and gastrointestinal tract. It can even spread to the fetus.

Patients present with symptoms that reflect the organs involved such as vaginal bleeding, hemoptysis, convulsions and hematuria. Thus, choriocarcinoma is a great imitator of other disease processes. The antecedent pregnancy is a hydatidiform mole in 50 percent of the cases, abortion in 25 percent and ectopic pregnancy in about 23 percent. Choriocarcinoma follows a term gestation once in 40,000 cases. In a patient with delayed postpartum bleeding or any atypical postpartum illness, serum β–hCG levels should be tested to exclude a choriocarcinoma.

PLACENTAL SITE TROPHOBLASTIC TUMOR

Placental site trophoblastic tumor (PSTT) is very rare. It is an unusual variant of gestational trophoblastic neoplasia usually confined to the uterus, although 10 percent of patients have metastases. Patients are around 30 years old and present with vaginal bleeding after an amenorrhea of variable duration. The uterus is 8 to 16 weeks in size however, the serum β–hCG may be normal or slightly elevated (< 3000 mIU/ml). The tumor grows in a polypoid fashion filling the uterine cavity or extensively infiltrating the myometrium. It is composed of round mononuclear intermediate trophoblast cells.

SURVEILLANCE AFTER A MOLAR PREGNANCY

In patients with risk factors such as postevacuation bleeding, uterus larger than 20 weeks in size, large theca-lutein cysts, postevacuation acute pulmonary insufficiency and serum β–hCG levels over 100,000 mIU/ml, the risk of persistent trophoblastic disease is 50 to 75 percent. In patients without any risk factor the risk is around 4 percent. Thus, every patient should be followed up after a molar pregnancy.

Serial β–hCG estimations are the most important part of surveillance. All patients should be asked about vaginal bleeding and hemoptysis and examined vaginally a week after evacuation at which time blood is also taken for β–hCG estimation. Serum β–hCG is then taken at weekly intervals initially till the regression pattern is normal and then fortnightly. Once levels are normal (< 5 mIU/ml), it is repeated every month for at least 6 months to complete the follow-up. If there is any abnormality in the regression of β–hCG or lutein cysts, patients are not released from medical supervision for 12 months. Patients are advised not to become pregnant and given oral contraceptive pills early in the follow-up period (after 3 weeks).

The WHO criteria for starting treatment for GTN are:
1. serum β-hCG > 20,000 mIU/ml more than 4 weeks after evacuation
2. progressively increasing levels of serum β-hCG in the absence of another pregnancy
3. histologic evidence of choriocarcinoma
4. metastases.

A more liberal attitude to starting treatment exists in several parts of the world where post-evacuation bleeding in spite of complete evacuation, plateau of serum b-hCG levels and, persistently high levels beyond 12 weeks are taken as evidence for GTN.

MANAGEMENT OF GTN

The staging work up would include a complete history and physical examination, chest radiograph, abdominal and pelvic ultrasonograms, serum β–hCG, liver and renal function test, urine microscopy, complete blood count, platelet count and CT or MRI of the brain. CT of the thorax and abdomen, in selected patients, can also be done to rule out metastasis that might otherwise be missed.

Although there are several staging systems available, the most useful is the WHO/Charing Cross Hospital prognostic scoring system shown in Table 23.2.

CHEMOTHERAPY IN GTD

All cases of low risk nonmetastatic GTN are considered to be curable. Single agent therapy with methotrexate can achieve primary remission in 90 percent of cases. Drug resistance or toxicity may warrant a change of therapy in the remaining with an overall cure rate of 99.5 percent. There are several regimens for single agent chemotherapy. In patients who have abnormal β–hCG regression after evacuation of a molar pregnancy, 40 mg/m^2 methotrexate can be given intramuscularly every week in the outpatient clinic till three weekly serum β–hCG levels are normal. Alternative regimens are the 5 day methotrexate (16 mg/m^2) or actinomycin D (10-13 µg/kg/m^2) repeated every fortnight (9 day gap), methotrexate (1 mg/kg) and folinic acid rescue (0.1 mg/kg) and, actinomycin D (10-13 µg/m^2) IV push every 2 weeks (Table 23.3). Before

Table 23.2: WHO scoring system based on prognostic factors				
Prognostic factor	*0*	*1*	*2*	*4*
Age (years)	< 39	> 39		
Antecedent pregnancy	Mole	Abortion	Term	
Interval to start chemo-therapy (months)	< 4	4-6	7-12	>12
Serum β-hCG (mIU/ml)	< 1000	1000-10,000	10,000-100,000	>100,000
Blood group (female × male)	O × A,	A × O	B, AB	
Largest tumor mass (cm)	3-5	> 5		
Site of metastasis	Lung, vagina	Spleen, kidney	GI tract, liver	Brain
Number of metastases	1-3	4-8	> 8	
Prior chemotherapy	Single	Two or more		
Low Risk: Total score of 4 or less	Medium risk: 5-7	High risk: 8 or more		

Table 23.3: MAC regimen for poor prognosis metastatic GTN	
Methotrexate	0.3 mg/kg/day IV on days 1-5
Actinomycin D	8-10 µg /kg/day IV on days 1-5
Cyclophosphamide	3-5 mg/kg/day IV on days 1-5

each course, complete blood counts, creatinine and liver function should be checked. When the β–hCG fails to drop significantly during two consecutive treatment courses or if it takes more than 8 weeks to induce remission, a change of chemotherapy is necessary. If the family is complete, then hysterectomy should be done as primary therapy or later if drug resistance occurs. About 10 percent of patients develop drug resistance and will require combination chemotherapy.

Patients with a moderate risk score (5 to 7) are best treated by combination therapy. Regimens available are:

1. EMA-CO,
2. methotrexate 0.4 mg/kg/day and actinomycin D 10 to 13 µg/kg/day i.v. for 5 days every three weeks, and
3. MAC.

Three courses of chemotherapy are given after the hCG level becomes less than 5 mIU/ml.

Patients with a high risk score (8 or more) should be given combination chemotherapy. MAC and CHAMOCA regimens give a 75 percent remission while Newlands et al reported a 93 percent success rate with the EMA-CO regimen, which has now become the standard of therapy. Pregnancy should be avoided for two years after remission (Table 23.4).

If brain metastases present, radiation therapy is given concurrently with the MAC regimen. If the EMA-CO regimen is used, then the dose of methotrexate is increased to 1 gm/m^2 and the folinic acid rescue is given for 9 doses. In addition, intrathecal methotrexate, 15 mg, is given on day 8. If response is only partial, then cisplatin 75 mg/m^2 and etoposide 150 mg/m^2 are given on day 8 instead of cyclophosphamide and oncovin.

The patients who fail on the above regimens can be salvaged with cisplatin, bleomycin, viniblastine (or doxorubicin) and etoposide. When

Table 23.4: EMA-CO regimen for high-risk GTN	
Etoposide	100 mg/m^2 IV over 30 minutes on day 1 and 2
Methotrexate	300 mg/m^2 IV infusion over 6 hours on day 1
Actinomycin D	0.5 mg IV push on day 1 and 2
Folinic acid	15 mg orally every 6 hours beginning 24 hours after methotrexate
Cyclophosphamide	600 mg/m^2 IV infusion over 2 hours on day 8
Vincristine (Oncovin)	1 mg/m^2 IV push on day 8

there are isolated drug-resistant foci of tumor, surgical extirpation along with chemotherapy or radiation may be beneficial. Most intracranial metastatic foci occur in superficial neurosurgically accessible sites. Hysterectomy, partial pneumonectomy or partial liver resection could salvage patients with drug-resistant disease.

The prognosis for high-risk GTN is about 70 percent cure. Many of these patients do get pregnant once they are cured. Death is usually due to delayed diagnosis or inappropriate therapy and development of drug resistance. The treatment has to be done in a specialized center that can handle the complications of high-dose antineoplastic therapy since life-threatening neutropenia occasionally occurs.

FURTHER READING

1. Berek JS, Hacker NF (Eds). Practical Gynecologic Oncology (3rd ed). Philadelphia: Lippincott, Williams and Wilkins, 2000.
2. Di Cintio E, Parazzini F, Rosa C, et al. The epidemiology of gestational trophoblastic disease. Gen Diagn Pathol 1997;143:103-08.
3. Di Saia PJ, Creasman WT. Clinical Gynecologic Oncology (5th ed). St Louis: Mosby, 1997.
4. Kendall A, Gillmore R, Newlands E. Chemotherapy for trophoblastic disease: Current standards. Curr Opin Obstet Gynecol 2002;14:33-38.
5. Kohorn EI. Negotiating a staging and risk factor scoring system for gestational trophoblastic neoplasia: A progress report. J Reprod Med 2002;47:445-50.
6. Lurain JR. Advances in management of high-risk gestational trophoblastic tumors. J Reprod Med 2002;47:451-59.
7. Newlands ES, Holden L, Seckl MJ, et al. Management of brain metastases in patients with high-risk gestational trophoblastic tumors. J Reprod Med 2002;47:465-71.
8. Papadopoulos AJ, Foskett M, Seckl MJ, et al. Twenty-five years' clinical experience with placental site trophoblastic tumors. J Reprod Med 2002;47:460-64.
9. Schorge JO, Goldstein DP, Bernstein MR, Berkowitz RS. Recent advances in gestational trophoblastic disease. J Reprod Med 2000;45:692-700.
10. Shapter AP, McLellan R. Gestational trophoblastic disease. Obstet Gynecol Clin North Am 2001;28:805-17.

Endometrial Cancer

24

Alice George

INCIDENCE

Endometrial carcinoma is the commonest genealogical malignancy in white women. Developing countries have a much lower incidence. The lowest rates are seen in India and South Asia.

ETIOLOGY

Unopposed estrogen increases the risk of endometrial cancer and progesterone lowers the risk. Therefore, unopposed estrogen therapy, obesity, anovulatory cycles and estrogen-secreting tumors are predisposing factors. Combined oral contraceptives and smoking reduce the risk.

SYMPTOMS

Postmenopausal bleeding is the best known symptom of cancer of endometrium. Irregular vaginal bleeding in a perimenopausal woman may also indicate endometrial cancer.

SIGNS

Abdominal examination may reveal ascites hepatomegaly or omental masses in advanced cases. The uterus may be bulky and there may be adnexal masses indicating metastasis or a coexisting ovarian tumor.

DIAGNOSIS

Hysteroscopy and curettage or a fractional curettage will confirm the diagnosis.

Preoperative investigations: Hemoglobin, serum creatinine, blood sugar, chest X-ray and ECG are the routine preoperative investigations. Advanced cases may necessitate CT scan or magnetic resonance imaging and liver function tests. A barium enema may be performed if there is a family history of bowel cancer.

SURGICAL STAGING OF CANCER OF ENDOMETRIUM

This type of staging was introduced by FIGO in 1988. When a patient does not undergo surgical staging, the clinical staging introduced by FIGO in 1971 can be used. For surgical staging, a laparotomy is performed through a median subumbilical or Maylard's incision (Table 24.1). Peritoneal washings are taken and all the abdominal viscera are inspected. Thereafter, a total abdominal hysterectomy and bilateral salpingo-oophorectomy are performed. Lymph nodes are sampled from all the pelvic groups and the para-aortic region. The pitfall of surgical staging is that the extent of lymphadenectomy is not specified.

Prognosis: The prognostic variables other than surgical staging are given in (Table 24.2).

Table 24.1: Staging: The staging of cancer of endometrium is surgical	
Stage IA G123	Tumor limited to endometrium
Stage IB G123	Invasion to less than one-half the myometrium
Stage IC G123	Invasion to more than one-half the myometrium
Stage IIA G123	Endocervical glandular involvement only
Stage IIB G123	Cervical stromal invasion
Stage IIIA G123	Tumor invades serosa and/or adnexa, and/or positive peritoneal cytology
Stage IIIB G123	Vaginal metastases
Stage IIIC G123	Metastases to pelvic and/or para-aortic lymph nodes
Stage IV A G123	Tumor invasion of bladder and/or bowel mucosa
Stage IV B	Distant metastases including intra-abdominal and/or inguinal lymph nodes

Table 24.2: Prognostic variables in endometrial cancer other than FIGO staging
Age
Histologic type
Histologic grade
Nuclear grade
Myometrial invasion
Vascular space invasion
Tumor size
Peritoneal cytology
Hormone receptor status
DNA ploidy
Type of therapy (surgery vs radiation)

TREATMENT

The initial treatment for all patients with carcinoma endometrium is total abdominal hysterectomy and bilateral salpingo-oophorectomy.

Postoperative pelvic irradiation or vaginal vault irradiation prevents recurrence in the pelvis, but does not affect overall survival. Patients with disseminated disease may be treated with a combination of surgery, radiation therapy and progestins.

UTERINE SARCOMAS

Uterine sarcomas constitute 3 percent of uterine cancers. Pelvic radiation may be a predisposing factor. The three common uterine sarcomas are leiomyosarcoma, endometrial stromal sarcoma and mixed mesodermal sarcoma.

Staging: The FIGO staging for carcinoma of the uterus is used.

TREATMENT

The mainstay of the treatment is surgery consisting of total abdominal hysterectomy and bilateral salpingo-oophorectomy. The ovaries may be preserved in young women with leiomyosarcoma. Postoperative radiation therapy improves local control in the pelvis but does not improve the final outcome. Chemotherapy is not found to be of benefit.

FURTHER READING

1. Barkat RR, Greven K, Muss HB. Endometrial cancer. In: Pazdar R, Coia LR, et al. (Eds): Cancer Management: A Multidisciplinary Approach (3rd ed). New York: PRR Melville, 1999;269-85.
2. DiSaia PJ, Creasman WT. Clinical Gynecologic Oncology (5th ed). St. Louis: Mosby, 1997.
3. Sabbatini P, Aghajanian C. Chemotherapy in gynecologic cancers. Curr Opin Oncol 1998;10:429-33.
4. Yamada SD, McGonigle KF. Cancer of the endometrium and corpus uteri. Curr Optin Obstet Gynecol 1998;10:57-60.

Ovarian Cancer

25

Alice George

Ovarian tumors are classified as follows:
1. epithelial
2. germ cell
3. sex cord-stromal
4. metastatic

Epithelial ovarian tumors are classified as follows:
1. Serous tumors
   Serous cystadenoma
   Serous tumor of low malignant potential
   Serous cystadenocarcinoma (40-50% of ovarian cancers)
2. Mucinous tumors
   Mucinous cystadenoma
   Mucinous tumor of LMP
   Mucinous cystadenocarcinoma (10% of ovarian cancers)
3. Endometrioid tumors
   Benign endometrioid tumor
   Endometrioid tumor of LMP
   Endometrioid carcinoma (25% of ovarian cancers)
4. Transitional cell tumors
   Benign transitional cell tumor (Brenner)
   Transitional cell tumor of LMP
   Transitional cell carcinoma
5. Clear cell tumors
   Benign clear cell tumor (adenofibroma)
   Clear cell tumor of LMP
   Clear cell carcinoma
6. Mixed carcinomas
   They contain two or more different carcinomas with each component being at least 10 percent of the whole tumor.
7. Undifferentiated carcinomas

INCIDENCE

Epithelial ovarian cancer is the sixth most common cancer of women worldwide particularly among women above the age of 55 years. Low parity and infertility increase the risk and

Plate 2

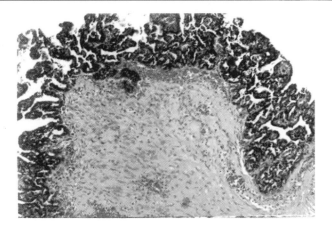

Figure 25.1: Papillary serous cyst adenocarcinoma of ovary: Low power view with complex arborising papillary structures lining a cyst. H and E × 90

the oral contraceptive pills protect against it. CA 125 levels and transvaginal ultrasound are used for screening, but their specificity is low and therefore these tests are not cost effective for routine screening. About 5-10% of malignant ovarian tumors may be familial.

SYMPTOMS AND SIGNS

The symptoms of ovarian cancer are nonspecific and include abdominal distension, bloating, nausea, anorexia and early satiety. Physical examination may reveal a hard, fixed pelvic mass, which may be associated with an upper abdominal mass or ascites (Fig. 25.1, Plate 2).

STAGING

The staging of ovarian cancer is surgical. The FIGO staging of 1987 is as given in Table 25.1.

Table 25.1: FIGO staging for primary carcinoma of the ovary	
Stage I	Growth limited to the ovaries
Stage I A	Growth limited to one ovary, no ascites containing malignant cells. No tumor on the external surface; capsule intact
Stage I B	Growth limited to both ovaries; no ascites containing malignant cells. No tumor on the external surfaces; capsules intact
*Stage I C**	Tumor either Stage I A or I B but with tumor on the surface of one or both ovaries; or with capsule ruptured; or with ascites present containing malignant cells or with positive peritoneal washings.
Stage II	Growth involving one or both ovaries with pelvic extension
Stage II A	A Extension and/or metastases to the uterus and/or tubes
Stage II B	Extension to other pelvic tissues
*Stage II C**	Tumor either Stage II A or II B but with tumor on the surface of one or both ovaries; or with capsule(s) ruptured; or with ascites present containing malignant cells or with positive peritoneal washings.
Stage III	Tumor involving one or both ovaries with peritoneal implants outside the pelvis and/or positive retroperitoneal or inguinal nodes. Superficial liver metastasis equals Stage III. Tumor is limited to the true pelvis, but with histologically proven malignant extension to small bowel or omentum.
Stage III A	Tumor grossly limited to the true pelvis with negative nodes but with histologically confirmed microscopic seedling of abdominal peritoneal surfaces.
Stage III B	Tumor of one or both ovaries with histologically confirmed implants of abdominal peritoneal surfaces, none exceeding 2 cm in diameter. Nodes negative.
Stage III C	Abdominal implants > 2 cm in diameter and/or positive retroperitoneal or inguinal nodes.
Stage IV	Growth involving one or both ovaries with distant metastasis. If pleural effusion is present, there must be positive cytologic test results to allot a case to Stage IV. Parenchymal liver metastasis equals Stage IV.

STAGING LAPAROTOMY

Staging laparotomy is performed through a midline abdominal incision. The ovarian tumor should be removed intact and sent for frozen section. Any free fluid should be sent for cytological evaluation. If no free fluid is present, peritoneal washings should be performed. All intra-abdominal surfaces and viscera should be examined. Any suspicious area or adhesion should be biopsied. The pelvic and para-aortic lymph nodes should be evaluated. An infracolic omentectomy should be performed. The treatment for early stage ovarian cancer is staging laparotomy, total abdominal hysterectomy and bilateral salpingo-oophorectomy and infracolic omentectomy. Patients with advanced stage ovarian cancer should have primary cytoreductive surgery, if optimal cytoreduction is thought to be possible (the smaller the lesions left behind, the better the survival). If optimal cytoreduction is unlikely to be possible because of bulky disease in the under surface of the diaphragm or root of the mesentery, the patient should be given chemotherapy, followed by interval cytoreduction, if there is response to chemotherapy.

ADDITIONAL THERAPY

Patients with stages Ia and Ib grades 1 and 2 cancer do not require any further treatment. Patients with stage I grade 3 and stage II tumors should be treated with three to six cycles of carboplatin and paclitaxel.

Patients with advanced stage epithelial ovarian cancer should have combination chemotherapy with carboplatin and paclitaxel for six cycles. Patients resistant to these drugs are treated with second line drugs like topotecan, etoposide, gemcitabine, ifosfamide and hexamethylamine. Dose intense chemotherapy, intraperitoneal chemotherapy, hormonal therapy, immunotherapy and whole abdominal irradiation are not found to be of definite benefit. Gene therapy has reached the stage of Phase I clinical trials.

Survival is dependent on the age, performance status, stage and grade of the tumor and residual disease after primary cytoreduction. The five-year survival is 93 percent for Stage I, 70 percent for Stage II, 37 percent for Stage III and 25 percent for Stage IV.

GERM CELL TUMORS OF THE OVARY

These arise from the primordial germ cells of the ovary and are classified as follows:

Ovarian germ cell tumors
1. dysgerminoma
2. teratoma
   a. immature

  b. mature
  solid
  cystic (dermoid cyst)
  c. monodermal and highly specialized
  struma ovarii
  carcinoid
  others
3. endodermal sinus tumor
4. embryonal carcinoma
5. polyembryoma
6. choriocarcinoma
7. mixed forms

They occur during the first three decades of life and secrete tumor markers, which are useful in diagnosis and follow up. Many patients present with abdominal pain because of the rapid growth of the tumor. The staging is surgical. Many of these patients are young and would like to retain their child-bearing potential. These tumors by and large are sensitive to chemotherapy. Therefore, the treatment consists of unilateral oophorectomy and accurate staging. The uterus and the contralateral ovary should be conserved even in the presence of metastatic disease, as these tumors are very sensitive to chemotherapy. The chemotherapeutic regimens commonly used for germ cell tumors are BEP (Bleomycin, Etoposide, Cisplatin), VBP (Vinblastine, Bleomycin and Cisplatin) and VAC (Vincristine, Actinomycin D and Cyclophosphamide).

SEX CORD-STROMAL TUMORS

Granulosa cell tumors can occur at any age. They secrete inhibin. The treatment is surgery. Chemotherapy and radiation therapy are ineffective. Granulosa cell tumors are characterized by late recurrence after many years. Sertoli-Leydig cell tumors secrete androgens and patients present with features of virilization. The treatment is surgery. VAC may produce some response in metastatic disease.

METASTATIC TUMORS

Tumors metastatic to the ovary usually arise from the female genital tract, the breast or the gastrointestinal tract.

FALLOPIAN TUBE CANCER

Fallopian tube cancer constitutes 3 percent of all cancers of the female genital tract. Their staging, spread, evaluation and treatment are the same as that of ovarian cancer.

CLINICAL FEATURES

They occur in women aged between 55 and 60. The commonest symptom is vaginal discharge or bleeding. Lower abdominal pain may also be present. On examination, a unilateral pelvic mass may be detected. Ascites may be present in advanced cases.

Spread is mainly transcoelomic or lymphatic.

The treatment is the same as that for ovarian cancer.

FURTHER READING

1. Alberts DS. Treatment of refractory and recurrent ovarian cancer. Semin Oncol 1999;26:8-14.
2. Hoskins WJ, McGuire WP, Brady MF, et al. The effect of diameter of largest residual disease on survival after primary cytoreductive surgery in patients with suboptimal residual epithelial ovarian carcinoma. Am J Obstet Gynecol 1994;170:974-79.
3. International Collaborative Ovarian Neoplasm. Lancet 2002;360:505-15.
4. Jacobs I, Bkates SJ, MacDonald N, et al. Screening for ovarian cancer: A pilot randomised controlled trial. Lancet 1999;353:1207-10.
5. Landis SH, Murray T, Bolden S, et al. Cancer statistics, 1999. CA Cancer Clin J 1999;49:8-32.
6. Ozols RF. Update of the NCCN ovarian cancer practice guidelines. Oncol Am 1997;11:95-105.
7. Rubin SC, Blackwood A, Bandera C, et al. BRCA1, BRCA2, and hereditary nonpolyposis colorectal cancer gene mutations in an unselected ovarian cancer population: Relationship to family history and implications for genetic testing. Am J Obstet Gynecol 1998;178:670-77.
8. Sabbatini P, Spriggs D. Salvages therapy for ovarian cancer. Oncology 1998;12:833-51.
9. Whitmore AS, Gong G, Intyre J. Prevalence and contribution of BRCA1 mutations in breast cancer and ovarian cancer: Results from three U.S. population-based case-control studies of ovarian cancer. Am J Hum Ganet 1997;60:496-504.
10. Young RC, Walton LA, Ellenberg SS, et al. Adjuvant therapy in stage I and stage II epithelial ovarian cancer. N Engl J Med 1990;332:1021-27.

APPENDIX 9

International comparison, India and five continents—AAR (ICMR and IARC).

CANCER OVARY

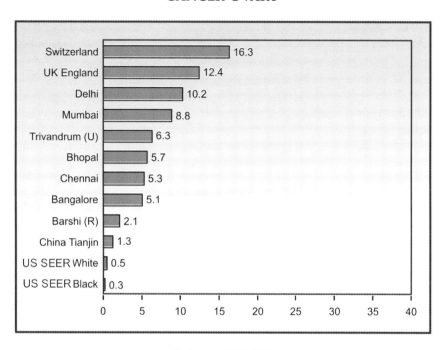

Rate per 100,000

Renal Tumors

26

Abraham Kurian
Iqbal S Shergill
Kim Mammen

Renal cell carcinoma (RCC) is a relatively uncommon solid tumor, accounting for 2 percent of all cancers worldwide. Renal tumors can be classified into primary (arising from the kidney) and secondary (metastatic), which are commoner than the former. Most renal tumors are malignant. Renal cell carcinoma is the most common malignancy of the kidney (90-95%) and accounts for approximately 3 percent of all adult malignancies. The incidence of kidney cancer is considerably higher in developed countries. It is relatively less common among Asians and African people. It usually occurs in the 4th-7th decade of life. Male: female ratio is 2:1.

ETIOLOGY

Various etiologic hypotheses have been suggested ranging from environmental and occupational exposure (petroleum products, heavy metals or asbestos) to the influence of diet (obesity), hormones (exogenous estrogens), chromosomal abnormality and oncogenes. Smoking is an important risk factor that increases the risk two fold. The risk of renal cell carcinoma is also increased in patients with acquired cystic kidney diseases that are associated with chronic renal insufficiency. Von Hippel-Lindau disease is strongly associated with RCC. Analgesic nephropathy (Phenacetin induced) also correlates with the development of RCC.

PATHOLOGY

RCC originates in the cortex (from proximal renal tubular epithelium) and tends to grow out into perinephric tissue. It may enlarge enormously to fill the retroperitoneal space. It has a characteristic yellowish to orange appearance owing to lipid content (especially the clear cell type). RCC is subdivided into conventional, papillary, chromophobe, oncocytoma, collecting duct, and medullary tumors. Conventional clear cell carcinoma is the most common histology, accounting for approximately 60 percent to 70 percent of RCC. Both papillary and chromophobe RCC are thought to be more indolent in nature, compared with conventional carcinoma. Oncocytoma is essentially benign, whereas collecting duct and renal medullary carcinoma, both accounting for less than 1 percent of RCC, are extremely aggressive tumors with poor prognosis. Transitional cell carcinoma accounts for 5-8 percent of kidney tumors and is derived from the renal pelvis transitional cell epithelium.

SPREAD

RCC is a vascular tumor that may spread by direct invasion through renal capsule, perinephric fat and adjacent visceral structures or by direct extension into renal vein. One-third of the patients have evidence of metastatic spread at presentation, the commonest site being the lung. Other sites are liver, bone, lymph nodes, brain and the opposite kidney.

SYMPTOMS AND SIGNS

The classical triad of hematuria, pain and abdominal mass is uncommon (<10%) and signifies a late presenting feature.

Hematuria

It is gross, intermittent and painless. The patient often ignores such intermittent hematuria. The patients may present with microscopic hematuria.

Pain

Pain occurs in late stage when the tumor invades the parenchyma and adjacent structures after crossing the capsule. Passage of clots may give rise to a ureteric colic.

Mass

A mass in the flank is the third most important feature of the clinical triad. However, nowadays with frequent routine ultrasonogram, RCC is diagnosed before the mass actually enlarges to a palpable size.

Fever

Pyrexia of unknown origin could be a presenting feature in 7-10 percent of patients. It is usually caused by endogenous pyrogens and is intermittent in nature.

Varicocele

Acute, non-reducible varicocele may be seen in 2 percent of male patients (left side usually). This is due to a thrombus occluding the left renal vein causing backpressure on testicular veins leading to dilatation of the pampiniform plexus.

Paraneoplastic Syndromes

Paraneoplastic syndromes are found in <5 percent of patients with RCC. Hypercalcemia, erythrocytosis, hypertension, and non-metastatic hepatic dysfunction (Stauffer's syndrome) are the common paraneoplastic syndromes encountered at presentation. Others are Cushing's syndrome, protein enteropathy, hypoglycemia, gynecomastia and hirsutism.

INVESTIGATION

Routine Blood Test

Anemia or erythrocytosis, raised ESR and other relevant lab parameters of paraneoplastic syndromes may also be present on examination.

IVU (Intravenous Urogram)

A kidney, ureter and bladder X-ray (KUB) helps in identifying areas of calcification in and around the kidney. Tumor may be identified by distortions of the renal or pelvic collecting system. It also helps in determining the function of the opposite kidney.

Ultrasound

It can pick up asymptomatic masses on routine test. It helps to differentiate a cystic mass from a solid mass. It also enables us to find the involvement of the parasitic lymph nodes, the liver and thrombus extension into the inferior vena cava.

CT Scan

A CT scan accurately reveals the size and extent of tumor, difference between solid or cystic tumor, the function of the opposite kidney (after contrast induction), evidence of metastasis and extension of thrombus into the vein.

Renal Angiogram

The classical features of renal tumor on angiogram are neovascularity, pooling of contrast media, arteriovenous shunting with premature venous opacification, puddling of contrast in necrotic areas of tumor, pseudoaneurysms, acclimation of capsular vessels.

Radionuclide Imaging

It may occasionally be useful in patients unable to receive contrast for IVU. Determination of metastasis to bones is more accurate by radionuclide scans.

MRI

This technique is equivalent to CT in staging the tumor. Its primary advantage is in the evaluation of patients with suspected vascular extension. MRI evaluation does not require either iodinated contrast material or ionizing radiation (unlike CT and angiography).

Fine-needle aspiration cytology (FNAC) is done only if there is evidence of metastatic disease and a histological diagnosis is required prior to consideration of non-surgical therapy.

STAGING

Based on the observation from the above mentioned investigations tumor staging is done (Tables 26.1 and 26.2).

TUMOR-NODE METASTASIS (TNM) SYSTEM (1997)

This system classifies the extent of tumor involvement more accurately. Distant metastases and stage grouping are given in Tables 26.3 and 26.4.

PROGNOSIS

The 5-year survival rate for stage I tumors is 75–85 percent, stage II is 65–70 percent, stage III is 35-40 percent and for stage IV it is 0 percent.

Table 26.1: Primary tumor	
T_x	Primary tumor cannot be assessed.
T_0	No evidence of primary tumor.
T_1	Tumor 7 cm or less limited to the kidney.
T_2	Tumor more than 7 cm limited to the kidney.
T_3	Tumors extend into major veins or invade adrenal gland or perinephric tissues but not beyond Gerota's fascia.
T_{3a}	Tumor involves adrenal gland or perinephric tissues but not beyond Gerota's fascia.
T_{3b}	Tumor grossly extends into renal vein or vena cava below diaphragm.
T_{3c}	Tumor extension into vena cava above diaphragm.
T_4	Tumor invades beyond Gerota's fascia.

Table 26.2: Regional lymph nodes	
N_x	Regional lymph nodes cannot be assessed.
N_0	No regional lymph node metastasis.
N_1	Metastasis in single lymph.
N_2	Metastasis in two or more lymph nodes.

Table 26.3: Distant metastasis	
M_x	Presence of distant metastasis cannot be assessed.
M_0	No distant metastasis.
M_1	Distant metastasis present.

Table 26.4: Stage grouping			
Stage I	T_1	N_0	M_0
Stage II	T_2	N_0	M_0
Stage III	T_1	N_1	M_0
	T_2	N_1	M_0
	T_3	N_0, N_1	M_0
Stage IV	T_4	Any N	M_0
	Any T	N_2	M_0
	Any T	Any N	M_1

TREATMENT

Radical Nephrectomy

Radical nephrectomy is the treatment of choice for localized non-metastatic RCC. The structures removed along with the kidney include its surrounding perinephric fat and Gerota's fascia, the adrenal gland and regional hilar lymph nodes.

Partial Nephrectomy (Nephron-Sparing Surgery)

Though radical nephrectomy is the treatment of choice for RCC, there are conditions when a partial nephrectomy has to be considered. When a tumor occurs in a solitary functioning kidney, bilateral renal tumors, a small tumor (<4 cm), and von Hippel-Lindau disease where multiple tumors usually occur, partial nephrectomy has to be considered.

Radiotherapy

Studies of adjuvant radiotherapy to the renal bed after resection have shown no survival benefit; however, it has shown significant toxicity. But one point to be remembered is that all these studies were done using older radiation techniques. Pain from bone metastasis can be controlled with radiotherapy.

Disseminated Disease

Surgery. In patients with solitary metastasis, that is accessible to surgery a combined nephrectomy and metastatic resection can be performed. In disseminated disease, palliative nephrectomy forms an important mode of palliative treatment.

Chemotherapy: RCC is resistant to chemotherapy due to the high level of expression of MDR genes. 5-Fluorouracil, vinblastine and gemcitabine have been tried with response rates of approximately 10 percent.

Biological Therapy

Interferon: It induces responses in 10-15 percent of patients. Two randomized controlled trials showed improved response rates and survival. Regarding those who respond to interferon, the response lasts for 4-6 months; at times the response can last for several years.

IL-2: High dose IL-2 induces response rates of 15 percent, with 50 percent of the responders having complete remission and most of these patients have never relapsed. Unfortunately high dose IL-2 is very toxic. Combination of cytokines has also been tried, however response rates are not much different. A variety of biologic agents are under investigation, e.g. Lymphokine activated killer cells, tumor infiltrating lymphocytes and dendritic cell vaccines.

Allogenic bone marrow transplantation: The fact that RCC is susceptible to manipulation of immune system is the basis for allogenic BMT. Allogenic BMT with HLA matched sibling donors using non-myelo-ablative conditioning regimen with fludarabine and cyclophosphamide has shown promising results.

SECONDARY RENAL TUMORS

Secondary metastasis in kidneys is usually a late presentation of a disease and typically invades the capsule and the stroma sparing the renal pelvis. The most frequent primary site of cancer is the lung, breast, stomach and opposite kidney. Bilateral involvement is found in approximately 50 percent of cases. Albuminuria and hematuria are frequent. The treatment is based upon responsiveness of the primary neoplasm. Patients with renal metastasis have a poor prognosis (since it usually occurs as an end stage of the primary neoplasm).

FURTHER READING

1. Fiori E, De Cesare A, Galati G, Bononi M, D'Andrea N, Barbarosos A. Prognostic significance of primary-tumor extension, stage and grade of nuclear differentiation in patients with renal cell carcinoma. Exp Clin Cancer Res 2002;21:229-32.
2. Gilbert SM, Russo P, Benson MC, et al. The evolving role of partial nephrectomy in the management of renal cell carcinoma. Current Oncology Reports 2003;5:239-44.

3. Javidan J, Stricker HJ, et al. Prognostic significance of the 1997 TNM classification of renal cell carcinoma. J Urol 1999;162:1277-81.

4. Marshall FF. Laparoscopic nephron-sparing surgery for renal tumors. J Urol 2002;168:876.

5. Martel CL, Lara PN. Renal cell carcinoma: Current status and future directions. Cit Rev Oncol/Hematol 2003;45:177-90.

6. Motzer RJ, Russo P. Systemic therapy for renal cell carcinoma. J Urol 2000;163:408-17.

7. Motzer RJ, Mazumdar M, et al. Survival and prognostic stratification of 570 patients with advanced renal cell carcinoma. J Clin Oncol 1999;17:2350-2540.

8. Parkinson DR, Snozl M. High-dose interleukin-2 in the therapy of metastatic renal cell carcinoma. Semin Oncol 1999;22:51-55.

Urothelial Tumors

27

Abraham Kurian, Iqbal S Shergill
Kim Mammen

Transitional cell carcinoma (TCC) accounts for 90 percent of upper tract urothelial tumors. Squamous cell carcinoma accounts for 0.7 to 7 percent of upper tract tumors. Adenocarcinoma of the renal pelvis is extremely rare and is usually associated with a long-standing infected staghorn calculus. Renal transitional cell carcinoma is a malignant tumor arising from the transitional epithelium lining of the renal pelvis. Patients with primary bladder cancer develop uppertract TCC in 2-4 percent of cases. Patients with upper tract urothelial tumors are at risk of developing bladder tumors, with an estimated occurrence of 30-75 percent.

SYMPTOMS AND SIGNS

Patients with renal TCC are rarely asymptomatic. Gross hematuria is the most common presenting symptom. Pain may be present and is usually dull and is caused by the gradual obstruction of the collecting system. Renal colic also may occur with the passage of blood clots. A palpable flank mass may be noted. The classic clinical triad of hematuria, pain, and mass is also rare (10%) and is usually an indicator of advanced disease.

INVESTIGATIONS

Voided-urine cytology is a convenient and noninvasive method of diagnosis, but it lacks the necessary sensitivity for diagnosing low-grade upper tract urothelial tumors.

Intravenous urogram can demonstrate a filling defect in the upper urinary tract in 50-75 percent of patients. Other common causes of filling defects (e.g. non-opaque stones, blood clots, papillary necrosis with sloughing, fungus balls) should be ruled out. Non-visualization of the affected kidney may occur in 13-31 percent of cases.

CT scan is useful in the diagnosis and staging of renal urothelial tumors. It can distinguish between uppertract urothelial tumors and radiolucent renal stones.

Cystoscopy is useful to rule out or confirm concomitant bladder lesions. It also helps to localize the bleeding side (left, right).

Retrograde pyelography (RPG) is useful when the kidney cannot be visualized by IVU, or when IVU cannot be performed because of renal insufficiency or severe contrast allergy.

With the development of the rigid and flexible ureteroscopes, ureteroscopy is used routinely in the diagnosis of upper tract urothelial tumors.

TREATMENT

Surgical intervention is the main form of radical treatment for localized disease. It consists of total nephroureterectomy with excision of a bladder cuff around the ureteral orifice.

Upper ureteral and midureteral tumors may be treated with segmental resections if they are low-grade, solitary lesions. For distal ureteral tumors, distal ureterectomy and ureteral reimplantation are the preferred treatments. In these cases, distal ureterectomy may be as successful as total nephroureterectomy.

Urothelial tumors of the upper urinary tract can be excised using an endoscope, similar to superficial bladder tumors. Electrocautery and fulguration are used most commonly in the endoscopic setting. Currently, lasers are being used for management of uppertract urothelial tumors.

Indications for endoscopic and conservative resection include low-grade tumors, bilateral involvement and compromised renal function that necessitates a nephron-sparing approach.

FURTHER READING

1. Lev-Chelouche D, Keidar A, Rub R, Matzkin H, Gutman M. Hydronephrosis associated with colorectal carcinoma: Treatment and outcome. Eur J Surg Oncol 2001;27(5):482-86.
2. Okubo K, Ichioka K, Terada N, Matsuta Y, Yoshimura K, Arai Y. Intrarenal Bacillus Calmette-Guérin therapy for carcinoma in situ of the upper urinary tract: long-term follow-up and natural course in cases of failure. BJU Int 2001;88(4):343-47.
3. Ureteroileoneocystostomy: The use of an ileal segment for ureteral substitution in gynecologic oncology. Gynecol Oncol 2002;84(1):110-14.

Bladder Cancer

28

Abraham Kurian
Iqbal S Shergill
Kim Mammen

INCIDENCE

Bladder cancer is the second most common urinary malignancy after cancer of the prostate. The peak incidence is in the age group of 50–70 years with a male-to-female predominance of 3:1. At the time of diagnosis approximately 85 percent are localized to the bladder while the rest have metastasized.

ETIOLOGY

Various factors have been implicated in the etiology of bladder cancer. Continuous contact with aniline dyes, 2-naphthylamine and benzidine used in the rubber, leather, textile and dye industries may account for significant number of bladder cancers. There is a four-fold increase of bladder tumors in cigarette smokers. Squamous cell carcinoma is more common in countries where schistosomiasis is endemic. The other factors implicated are pelvic irradiation, phenacetin, cyclophosphamide, and presence of chronic indwelling catheter or stones.

TYPES OF TUMORS

Most bladder tumors arise from the transitional epithelium (urothelium). Transitional cell carcinoma accounts for nearly 90 percent of all cases of bladder cancers. Squamous cell carcinoma accounts for approximately 8 percent of cases of bladder cancer and is usually associated with chronic irritation of the epithelium as in cases by stones, foreign bodies like long standing indwelling catheter, bladder diverticula and schistosomiasis. Adenocarcinoma accounts for 1 percent to 2 percent of cases and is associated with chronic infection, bladder exstrophy or urachal remnants in the dome of the bladder. Metastatic adenocarcinoma can occur in the bladder as a spread from tumors in the rectum, prostate, ovaries and stomach. Other types including melanoma, carcinoid and sarcoma are very rarely seen.

MACROSCOPIC APPEARANCE

Bladder cancer is more commonly seen as a papillary growth. Bladder cancer also can present as a sessile growth or as an ulcer. Carcinoma *in situ* appears as a flat, non-papillary, erythematous epithelium. When carcinoma *in situ* is seen associated with a growth, the likelihood of recurrence or tendency for invasion is much higher. Carcinoma *in situ* in bladder carcinomas is usually a poorly differentiated transitional carcinoma confined to the mucosa of the bladder.

SIGNS AND SYMPTOMS

Hematuria is the most common complaint. The hematuria is usually gross and painless. It can be intermittent. Dysuria and irritative symptoms may be present in some of the patients. Often these symptoms mislead the physician into a diagnosis of urinary tract infection or prostatic symptoms. Carcinoma *in situ* has a tendency to cause these irritable symptoms. Approximately 20 percent of patients will present solely with microscopic hematuria. Ten percent of patients present with symptoms secondary to metastasis.

INVESTIGATIONS

Anemia may be present owing to chronic blood loss or replacement of bone marrow with metastatic disease. The most common finding in a routine examination of the urine is hematuria. Pus cells may also be seen in the urine, as there can be concomitant urinary tract infection. Urine cytology to check for malignant cells should be done on freshly voided samples of urine. Exfoliated cells from both normal and neoplastic urothelium can be identified in voided urine. Larger quantities of cells can be identified by gently irrigating the bladder with isotonic saline solution through a urethral catheter. Bladder tumor antigen (BTA, Bard) is a latex aggregation assay that detects high molecular weight basement membrane complexes, which are present when the tumor cells become invasive. Studies show this test to be highly sensitive but low in specificity with a high incidence of false positives. Flow cytometry measures the DNA content of cells and helps in differentiating an aneuploid cell population from a diploid cell population. Flow cytometry detects up to 80 percent of bladder cancers. Flow cytometry is expensive compared to the much cheaper cytology. Intravenous urogram (IVU) usually shows a filling defect in the bladder. But in approximately 40 percent of the time a filling defect may not be seen, hence a negative IVU does not rule out a bladder cancer. IVU can delineate any tumor elsewhere in the urinary tract, which occurs in about 10 percent of cases. It is important to visualize the upper urinary tracts and the function of both the kidneys before contemplating any major surgery or chemotherapy. Upper urinary tract obstruction is rare in the initial presentation but suggests advanced disease in 50 percent of patients. Spiral CT scan with contrast has a similar sensitivity as IVU in detecting bladder cancers.

Cystoscopy is the most important investigation to confirm or exclude the diagnosis of bladder cancer. A rigid cystoscope remains the instrument of choice to examine the patient under anesthesia enabling the urologist to take biopsies as well as assess the bladder bimanually. A flexible cystoscope is essentially an office instrument to enable visualization of the bladder interior under local anesthesia.

STAGING PROCEDURES (TABLE 28.1)

Transurethral resection of bladder tumor (TURBT) performed under anesthesia removes as much tumor as possible and assesses the degree of muscle invasion, confirmed by the pathologist. Except when the tumor is obviously large and invasive it is wise to acquire four quadrant biopsies from the urothelium, elsewhere to detect carcinoma *in situ*. Under anesthesia bimanual examination of the bladder tumor before and after TURBT allows for assessment of the tumor size and contiguous invasion. A CT scan of the abdomen will be valuable in assessing the pelvis and abdomen for nodal involvement (> 2 cm) and determine the extent of local invasion of the tumor. Any liver metastasis may also be detected. An MRI may be superior to CT scan in detecting muscle invasion. Chest X-ray, bone scan, alkaline phosphatase and liver function tests are useful in diagnosing metastatic disease.

Table 28.1: The TNM staging system of bladder carcinoma is steadily gaining popularity over the older Jewett classification	
Bladder cancer-TNM staging system	
T_0	No tumor
T_{is}	Carcinoma in situ
T_a	Papillary non-invasive
T_1	Submucosal invasion
T_2	Superficial muscle invasion
T_{3a}	Deep muscle invasion
T_{3b}	Perivesical fat invasion
T_4	Invasion of contiguous organs
N_1	Single node < 2 cm
N_2	Multiple < 5 cm / single 2-5 cm
N_3	Node > 5 cm
M_0	No distant metastasis
M_1	Distant metastasis

TREATMENT

Further treatment primarily depends upon whether the tumor is muscle invasive or not. Superficial transitional carcinoma (not involving the muscle layer) has a tendency for recurrence mainly in the first year following resection. Intravesical chemotherapy following TURBT may help reduce further recurrence. "Intravesical BCG Instillation" has been used successfully with a good response. The mechanism of action of BCG against bladder cancer is not well understood, but it appears to be immunologically based because interleukin-1, interleukin-2 and tumor necrosis factor have been found in the urine of patients who responded to the treatment. 120 mg of BCG dissolved in 100 ml of normal saline solution is instilled into the bladder via a urethral catheter. The patient retains the solution for about 2 hours. BCG is instilled weekly for six weeks. Following the primary instillation, the need of maintenance therapy is debatable. Recent studies have confirmed the efficacy of maintenance therapy for carcinoma *in situ* in which BCG is instilled once a week three times at 3 months, 6 months and every 6 months to 3 years. The complications of BCG therapy include primarily irritative bladder symptoms. Some patients manifest with a systemic disease "BCG-osis" characterized by fever and pulmonary infiltrates requiring antituberculous treatment.

The other chemotherapeutic agents used for intravesical therapy are mitomycin C, thiotepa and adriamycin.

The treatment of choice for muscle invasive bladder tumor is radical cystectomy with urinary diversion. In men the bladder with its surrounding fat, peritoneal attachments, the prostate and the seminal vesicles are resected. In women the bladder, surrounding fat and peritoneal attachments are removed along with the uterus, cervix, anterior vaginal vault, urethra and ovaries. A bilateral pelvic node dissection is performed simultaneously. Lymph node metastases are found in approximately 30 percent. Urinary diversion may be achieved using a variety of techniques. Methods have been perfected that allow construction of reservoirs that are continent and do not require the patient to wear external appliances for collection of urine. Partial cystectomy may be done when a solitary tumor is found in the dome of the bladder so that a safe resection with a 2 cm margin is achieved.

Patients who have undergone radical cystectomy and are found to have microscopic evidence of nodal metastasis or infiltration of tumor into the perivesical fat will benefit from adjuvant chemotherapy. Current chemotherapeutic regimens include methotrexate, vinblastine, adriamycin and cisplatinum (M-VAC), methotrexate and vinblastine (CMV). Studies have suggested a longer recurrence-free survival with the given adjuvant therapy. If a preoperative decision is made to use chemotherapy, radical cystectomy and diversion are justified in node positive patients.

Radiotherapy can be offered to patients who are poor surgical candidates or to those who refuse surgery. However, the survival with radiotherapy is not as good as surgery.

For those patients with metastatic disease palliative measures should be undertaken for relief of symptoms. Chemotherapy may be administered.

FURTHER READING

1. Droller MJ. Tumor progression and survival in patients with T1G3 bladder tumors: multicentric retrospective study comparing 94 patients treated during 17 years. J Urol 2002;168(2):855-56.
2. Fradet Y. Recent advances in the management of superficial bladder tumors. Can J Urol 2002;9(3):1544-50.
3. Samaratunga H, Makarov DV, Epstein JI. Comparison of WHO/ISUP and WHO classification of noninvasive papillary urothelial neoplasms for risk of progression. Urology 2002;60(2):315-19.
4. Zhou JH, Rosser CJ, Tanaka M, Yang M, Baranov E, Hoffman RM, Benedict WF. Visualizing superficial human bladder cancer cell growth in vivo by green fluorescent protein expression. Cancer Gene Ther 2002;9(8):681-86.

Cancer of the Prostate

29

Abraham Kurian
Iqbal S Shergill
Kim Mammen

Prostate cancer is one of the most common cancers among males. Due to continuous advances, the diagnosis and treatment of prostate cancer is constantly evolving into an optimal state. With the development of prostate-specific antigen (PSA) screening, more men, having prostate cancer are identified earlier. While prostate cancer can be a slow-growing cancer, many men die of the disease each year.

ANATOMY

The prostate lies below the bladder and encompasses the prostatic urethra. It is surrounded by a capsule and separated from the rectum by a layer of fascia called the Denonvilliers fascia. The blood supply to the base of the bladder and the prostate is from the inferior vesical artery, which is derived from the internal iliac artery. The neurovascular bundle lies on either side of the prostate on the rectum. It is derived from the pelvic plexus and is important for erectile function.

INCIDENCE

Prostate cancer is currently the most frequently diagnosed malignancy among men and the second leading cause of cancer death. Prostate cancer is rarely diagnosed in people below 40 years, and it is uncommon in people below 50 years. Prostate cancer is found also during autopsies carried out following other causes of death. The incidence of this latent or autopsy cancer is much greater than cases of clinical cancer. In fact, it may be as high as 80 percent by the age of 80 years.

The incidence of clinical cancer varies regionally, and these differences may be due to some of the genetic, hormonal, and dietary factors.

They are discussed below:
- High in northern Europe and North America.
- Intermediate in southern Europe and Central and South America.
- Low in eastern Europe and Asia.

ETIOLOGY

GENETICS

Genetic studies suggest that a strong familial predisposition may be responsible for as many as 10 percent of prostate cancer cases. Alteration of genes on chromosome 1 and the X chromosome have been found in some patients with a family history of prostate cancer.

RACE

African Americans have a higher incidence and more aggressive type of prostate cancer than white men, who in turn have a higher incidence than men of Asian origin. Studies have found that young African men have testosterone levels 15 percent higher than those of young white men. Furthermore, evidence that 5-alpha reductase may be more active in African Americans than in whites, implying that hormonal differences may play a role.

DIET

A high-fat diet may lead to increased risks while a diet rich in soya may be protective. These observations have been proposed as reasons for the low incidence of this cancer in Asia. Vitamin E may have some protective effects by virtue of being an antioxidant. Decreased levels of Vitamin A may be a risk factor since normal levels of Vitamin A can promote cell differentiation and stimulate the immune system. Vitamin-D deficiency was suggested as a risk factor, and studies show an inverse relation between ultraviolet exposure and mortality rates of prostate cancer. Selenium may have a protective effect based on epidemiological studies, and it also is believed to extend its effect via its antioxidant properties.

HORMONES

Hormonal causes also have been postulated because androgen ablation causes regression of prostate cancers, and eunuchs do not develop adenocarcinoma of the prostate.

PATHOPHYSIOLOGY

Prostate cancer develops when the rates of cell division and cell death are no longer equal, leading to uncontrolled tumor growth. Most prostate cancers are adenocarcinomas (95%). About 4 percent cases of prostate cancer have transitional cell morphology. Few cases have neuroendocrine morphology. Out of the cases of prostate cancer, 70 percent arise in the peripheral zone, 15-20 percent arise in the central zone, and 10-15 percent arise in the transitional zone. Most prostate cancers are multifocal with synchronous involvement of multiple zones of the prostate.

LOCAL SYMPTOMS

The common local symptoms include urinary retention, back or leg pain, hematuria, urinary frequency, decreased stream and urgency. Currently by screening with PSA and digital rectal examination, prostatic cancer is being detected in patients with minimal lower urinary tract symptoms or sometimes with no symptoms.

METASTATIC SYMPTOMS

Metastatic symptoms include weight loss and loss of appetite, bone pain, with or without pathologic fracture (because prostate cancer, when metastatic, has a strong predilection for bone); and lower extremity pain and edema from nodal metastasis obstructing venous and lymphatic tributaries. Uremic symptoms can occur from ureteral obstruction caused by local prostate growth or retroperitoneal adenopathy secondary to nodal metastasis.

NATURAL HISTORY

The natural history of clinically localized disease is variable, with lower-grade tumors having a more indolent course, while some high-grade lesions are aggressive and progress to metastatic disease with relative rapidity.

Evidence suggests that most prostate cancers are multifocal and heterogeneous. Cancers can start in the transitional zone or more commonly, the peripheral zone. When these cancers are locally invasive, the transitional zone tumors spread to the bladder neck, while the peripheral zone tumors extend into the ejaculatory ducts and seminal vesicles. Penetration through the prostatic capsule and along the perineural or vascular spaces is a relatively late event.

The mechanism for distant metastasis is poorly understood. There is early spread to bone, occasionally without significant lymphadenopathy.

DIAGNOSIS AND STAGING

Digital Rectal Examination (DRE)

Various factors are taken into consideration when performing the DRE. A nodule is important, but findings such as asymmetry, difference in texture, and bogginess are important clues. Cysts or stones cannot be accurately differentiated from a cancer by DRE alone. Hence a high level of suspicion should be held, if the DRE is abnormal. In addition, if cancer is detected, the DRE forms the basis of the clinical stage of the primary tumor [i.e. T stage in the tumor, node, metastasis (TNM) staging system] (Table 29.1).

Prostate-specific Antigen

PSA is a single-chain glycoprotein that has chymotrypsin-like properties. PSA slowly hydrolyzes peptide bonds, thereby liquefying semen. The upper limit of the normal PSA level is 4 ng/ml. Some advocate age-related cut-off, such as 2.5 ng/ml for the fifth decade of life, 3.5 ng/ml for the sixth decade of life, and 4.5 ng/ml for the seventh decade of life.

In patients who have a PSA in the range of 4-10 ng/ml, the percentage of free PSA can be estimated. The measurement of bound and free PSA

Table 29.1: The 1997 tumor, node, metastases (TNM) staging system stages prostate cancer	
TX	Primary tumor cannot be assessed
T0	No evidence of primary tumor
T1	Clinically unapparent tumor not palpable or visible by imaging
T1a	Tumor incidental histological finding in less than or equal to 5 percent of tissues resected
T1b	Tumor incidental histological finding in greater than 5 percent of tissues resected
T1c	Tumor identified by needle biopsy (because of elevated PSA); tumors found in 1 or both lobes by needle biopsy but not palpable or reliably visible by imaging
T2	Tumor confined to prostate
T2a	Tumor involving 1 lobe
T2b	Tumor involving both lobes
T3	Tumor extending through the prostatic capsule; no invasion into the prostatic apex or into, but not beyond, the prostatic capsule
T3a	Extracapsular extension (unilateral or bilateral)
T3b	Tumor invading seminal vesicle(s)
T4	Tumor fixed or invading adjacent structures other than seminal vesicles (e.g. bladder neck, external sphincter, rectum, levator muscles, pelvic wall)
NX	Regional lymph nodes (cannot be assessed)
N0	No regional lymph node metastasis
N1	Metastasis in regional lymph node or nodes
MX	Distant metastasis cannot be assessed
M0	No distant metastasis
M1	Distant metastasis
M1a	Nonregional lymph node(s)
M1b	Bone(s)
M1c	Other site(s)
PM1c	More than 1 site of metastasis present

can help discriminate between patients with cancer and those with benign prostatic hyperplasia (BPH). The lower the ratio of free-to-total PSA, the higher the likelihood of cancer. A cut-off of 22 percent prompts different techniques in cancer detection and minimizes unnecessary biopsies.

Men with PSA levels less than 10 and low or moderate grade histology (Gleason <7) with no findings or minimal findings on physical examination may proceed to surgery or brachytherapy without further studies.

PSA levels greater than 10, high-grade histology (Gleason score of 7 or higher), or physical findings suggesting stage T3 disease probably should undergo a staging CT scan and bone scan.

PROSTATIC ACID PHOSPHATASE

It was a widely used tumor marker in the past but is rarely used today. It lacks the specificity and sensitivity required for a reliable screening test.

PROSTATE BIOPSY OR FINE-NEEDLE ASPIRATION CYTOLOGY

Prostate biopsy or FNAC may be done through a transrectal or a transperineal approach. The use of a transrectal ultrasound has improved the localization of the nodule and increases the accuracy of the procedure. Ultrasound-guided transrectal core needle biopsy of the prostate can be done using, either a tru-cut needle or a biopty gun. Most urologists carry out 8 to 10 biopsies from different areas of the gland.

When patients have a persistently elevated PSA in the face of negative biopsy results, the literature supports repeating the biopsy 1 or 2 times.

Histologically prostatic cancer is classified as well differentiated, moderately differentiated and poorly differentiated. The most commonly used system of classifying the histological characteristics of prostate cancer is the Gleason score. The glandular architecture and growth factor within the tumor determine the classification. The system assigns a grade from 1-5 to the predominant pattern and the second is the most common pattern in the tumor. The sum of these 2 grades is referred to as the Gleason score. Scoring based on the second most common pattern, is an attempt to correlate with the considerable heterogeneity that is seen within prostate cancers. Grades 2-4 are considered low grade, Grades 5-7 are considered moderate, and Grades 8-10 are considered high grade. This scheme of grading histological features is highly dependent on the skill and experience of the pathologist and, thus, is subject to some degree of individual variation.

TRANSRECTAL ULTRASOUND (TRUS)

TRUS is used to examine the prostate for hypoechoic areas, which are commonly found with cancers but are not specific enough for diagnostic purposes. Systematic biopsies of peripheral and, occasionally, transitional zones are taken under ultrasound guidance. This procedure is an accurate one as it assesses the capsular invasion, especially into the seminal vesicles.

BONE SCAN

Bony metastases occur in 80 percent of patients with advanced disease. The lesions are mostly osteoblastic but may also be osteolytic. Bone scanning is more sensitive but less specific than skeletal radiography. Bone scan may be omitted if the PSA level is below 10 ng/ml in a patient with cancer of the prostate.

CT SCAN OR MRI

CT scan of the abdomen and pelvis or an MRI in patients suggested to have locally advanced disease may give an indication of extracapsular extension, seminal vesicle involvement, pelvic lymph node enlargement, liver metastases, and hydronephrosis as a result of distal ureteral obstruction. The CT scan can help stage the patient or to consider lymph node sampling prior to treatment.

MRI is superior to bone scan in evaluating bone metastasis, but it is impractical for routine total body surveys. Instead, it is used to determine the etiology of questionable lesions found on bone scans.

Neither CT scan nor MRI can be used to determine if lymph nodes are reactive or contain malignant deposits unless the nodes are much enlarged and a percutaneous biopsy can be undertaken.

DIFFERENTIAL DIAGNOSIS

— Benign Prostatic Hypertrophy (BPH)
— Calculi
— Prostatic cysts
— Prostatic tuberculosis
— Prostatitis

TREATMENT

NON-SURGICAL THERAPY

Early localized disease (clinical stage T1-2N0M0)
- Watchful waiting
  — This is a program of regular examinations, PSA monitoring, and digital rectal examination (DRE) monitoring. This approach is considered in patients of advanced age who have significant life-limiting morbidity. In addition, it is rarely appropriate in patients who do not harbor well-differentiated tumors.
- External-beam radiation
  — This is used with curative intent for patients with clinically localized cancer.

— Conventional external beam (4-field box).
— Conformal external beam, which delivers higher doses of radiation to the prostate while sparing adjacent tissues, is much better than the conventional approach.
• Brachytherapy/Interstitial radiation
— Radioactive palladium or iodine seeds are placed into the prostate.
— This therapy may be used alone or in combination with external-beam radiotherapy.
• Androgen ablation combined with radiation

This procedure offers improved disease-specific survival and increased time for tumor recurrence in patients with locally advanced prostate cancer. The advantage of this approach in patients with early disease remains to be determined, but it could offer significant advantages when used in younger patients with significant longevity (>20 y). Androgen ablation traditionally has been achieved by the use of luteinizing hormone-releasing hormone (LHRH) agents combined with antiandrogens, though variations on this theme have been described. Androgen ablation commonly begins several months before radiation is initiated and continues for several months more.

LOCALLY ADVANCED DISEASE (T3-4N0M0)

• Treat patients with radiation as above.
• Combining radiation with hormones improves local control and allows longer freedom from metastasis and disease-free survival.
• Watchful waiting is an option only in highly selected patients because of the aggressive nature of these tumors.

METASTATIC DISEASE (STAGE N+ M+)

The androgen dependency of the prostate gland is well known. Any agent or procedure that interferes with the production, release, binding or action of androgens will potentially inhibit the growth of the prostate cancer cell. Hormonal therapy is associated with significant responses. Its curative potential is limited due to the inherent heterogeneity of prostate cancer and due to the inability of hormones to eradicate all prostate cancer clones, the androgen-dependent and androgen-independent components.

BILATERAL ORCHIDECTOMY

This appears to be the most consistent procedure in endocrine manipulation. Results are immediate with virtually no operative morbidity.
Medical castration
• LHRH agonists

They are synthetic analogs of the gonadotrophin-releasing hormones. They are available as depot forms that enable 3-monthly or 4-monthly injections.

— Leuprolide acetate-30 mg q16 wk
— Goserelin acetate - 10.8 mg q12 wk
- Non-steroidal antiandrogens
They inhibit androgens on the target cell.
— Flutamide-250 mg tid
— Bicalutamide-50 mg qd
- Estrogens
It suppresses the pituitary gonadotrophin.
— Diethylstilbestrol-1 to 3 mg qd
— Estradiol-1 mg tid
- Adrenal steroid inhibitors
They can be used to lower serum testosterone levels quickly in cases involving spinal cord compression secondary to metastases.
— Aminoglutathimide-1 to 2 gm qd
— Ketoconazole-400 mg tid
Combined androgen blockade
- Androgen ablation is achieved by bilateral orchidectomy or by the use of LHRH agents. But they have no effect on adrenal androgens, which contribute as much as 40 percent of prostatic dihydrotestosterone.
- Combined androgen blockade combines surgical or medical castration with peripheral androgen blockade.

BISPHOSPHONATES

Bisphosphonates, which are stable analogs of calcium pyrophosphate, inhibit osteoclastic activity in bone, relieving bone pain. In addition, they also may have a beneficial effect on the progression of prostate cancer. They also are being studied for the treatment of osteoporosis induced by androgens.

RADIATION THERAPY

- External beam radiation therapy is used to palliate painful isolated bone metastasis in patients with hormone-refractory prostate cancer and in patients with impending spinal cord compression.
- Certain radiopharmaceutical agents, such as strontium chloride 89 and samarium 153, relieve pain by delivering beta ray irradiation at new bone formation sites.

SURAMIN

- Suramin acts via growth factor inhibition. Suramin is an active drug in patients with hormone-refractory prostate cancer and can be used in combination with other agents.

- Adverse effects include edema, leukopenia, infection, hyperglycemia, anemia, anorexia, dyspnea, platelet abnormalities, elevated creatinine, malaise, arrhythmias, and prothrombin abnormalities.

CHEMOHORMONAL THERAPY

- The rationale behind chemohormonal regimens for hormone refractory prostate cancer (HRPC) is based on exposing prostate cancer cells to cytotoxic chemotherapy earlier, before clonal expansion of androgen independent cells or constitutive overexpression of cell survival genes becomes established and before patients develop hormone-refractory prostate cancer.
- Various agents identified are Doxorubicin, Methotrexate, Cis-platinum, Cyclophosphamide and 5-FU. No significant survival advantage without affecting quality of life has been documented until now.

SURGICAL THERAPY

Early localized disease (T1-2N0 M0)

Radical prostatectomy is removal of the prostate and seminal vesicles. Pelvic lymphadenectomy includes the medial half of the external iliac vessels and obturator fossa, from the bifurcation of internal and external iliac vessels to the node of Cloquet. Currently, the following approaches are used to remove the prostate gland:

- Radical retropubic prostatectomy
- Radical perineal prostatectomy
- Laparoscopic prostatectomy

The following criteria are general suggestions for any candidate for radical prostatectomy:

- Patient below 70-75 years.
- Multiple morbidities, with life expectancy longer than 10 years.
- Histologically, Gleason score of 7 or less.
- PSA less than 20 ng/mL.

Complications may include the following:

- Impotence rates vary greatly and depend on patient age and whether surgery is nerve sparing (unilateral or bilateral) or non–nerve sparing.
- Incontinence (4-30%) also depends on the patient's age and whether the surgery is nerve sparing or non–nerve sparing.
- Strictures (10%) and rarely, fecal incontinence occur; the latter occurs more commonly with perineal prostatectomy.

METASTATIC DISEASE (STAGE N+ M+)

Patients diagnosed with impending paralysis due to spinal cord compression or patients with pathologic fractures should be immediately immobilized until appropriate consultations are obtained. Spinal cord decompression for patients with spinal cord compression must be performed immediately. Similarly, pinning/plating of weight-bearing bones involved in pathological fractures is mandatory.

FURTHER READING

1. Amato RJ, Ellenhorst J, et al. Treatment of prostatic cancer with low dose prednisone: Evaluation of pain and quality of life as pragmatic indices of response. J of Clin Oncol 1989;7:590-97.
2. Berawley OW, Knopf K, Merrill R. The epidemiology of prostate cancer. Descriptive epidemiology. Semin Urol Oncol 1998;16:187-92.
3. Boola M, Gonzalez D, Warde P, et al. Improved survival in patients with locally advanced prostate cancer treated with radiotherapy and goserelin. N Engl J Med 1997;337:295-300.
4. Brawley OW, Knopf K, Thompson I. The epidemiology of prostate cancer: The risk factors. Semin Urol Oncol 1998;16:193-201.
5. Esinberger MA, Blumenstein BA, et al. Bilateral orchidectomy with or without flutamide for metastatic prostatic cancer. New Eng J Med 1998;339:1036-42.
6. Goharderakhshan RZ, Sudilovsky D, Carroll LA, Grossfeld GD, Marn R, Carroll PR. Utility of intraoperative frozen section analysis of surgical margins in region of neuromuscular bundles at radical prostatectomy. Urology 2002;59(5):709-14.
7. Oh WK, Kantoff PW. Management of hormone refractory prostatic cancer: Current status and future prospects. J of Urol 1998;160:122-39.
8. Pienta KJ, Redman B, Hussein M, et al. Chemotherapy with mitoxantrone plus prednisone for hormone resistant prostatic cancer: A Canadian randomized trial with palliative end products. J of Clin Oncol 1996;14:1256-64.
9. Pound CR, Partin AW, et al. Natural history of progression after PSA elevation following radical prostatectomy. JAMA 1999;281:1591-97.
10. Wareing M. Reflective, holistic care after radical prostatectomy. Nurs Times 2002;98(14):34-36.

APPENDIX 10

International comparison, India and five continents—AAR (ICMR and IARC).

CANCER PROSTATE

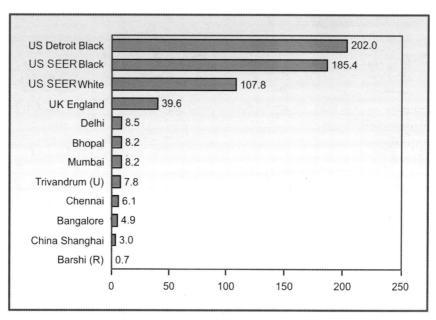

Rate per 100,000

Testicular Carcinoma

30

Abraham Kurian
Iqbal S Shergill
Kim Mammen

Testicular cancer primarily affects people of the younger age group between 15 and 35 years. Available data suggest that more than 90 percent cure rate can be achieved in testicular cancers in the initial stages owing to effective advances in multimodality treatment. Patients with cryptorchidism have approximately 50 times greater chance of developing testicular cancer regardless of whether orchidopexy was carried out. Additionally these patients with undescended testis have a higher risk (about 5% to 10%) of developing a cancer in the opposite normally descended testis. So a patient with undescended testis should be followed up closely after orchidopexy for any palpable mass. This is also where testicular self-examination attains importance.

Approximately 5 percent of germ cell tumors arise in the extragonadal location, particularly in the mediastinum and retroperitoneum.

A previous history of trauma is common in men with testicular tumors. It might be possible that an unnoticed lump was brought to the attention of the patient because of the injury.

Hormones may be implicated in the etiology of testicular cancer. Stilbesterol in pregnancy increases the risk of maldescent and testicular cancer in the offspring.

Genetic influences affect the incidence of testicular cancer. It is virtually unknown in black men in Africa, West Indies and America.

A person with testicular cancer has a 500 fold increased chance for the development of a contralateral tumor than the general male population. Simultaneous bilateral tumors are seen in only 1 to 2 percent.

AGE DISTRIBUTION

In neonates embryonal cell carcinoma and yolk sac tumor are the most common types. In the young adults from 15 to 35 years germ cell tumors of different varieties occur. In the older age group above 50 years, spermatocytic seminomas and lymphomas are the most common. Germ cell tumors occurring in the young adult are the commonest type of testicular tumors seen in clinical practice.

HISTOPATHOLOGY AND CLASSIFICATION

Testicular tumors can be broadly classified into germ cell tumors (seminomas and non-seminomas), gonadostromal tumors and metastatic tumors.

Germ cell tumors comprise nearly 95 percent of the tumors.

Seminoma (classical, anaplastic and spermatocytic types) constitutes about 40 percent. The other types of germ cell tumors are all clubbed together to form the non-seminomas. Embryonal cell carcinoma and teratocarcinoma (combination of embryonal and teratoma) are found in 20 to 25 percent of the population each. Teratomas constitute about 5 to 10 percent. Choriocarcinomas constitute about 1 to 3 percent. Both seminomatous and non-seminomatous elements can be found in approximately 6 percent of all testicular tumors. The treatment of these mixtures of seminoma and non-seminomatous germ cell tumors is similar to that of non-seminoma alone.

Testicular tumors arising from the stromal elements of the testis are called gonadostromal tumors like the Leydig cell, Sertoli cell and Granulosa cell tumors. Secondary (metastatic) tumors from lymphoma, leukemia, melanoma, carcinoma lung and prostatic cancer are seen in the testis.

CLINICAL FINDINGS

The commonest presenting symptom of a testicular tumor is a painless testicular mass. All masses arising from the testis should be considered carcinoma until proved otherwise. As the mass increases in size it may produce heaviness or a dragging sensation. Testicular pain is a presenting symptom in about 10 percent of the patients and may be the result of intratesticular hemorrhage or infarction. Approximately 10 percent of patients present with symptoms related to metastasis. Back pain (retroperitoneal metastasis), cough with or without hemoptysis, dyspnea (pulmonary/mediastinal metastases), bone pain (bony metastasis), pedal edema (vena caval compression), supraclavicular mass, a large abdominal mass, etc. are the more common presenting features. Approximately in 10 percent of instances the patient is asymptomatic and the tumor may be detected incidentally following trauma or may be detected by the sexual partner. Gynecomastia occurs in less than 5 percent of patients and is usually associated with increased human chorionic gonadotrophin stimulation of the Leydig cells, which produce estradiol as commonly seen with choriocarcinoma. Often a testicular tumor is misdiagnosed as epididymo-orchitis and the patient is treated chronically with antibiotics. It is essential to remember that any case of epididymo-orchitis should be called back after a period of about 3 weeks to reassess the testis and see if the swelling has regressed. Occasionally a hydrocele may hinder the palpation of the testis. A scrotal ultrasound can be very useful in differentiating a testicular tumor from other scrotal pathologies.

DIAGNOSIS

The diagnosis of a testicular tumor is histopathologically obtained by an inguinal orchiectomy. If there is a doubt regarding the diagnosis, tumor markers may be sent and the patient may be reassessed following a course of antibiotics. If clinically the mass appears to be a tumor, time should not be wasted to do an orchiectomy. Whenever there is a doubt it is safer to remove the testis rather than leave a testis with a tumor behind. A biopsy should never be done through a scrotal incision. This violates the scrotal lymphatics. Testicular tumor will spread along the scrotal lymphatics into the inguinal lymph nodes. The incision for an inguinal orchiectomy is made as for an inguinal hernia repair. The spermatic cord and the vas deferens should be tied separately before delivering the testis into the wound. If the surgeon still has a doubt regarding the diagnosis, a soft clamp may be applied on the cord and the testis is delivered into the canal. The testis can be closely examined and if necessary a frozen section biopsy can be done (Table 30.1).

In the more commonly used clinical staging of Memorial Sloan-Kettering, Stage A is tumor confined to the testis. Stage B is tumor in the retroperitoneum. Stage C is tumor spread into the supradiaphragmatic nodes or visceral involvement (Table 30.2).

Table 30.1: TNM staging for testicular cancer	
To	No evidence of tumor
Tis	Intratubular, preinvasive
T1	Confined to testis
T2	Invades beyond tunica vaginalis or into Epididymis
T3	Invades spermatic cord
T4	Invades scrotum
N1	Single < 2 cm
N2	Multiple < 5 cm/Single 2-5 cm
N3	Any node > 5 cm
Mo	No distant metastasis
M1	Distant metastasis

Table 30.2: Memorial Sloan-Kettering staging (clinical staging)	
A (I)	Confined to testis, epididymis or spermatic cord.
B1 (II A)	Retroperitoneal lymph node involvement, < 2 cm in diameter and/or 5 or fewer nodes involved.
B2 (II B)	Retroperitoneal lymph node involvement, none 2 cm to 5 cm in diameter and/or more than 5 nodes involved.
B3 (II C)	Large bulky palpable retroperitoneal nodes greater than 5 cm.
C (III)	Mediastinal or visceral involvement.

TUMOR MARKERS

For testicular tumors the markers in the serum are Alpha-fetoprotein and Beta subunit of human chorionic gonadotrophin. Other markers, which are used occasionally, are Lactic acid dehydrogenase (LDH) and Placental alkaline phosphatase (PLAP). Even though they are useful in staging, the primary role of tumor markers is not in staging but in monitoring disease progression or response to therapy.

- AFP is a glycoprotein produced by fetal yolk sac and liver. AFP is not elevated in pure seminoma or choriocarcinoma. So a testicular malignancy with raised AFP suggests a non-seminomatous histopathology. The half-life is seven days. Persistence of levels four weeks after orchiectomy indicates a metastatic disease. False positive elevations can occur with hepatitis, hepatoma, bronchogenic cancer, pancreatic cancer and other gastrointestinal malignancies.
- B-hCG is produced by syncytiotrophoblastic cells. Normal males do not produce significant amounts of B-hCG except from testicular tumors. Its half-life is 24 to 36 hours. Persistence of high level of B-hCG seven days after orchiectomy indicates metastatic disease. Only 7 percent of patients with pure seminoma have elevated B-hCG levels.
- LDH, particularly its isoenzyme-1, is elevated in large volume (bulky) testicular tumors of any histology. It is useful when the AFP, B-hCG levels have normalized or are normal. LDH levels when elevated correlate well with the volume of the tumor.
- PLAP is the most sensitive indicator for metastatic seminomatous disease. It is detected in 65 percent of seminomas.

Tumor markers do help in the staging of the disease. Following an orchiectomy if the tumor markers continue to be elevated it indicates a Stage II or III disease. Following a retroperitoneal lymph node dissection, if the tumor markers continue to be elevated it indicates a Stage III disease. Negative tumor markers becoming positive on follow up suggest a recurrent tumor. Markers are also useful in the histologic classification of the disease. If in a seminomatous disease, AFP is raised, it indicates non-seminomatous elements and the treatment should be according to a non-seminomatous tumor protocol.

PATTERN OF METASTATIC SPREAD

With the exception of choriocarcinoma, which demonstrates early hemato-genous spread, germ cell tumors spread mostly through the lymphatics. The retroperitoneum is the first area of spread of the testicular tumors. From a tumor in the right testis the primary drainage area is into the inter-aortocaval nodes at the level of the right renal hilum and then the spread can occur into pre-caval nodes, paracaval nodes, right common and external iliac nodes. From a left testicular tumor the initial node of spread is the para-aortic nodes at the level of the left renal hilum followed by the preaortic nodes, para-aortic nodes, left common and external iliac nodes. Certain factors can alter the pattern of spread of a testicular tumor. Scrotal violation (scrotal biopsy) may result in inguinal metastasis. Invasion of the epididymis or spermatic cord may allow spread to the distal external iliac nodes and obturator nodes. Occasionally the tumor invades the vascular structures and spreads to the lungs. It can also spread to other organs like the liver, brain, bone, kidney and adrenal glands.

As mentioned previously choriocarcinoma is the exception to the rule and is characterized by early hematogenous spread mainly to the lungs.

INVESTIGATIONS

The three main groups of investigations are: (1) tumor markers, (2) CT scan of the abdomen to visualize the retroperitoneal spread, (3) chest X-ray or CT scan of the chest to look for pulmonary and mediastinal metastasis.

Other imaging modalities available are Magnetic Resonance Imaging (MRI) and Positron Emission Tomography (PET) scanning.

TREATMENT

Radical inguinal orchiectomy is the first line of therapy. If a scrotal biopsy is done in the initial diagnosis of the cancer a hemiscrotectomy should also be done in the same sitting. Depending on the histopathology and the stage of the tumor the following treatment schedule is generally followed (Tables 30.3 and 30.4).

The limits and boundaries of retroperitoneal dissection vary with the side of the tumor. For right-sided tumors the main group of lymph nodes removed are para-caval, pre-caval, inter-aortic caval and the right iliac nodes. For the left-sided tumor the main group of lymph nodes removed are para-aortic, pre-aortic, inter-aortic caval and the left iliac nodes. The main drawback of retroperitoneal lymph node dissection is the loss of ejaculation and emission resulting in infertility. This has led many surgeons to follow modified, nerve sparing protocols to encompass smaller fields of dissection. In Stage I non-seminomatous disease some surgeons believe

Table 30.3: Seminoma		
Stage I	Radiation (2500 rads) to the retroperitoneum and ipsilateral iliac group of nodes.	
Stage II A, II B and II C (non-bulky, less than 10 cm in size).	As above plus 1000 rads boost to the mass.	
Stage III (bulky, more than 10 cm in size).	Chemotherapy (platinum based regimens).	Residual mass if present is resected. Further chemotherapy if viable tumor is present.

Table 30.4: Non-seminoma		
Stage I, II A	Retroperitoneal lymph node dissection	
Stage II B	Retroperitoneal lymph node dissection	Adjuvant or neo-adjuvant chemotherapy may be given.
Stage II C and Stage III	Neo-adjuvant chemo-therapy followed by retroperitoneal lymph node dissection.	Further chemotherapy if viable tumor still present.

in a watchful, waiting or surveillance protocol. But this requires a willing patient with regular follow-ups, with frequent evaluation by tumor markers and imaging by CT scan.

FURTHER READING

1. An oncological view on the blood-testis barrier. Lancet Oncol 2002;3(6):357-63. Review.
2. Evans CP. Follow-up surveillance strategies for genitourinary malignancies. Cancer 2002;94(11):2892-905.
3. Fizazi K, Prow DM, Do KA, Wang X, Finn L, Kim J, Daliani D, et al. Alternating dose-dense chemotherapy in patients with high volume disseminated non-seminomatous germ cell tumors. Br J Cancer 2002;86(10):1555-60.
4. Hennessy B, O'Connor M, Carney DN. Acute vascular events associated with cisplatin therapy in malignant disease. Ir Med J 2002;95(5):145-46.
5. Kasahara T, Hara N, Bilim V, Tomita Y, Tsutsui, et al. Immunohistochemical studies of caveolin-3 in germ cell tumors of the testis. Urol Int 2002;69(1):63-68.
6. Marty C, Odermatt B, Schott H, Neri D, Ballmer-Hofer K, Klemenz R, Schwendener RA. Cytotoxic targeting of F9 teratocarcinoma tumors with antibody modified liposomes. Br J Cancer 2000;87(1):106-12.

7. Mature teratoma arising in intraabdominal undescended testis in an infant with previous inguinal exploration: Case report and review of intraabdominal testicular tumors in children. J Pediatr Surg 2002;37(8):1236-38.

8. Middleton WD, Teefey SA, Santillan CS. Testicular microlithiasis: prospective analysis of prevalence and associated tumor. Radiology 2002;224(2):425-28.

9. Price KS, Castells MC. Taxol reactions. Allergy Asthma Proc 2002;23(3):205-08.

Penile Cancer

31

Abraham Kurian
Iqbal S Shergill
Kim Mammen

Penile lesions can be categorized as benign non-cutaneous, benign cutaneous, premalignant cutaneous, virus related dermatological lesions, carcinoma *in situ* and invasive carcinoma.

Benign non-cutaneous lesions include: congenital inclusion cyst, acquired inclusion cyst, retention cyst, angioma, neuroma, myoma, etc.

Benign cutaneous lesions include: cutaneous nevi, hirsute papilloma, pearly penile papules or coronal papillae.

Pre-malignant cutaneous lesions include: cutaneous horns, balanitis xerotica obliterans and leukoplakia.

Leukoplakia presents as solitary or multiple, whitish plaques, which often involve the meatus. Leukoplakia has been associated with squamous cell carcinoma.

Balanitis xerotica obliterans is a variation of lichen sclerosis et atrophicus and presents as a white patch on the prepuce or glans where it usually involves the urethral meatus.

Viral-related dermatological lesions include: condyloma acuminatum, Bowenoid papulosis, Kaposi's sarcoma and Buschke-Lowenstein tumor (giant condyloma acuminatum, verrucous carcinoma).

Condyloma acuminata are soft papillomatous growths. They are known as venereal warts and have a predilection for the genital and perineal regions. These lesions are usually sexually transmitted by the human papillomavirus (HPV).

Giant condyloma acuminata or Buschke-Löwenstein tumor differs from the standard condyloma in that it displaces, invades, and destroys adjacent structures by compression, whereas the standard condyloma remains superficial and never invades. Despite their large size and invasive potential, the Buschke-Löwenstein tumors show no signs of malignant change on histological examination.

CARCINOMA IN SITU-ERYTHROPLASIA OF QUEYRAT OR BOWEN'S DISEASE

The diagnosis depends on their appearance and the site of origin. Erythroplasia of Queyrat involves the glans, prepuce, or penile shaft, while similar lesions on the remainder of the genitalia and perineum are called Bowen's disease. Carcinoma *in situ* can precede and progress to invasive carcinoma.

INVASIVE CARCINOMA

Incidence

Carcinoma of the penis constitutes up to 10 percent of all male malignancies in developing countries. Penile cancer is commonly diagnosed during the 6th to 7th decades of life. However, the tumor is not unusual in younger men.

Etiology

The disease is almost never seen in individuals who are circumcised in the neonatal period. Adult circumcision offers little or no protection.

Smegma, a by-product of bacterial action on desquamated cells that are retained within the preputial sac, is widely believed to act as a carcinogen by its chronic irritative effects. This is accentuated by the presence of phimosis.

Human papillomaviruses 16 and 18 have been found in one-third of men with penile cancer. Whether or not these viruses are involved in the causation of the cancer or are found as saprophytes has not been proved.

Natural History

Penile cancers begin as small lesions on the glans or prepuce. They gradually grow laterally along the surface, covering the entire glans and prepuce and invading the corpora and shaft of the penis. The cancers may be papillary and exophytic or flat and ulcerative. Buck's fascia, which surrounds the corpora, acts as a temporary barrier. Eventually, the cancer penetrates Buck's fascia and the tunica albuginea where the cancer has access to the vasculature and systemic spread is possible. Metastases to the superficial and deep inguinal lymph nodes are the earliest path for tumor dissemination. From here, the drainage is to the pelvic nodes. Multiple cross connections exist at all levels, permitting penile lymphatic drainage to proceed bilaterally. Untreated, metastatic enlargement of the regional nodes leads to skin necrosis, chronic infection, and eventually, death from sepsis or hemorrhage secondary to erosion into the femoral vessels. Clinically apparent distant metastases to the lung, liver, bone, or brain are unusual until late in the course of the disease, often after the primary has been treated. Distant metastases are usually associated with regional node involvement. Most penile cancers are low grade, but there has been a lack of correlation between grade and survival. There is an association between high-grade disease and the presence of regional lymph node metastases. The strongest predictor for survival is the presence or absence of nodal metastases.

Signs and Symptoms

Penile tumors can originate anywhere on the penis but are most commonly found on the glans, prepuce and coronal sulcus. The common sites of origin may be related to constant exposure to smegma and other irritants within the preputial sac. 15-50 percent of patients delay seeking medical attention for more than 1 year. This delay is attributed to embarrassment, fear and personal neglect. Patients present with a 'sore' that has failed to heal, a subtle induration in the skin, a papule, pustule, warty growth, or a large exophytic growth. Because most of these patients are uncircumcised, they may have a phimosis that obscures the tumor and allows it to grow undetected. Rarely, a mass, ulceration, suppuration, or hemorrhage may present in the inguinal area because of nodal metastases. Rarely patients may present with autoamputation. Pain is usually not a presenting complaint.

Diagnosis and Staging (Table 31.1 and 31.2)

The most important diagnostic test is the biopsy and it is mandatory before any therapy. This may be an excision biopsy if the cancer is small and a circumcision is acceptable. Most commonly the histology shows squamous cell carcinoma. Very rarely the histology shows basal cell carcinoma and malignant melanoma.

MRI, CT scan and ultrasonography are useful for local cancer staging and to assess the lymph nodes. MRI produces sharp images of the penile structures and is accurate in demonstrating invasion of the corpora and can determine the extent of the tumor. Both MRI and CT scan can demonstrate enlarged pelvic and retroperitoneal lymph nodes.

Table 31.1: Jackson staging system	
Stage I (A)	Tumors confined to the glans, prepuce or penile skin
Stage II (B)	Tumors extending onto the shaft of the penis
Stage III (C)	Tumors with inguinal metastases that are operable
Stage IV (D)	Tumors involving adjacent structures and tumors associated with inoperable inguinal metastases or distant metastases

	Table 31.2: TNM staging system
Tx	Primary tumor cannot be assessed.
T0	There is no evidence of primary tumor.
Tis	There is carcinoma *in situ*.
Ta	There is noninvasive verrucous carcinoma.
T1	Tumor invades subepithelial connective tissue.
T2	Tumor invades corpora spongiosum or cavernosum.
T3	Tumor invades urethra or prostate.
T4	Tumor invades other adjacent structures.
N1	Single superficial inguinal node
N2	Multiple or bilateral superficial inguinal nodes
N3	Deep inguinal or pelvic nodes
M0	No distant metastasis
M1	Presence of distant metastasis

TREATMENT OF THE PRIMARY TUMOR

The standard of therapy for the primary cancer is either partial or total penectomy.

In patients with small tumors confined to the prepuce, a circumcision may be adequate. Margins of 2 cm are necessary to reduce local recurrences. Attempts to treat cancers larger than 1.5 cm have led to a high recurrence rate.

A partial amputation is appropriate when the cancer involves the glans and distal shaft. A 2 cm margin is necessary. If partial penectomy does not provide an adequate margin, a total penectomy should be considered. The penile stump following a partial penectomy should be sufficiently long to allow the patient to urinate while standing. A perineal urethrostomy is necessary along with total amputation. There are a few surgical complications involved in partial or complete penectomy. They include infection, edema, or urethral stricture if a new urethral meatus needs to be constructed.

Another surgical technique is the Mohs' micrographic surgery (MMS), which is applicable to some patients with noninvasive disease. This involves removing the skin cancer by excising thin layers of tissue and examining them microscopically. With an experienced surgeon, of this technique, the ability to remove the cancerous tissue while preserving normal structures makes this an attractive procedure because the results are similar to those obtained from more radical surgery.

Laser surgery has been used for patients with Tis, Ta, T1 and some T2 penile cancers. Two types of lasers have been used. They include the CO_2 (carbon dioxide) and ND:YAG. The CO_2 laser vaporizes tissues but penetrates only to a depth of 0.01 mm and can coagulate blood vessels < 0.5 mm. The ND:YAG laser can penetrate 3-6 mm depending on the power and can coagulate vessels up to 5 mm. Close follow up is essential for these patients undergoing laser therapy to detect tumor recurrences demanding further therapy.

Radiation therapy can be used as an alternative modality in selected patients. The psychological trauma associated with partial or complete penectomy has encouraged radiation therapists to explore various techniques of treatment for this disease. High tumor dose (60cGy) necessary to treat the tumor may cause urethral fistula, strictures, penile necrosis, pain and edema. Candidates for radiation therapy include young men with small (< 3 cm), superficial, exophytic lesions or noninvasive cancers on the glans or coronal sulcus. Other candidates are those who refuse surgery or have metastatic disease and need some form of palliative therapy. The use of external beam therapy and brachytherapy has been reported on patients with penile cancers.

TREATMENT OF INGUINAL NODES

Cancers that have invaded through the basement membrane are much more likely to have nodal metastases than superficial tumors. Nodal metastases are more frequently associated with high-grade or invasive histology.

Following the treatment of the primary tumor, consideration is given to the management of the inguinal lymph nodes. These nodes may be enlarged because of cancer or infection. They are better assessed after a course of antibiotic therapy.

Bilateral inguinal lymphadenectomy should be performed if palpable lymph nodes are present after the primary tumor has been treated and the patient has been on antibiotics. This surgery is usually performed several weeks after the primary tumor has been removed and the penile wound has healed. Bilateral inguinal lymphadenectomy is also advocated in patients with no palpable lymph nodes but with a higher tumor stage (T2, T3).

The decision to resect the inguinal nodes in patients with no evidence of adenopathy, either clinically or on imaging studies, with a low tumor stage (Ta, Tis, T1) is controversial. Because of the morbidity associated with this surgery, some urologists have contended that it is safe to observe these patients. If on follow-up there is appearance of unilateral lymph node enlargement, a unilateral node dissection might suffice.

Superficial dissection has been employed for patients with no palpable nodes, but the procedure is extended to the deep fascia and femoral canal if any nodes are positive for cancer. Catalona, in 1988, described a superficial and deep inguinal node dissection technique employing limited boundaries to minimize morbidity. Cabanas, in 1977, suggested that there is consistent drainage of lymphatics of the penis, into a sentinel node or group of nodes located superiomedial to the junction of the saphenous and femoral veins in the area of the superficial epigastric vein. Metastasis to this node indicated the need for a complete superficial and deep inguinal dissection. But many authors feel this procedure is too limited and often inaccurate in predicting the extent of the cancer.

The indications for pelvic lymphadenectomy have not been clearly delineated. Patients with negative inguinal lymph nodes rarely have pelvic node involvement. When 2 or more inguinal nodes contain cancer, there is an increased probability of pelvic node involvement.

Complications associated with inguinal node dissections are common and are generally connected with more extensive dissections. Early complications include wound infection, skin flap necrosis, seromas, phlebitis, and pulmonary embolus. Late complications include lymphedema of the lower extremities. Mortality due to sepsis has been reported in situations where surgery was performed when the nodes were infected.

FURTHER READING

1. Burgers JK. Penile cancer: Clinical presentation, diagnosis and staging. Urol Clin North Am 1992;19:267-73.
2. Dechev IY, Banchev AB, Kadim MN, Zdravchev SA. Penile cancer—surgical treatment of the primary tumor. Folia Med 2001;43(4):46-50.
3. Gerber GS. Carcinoma in situ of penis. J Urol 1994;151:829-36.
4. Khandpur S, Reddy BS, Kaur H. Multiple cutaneous metastases from carcinoma of the penis. J Dermatol 2002;29(5):296-99.
5. Lopes A, Bezerra AL, Pinto CA, Serrano SV, de MellO CA, Villa LL. p53 as a new prognostic factor for lymph node metastasis in penile carcinoma: Analysis of 82 patients treated with amputation and bilateral lymphadenectomy. J Urol 2002;168(1):81-86.
6. Ono Y, Ozawa M, Tamura Y, Suzuki T, Suzuki K, et al. Tumor-associated tissue eosinophilia of penile cancer. Int J Urol 2002;9(2):82-87.
7. Tanis PJ, Lont AP, Meinhardt W, Olmos RA, et al. Dynamic sentinel node biopsy for penile cancer: Reliability of a staging technique. Urol 2002;168(1):76-80.

Brain Tumors

32

M Nageswara Rao

INTRODUCTION

History mentions that some form of neurosurgery was practiced in India in ancient times. It was mainly concerned with head injuries sustained in battles. Susrutha and Charaka (5th century AD), two ancient Indian surgeons, were pioneers in this field. In fact, Susrutha mentions in his surgical treatise '*Susrutha Samhita*' about burr holes placed in the skull to relieve intracranial pressure. It was Jivaka, the personal physician of Gautama Buddha (BC 566-480) who was known as the earliest Indian neurosurgeon. It was he who applied trephine holes and removed intracranial tumors during Buddha's time. Two physicians working together removed the pearly intracranial tumor on King Bhoja of Dhar and relieved him of his headache.

The development of modern neurosurgery is intimately connected with diagnosis and the treatment of brain and spinal cord tumors. In the earlier years the cerebral localization was a great challenge, and it was made possible by the tireless endeavor of many great neurologists like David Firier, William Grover, Leopole Goltz, Victor Horsley, Paul Broca, John Hughlings Jackson and Sir Charles Sherrington.

The recent advances in imaging sciences like CT scan, MRI, etc, modern techniques in surgery like the endoscopic instruments, radiotherapy and chemotherapy have helped the neurosurgeon to achieve the lowest morbidity and mortality in patients with brain tumors. The pioneers in this field of neurosurgery whose contributions shall ever be remembered are men like Sir Victor Horsley (1857-1916), Sir William Macewen (1848-1924), Harvey Cushing (1869-1939), Egaz Monitz, Walter Dandy and Norman Dott. In India Jacob Chandy, Baladev Singh and Ramamoorthi were the pioneers in modern neurosurgery.

Computed axial tomography: (Popularly called CT scan or CAT scan) it has brought revolutionary changes in the management of neurological disorders and in fact neurosurgical period can be divided into 'Pre Scan and Post Scan era'. The combined efforts of Hounsfield, Cormack and Ambrose successfully applied this new modality in clinical practice. Hounsfield was awarded the Nobel Prize for medicine for the discovery of CT scan.

Magnetic resonance imaging: The concept of MRI (initially called Nuclear Magnetic Resonance) was originated by the Dutch physicist Gorier in 1936. Lauterbus suggested that MRI can be used on humans and in January 1977 a team from Nottingham University produced the first human images in clinical medicine.

The other advances in the field of imaging sciences are:

MRI spectroscopy, MRI angiography, digital subtraction angiography (DSA), single photo emission computed tomography (SPECT), positron emission tomography (PET), Biomagnetography, etc.

NEUROELECTROPHYSIOLOGICAL INVESTIGATIONS

1. EEG
2. Sensory evoked potentials: somatosensory evoked potentials (SSEP) visual evoked potentials, auditory evoked potentials.

HUMAN NERVOUS SYSTEM

Human nervous system is divided into central nervous system (brain and spinal cord) and peripheral nervous system (cranial and spinal nerves and their associated ganglia). Autonomic nervous system is concerned with the control of cardiac muscle, smooth muscle and glands and it is part and parcel of both central and peripheral nervous system.

The central nervous system comprising brain and spinal cord is composed of three basic elements:

1. neuron
2. neuralgia (astrocytes, oligodendrocytes, ependymal cells and microglial cells)
3. blood vessels

Neuroglial cells outnumber the neurons and constitute only 50 percent of the total volume and weight of the brain and spinal cord. Literally neurons are in the sea of glial cells. Depending upon the region, glial cells outnumber the neurons 10 to 100 times.

Astrocytes, oligodendrocytes and ependymal cells are derived from the neuroectoderm, whereas microglia, the scavengers of the central nervous system are derived from the bone marrow. Glial cells are astrocytes, oligodendrocytes and ependymal cells.

MAGNITUDE OF THE PROBLEM

Cancer is the leading cause of death next to cardiovascular diseases in developed countries. The incidence of malignant tumors of the central nervous system ranges from 5.1 (Chandigarh) to 3.7 (Thiruvanantha-puram) per 1,00,000 population (NCRP 1984-1993, page No.5). Primary central nervous system tumors account for 9 to 10 percent of all cancer deaths. About 10 percent of all nervous system disorders are neoplasms, 50 percent are gliomas and out of 100 gliomas 55 percent are glioblastoma multiforme, 20 to 30 percent are grade I to grade III and the rest is grade IV. Astrocytomas and oligodendrogliomas form another 20 percent and the rest are other types of tumors, such as meningiomas, ependymomas and secondary brain tumors. Hence 25 percent of all intracranial tumors are glioblastoma multiforme the most common and most malignant tumor of the brain. In general 70 percent of the tumors in adults are supratentorial while in children 70 percent are infratentorial. In children 20 percent of cancer deaths are due to the central nervous system tumors.

In India the incidence of all cancers ranges from 106.2 to 130.4 for men and from 100 to 140.7 for women per 1,00,000 population.

GENETIC CHANGES IN CNS TUMORS

Molecular Genetics of Gliomas

Genetic alterations form a continuum of progressive anaplasia in gliomas. Whereas secondary or progressive gliomas seldom show epidermal growth factor receptor (EGFR) amplification, primary or *de novo* glioblastoma multiforme (GBM) usually lacks p53 mutations and contains an amplified EGFR. However, none of the molecular parameters has demonstrated any significant association with patient survival in GBM (Table 32.1).

CLASSIFICATION OF BRAIN TUMORS

Classification of brain tumors dates back to Virchow who studied cerebral and spinal tumors based on a combination of naked eye and microscope examinations. Tooth (1912) after studying the neoplasms, collected at the National Hospital, Queen Square, London attempted to link the course

Table 32.1: Different stages of genetic alteration		
Genetic alteration	*Anaplasia*	*Glioma variants*
TP53 mutation astrocytoma PDGF overexpression Loss of chromosome 17p and 22q	Low grade	Low-grade
CDKN2/p16 deletion RB mutation CDK4 amplification Loss of chromosome 9p, 19q, 11p	Anaplastic astrocytoma	
MDM2 amplification/overexpression EGFR amplification rearrangements PTEN mutation Loss of chromosome 13GBM, glioblastoma multiforme	High grade	GBM

of the disease observed clinically with morphology of the underlying growths.

Bailey and Cushing classified the brain tumors based on embryogenesis of the various cellular components of the central nervous system and attempted to classify the tumors observed in terms of morphological stages through which these cells pass on oncogenesis. Even the modern classification of brain tumors is based on the Bailey and Cushing's classification. Kermohan and Sayre (1952) divided the gliomas into 7 groups depending upon:

1. Cellularity
2. Pleomorphism
3. Presence of giant cells
4. Vascularity
5. Endothelial proliferation
6. Mitosis
7. Necrosis and infiltration zone

They have also graded them into 4 grades: grade I and II low-grade, grade III anaplastic, grade IV highly malignant glioblastoma multiforme.

Ringers objected to this type of grading, as he hardly noticed any difference of survival rate between grade III and grade IV Zulch supported the Kemohan's grading as he noticed difference in survival rates in different grades of the gliomas.

Hart and Earle classified certain supratentorial tumors in infancy as Primitive neuroectodermal tumors (PNET). Rorke and Becker proposed to include all CNS neoplasms of embryonal neuroectodermal origin as PNET.

Revised WHO classification is given in Tables 32.1 to 32.6.

CLINICAL FEATURES OF INTRACRANIAL TUMOR

An expanding intracranial tumor may present in two ways.

1. General (non-localizing)
   a. *Signs and symptoms of raised intracranial tension.* Raised intracranial tension may be due to tumor itself or tumor related epiphenomenon, e.g. Peritumoral edema, intratumoral bleed and hydrocephalus in case of posterior fossa and midline tumors.
   Headache is the commonest symptom in most of the gliomas followed by vomiting, and diplopia due to the sixth cranial nerve involvement. Papilledema is the commonest clinical sign of raised intracranial tension. Change in mental status occurs from minor deficits in higher intellectual functions to psychomotor asthenia, and depressed consciousness. Alteration in intellectual functions may be in the form of loss of memory, judgement and reasoning. Patients with intracranial tumors usually present with chronic

Table 32.2: Revised WHO classification (Kleihues and Cavenee 2000)

Tumors of the neuroepithelial tissue
Astrocytic tumors
Diffuse astrocytoma (grade II)
Fibrillary astrocytoma
Protoplasmic astrocytoma
Gemistocytic astrocytoma
Anaplastic astrocytoma (grade III)
Glioblastoma (grade IV)
Giant cell glioblastoma
Gliosarcoma
Pilocytic astrocytoma (grade I)
Pleomorphic xanthoastrocytoma (grade II)
Oligodendroglial tumors
Oligoastrocytoma (grade II)
Anaplastic oligodendrogliomas (grade III)
Mixed gliomas
Oligoastrocytoma (grade II)
Anaplastic oligoastrocytoma (grade III)
Ependymal tumors
Ependymoma (grade II)
• cellular
• papillary
• clear cell
• tanycytic
Anaplastic ependymoma (grade III)
Myxopapillary ependymoma (grade I)
Subependymoma (grade I)
Choroid plexus tumors
Choroid plexus papilloma (grade I)
Choroid plexus carcinoma
Glial tumors of uncertain origin
Astroblastoma (grade not assigned)
Gliomatosis cerebra (grade III)
Choroid glioma of the third ventricle (grade II)
Neuronal and mixed neuronal glial tumors
Gangliocytoma (grade I)
Dysplastic gangliocytoma of cerebellum (Lhermitte-Duclos)
Desmoplastic infantile astrocytoma/ganglioglioma (grade I)
Dysembryoplastic neuroepithelial tumor (DNT) (grade I)
Ganglioglioma (grade I or II)
Anaplastic ganglioglioma (grade III)
Central neurocytoma (grade III)
Cerebellar liponeurocytoma (grade I or II)
Paraganglioma of the filum terminal (grade I)
Neuroblastic tumors
Olfactory neuroblastoma (esthesion-neuroblastoma)
Olfactory neuroepithelioma
Neuroblastoma of the adrenal gland and sympathetic nervous system

contd...

Table 32.2: contd...

Pineal parenchyma tumors
Pineocytoma (grade II)
Pineoblastoma (grade IV)
Pineal parenchymal tumor of intermediate differentiation
Embryonal tumors
Medulloepithelioma
Ependymoblastoma
Medulloblastoma (grade IV)
- desmoplastic medulloblastoma
- large cell medulloblastoma
- medullomyoblastoma
- melanotic medulloblastoma
- supratentorial primitive neuroectodermal tumor (PNET) (grade IV)
- neuroblastoma
- ganglioneuroblastoma
Atypical treated/rehabbed tumor (grade IV)
Tumors of peripheral nerves
Schwannoma (grade I)
(neurilemmoma, neurinoma)
- cellular
- plexiform
- melanotic
Neurofibroma (grade I)
- plexiform
Perineurioma (grade I)
- intramural perineurioma
- soft tissue perineurioma
Malignant peripheral nerve sheath tumor (MPNST) (grade III or IV)
- epithelioid
- MPNST with divergent mesenchymal and/or epithelial differentiation
- melanotic
Melanotic psammomatous

Table 32.3: Tumors of the meninges

Tumors of the meningothelial cells
Meningioma (Grade I)
Meningothelial (Grade I)
Fibrous (Fibroblastic) (Grade I)
Psammomatous (Grade I)
Angiomatous (Grade I)
Microcystic (Grade I)
Secretory (Grade I)
Lymphoplasmacyte–Rich (Grade I)
Metaplastic (Grade I)
Clear Cell (Grade I)
Choroid (Grade II)
Atypical (Grade I)
Papillary (Grade I)
Rhabdoid (Grade I)
Anaplastic meningiomas (Grade III)

Table 32.4: Mesenchymal, non-meningothelial tumors

Lipoma
Angiolipoma
Hibernoma
Liposarcoma (Intracranial)
Solitary fibrous tumor
Fibrosarcoma
Malignant fibrous histiocytoma
Leiomyoma
Leiomyosarcoma
Rhadomyoma
Rhadomyosarcoma
Chondroma
Chondrosarcoma
Osteoma
Osteosarcoma
Osteochondroma
Hemangioma
Epithelioid hemangioendothelium
Hemangiopericytoma (Grade II Or III)
Angiosarcoma
Kaposi's sarcoma
Primary melanocytic lesions
Diffuse melanocytosis
Melanocytoma
Malignant melanoma
Meningeal melanomatosis

Table 32.5: Tumors of the uncertain histiogenesis

Hemangioblastoma
Lymphomas and hemopoietic neoplasms
Malignant lymphomas
Plasmocytoma
Granulocytic sarcoma
Germ cell tumor
Germinoma
Embryonal carcinoma
Yolk sac tumor
Choriocarcinoma
Teratoma
Mature
Immature
Teratoma with malignant transformation
Mixed germ cell tumors

Table 32.6: Tumors of the sellar region

Craniopharyngioma

Adamantinomatous

Papillary

Granular cell tumor

Metastatic tumor

intracranial hypertension. Acute onset may be seen in intratumoral bleeding which can occur without any warning, e.g. secondaries from choriocarcinoma, malignant melanoma etc.

In late stages the patient may present with various herniation syndromes (tentorial, subfalcine, tonsillar, foramen magnum herniation).

In case of intraventricular tumors of the brain the patient will present with raised intracranial tension due to hydrocephalus without any localizing signs. Sometimes the patient may present with false localizing signs.

b. *Seizures* Seizure is the commonest symptom next to headache.

The definition of seizure: It is paroxysmal abnormal synchronized neuronal discharge in the brain resulting in disturbances of movement, sensation, behavior perception and/or consciousness. Characteristics of seizures, which signify the intracranial tumor are the following:

1. Late onset of seizure: It is the first episode of seizure occurring after the age of 18 years. It is very important and any patient presenting with late onset seizures should be investigated to rule out intracranial tumor.
    i. Change in character and frequency of the seizures
    ii. Status epilepticus
   iii. Postictal paralysis
    iv. Resistance to anticonvulsant therapy
    v. Seizures associated with raised intracranial tension and focal neurological deficits. Two percent of the seizures are caused by brain tumors in all age groups and in children 0.5 percent of seizures are by brain tumors.
    Brain tumor may occasionally present with systemic manifestations.
2. Focal neurological signs and symptoms
   Focal neurological deficits are due to alteration in brain function adjacent to tumor or tumor itself. They may be in the form of:
    i. Motor or sensory deficits
    ii. Speech disturbances
   iii. Seizures

   iv. Cranial nerve involvement
    v. Visual disturbances
   vi. Endocrinal disturbances
  vii. Syndromes associated with lobes of the brain
 viii. Cerebellar deficits.

FOCAL NEUROLOGICAL DEFICITS

A tumor located in the motor area will give rise to contralateral hemiparesis, hemiplegia, monoparesis or monoplegia. Tumor located in the sensory area may give rise to sensory deficits in the form of paresthesia etc. and a tumor located in the motor speech area will give rise to confluent aphasia. Sensory aphasia results from tumor located in the Wernick's area.

Seizures: The type of seizure may localize the location of the tumor. Absence of seizures in children may be associated with tumors located in the frontal and temporal components of the limbic system.

Complex partial seizures (psychomotor epilepsy) consist of disorders of awareness, perception, emotion and movement. It indicates medial temporal lobe involvement.

Somatosensory seizures consisting of paresthesias, numbness, a sense of extreme heaviness, or illusions of movement point to a lesion in the contralateral postcentral gyrus.

Focal motor seizures indicate tumor in the contralateral frontal lobe. *Involvement of cranial nerves:* It is seen in the initial stages of tumors like CP angle tumors, pituitary tumors and tumors involved in the cavernous sinus.

Visual disturbances: It manifests in the form of decrease in visual activity, field defects and blindness. Optical nerve involvement is either due to direct pressure over the optic nerve or chiasma resulting in primary optic atrophy, e.g. pituitary edema, craniopharyngioma or increased intracranial tension results in papilledema followed by the secondary optic atrophy leading to blindness in late stages.

Endocrinal disturbances are discussed in pituitary disorders.

SYNDROMES ASSOCIATED WITH LOBES OF THE BRAIN

Effect of Frontal Lobe Involvement

Unilateral frontal lobe lesions give rise to contralateral motor paralysis, lack of initiative, difficulty in adaptation, lack of tact, elevated mood, tendency to joke, and increased talkativeness.

If the lesion is in entirely prefrontal region no motor paralysis but revival of elementary reflexes are seen (grasping and suckling reflexes). Pure motor area lesion results in flaccid paralysis. If the lesion involves both premotor and motor areas it results in spastic paralysis.

Bilateral frontal lobe involvement results in bilateral hemiplegia and spastic bulbar palsy.

If prefrontal lobes are involved diffusely the following features are seen: abulia, akinetic mutism, lack of restraint with hyperactivity, flight of ideas, distractibility, failure to realize impairment in memory and social sense.

Effects of Parietal Lobe Involvement

Somatosensory area involvement manifests in focal sensory epilepsy, parietal hemianesthesia, disturbances in two-point discrimination, loss of position sense, fine touch, pain and temperature and vibrations and objective recognition disturbance, astereognosis and graphesthesia. Involvement of dominant parietal lobe results in transcortical aphasia, apraxia, agnosia and Gestman syndrome. Gestman syndrome includes right and left disorientation, finger agnosia, acalculia and agraphia.

Involvement of nondominant parietal lobe results in:
1. Anosognosia (loss of recognition of side of the limb)
2. Autotopognosia (patient believes that part of his body actually does not exist and belongs to someone else)
3. Constructional apraxia
4. Dressing apraxia
5. Visuospatial disorientation
6. Hemispatial neglect and loss of topographic memory. Visual field defects in the form of homonymous hemianopia with macular sparing.

Effects of Temporal Lobe Involvement

Effects of involvement of either of the temporal lobe results in:
1. Auditory, visual, olfactory and gustatory hallucinations. Well-formed visual hallucinations are characteristic features of temporal lobe involvement.
2. Dreamy states with uncinate seizures.
3. Emotional and behavioral changes.
4. Disturbances in time perception.

Involvement of dominant lobe results in Wernick's aphasia, amusia and visual agnosia.

Effects of involvement of nondominant hemisphere results in agnosia for sounds and inability to judge spatial relationships in some cases.

Bilateral temporal lobe involvement manifests as Korsakoff amnesic effect and Kluver-Bucy syndrome (hyperorality, hypersexuality, blunted emotional reactivity).

Visual field defects are in the form of upper quadrant hemianopia.

Effects of Occipital Lobe Involvement

Involvement of either of the lobes results in unformed visual hallucinations and contralateral homonymous hemianopia. Involvement of left occipital lobe results in visual object agnosia and involvement of right occipital lobe results in visual illusions, visual hallucinations and loss of topographic memory and visual orientation.

Bilateral occipital disease manifests as:
1. Cortical blindness
2. Denial of cortical blindness (Anton syndrome)
3. Loss of perception of color and Balint syndrome.

Bilateral destruction of primary visual areas (striate area) results in total blindness.

CLINICAL FEATURES OF CEREBELLAR LESIONS

1. Disorders of postural fixation
   a. Hyptomia
   b. Pendular knee jerk
2. Disorders of movement
   a. Intention tremors
   b. Dysmetria
   c. Dyssynergia
   d. Dysdiadochokinesia
   e. Rebound phenomenon
3. Disorders of gait
   a. Swaying towards side of the lesion
   b. Truncal ataxia
   c. Titubation
4. Ocular signs
   a. Nystagmus
5. Speech disturbances
   a. Dysarthria in the form of scanning or explosive or staccato speech.

TREATMENT OF BRAIN TUMORS (GENERAL PRINCIPLES)

The ultimate aim in the treatment of brain tumors is to reduce the morbidity and mortality of patients affected by this serious malady. Advances in neuroimaging, surgical techniques, modern equipments and adjuvant therapy are complementary to each other and no single method of treatment is complete or ideal. It is always a multimodality approach. In malignant lesions, even multimodality approach achieves a palliation. First operation for glioma was performed in 1884 by Godlee and interstitial brachytherapy was started by Madame Curie in 1898. Though the surgical treatment and radiation therapy started more than 100 years ago and even with the latest developments in the neurosurgical and allied fields, there is no cure for glioblastoma multiforme (GBM). The treatment of low-grade gliomas, brainstem gliomas, intracranial metastasis, etc. still remains controversial. On the contrary, benign tumors of the brain on proper treatment are associated with gratifying results. Peroperative use of ultrasound to localize the tumor and CUSA (Cavitron Ultrasonic Aspirator) to decompress and coagulate the tumor are widely accepted. Lasers are also made use of in the treatment of brain tumors.

The treatment of brain tumors falls into four main types:
1. Medical
2. Surgical
3. Radiotherapy
4. Chemotherapy
   Radiotherapy and chemotherapy are together called *Adjuvant therapy.* Adjuvant therapy is applied in an attempt to prevent recurrence after surgical treatment or to treat recurrence after it arises.

Medical Therapy

a. Steroids (dexamethasone and methyl prednisolone): These are administered to reduce the size of the tumor and peritumoral edema.
b. Diuretic is commonly used during surgery to prevent the brain swelling and in case of emergencies to decrease the intracranial pressure.
c. Anticonvulsant drugs are indicated in any supratentorial lesions especially where there is high incidence of seizures, as in meningioma and oligodendroglioma, etc. They are continued postoperatively to a certain period.
d. Hormone therapy is particularly important in pituitary tumors with endocrinal dysfunction during both pre- and postoperative periods. Hormone therapy is also indicated in case of hormone dependent carcinoma breast with intracranial metastasis.

Surgical Therapy

It is most crucial when compared to other modalities. Cytoreduction is the basis of this treatment. It helps in histopathological examination so as to know the type of the tumor, its grade and thus to assess the prognosis. Surgery decreases the intracranial pressure and is complementary to adjuvant therapy by removing non-dividing cells and synchronizing with phases of cell cycles.

It is important to remember that posterior fossa lesions are associated with hydrocephalus due to the fourth ventricular obstruction, e.g. CP angle tumors, medulloblastoma, ependymoma and cerebellar hemispheric lesions. Performing V-P shunt is helpful in these tumors.

Operative procedures include: 1. Closed tumor biopsy, 2. Stereotactic procedures.

Open Operation

Stereotactic procedures are valuable both for diagnosis (diagnostic biopsy) and therapeutic management (tumors, cyst aspiration and brachytherapy implantation).

Steps in open operation:

1. Documentation of neurological deficits and discussion on prognosis with patient and relatives are absolutely important and consent is taken for surgery.
2. Pre-anesthetic evaluation is done.
3. Preparation of the head and a single dose of antibiotic are provided.
4. Blood reservation is essential.
5. Open operation is done under general anesthesia. In some centers awake-craniotomy is practiced in case of lesions in eloquent areas.
6. Indwelling urinary catheter is passed due to long duration of surgery and use of diuretics during surgery.
7. The position of the patient is important. Keeping the head 10 to 15 degrees above the level of the heart favors the venous drainage of the head preventing brain swelling. Brain swelling is also a complication of endotracheal tube obstruction and preoperation overhydration.

   Supine, prone lateral, sitting and semisitting positions are commonly followed. In case of sitting and semisitting positions, developments of hypotension and air embolism and pneumocephalus are to be kept in mind.
8. Marking the craniotomy flap is of paramount importance. After the advent of CT scan and MRI, the classical frontal, parietal, temporal and occipital craniotomies are tailored depending on the extent of the tumor as the tumor need not be confined to anatomical divisions of the brain.
9. Osteoplastic bone flap is preferred to free bone flap.

   In case of posterior fossa lesions, midline, lateral or extreme lateral craniectomies are performed.
10. Dura is opened, when brain is lax.
11. Tumor decompression, radical excision and lobectomies are the procedures usually followed.
12. Hemostasis is secured.

Postoperative care includes placement of patient on ventilator and administration of antibiotics, anticonvulsant, antiedema measures and ancillary drugs (analgesics).

RECENT ADVANCES IN TREATMENT OF BRAIN TUMORS

Neuroendoscopy (Video Endoscopic Neurosurgery-VENS)

Lespinasse (a urologist) started the treatment of hydrocephalus by endoscopic approach in 1910. Applying the same principle, Dandy in 1922 coagulated the choroid plexus to treat hydrocephalus. Since 1962, Bosma of Holland pioneered the various applications of neuroendoscopy.

The main indications with reference to brain tumors are:

a. Cystic tumors (biopsy, partial and total removal and fenestration).

b. Tumor biopsy, partial or total removal of the tumors, e.g. intraventricular tumors and craniopharyngioma.

c. Endoscopy-assisted microsurgery-acoustic neuroma, transsphenoidal pituitary surgery.

CT/MRI based computer-assisted volumetric stereotactic resection of intracranial lesions.

With this volumetric stereotactic assessment, the surgeon visualizes the border between tumor and normal brain. Hence this form of assessment, guides the surgeon to excise only tumor tissue avoiding manipulation of adjacent normal brain. It is particularly effective in deep-seated lesions (thalamic glioma).

Radiotherapy (Refer Chapter 48)

Radiosurgery

Lars Leksell introduced the term radiosurgery in 1951. It is the treatment of tumor without surgery. At the same time, the radiation dose given affects later surgical treatment. It is a noninvasive procedure. In this modality, multiple intersecting radiation waves are given stereotactically in a single session. A total dose of 60 Gy is delivered in 30-33 fractions to a small target area. Radiosensitivity of the tumor is not essential. The physical property of the radiation dose results in tumor necrosis. The tumorocidal effect is due to damage of DNA or intravascular thrombosis leading to ischemia and necrosis. The goal of any radiosurgical procedure is to deliver accurately high dose of radiation to a small target in a single session with minimal exposure to surrounding normal brain. Stereotactic radiosurgery is different from stereotactic radiotherapy. In stereotactic radiosurgery only physical properties of radiation are utilized whereas in stereotactic radiotherapy biological property of the tumor is important.

There are three sources of radiation in radiosurgery:

1. Cobalt-machines provide gamma rays and the knife is called gamma knife (In gamma knife, 100 to 400 cGy per minute is given).

2. X-rays from linear accelerator are used and is known as X-knife.

3. Charged particle radiation (very expensive).

Radiosurgery is applicable only to non-infiltrative and well-localized tumors and it is applied in cases where surgery and radiotherapy have failed.

STEREOTACTIC INTERSTITIAL RADIOSURGERY IN THE MANAGEMENT OF BRAIN TUMORS

Interstitial brachytherapy means placement of radioactive source within the tumor tissue. Radiosurgery means high dose of radiation given in a single session non-invasively. Interstitial radiosurgery implies the delivery of ionizing radiation interstitial to the tumor (as in brachytherapy) and in a high dose fraction (as in radiosurgery)-hence the name interstitial radiosurgery. The equipment is called Photon Radio Surgical system (PRS). It is a novel device for the treatment of intracranial metastases and possibly for other tumors.

It consists of a portable miniature X-ray generator capable of delivering a prescribed therapeutic radiation dose directly into the tumor of a small size. The PRS is mounted on the carrier of the CRW frame that stereotactically places the probe tip at the target center. After the device has been activated, a low-energy X-ray beam emanates from the tip of the probe to irradiate the lesion target.

Technique: A burr hole is made under local anesthesia and sedation for stereotactic biopsy. If frozen section proves malignancy, dilators are passed to introduce the probe of 3 mm diameter.

The probe of PRS system is passed through the same path into the center of the tumor and radiation is given for a few minutes.

After radiation, the probe is removed and the wound is closed.

PRIMARY BRAIN TUMORS

The annual incidence of intracranial tumors is 16.5 per 1,00,000 population (US Statistics). Half of them are primary and the rest are secondary deposits. Incidence of primary intracranial tumors is 8.2 per 1,00,000 population per year. The tumors which originate—neuronal, glial or neuroglial cells—are grouped as neuroepithelial tumors. They are incompletely removable with recurrent tumor growth having poor prognosis. Gliomas are subgroups of neuroepithelial tumors (i.e. astrocytoma, oligodendroglioma and ependymoma).

Neuroepithelial tumors account for 50 to 60 percent of primary intracranial tumors in adults. The ratio of glial tumors to that of neuronal tumors is about 100:1. Among 100 cases of neuroepithelial tumors, 50 percent are glioblastoma multiforme, 30 percent anaplastic astrocytomas, 6 percent oligodendrogliomas, 5 percent non-anaplastic astrocytomas, 4 percent ependymal cell tumors, and 2 percent medulloblastomas as well as 3 percent nerve cell tumors. Neuroblastomas, pineal cell tumors, subependymal giant cell astrocytomas, pilocytic astrocytomas and choroid plexus tumors account for 1 percent each.

CLASSIFICATION OF NEUROEPITHELIAL TUMORS

Neuroepithelial tumors are categorized into:
1. Astrocytic tumors
2. Oligodendroglial tumors (low grade and malignant)
3. Ependymal cell tumors (ependymoma, anaplastic ependymoma, etc.)
4. Mixed gliomas

5. Tumors of choroid plexus
6. Neuroepithelial tumors of uncertain origin
7. Neuronal and mixed neuronal glial tumors (gangliocytoma, dysplastic gangliocytoma, ganglioglioma, central neurocytoma, olfactory neuroblastoma, etc.)
8. Pineal tumors
9. Tumors with neuroblastic or glioblastic elements (embryonal tumors, medulloepithelioma and PNET-medulloblastoma).

Astrocytic tumors are further divided into six groups:
   a. Astrocytoma (protoplasmic, gamistocytic, fibrillary and mixed)
   b. Anaplastic astrocytoma (malignant)
   c. Glioblastoma multiforme
   d. Pilocytic astrocytoma
   e. Subependymal giant cell astrocytoma
   f. Pleomorphic xanthoastrocytoma.

Astrocytic Tumors

They constitute 75 percent of gliomas. Astrocytomas vary histologically from low-grade tumors to highly malignant glioblastoma multiforme. The rate of cell growth to turn into glioblastoma multiforme is highly variable. Glioblastoma multiforme may develop from preexisting low-grade astrocytoma or rarely from oligodendroglioma or ependymoma or *de novo*.

Astrocytoma

Age incidence is 25 to 45 years with no sex predilection. The most common site is frontal lobe and the least is occipital lobe. Histologically they are divided into protoplasmic astrocytoma, fibrillary astrocytoma and gamistocytic astrocytoma. Gamistocytic astrocytomas are considered anaplastic variety and 80 percent of them turn malignant. Fibrillary astrocytomas have poor prognosis particularly with infiltration to surrounding parenchyma.

Diagnostic Studies

Magnetic resonance imaging is superior to CT scan. The infiltrating limits of the tumor are well-delineated and no-contrast enhancement is noted with MRI. Astrocytoma is isointense on T1 and hyperintense on T2 weighted images. The contrast enhancement with CT-Scan is not conclusive.

Low-Grade Astrocytoma (Figs 32.1 and 32.2)

Low grade astrocytoma is a separate entity and their management is highly controversial. The low-grade tumors will turn into glioblastoma multiforme. The rate of growth of the tumor and biological behaviour of these

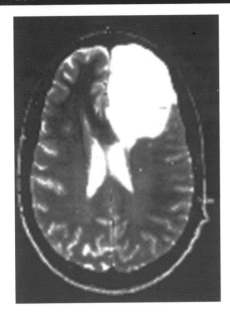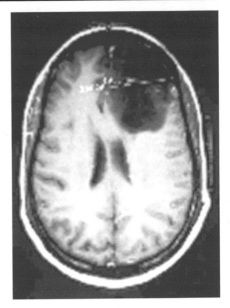

Figures 32.1 and 32.2: MRI of low-grade astrocytoma of the right frontal lobe

tumors are highly unpredictable. Under the heading of low-grade, glioma pilocytic astrocytomas, gangliogliomas, oligodendrogliomas, pleomorphic xanthocytomas, subependymal giant cell astrocytomas, and low-grade ependymomas are included. The management of low-grade gliomas depends on the clinical picture and the radiological evidence.

The options are:
1. Observation with periodical neurological examination and neuroimaging studies
2. Radiation
3. Resection with or without radiation.

Anaplastic Astrocytomas

The age incidence is 35 to 60 years with male preponderance and the frontal lobe is the commonest site of involvement.

Diagnostic Studies

They are hypointense on T1 and hyperintense on T2 weighted images with definite contrast enhancement. They show mass effect, brain edema and macrocystic changes.

The treatment of anaplastic astrocytoma is radical resection followed by radiotherapy and frequently chemotherapy.

Glioblastoma Multiforme (GBM)

GBM is the most common and most malignant tumor of the brain. It constitutes 50 to 55 percent of all gliomas and 25 percent of all intracranial tumors in adults.

The common age is 45 to 65 with male and female ratio 3:2. Glioblastoma multiforme most commonly occurs in the frontotemporal region and rarely occurs in posterior fossa. GBM may develop from pre-existing low-grade astrocytomas, oligodendrogliomas, ependymomas or anaplastic astrocytomas or *de novo*. It is considered the extreme of the continuum of astrocytic tumors. GBM shows all malignant features histologically (hypercellularity, cellular pleomorphism, nuclear pleomorphism, frequent mitosis, coagulative necrosis, capillary endothelial proliferation and pseudopalisades). The name multiforme is given due to heterogeneity of histological picture. They are highly infiltrating and due to this multi-centric nature is seen. In 2 to 5 percent of cases they are multifocal (independent sites of origin).

They extend and infiltrate to basal ganglia and brainstem regions. In case of corpus callosal gliomas due to bilateral extension they are called butterfly gliomas (Fig. 32.3). Metastatic spread occurs intracranially and extracranially. Lungs, lymph nodes and bone marrow are the commonest sites of secondary deposits.

Diagnostic Studies

MRI is the investigation of choice. It illustrates the variegated composition of the tumor with distortion and mass effect on neighboring structures. It is hypointense on T1 and hyperintense on T2 weighted images. Solid

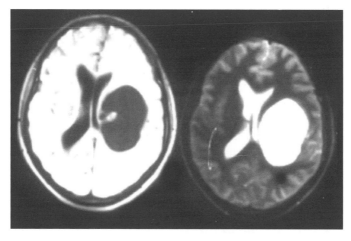

Figure 32.3: MRI of the cystic glioma with mural nodule of left parietal lobe (T1 and T2 weighted images)

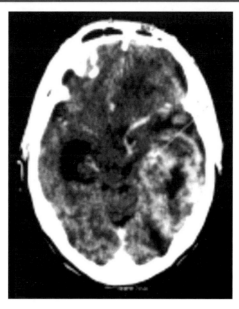

Figure 32.4: CT scan of glioblastoma multiforme of right temperoparietal lobe images

component of the tumor gets brightly enhanced with contrast. On CT scan they are heterogeneous. The image can be hypodense or isodense. Heterogeneous enhancement is noted on contrast administration, with significant edema and necrotic areas (Fig. 32.4).

Treatment

There is not a possibility of cure. Even with multimodality approach it is only palliative treatment. The treatment is radical resection followed by radiotherapy and chemotherapy. In some of the cases re-operation is frequently indicated.

Prognosis

The prognosis is very poor. It depends on the age of the patient, duration of the symptoms, clinical presentation, preoperative scoring and site of the tumor. If untreated, (after biopsy) the patient will die within three months. Only 10 percent will survive for 2 years after aggressive resection, irradiation and chemotherapy.

Oligodendrogliomas

The main cell type is oligodendrocyte. When compared to astrocytomas, they have got favorable prognosis. They constitute 4 percent of intracranial gliomas. The commonest age is 3rd to 5th decade. Occasionally it is seen in children. It is more commonly seen in males and the frontal lobe is the commonest site. Less than 10 percent occur in posterior fossa.

Microscopically the cells are monotonous sheets of small rounded cells. Perinuclear halo gives appearance like fried eggs and sheets of cells resemble honeycomb. Calcification occurs in 1/2 to 2/3 of cases.

Clinical Course

Patients with oligodendrogliomas present with long duration of symptoms. 50 percent of patients will present with seizures as an initial symptom and the incidence of seizures is 85 percent. The other manifestations are increased intracranial pressure and focal neurological deficits, etc.

Diagnostic Studies

MRI shows hypointense on T1 and hyperintense on T2 weighted images except in the regions of calcification. On CT scan they are hypodense or iso-dense without contrast enhancement. Calcification is seen in 90 percent cases.

Treatment: Craniotomy and decompression followed by radiotherapy depending on histological evidence of malignancy. Chemotherapy with procarbazine lomistine and vincristine has a role in anaplastic and aggressive oligodendrogliomas.

Ependymomas

These arise from the ependymal cells lining the ventricles and central canal of the spinal cord. Occasionally intraparenchymal location is seen due to ependymal cell rests.

Ependymomas constitute 5 percent of all intracranial gliomas. One-third of them are seen supratentorially and two-thirds infratentorially. Supratentorial tumors are more common in adults. Seventy-five percent of infratentorial tumors are seen in children and 25 percent in adults. Age incidence is in two peaks. One at the age of 5 years and the other at between 30 and 40 years. The commonest location is the fourth ventricle followed by lateral and third ventricles. Tumors may be seen totally or partially in the ventricular cavities. Infratentorial ependymomas arise from the floor of the fourth ventricle. Macroscopically, they are soft reddish gray masses, occasionally granular and microscopically, highly cellular, occasionally interrupted by papillary structure. Clusters of uniform polygonal cells separated by collagen containing stoma form most of the anaplastic ependymoma. Ependymal rosettes and pseudorosettes are also seen. About one-third to half of the cases show pseudo calcification.

Malignant conversion is seen in 10 percent of cases and the incidence of spinal seeding is less than 5 percent.

Clinical Picture

Headache is the commonest presentation. The patient may present with acute or progressive symptoms. Patients with posterior fossa tumors present with short duration of symptoms, with cerebellar and brainstem dysfunction. Other features of raised intracranial pressure also are seen.

Investigations

Plain X-ray may show features of raised ICP and calcification.

CT scan shows isodense to hyperdense mass with irregular contrast enhancement.

MRI shows hypointense and hyperintense in T1 and T2 weighted images respectively. Calcification also is seen. Irregular contrast enhancement is seen due to necrosis and cyst formation.

In brief, irregular enhancement with cyst formation and areas of calcification are more in favor of an ependymoma than medulloblastoma.

Ventriculoperitoneal shunt is performed to relieve ventriculomegaly (Fig. 32.5).

Treatment

Suboccipital craniotomy and total excision reduce the bulk of the tumor. Tissue diagnosis is followed by establishment of CSF pathways. Infiltration into brainstem may warrant total excision.

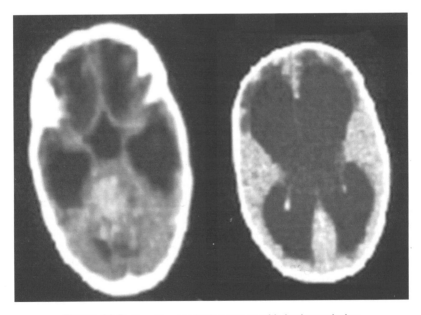

Figure 32.5: Fourth ventricular tumor with hydrocephalus

Ependymomas are radiosensitive. 4.5 to 5.4 Gy of external beam radiation is given with wide tumor margin. Spinal irradiation is controversial.

Prognosis

Five-year survival rate is 49 to 83 percent in adults with surgery followed by radiotherapy.

Medulloblastoma

Bailey and Cushing coined the term Medulloblastoma in 1925. Under WHO classification it is included in PNET and constitutes 3.7 percent of all intracranial tumors. 18 percent of all pediatric brain tumors and 29 percent of all posterior fossa tumors in children are medulloblastomas.

It is commonly seen in the first decade of life but can occur at any age. Males are more affected than females.

Pathology

Macroscopically they are solid, purple, friable and necrotic and may have pseudocapsule. In 90 percent of cases it is seen in vermis (posterior medullary velum) and 10 percent cases in the cerebellar hemisphere. They occupy the 4th ventricle frequently invading brainstem and cerebellar hemispheres. Microscopically they are highly cellular with hyperchromatic elongated or round nuclei with scanty cytoplasm. Fine fibrillary background is also seen. Presence of Homer-Wright's type of rosettes indicates neuroblastic differentiation. Desmoplastic variety seen in cerebellar hemisphere occurs in 20 years of age. They are made up of islands of cells surrounded by a network of fibrous and connective tissue. The cell of origin is controversial and is presumed to arise from medulloblast or germinative cell of external granular layer or from neuroblast.

Clinical Features

The commonest presentation is symptoms of increased intracranial tension (early morning headache, vomiting and papilledema). 80 percent of them are associated with hydrocephalus. Other manifestations are truncal ataxia, nystagmus and cranial nerve palsies. Occasionally they may present with spinal compression and cerebral hemispheric signs due to secondaries. The incidence of extra cranial spread is about 19 percent.

Radiology

Plain X-ray skull may show separation of sutures.

CT scan shows hyper or isodense oval or lobulated well circumscribed mass with homogeneous contrast enhancement and ventriculomegaly. Reconstruction studies are done to differentiate it from the 4th ventricular ependymoma. MRI shows homogeneous mass with prolonged T_1 and T_2 relaxation and contrast enhancement and ventriculomegaly.

Treatment

1. Treatment of hydrocephalus—ventriculoperitoneal shunt (VP shunt). These shunts are provided into filtering devises. CSF diversion is controversial due to peritoneal dissemination and shunt malfunction.
2. Treatment of tumor—Suboccipital craniotomy and macroscopic excision followed by radiotherapy is the accepted protocol. Radiotherapy is given in the following doses. 5000 – 5500 rads for posterior fossa, 4000—4500 rads for whole cranial cavity and 3000 – 3500 rads for spinal axis.
3. CCNU, lomustine and vincristine are commonly used as chemotherapeutic agents.

Brainstem Gliomas (Fig. 32.6)

Brainstem gliomas comprise 30 percent of pediatric posterior fossa tumors, 10 percent of all pediatric brain tumors and 1 percent of adult brain tumors.

Till 1980, based on clinical examination and CT scan, they were treated by radiotherapy and rarely operated on, assuming uniformly poor prognosis. After the advent of MRI, it was proved that brainstem gliomas are a heterogeneous group of lesions with variable prognostic importance.

Brainstem gliomas are classified by various authors but according to Albright AL, brainstem gliomas are classified as diffuse and focal. The diffuse type constitutes 75 percent and the focal type 25 percent. Focal tumors occur in midbrain (7 to 8%), in the pons as dorsally exophytic pontine gliomas (5%) and in the medulla (10 to 15%). Pontine tumors infiltrate entire pons and involve adjacent structures. The exophytic growth may extend up to the fourth ventricle or even up to cerebellopontine angle presenting as cerebellopontine angle tumors.

Clinical features: The commonest age is between 6 and 10 years.

Diffuse tumors: Diffuse tumors show classical signs of brainstem involvement, multiple asymmetric bilateral cranial nerve involvement. and long tract signs (hemiparesis, quadriparesis). Internuclear ophthalmoplegia (INO), nystagmus and ataxia are found in these tumors. Diffuse type is usually seen between 6 and 10 years of age with less than 2 months duration of symptoms. Children with symptomatology of less than 2 months with cranial nerve involvement have poor prognosis.

Focal Tumors

Mesencephalic (Midbrain)
  They are of two types:
  Non-enhancing periaqueductal gliomas have got indolent course and may present with hydrocephalus and the Perinaud's syndrome.

Enhancing focal lesions may manifest with third nerve palsy, hemiparesis and hydrocephalus.

Pons: Focal intrapontine (endophytic) tumors present with seventh nerve palsy, facial myokymia, hearing loss and motor weakness.

Medulla: They may be confined to medulla or extend up to cervical spinal cord. They may present with symptoms of lower cranial nerve palsies (difficulty in swallowing, hoarseness of voice and motor weakness).

Some consider dorsally exophytic group tumors are a subgroup of brainstem gliomas.

TREATMENT OF BRAINSTEM GLIOMAS (FIG. 32.6)

Patients with diffuse brainstem gliomas carry a bad prognosis. Hence both radiotherapy and chemotherapy are justified. Chemotherapy is started before starting of radiotherapy and is continued for one year after completion of radiotherapy. Recently hyperfractionated radiotherapy with total dose of 7600 cGy has been started and is found to be effective.

For focal cystic lesions cyst is evacuated followed by focal radiotherapy.

For focal solid tumors resection is the treatment of choice. Radiotherapy is indicated only when there is recurrence. For patients with malignant focal intrinsic lesions both chemotherapy and focal radiotherapy are given.

For dorsally exophytic tumors in the fourth ventricle resection is the treatment of choice and they are usually low grade astrocytomas and gangliogliomas.

Ventriculoperitoneal shunt is performed in cases associated with hydrocephalus.

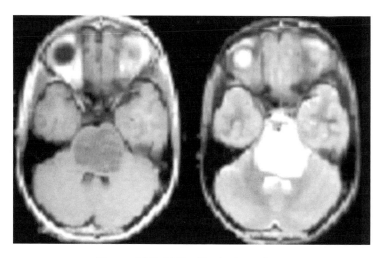

Figure 32.6: MRI of brainstem glioma

PINEAL TUMORS

They constitute 1 percent of intracranial tumors. They are called posterior third ventricular tumors. These tumors usually produce symptoms by compressing the midbrain or obstructing the aqueduct of Sylvius resulting in hydrocephalus. Perinad's syndrome includes:
1. Disturbances of vertical gaze
2. Pupillary abnormalities
3. Disturbance of accommodation
4. Convergence insufficiency
5. Lid retraction and
6. Retraction nystagmus

Pineal tumors can also extend anteriorly to involve hypothalamus causing diabetes insipidus and precocious puberty or the optic pathways. The common tumors are germinoma, pineocytoma, pineoblastoma, astrocytoma, ganglioneuroma and epidermoid cysts.

TREATMENT

The treatment is:
1. Treatment of hydrocephalus by ventriculoperitoneal shunt
2. Surgical excision of the tumor and radiotherapy
3. Chemotherapy has its correct role in pineal tumors especially germinoma, nongerminomatous germ cell tumors.
4. Stereotactic procedures: They are useful in arriving at the etiology of the tumors, therapeutic aspiration of the cystic tumors and for the placement of catheter in case of brachytherapy.

PITUITARY TUMORS

Pituitary tumors constitute 8 to 12 percent of all intracranial tumors. In 1543 Vesalius named pituitary gland ('pituita' in Latin meaning 'thick nasal mucus'), as he thought, this gland clears noxious secretions from the brain.

Pituitary otherwise called hypophysis is derived from a Greek word meaning undergrowth. Hypophysis is divided into anterior (adenohypophysis) and posterior (neurohypophysis) parts. Anterior and posterior parts of the hypophysis are different embryologically, anatomically and functionally. Anterior hypophysis, the glandular part, is derived from the stomodeum or Rathke's pouch (ectodermal origin) which grows cephalad and joins the neurohypophysis, which is derived from the diverticulum, of the floor of the third ventricle.

A stalk composed of glandular, vascular and neural elements connects pituitary gland and hypothalamus. The hypothalamus and pituitary gland function as one unit having two systems: 1. hypothalamic adenohypophysial system, 2. hypothalamo-neurohypophysial system. Releasing and inhibitory factors from hypothalamus are transported to anterior hypophysis through portal vessels of the pituitary stalk. Vasopressin and oxytocin are secreted by nuclei of the hypothalamus and transported in granules through neurons. They are stored and released from the posterior pituitary.

Anterior pituitary secretes the following hormones:
1. Prolactin (PRL)
2. Growth hormone (GH)
3. Adrenocorticotropic hormone (ACTH)
4. Thyroid stimulating hormone (TSH)
5. Gonadotrophic hormone which is the follicle stimulating hormone (FSH) and the luteinizing hormone (LH).

The pituitary gland lies in its fossa sella turcica (sella turcica means a Turkish saddle) and weighs about 0.5 to 0.6 gm. It measures 12 to 15 mm in transverse diameter and 8 to 10 mm in anteroposterior diameter.

The pituitary tumors can be classified according to:
1. Size as
    a. micro (less than 1 cm in size)
    b. macro (more than 1 cm in size)
2. Functional
    a. functioning
    b. non-functioning
3. Radiological

Radiological classification (Fig. 32.7)

Grade I: Intrapituitary adenoma, less than 1cm in diameter with normal sella, minimal configurational changes.

Grade II: Intrasellar adenoma, more than 1 cm in diameter, enlarged sella with no erosion.

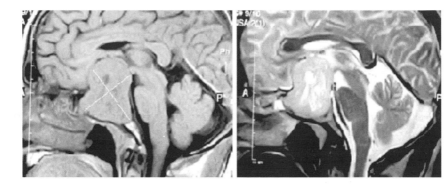

T1 Weighted   **T2 Weighted**

Figure 32.7: MRI of pituitary adenoma

Grade III: Diffuse adenoma, enlarged sella localized erosion.

Grade IV: Invasive adenoma, extensive destruction of the bony structures (ghost sella).

Classification according to cytogenesis:

1. Prolactin cell adenoma	29 percent
2. Null cell adenoma	18.2 percent
3. Growth hormone cell adenoma	16 percent
4. Crotch tropic cell adenoma	15 percent approx.
5. Plurihormonal adenoma	12 percent
6. Gonadotrophic cell adenoma	3.3 percent
7. Thyrotrophic cell adenoma	0.5 percent
8. Oncocytoma	6.7 percent

CLINICAL FEATURES

They depend on: 1. size of the tumor. 2. extent of the tumor. 3. functioning of the tumor. A microadenoma may be hyperfunctioning or hypofunctioning and when it increases in size it may compress the rest of the gland and result in hypofunction. When it enlarges the sella, it causes headache due to stretching of diaphragm sella. When the tumor expands out of the sella, there may be temporary relief in headache (due to rupture of the diaphragm). When it further extends to suprasellar region (upwards), it compresses the most important structure-the optic chiasma resulting in classical bitemporal hemianopia and even leading to total blindness. When it further extends higher, it obstructs the anterior third ventricle region, resulting in hydrocephalus (raised ICP signs) and hypothalamic disturbances. When it extends to parasellar region (laterally), the tumor involves the cavernous sinus resulting in cranial nerve deficits and temporal lobe compression resulting in seizures. The symptoms and signs of individual pituitary tumor will be discussed later. In a broad sense, signs and symptoms of pituitary tumor may be divided into:

- Endocrinal dysfunction
- Mechanical pressure effects on the neighboring neural structures
- Increased ICP
- Combined effects.

TREATMENT OF PITUITARY ADENOMAS

The modalities available are:

1. surgery
2. medical management
3. radiotherapy and radiosurgery

Surgery: There are two surgical approaches—the transsphenoidal and the transcranial. The former is the most accepted approach and the routes to sphenoid sinus are sublabial, transnasal and transethmoidal. The endoscopic transsphenoidal approach is a recent development. For a given case, either transcranial or transsphenoidal approaches can be adapted. The transcranial route is indicated when the tumor extends to the temporal, sub frontal and posterior regions.

Medical management and *radiotherapy* are dealt with in respective syndromes.

PROLACTINOMAS

This is the most common pituitary tumor, that accounts for 25-40 percent of the total number of pituitary tumors. It may be a micro- or a macroadenoma.

SIGNS AND SYMPTOMS

Signs and symptoms depend on the functional status of the tumor, hypersecretion of the prolactin, size and extent of the tumor. They differ in men and women.

In women the commonest features are: 1. menstrual disturbances like amenorrhea, oligomenorrhea and irregular periods. 2. galactorrhea and infertility.

In men, the symptoms are loss of libido, oligospermia and occasionally galactorrhea. Microadenoma is more common in females and present with endocrinal disturbances whereas in men macroadenoma is less common and they present with signs and symptoms related to the size of the tumor (mechanical pressure on the neighboring structures).

ENDOCRINOLOGY

Normal prolactin level is 10-20 mg/ml. Between 30-100 mg/ml may be associated with:
1. pregnancy
2. renal failure
3. hypothyroidism
4. intake of drugs like phenothiazine, tricyclic antidepressants, etc.
5. stalk effect (due to compression of the nonfunctioning tumor on pituitary stalk and hypothalamus leading to decreasing levels of dopamine). Prolactin levels above 150 mg/ml are strongly suggestive of prolactinomas and levels above 1000 mg/ml indicate invasive prolactinoma.

MANAGEMENT

The recent trend is to treat medically both micro- and macroadenomas. The drugs commonly used are bromocriptine, pergolide, cabergolide and quinagolide.

Bromocriptine is an ergot derivative and it is a dopamine agonist. The dosage is 5-20 mg/day. Bromocriptine lowers the prolactin levels, reduces the size of the tumor and restores the gonadal dysfunction. Bromocriptine has to be used indefinitely because discontinuation of the drug may result in expansion of the tumor with relapse of the signs and symptoms. Bromocriptine should be continued especially during pregnancy to prevent pituitary apoplexy.

SURGERY

Surgery is indicated in the following cases:
1. no response of tumor to medical line of treatment
2. intolerance of the drug by patient
3. progressive visual loss
4. increasing size of the tumor even with bromocriptine therapy
5. pituitary apoplexy

Acromegaly and gigantism: Pirre Marie described acromegaly in 1886 as a medical syndrome. Cushing in 1909 regarded this condition as a disease of pituitary hypersecretion. In 1927 Cushing and Davidoff attributed this to hyperplasia or adenomatous enlargement of pituitary gland composed of acidophilic cells responsible for the growth hormone secretion.

Acromegaly represents the somatic manifestations of pathological excess of the growth hormone secretion. The term gigantism is applied when there is hypersecretion of the growth hormone before the closure of epiphysis resulting in proportional increase in the size of all parts of the body.

Pathology : It is of two types:
1. Abnormal growth hormone secretion.
2. Abnormal growth hormone releasing hormone (ghrh) resulting in increasing growth hormone secretion.

Growth hormone or ghrh can be released either from primary sources or from ectopic sources.

Acromegaly may result from increase in the level of the growth hormone or increased activity of growth hormone or increased response of tissues to growth hormone.

Causes

1. Pituitary tumors:
   a. The growth hormone producing adenoma is the most common cause of acromegaly.
   b. Acidophil hyperplasia
   c. Plurihormonal adenoma
   d. Ghrh cell carcinoma
   e. Mammosomatotrophic cell adenoma
2. Extrapituitary tumors:
   a. Ectopic Gh cell adenoma of sphenoid origin, parapharyngeal.
   b. Ectopic Gh producing tumors: lung, ovary and breast.

3. Excess Gh releasing factor secretion (Ghrh)
4. Ectopic-Hamartoma, Choristoma, Pancreatic islet cell tumors

CLINICAL FEATURES

Acromegaly manifests between the third and the fourth decades of life and gigantism before closure of epiphysis.

Acral and facial enlargement is a regular feature of this disease. Alterations in bones and soft tissues are more marked in hands, feet, and skull. Hands are described as 'spadelike' characterized by marked thickening of the digits and tufting of distal phalanges of the hands and feet on X-ray examination. Increase in the length and thickness of the mandible produces characteristic 'lantern jaw' (prognathism). Overgrowth of the facial soft tissues and cartilage gives a classical clinical picture. Extensive enlargement of the frontal air sinuses gives 'beetle brow' appearance on X-ray examination.

There will be enlargement of the viscera (liver, spleen, kidney, lung and heart), thickening of the heel and heel pads.

Abnormal glucose metabolism is common and the patients may present with diabetes mellitus. About 20 percent of acromegalic patients may present with diabetes mellitus. About 20 percent of acromegalic patients also have hyperprolactinemia. Premenopausal women may develop menstrual disturbances, galactorrhea and males may present with loss of libido and impotence.

Large tumor may produce hypopituitarism. Compression over the optic nerves and chiasma may produce photophobia, decreased visual activity, bitemporal hemianopia, optic atrophy and sudden loss of vision due to apoplexy. Lateral extension may produce cavernous sinus involvement causing trigeminal pain and diplopia. Acromegaly patients may present with neuropathies, myopathies, epilepsy and dementia due to abnormalities in peptide neurotransmitters.

Treatment

The modalities available are surgery, medical therapy and radiotherapy.

Surgery: Trans-sphenoidal microsurgery is the treatment of choice.

Medical treatment: Octreotide and bromocriptine are the drugs used in case of persistent high levels of growth hormone after surgery or in case of tumor recurrence.

Cushing's disease and Nelson's syndrome:

Harvey Cushing gave a detailed report in 1932. Howard Naffziger performed the first craniotomy for the removal of the pituitary tumor with Cushing's disease in 1933.

Pituitary dependent adrenocorticotropic hormone (ACTH) results in two conditions:

1. Pituitary tumor produces a high amount of ACTH causing bilateral adrenal cortical hyperplasia resulting in hypercortism.
2. Bilateral adrenalectomy for the treatment of Cushing's disease causes high amount of ACTH. Since there is no adrenal glands hypercortism cannot occur. But there may be hyperpigmentation, which is known as 'Nelson's syndrome'.

Pathogenesis: Two-thirds of Cushing's syndrome develop from pituitary tumor while one-third can develop either from ectopic ACTH producing non-pituitary and non-endocrine tumors from adrenal tumors. In the group of ectopic ACTH tumors small cell carcinoma of the lung is the most common type of tumors and in case of adrenal tumors, it is commonly the adrenal adenoma.

Clinical Features

Cushing's disease in women is due to ACTH producing pituitary tumor in 75 percent of cases. In males 60 percent is due to ectopic non-pituitary sources. In children 65 percent are due to adrenal tumor (primary). No single feature is diagnostic and clinical diagnosis is possible only in less than 50 percent of cases.

Moon face, centripetal obesity, buffalo hump, hypertension, thin skin, purple abdominal striae, ecchymosis, emotional disturbances (depression, psychosis), menstrual irregularities, impotence, osteoporotic back pain and glucose intolerance are the common clinical features.

The cause of these symptoms is mainly increased adrenal production of cortisol. This increased production to a great extent (80 to 90%) is due to the ACTH producing pituitary tumor. The rest of the Cushing's syndrome is due to the releases of ACTH from ectopic non-pituitary areas and tissues. It must be understood that when the term Cushing's disease is used, it means that the etiology of this disease is ACTH producing pituitary tumor.

Treatment

The treatment includes surgical, medical and radiotherapy.

Transsphenoidal microsurgical excision is the treatment of choice. Radiotherapy is used as an adjuvant therapy in case of recurrence and when there is no initial cure by surgery.

Medical treatment is followed in case of failure of surgery or if the patient is unfit for surgery. The common drugs used are metyrapone, aminoglutethemide and mitotane.

Craniopharyngiomas

Rathke's pouch tumor (suprasellar epidermoid)

Craniopharyngioma constitutes 2.5 to 4 percent of intracranial tumors in general.

In children, it constitutes 12 to 15 percent and in adults 2 to 3 percent of all intracranial tumors.

INTRODUCTION

Small rests of squamous cells are commonly found along the pituitary stalk on routine examination. These rests are from the Rathke's pouch, a diverticulum that proceeds upwards from the roof of the pharynx to meet the downgrowing projection from the floor of the third ventricle. Developmental tumors arising from these cells are known as craniopharyngiomas. It is a tumor of suprasellar area.

Signs and Symptoms

Age incidence—Two-thirds present below 20 years of age. It is seen in two peaks of age groups. More than 50 percent present in the first and second decades followed by the fourth and fifth decades.

Suprasellar tumor can grow in different directions causing various signs and symptoms. It may extend in a superior direction causing disturbances of hypothalamus and obstruction to third ventricle leading to hydrocephalus, laterally to parasellar region, and posteriorly, i.e. to retrosellar region causing brainstem compression and anteriorly to presellar regions and to an inferior direction to pituitary gland.

Signs and symptoms in a broad sense are divided into increased intracranial tension due to tumor mass itself or due to hydrocephalus. *Visual*: Various field defects due to direct pressure on optic chiasm or due to hydrocephalus leading to secondary optic atrophy.

Endocrinal dysfunction: May result from pressure over the hypothalamus, pituitary stalk or pituitary gland.

Seizures

Cerebellar signs: Retrosellar extension compressing over the brainstem or its peduncles resulting in ataxia and limb weakness.

Anatomy of Hypothalamus

Anatomically hypothalamus can be divided into anterior and posterior parts by coronal plane and medial and lateral parts by a parasagittal plane passing through fornix.

Functionally it is divided into four groups of areas associated with different nuclei.
  – Preoptic area
  – Supraoptic area

  – Tubercinerium (tubular nuclei)
  – Mamillary area (bodies)

Each area is further divided into 3 zones: paraventricular, medial and lateral. Hence hypothalamic nuclei functionally can be divided into 12 zones (4 areas × 3 zones). Clinical findings with lesions in different regions of hypothalamus or pituitary gland are as follows:

• Anterior hypothalamus (par sympathetic area) on disturbance results in hypothermia, insomnia, diabetes insipidus and emaciation.
• Posterior hypothalamus (sympathetic area) results in hypothermia, poikilothermia, hypersomnia, coma and apathy.

Medial hypothalamus results in hyperdipsia, diabetes insipidus (SIADH), obesity, amnesia, rage and dwarfism (excessive intake of water and food).

• Lateral hypothalamus (decreased intake of water), emaciation and apathy.
• Arcuate nucleus or infundibulum results in hypopituitarism.

Signs and symptoms are different in children and adults. Endocrine dysfunction in the form of growth retardation, papilledema, headache, etc. are more common in children whereas visual field defects, mental disturbances, etc. are more common in adults.

In adults, mental disturbances in the form of memory loss, apathy, depression, hypersomnia and incontinence can develop in the course of the disease. Endocrine dysfunction is also seen in adults in the form of decreased sexual drive in males and primary or secondary amenorrhea in females.

Investigations

Plain X-ray of the skull: It shows features of raised ICP, areas of calcification, enlargement of sella or erosion of dorsum sellae or anterior clinoids.

CT scan: Heterogeneous suprasellar mass is found with irregular margins and cystic portions. Cystic portions are mostly hypodense. The area of calcification is a prominent feature. Calcification may be in the form of punctate dots or densely calcified mass. When the mass extends into third ventricle or foramen of Monro, dilatation of the ventricles is seen. Coronal CT scan is essential to visualize the superior limit of the tumor and relation to the sellar and hypothalamic regions.

MRI: Cystic component is hypointense to hyperintense depending upon keratin or cholesterol content. MRI helps in delineating anatomical extent and relations of the tumor with adjacent structures, e.g. optic chiasma, etc.

Treatment: The treatment is divided into four types:

Surgical management: The aim is to do total excision with minimal damage to adjacent structures and to decompression of the visual pathways.

Radiotherapy: Radiotherapy is indicated in case of residual and recurrent tumors.

Intracystic irradiation: In case of large cystic components total removal is not possible. Hence intracystic irradiation is done either by stereotactic method or catheter placement after craniotomy.

CEREBELLO-PONTINE ANGLE MASSES

Anatomy

Cerebello-pontine angle is an inverted triangular cistern bounded laterally by the backwall of petrous temporal bone, medially by the pons and cephalad by the tentorium which forms the base of the triangle. The contents of the CP angle are trigeminal nerve, facial nerve, vestibulo-cochlear nerve and anterior interior cerebellar artery.

The following discussion will be on vestibular schwanomas (acoustic schwanomas) since they constitute 80 to 90 percent of the CP angle masses.

History

Henneberg and Koch introduced the term cerebellopontine angle. Cushing in 1917 elaborated the clinical picture and diagnosis and demonstrated the value of intracapsular decompression and decapping of the cerebellum.

Dandy demonstrated the value of total excision. First successful removal of the tumor was done by Balance (1884). Pens introduced translabyrinthine approach but it was later abandoned by Harvey Cushing and Dandy. William House and John Doyle (Jr) in 1961 reintroduced the translabyrinthine approach with microscope.

Incidence

They constitute 8 percent of all intracranial tumors. About 2.5 percent are bilateral. It is seen between the third and the fifth decades of life with female preponderance.

Signs and Symptoms

Signs and symptoms of acoustic schwanoma are broadly divided into:
1. Cranial nerve involvement
2. Brainstem involvement
3. Cerebellar involvement
4. Increased intracranial tension (hydrocephalus)

Cranial Nerve Involvement

Signs and symptoms of the eighth nerve involvement are the earliest and the commonest. Deafness is seen in 70 percent of cases and tinnitus in about 30 percent of cases. Vestibular symptoms are seen in 83 percent of cases in the form of unsteadiness.

Trigeminal nerve is the second commonest to be involved. In about 80 to 90 percent of cases sensory and 10 to 15 percent of cases trigeminal motor deficit is seen. The commonest finding is impairment of corneal reflex. According to Dandy ipsilateral deafness, incomplete closure of the eye (seventh nerve involvement) and decreased corneal reflex make the clinical diagnosis certain. Trigeminal nerve involvement is seen when the tumor size is more than 3 cm in diameter. Facial nerve is involved less commonly and in late stages. It is involved in about 70 to 80 percent of cases.

In about 20 percent of cases lower cranial nerves are involved in the form of palatal palsy, hoarseness of voice and dysphagia.

Cerebellum is involved in about 65 to 75 percent of cases in the form of ataxia of gait and nystagmus.

Signs and symptoms of raised intracranial pressure are seen in about 90 percent of the cases due to obstructive hydrocephalus.

Dementia, sudden onset of deafness, trigeminal neuralgia, decreased sense of taste, contralateral facial nerve involvement, etc. are rare presentations of CP angle tumors.

Investigations:
1. Radiological
2. Audiological
3. Electroneurophysiological

In the order of frequency CP angle masses are:
1. Acoustic neurinoma 80 to 90 percent
2. Meningioma 5 to 10 percent
3. Epidermoid and dermoid 5 percent
4. Metastasis
5. Trigeminal neuroma
6. Arachnoid cyst
7. Aneurysm
8. Dolichobasilar ectasia
9. Extensions from brainstem growth, pituitary adenoma, craniopharyngioma, chordoma, fourth ventricular tumors, tumors of lower cranial nerves, glomus, jugular tumors and primary temporal bone tumor may extend into the CP angle region.

RADIOLOGICAL

Plain X-ray

50 percent of the cases show positive finding in the form of widening of the internal canal or erosion of the meatus of the canal and widening of the basal foramina. Town's view to assess internal auditory canal and Server's view to see the erosion of the meatus of the canal are taken.

CT Scan

Both plain and contrast studies are done. It can detect the tumor particularly when the extracanalicular component is greater than 1.5 cm. Homogeneous enhancement is seen in 75 percent of cases.

MRI

MRI brain scan with contrast study is presently the gold standard to detect the earliest stages of CP angle masses (intracanalicular lesion). MRI findings in acoustic neuroma hypo- or isointense is noticed on T1 weighted images whereas in meningiomas both T1 and T2 weighted images are isointense.

Acoustic neurinoma

1. Eighth nerve involvement followed by fifth nerve, lower cranial nerves
2. Abnormal internal auditory canal is seen in the X-rays
3. Narrow angle with the petrous bone.
4. No dural tail signs in MRI

Meningioma

1. Early involvement of facial nerve and sparing of the eighth nerve is characteristic
2. Intracanal extension not seen in plain X-rays
3. Broad based angle with the petrous bone
4. Dural tail sign present

AUDIOLOGICAL TESTS

An acoustic neurinoma produces retrocochlear type of sensorineural hearing defect characteristic of the eighth nerve involvement.

1. Elevated auditory threshold
2. Reduced speech discrimination
3. Absence of loudness recruitment
4. Abnormal tone decay
5. Decreased differential sensitivity for intensity
6. Absent acoustic reflex

NEURO ELECTRO PHYSIOLOGICAL TESTS

Brainstem auditory evoked potential response (BSAER) are done. It is preoperatively done in suspected bilateral CP angle masses and its sensitivity is about 80 to 90 percent. There are 7 waves in BSAER studies. The first wave is from action potentials of the acoustic nerve, the second is from the cochlear nucleus, the third is from superior olivary nucleus, the fourth from the nucleus of lateral lemniscus, the fifth from inferior colliculus, the sixth and the seventh from medical geniculate nucleus and geniculocortical pathway.

Waves I and III are preserved and inter peak latency I to III are often prolonged as a result of pontine compression characteristic of CP angle tumor. In advanced centers peroperative motoring of BSAER, facial nerve function, and auditory functions are available.

TREATMENT OF CEREBELLOPONTINE ANGLE TUMORS

Ventriculoperitoneal shunt is performed as an initial procedure, opposite to the side of the lesion since shunt tube will come in the way of the surgical field.

TREATMENT OF TUMOR

It is one of the challenging fields for the neurosurgeon.

SURGICAL APPROACHES

1. Suboccipital transmeatal approach-the most accepted
2. Suboccipital translabyrinthine
3. Translabyrinthine
4. Middle fossa transtentorial translabyrinthine
5. Subtemporal-transtentorial
   Selection of the approach depends on
   a. Size of the tumor
   b. Radiological findings
   c. Neurological findings
Cerebello-pontine angle tumor is classified according to the size of the tumor.
1. Small (less than 2 cm)
2. Medium (2 to 3 cm)
3. Large (3 cm and above)

OPERATIVE STEPS IN A SUBOCCIPITAL TRANSMEATAL APPROACH

a. Patient under general anesthesia is kept in lateral or sitting position.
b. Retromastoid vertical incision is made.
c. Suboccipital craniotomy is performed.
d. Dura is opened usually in 'K' shaped fashion.
e. Cisterna magna is punctured and CSF is drained; lateral 1/3rd of the cerebellum may be excised.
f. Tumor is visualized; internal decompression is done followed by excision.
g. Using microdrills internal auditory canal is opened and intra-canalicular part is excised.

TRANSLABYRINTHINE APPROACH

It exposes the posterior fossa dura in the retromeatal trigone (Trautmann's triangle) formed by the sigmoid sinus, jugular bulb and superior petrosal sinus. This approach is usually reserved for medium size tumors that are 1 to 2.5 cm wide. One of the major disadvantages of this approach is loss of auditory function.

MIDDLE FOSSA APPROACH

This involves an extradural subtemporal approach with unroofing of the internal auditory canal. This approach is preferred for the tumors, which are confined to internal auditory canal. The advantage of this procedure is preservation of hearing.

MENINGIOMAS

Meningiomas account for 15 percent of all intracranial tumors in adults and 1 to 4 percent of all brain tumors in children. Harvey Cushing coined the term meningioma in 1922. Age incidence is 20 to 60 years of age. Females are more affected than males. Meningiomas can be classified in two ways.

1. By histological classification (Table 32.7)
2. By location

By location: 90 percent of them occur in supratentorial compartment. The most common locations are: 1. Parasagittal, 2. falx, 3. convexity, 4. sphenoid wing.

In one of the major series the following distribution of the meningiomas is found.

a. Parasagittal-10 percent
b. Falx-4 percent
c. Convexity-25 percent
d. Olfactory groove-4.5 percent
e. Tuberculum sella-9.1 percent
f. Sphenoid wing-15 percent
g. Anterior fossa-1 percent
h. Middle cranial fossa-1 percent
i. CP angle-14 percent
j. CP angle and middle fossa-1.5 percent
k. Cerebellar convexity-3 percent
l. Subtentorial-7.5 percent, Clival-1.5 percent, Intraventricular-1 percent, Foramen magnum-1.5 percent.
   1. Parasagittal meningiomas (involving the lateral wall of sagittal sinus, adjacent convexity dura and falx).
   2. Falx meningiomas–Often bilateral and completely concealed by covering cerebral cortex.
   3. Cerebral convexity meningioma:
      Convexity meningioma may arise from any point on dura, but most commonly are seen in parasagittal region along the coronal suture

Table 32.7: Histological classification		
Group	*Type*	*Variant*
Tumors of meningo-thelial cells	Meningioma Atypical papillary Anaplastic	Meningothelial, fibrous, transitional, psammomatous, angiomatous, microcytic, secretory, clear cell, choroid, lymphoplasmacyte-rich, metaplastic
Mesenchymal, Nonmeningothelial tumors, Benign Malignant	Osteocartilaginous tumors Lipoma fibrous Histiocytoma Hemangiopericytoma Chondrosarcoma Mesenchymal Malignant fibrosarcoma Histiocytoma, meningeal sarcomatosis Rhabdomyosarcoma Others	
Primary melanocytic lesions	Diffuse melanosis Melanocytoma malignant Melanoma meningeal Melanomatosis	
Tumor of uncertain histiogenesis	Hemangioblastoma	

and pterion (anterior sylvian region). About 70 percent of tumors lie anterior to rolandic fissure.

4. Olfactory groove meningioma:
   Tumors arise from the midline of anterior fossa between cristagalli and tuberculum sella. Usually bilateral but occasionally asymmetric, they attain large size before causing symptoms.
5. Sphenoidal wing meningioma :
   They are situated over the lesser wing of the sphenoid bone. As it grows it may expand medially to involve the cavernous sinus, anteriorly into the orbit, and laterally into the temporal bone.

Cushing divided these meningiomas into three types:
a. Clenoidal (inner)
b. Alar (middle)
c. Pterional (outer)

ETIOLOGY

"Meningiomas usually occur as isolated tumors which adhere to and involve the dura even though they do not actually arise from it.", Harvey Cushing and Louise Eisenhardt, 1938.

They arise from the arachnoid cells, arachnoid cap cells or both. Meningiomas can also arise from tela choroidea and choroid plexus. The following factors are thought to be the etiological factors:

1. Trauma: Controversial
2. Viruses: Both DNA and RNA viruses are capable of producing neoplasms within the central nervous system of rodents and nonhuman primates. Large T antigen of the Papova virus is found frequently in human meningiomas. But there is no evidence in experimental animals.
3. Radiation: Radiation is thought to be a proven cause of meningioma in some series.
4. Genetics: Most common genetic conditions associated with the development of meningiomas are neurofibromatosis type II (central neurofibromatosis). In these the loss of part of chromosome 22 is seen. Gorlia's syndrome (multiple basal cell carcinoma syndrome) is associated with medulloblastoma and meningioma.
5. Hormone and growth factor receptors: It has been proved that progesterone receptors are more commonly seen in meningioma cells than estrogen receptors.

CLINICAL FEATURES

They depend upon the size, location, and growth rate of the tumor. Generally they present as

a. seizures (50%)
b. increased intracranial signs (headache)
c. focal neurological deficit. It rarely present as intracranial vascular effect from venous sinus occlusion, intracranial hemorrhages and cerebral infarcts due to arterial obstruction.

INVESTIGATIONS

1. Plain X-rays:
   a. Local accumulation of calcium in tiny globular bodies over the surface of the brain. Incidence of calcification in plain X-rays is about 6 to 9 percent.
   b. Sclerosis of the inner table of the calvarium. Increasing number and tortuosity of the meningeal vessels grooving the inner table.
   c. Enlargement of the foramen spinosum.
2. CT scan (Figs 32.8 and 32.9):
   Both plain and contrast studies are essential. It will show brain anatomy, shift, calcification, and edema and bone changes. On plain CT 75 percent are hyperdense, 15 percent are isodense and 10 percent are hypodense. Hyperdensity on plain CT is due to compactness of the tumor cells, connective tissue collagen, hypervascularity of the tumor and presence of psammoma bodies. The incidence of

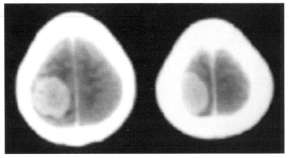

Figure 32.8: CT scan of left parietal convexity meningioma

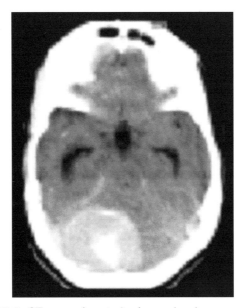

Figure 32.9: CT scan of posterior fossa showing a meningioma

calcification on CT scan is about 20 to 27 percent. 60 to 90 percent of meningiomas are associated with vasogenic edema. They will be homogeneous and intense enhancement with contrast administration. Buckling phenomenon is seen due to compression on the surface of the brain by extraaxial location of the tumor.

3. MRI:

All are isointense and all enhance with contrast.

Buckling effect, broad base over the dura, pseudo capsule with displaced vessels and CSF and peritumoral edema are the features on MRI. Dual tail sign is seen in 60 percent of meningiomas.

4. Angiogram:

It is done to confirm the encasement of carotid arteries, to consider preoperative embolisation of the feeding artery as an adjuvant to definitive surgery, to plan surgical approach, to establish patency of

dural sinuses and to identify the length of attachment of the tumor. The following are angiographic features:
1. Enlarged and tortuous feeding vessels.
2. Sunburst appearance of the arteries at the hilum or at attachments to the dura.
3. Corkscrew appearance of the small arteries in the tumor.
4. Enlarged draining veins.
5. Dense tumor capillary blush in the late venous phase.

TREATMENT OF MENINGIOMAS

Surgery is the treatment of choice. The objective is to do total removal of the meningioma including the dura and bone if possible. The aim is to preserve and improve the neurological function. Surgical approaches depend upon the location and the extent of the tumor.

Radiotherapy: Radiotherapy is given either by external beam radiation or by radiosurgery (Gamma knife or X knife). The indications of radiotherapy are residual, recurrent, surgically inaccessible and malignant meningiomas.

All patients with meningioma should be given anti-convulsant therapy in perioperative periods.

HEMANGIOPERICYTOMA

It accounts for 2.4 percent of meningiomas. It is considered as angioblastic meningioma. As it arises from the capillary pericytes it is also called meningeal hemangiopericytoma. It occurs between the ages of 30 and 40 years. Mostly it is supratentorial and usual locations are parasagittal, tentorium and sphenoid wing. It usually presents with headache, seizures and in case of posterior fossa gait disturbance.

It is considered equal to malignant meningioma, and lung, liver, bone and retroperitoneum are the usual sites of metastases.

TREATMENT

Complete excision followed by radiotherapy.

Malignant Meningioma

It accounts for 2 to 12 percent of meningiomas and it occurs in the sixth decade of life. Males are more affected than females and they are mostly in supratentorial location (parasagittal and convexity regions). Common presenting symptoms are headache, seizures, hemiparesis, personality changes and painless scalp or skull swellings. They metastasize to lung, liver, lymph node and bones.

CT scan: The following are the CT scan findings of aggressive meningiomas: 1. marked edema. 2. absence of visible calcium aggregates. 3. heterogeneous contrast enhancement. 4. non-enhancement of central hypodense areas. 5. mushrooming pattern of the intracranial tumor which is more than the dural attachment. 6. lobulated contour of the tumor. The cardinal feature of the malignant meningioma is invasion of brain parenchyma.

MRI: Increased intensity on T2 weighted images, invasion of brain with poorly defined margins between the tumor and brain. Extensive brain edema, destruction of the bone with extension through bony foramina.

Treatment: The prognosis is grim. Recurrence is extremely high. Surgery is followed by radiotherapy or chemotherapy. But results are controversial.

Multiple meningiomas: They account for 0.9 to 8.9 percent of meningiomas. Average age is 50 years. 93 percent of cases are women. Most common locations are convexity and parasagittal falx of the supratentorial compartment. In 50 percent of the cases one hemisphere is involved and in 70 percent of cases only two tumors are seen. Cushing and Eisenhardt recognized that neurofibromatosis type II and I are associated with multiple meningiomas.

Surgery is the treatment of choice.

MENINGIOMAS IN CHILDREN

61 percent of cases are seen between 11 and 20 years, and 39 percent seen in below the age of 10. 67 percent are seen supratentorial. 15 percent infratentorial and 9 percent are intraventricular.

The commonest presentation is focal neurological deficit followed by seizures, signs and symptoms of raised intracranial pressure, and in some cases scalp swelling and proptosis are also seen.

BRAIN METASTASES

Brain metastasis (secondary deposits) constitute 10 percent of all intracranial tumors. 20-40 percent of systemic cancer patients have secondary deposits in the brain.

In adults in the order of frequency, the most common primary is lung, breast, gastrointestinal tract, genitourinary tract and skin (malignant melanoma).

In the patients below 21, brain metastasis arises from sarcomas (osteogenic sarcoma, rhabdomyosarcoma, Ewing's sarcoma) and from germ cell tumors. The false positive rate for single brain metastasis is approximately 11 percent. Non-metastatic brain lesions are equally divided between primary brain tumors and infections. In patients with primary breast cancer with a dural based lesion, meningioma must be considered, as the frequency of this primary brain tumor is increased in breast cancer.

The method of spread, most commonly seen is hematogenous followed by adjacent bone and through CSF pathway.

80 percent of brain metastases are in cerebral hemispheres, 15 percent in cerebellum and 5 percent in brain stem. Metastases are seen just underneath the junction of gray and white matter and watershed areas of major arterial territories. Metastasis may be small or large in size. With the advent of newer radiological techniques, approximately 15 percent are found to be multiple.

Metastases from colon, breast, renal carcinoma etc. are single, whereas malignant melanoma, lung cancers etc. produce multiple deposits.

CLINICAL PRESENTATION

The clinical presentation is similar to that of any other intracranial space occupying lesions. Difficulty in localization arises in case of multiple lesions. Small size lesions are located in basal and non-eloquent areas. Headache is the commonest presenting symptom followed by seizures.

5-10 percent of patients will present with stroke-like presentation due to acute intratumoral hemorrhage, commonly seen in choriocarcinoma and malignant melanoma.

INVESTIGATIONS

The best modality is Contrast Magnetic Resonance Images of the brain. Contrast CT when compared to MRI is less sensitive. Lesions less than 5 mm and located adjacent to larger metastatic lesions may be missed.

Chest X-ray is mandatory in every case of brain metastasis. It may show either a primary or a secondary lesion in the lung, the latter due to the presence of malignancy in some other organ. More than 60 percent of X-ray chest shows a metastatic deposit in brain metastasis.

TREATMENT OF BRAIN SECONDARIES

General Principles

1. Tissue diagnosis is essential to plan the adjuvant therapy. In 10-15 percent of cases primary is not known. Biopsy is taken from open craniotomy or by stereotactic method.
2. If the intracranial masses are associated with intracranial tension with life threatening situation open craniotomy is done to relieve the intracranial tension.
3. If the life expectancy is less than two months due to uncontrolled systemic cancer, steroids with or without radiotherapy are given.

If it is a single mass, excision of the tumor followed by radiotherapy is the treatment of choice. If the lesion is surgically inaccessible, the options are:

1. stereotactic biopsy and stereotactic radiosurgery with or without whole brain radiotherapy.
2. sometimes radiosurgery followed by whole brain radiotherapy.

If the lesions are multiple surgery and whole brain radiotherapy or stereotactic radiosurgery followed by whole brain radiotherapy or surgery and stereotactic radiosurgery whole brain radiotherapy are followed. If the lesions are small, discrete and multiple, whole brain radiotherapy is the treatment of choice.

Cranial radiotherapy is the treatment of choice for many patients. It must not be forgotten that the treatment of secondaries of brain is only a palliative procedure. Chemotherapy may have a role in case of secondaries on the brain from small cell carcinoma of the lung, carcinoma of the breast and choriocarcinoma.

Stereotactic interstitial radio surgery (SIRS) is the new modality tried in secondaries of the brain.

FURTHER READING

1. Adams and Victor's Principles of Neurology, Nuance Victor, Alan Rooper (Eds), McGraw-Hill, New York, Tokyo, Medical Publishers Division.
2. Indian Clinical Neurosurgery, Volume II. Malignant Brain Tumors: Anil K Singh, (Ed). Delhi: CBS Publishers.
3. Kleihues P, Burger PC, Scheithauer BW (Eds): Histological typing of tumors of central nervous system. Springer-Verlag 1993:33-42.
4. Michael Swash (Ed). Hutchinson's Clinical Method (19th ed). London ELBS, Bailliere Tindall,
5. Neurological Surgery (3rd ed). Julian Youmanis (Ed). New York: WB Saunders.
6. Neurosurgery (2nd ed), Volume II. Robert H Wilkins, Setti S Rengachery (Eds). Delhi: McGraw– Hill, Medical Publisher Division.
7. Text book on Neurosurgery (2nd ed), Ramamurthi B, Tandom PN (Eds). New Delhi: Churchill Livingstone.
8. Textbook on Radiation Oncology. Gouda K Rath, Bindhu K Mohanti (Eds), New Delhi: BI Churchill Livingstone.

APPENDIX 11

International comparison, India and five continents—AAR (ICMR and IARC).

TUMOR BRAIN (MALE)

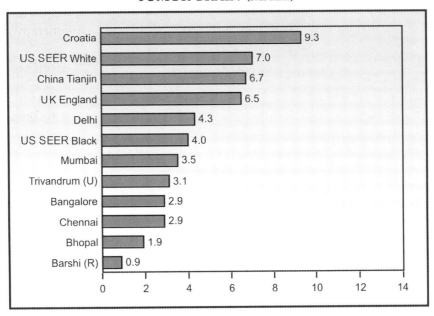

TUMOR BRAIN (FEMALE)

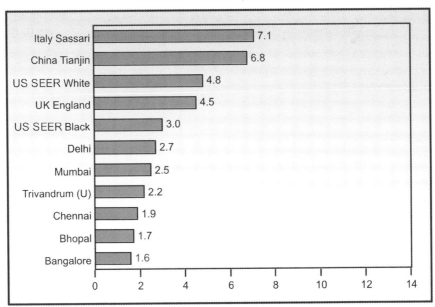

Rate per 100,000

Spinal Cord Tumors

33

M Nageswara Rao

Sir Victor Horsley is credited with the first successful removal of the spinal cord tumor in 1887, which was diagnosed by William Gowers. Harvey Cushing effected successful removal of the intramedullary ependymoma. Elsberg mastered the subject of surgery for spinal cord tumors.

Spinal cord tumors constitute 15 percent of all central nervous system tumors and depending on the site of origin they can be divided into: 1. tumors of the spinal cord 2. tumors of the spinal axis (vertebral column). In relation to the spinal cord, they also can be further divided into extradural and intradural tumors. Intradural tumors are again divided into: a. intradural extramedullary (Id-Em), b. intradural intra-medullary (Id-IM). A small number of tumors can exist as both intramedullary and extramedullary which communicate either through nerve root entry zone or at conus medullaris-filum terminal transition. Similarly tumor may have both extradural and intradural components (dumb bell tumor) extending through nerve root sleeve. All tumors of the spine may be primary or secondary and may be benign or malignant. Metastatic deposits are most commonly extradural in location.

Spinal cord tumors in relation to cell of origin: they may arise from:

1. cellular constituents of the spinal cord and filum terminal (astrocytoma and ependymoma).
2. nerve root (neurofibroma)
3. meninges (meningioma).

Cells involved in the production of primary bone tumors are osteoblast, chondroblast, fibroblast and osteoclast. Primary bone tumors may also arise from blood vessels of the vertebra, adipose tissue, bone marrow, nerve sheath and notochord.

Metastatic bone tumors of the spine are more common than primary bone tumors. Secondary deposits of the spine may arise from distant organs through tumor emboli or as a direct spread from the adjacent organs through intervertebral foramen, e.g. pulmonary malignancy, paraspinal sarcomas, etc.

CLASSIFICATION OF THE SPINAL CORD TUMORS

1. Intradural–extramedullary (84% of all intradural tumors)
   Neurofibroma–29%
   Meningioma–25%
   Exophytic ependymoma–13%
   Sarcoma–12%
   Exophytic astrocytoma–6%
   Other vascular, epidermoid and lipoma–15%
2. Intradural–intramedullary (16% of all intradural tumors)
   Ependymoma–56%
   Astrocytoma–29%
   Hemangioblastoma–3%
   Oligodendrogliomas–3%
   Lipoma–2%
   Metastatic
   Malignant glioma
   Dermal
   Epidermoid
   Teratoma
   Cavernous hemangioma

EXTRADURAL TUMORS

Mostly metastatic
Lesions of vertebral column
Lesions of extradural space
Traction on the cord and compression

PRIMARY TUMORS OF THE SPINE

True Bone Tumors

Osteoma, osteoid osteoma, osteoblastoma, osteosarcoma, chondroma, enchondroma, osteochondroma, chondroblastoma, chondrosarcoma, fibroma, fibrosarcoma, fibrous histiocytoma, giant cell tumor.

Associated Bone Tumors

Hemangioma, aneurysmal bone cyst, hemangiopericytoma, hemangio-endothelioma, angiolipoma, angiosarcoma, plasmacytoma, myeloma, Ewing's sarcoma, lipoma, angiolipoma, notochord tumors and chordoma.

CLINICAL SIGNS AND SYMPTOMS

Tumors of the spine may produce radiculopathy or myelopathy or both either by compression, traction or vascular impediment. There are two types of myelopathies: 1. non-compressive myelopathy usually due to neurological conditions (e.g. inflammatory conditions), 2. compressive myelopathy caused by neurosurgical conditions. Compressive myelopathy is characterized by: 1. progressive symptomatology, e.g. paraparesis may progress to paraplegia, 2. cumulative symptomatology. Involvement of one system followed by involvement of another system, e.g. Motor symptoms may be followed by sensory symptoms and then involvement of autonomic nervous system. There will be both bowel and bladder disturbances such as retention, incontinence and loss of sphincter control, 3. fairly clinical level of the lesion.

Due to disproportionate growth of the vertebral column spinal cord ends at the lower border of the first lumbar vertebra. Hence spinal cord segments do not correspond with the vertebra overlying them. To determine which spinal segment is related to a given vertebral body:

- For the cervical vertebrae, add 1
- For thoracic 1-6, add 2
- For thoracic 7-9, add 3
- The 10th thoracic arch overlies lumbar 1 and 2 segments.
- The 11th thoracic arch overlies lumbar 3 and 4 segments.
- The 12th thoracic arch overlies lumbar 5
- The first lumbar arch overlies the sacral and coccygeal segments.

The extent of the spinal cord lesion is in two ways: 1. vertical extent, e.g. A lesion extending from cervical to thoracic segments. 2. horizontal extent either i. extradural ii. intradural: (a) intradural intramedullary, (b) intradural extramedullary.

Extramedullary compression of the spinal cord is characterized by root pain, ascending sensory disturbance with no dissociation and Brown-Sequard type of clinical picture.

Intramedullary tumors of the spinal cord present with disanesthesia and paresthesia with descending sensory disturbance and dissociated sensory loss. Since sacral fibers are laminated in the outer part of the corticospinal tract, sacral sparing is a feature of intraspinal tumors. Lower motor neuron paralysis in the form of muscle wasting fasciculation, absent deep tendon reflexes at the level of lesion and upper motor neuron paralysis below the level of the lesion are seen. Sphincter disturbances are an early feature.

Lesions from the first cervical to the first thoracic segments of the cord involve both lower and upper limbs and lesion below the level of first thoracic segment results in paraperesis or paraplegia. Lesions from S3 to coccyx 1, regarded as conus medullaris and from L4-S2 as epiconus are described below. Cauda equina includes spinal segments from L3 root to coccyx 1.

SIGNS AND SYMPTOMS OF CONUS MEDULLARIS LESIONS

Conus medullaris involvement causes paralysis of the pelvic floor muscles, early sphincter dysfunction, autonomous neurogenic bladder, and symmetric saddle anesthesia with impaired erection and ejaculation.

CAUDA EQUINA LESIONS

They cause early unilateral or bilateral asymmetric radicular pain. Pain is aggravated in recumbent position and the patient will develop flaccid hypotonic and flaccid paralysis (LMN type). There may be asymmetric saddle anesthesia involving all modalities of sensations. Autonomous bladder is seen.

INVESTIGATIONS OF THE INTRADURAL SPINAL TUMORS

Plain X-rays

Plain X-rays of anteroposterior, lateral and oblique views are taken to see the following features:

1. Size, shape and mineral content of the vertebral body (Flattening of the medial convex border of the pedicle).
2. Interpedicular distance.
3. Configuration of the posterior surface of the vertebral body (Scalloping of the posterior surface of the vertebral body is seen in intraspinal tumors due to pressure on the surface).
4. Intervertebral foramen : Enlargement of the intervertebral foramen is seen in cases of dumb bell tumors (intraspinal tumors with extra extension).
5. Spinous process.
6. Lamina and transverse process.
7. Paravertebral shadow.
8. Presence of calcification in the tumor.

MRI (Fig. 33.1)

It is the investigation of choice for all spinal tumors. Gadolinium contrast studies are essential especially in cases of intramedullary tumors.

Myelogram

Before the advent of MRI and CT scan myelogram was the investigation of choice. With the advent of MRI, myelogram is occasionally done. Myelogram followed by CT scan (Myelo-CT) is done on special occasions.

INTRASPINAL TUMORS

Neurofibroma: It constitutes 30% of all intraspinal tumors and is the commonest intraspinal tumor. Males and females are equally affected but

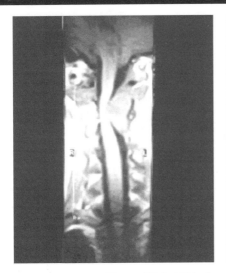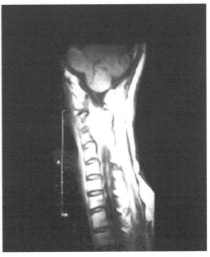

Figure 33.1: MRI of neurofibroma c2-c3 level

some authors regard the males as more affected than females. This tumor commonly occurs in middle aged persons. Thoracic spine is the commonest site followed by cervical spine and the least common region is lumbosacral spine. It arises usually from dorsal root. They are usually single, globoid in shape with increased vascularity. No calcification is seen. Multiple neurofibromas are seen in association with Von Recklinghausen's disease. 82 percent of them are intradural and extramedullary and the rest of them are in extradural locations and may coexist as intradural and extradural components (dumb bell tumors). Areas of cystic degeneration, necrosis and hemorrhage are seen on MRI.

MRI shows hypo- or isointensity on T1 weighted images and hyperintensity on T2 weighted images.

Treatment: Treatment is by total excision of the tumor along with its capsule.

Meningiomas: They account for 25 percent of intraspinal tumors. It is seen in the middle age. Females are more affected than males. The commonest site is thoracic spine and is located in the posterior or posterolateral segment of the spinal canal.

MRI shows hypointense on T1 and hypointense or isointense in T2 weighted images.

The treatment is by total excision of the tumor along with excision of the dura to which tumor is attached.

EPENDYMOMA (FIG. 33.2)

Spinal ependymomas constitute 50 percent of all central nervous system ependymomas. 50 percent of the spinal ependymomas are located at filum

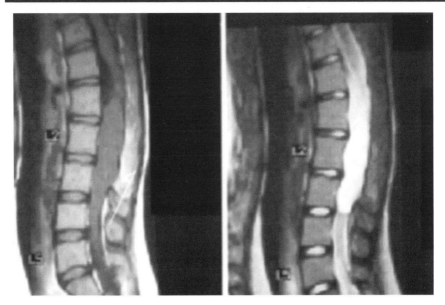

Figure 33.2: MRI of the intradural intramedullary tumor (ependymoma) of conus medullaris and filum terminale

terminale and conus medullaris region. They are seen in the third decade of life. Males are more affected than females. Tumor may be associated with intratumoral hemorrhage. MRI shows iso- or slightly hyperintense on both T1 and T2 weighted images. Treatment by surgical excision is followed by radiotherapy.

ASTROCYTOMA

Spinal astrocytomas constitute 3 percent of all central nervous system astrocytomas. The commonest site is thoracic spinal cord and it involves many segments of the spinal cord. The treatment is by surgical resection followed by radiotherapy depending on the histological grade.

TREATMENT OF INTRADURAL TUMORS

Almost all intradural extramedullary tumors are completely resectable and thus complete cure is possible. In case of intramedullary tumors, with 1. the introduction of operative microscope, 2. peroperative use of ultrasound to localize and to assess the extent of the tumor, 3. the use of bipolar CUSA applications, most of the tumors are resectable (subtotal resection) with low incidence of postoperative deterioration. Postoperative radiotherapy is given to prevent the recurrence of the intramedullary tumors.

SPINAL METASTASES

It indicates an ominous systemic cancer. Spinal metastasis is the most common tumor of the spine.

5-10 percent of cancer patients with systemic cancer will develop symptomatic spinal secondaries. Most common primary lesions are breast, lung and prostate. 10 percent of spinal metastases have no known primary. Most common spinal secondaries are extradural in location while intradural location is uncommon. But they may metastasize through spinal CSF pathways, e.g. medulloblastoma, ependymoma, etc. Intramedullary spinal metastases too are rare.

Spinal metastasis occurs in three ways:
1. Arterial emboli
2. Direct extension
3. Venous spread (Braxton's plexus).

SYMPTOMS AND SIGNS

Pain along the spinal nerves with local tenderness is the most common symptom. 90 percent of cases are followed by long tract signs with motor and sensory deficits and with sphincteric disturbances.

INVESTIGATIONS

Radiographic evaluation Plain X-ray of anteroposterior and lateral films of the affected spine will demonstrate abnormalities in 90 percent of cases. In one-third of cases multisegmental involvements are seen. Osteoblastic and osteosclerotic bony changes are seen in cases of cancer breast and prostate.

Common findings in plain X-rays are:
1. Pedicle erosion seen in 80 percent of cases (Winking Owl sign)
2. Paraspinal soft tissue shadow
3. Vertebral collapse
4. Pathological fracture, etc.

MRI

It is the investigation of choice and it demonstrates the location and extent in all three planes (axial, sagittal and coronal planes).

CT SCAN

CT scan is particularly useful in assessing bony abnormalities.

BONE SCAN

Radionucleotide scan is useful in the early stages but lacks specificity.

TREATMENT OF SPINAL METASTASIS

The treatment is aimed to relieve pain and to preserve and restore neurological function. Palliation is the realistic goal of treatment.

1. Steroids
2. Decompression with or without stabilization
3. Radiotherapy.

STEROIDS

Administration of steroids will reduce the edema of the spinal cord at the site of compression resulting in improvement in neurological function. As soon as diagnosis is made, 100 mg of dexamethasone is given followed by 4 mg 6 hourly, till definitive treatment is completed.

RADIOTHERAPY

It is particularly effective in metastasis of lymphoreticular origin, moderately effective in breast and prostatic origin and less effective in lung and melanoma.

Radiotherapy followed by surgical procedure is outdated. The modern trend is decompression followed by radiotherapy.

DECOMPRESSION

It can be done either by anterior or posterior approaches. Posterior approach is by laminectomy which is not advised as it is not adequate to decompress (except in intradural metastasis), and mechanical spinal instability is noted in this approach. Hence anterior approaches are preferred. After decompression, spinal instability is achieved either by bone graft in cases where life span is expected to be long or by metallic implants when life span is short. Various types of instruments are available both for anterior and posterior spinal fusion.

FURTHER READING

1. Ahamed Rasheed BK, Wiltshire RN, Bigner SH, et al. Molecular pathogenesis of malignant gliomas. Curr Opin Oncol 1999;11:162-67.
2. An atlas of tumors involving the ventral nervous system, Robin O.Barnard, Valenrine Loge, et al. London, Bailliere Tindal.
3. Kyritisis AP, Yung WKA, Bruner JB, et al. The treatment of anaplastic oligodendrogliomas and mixed gliomas. Neurosurgery 1993;32: 365-70.
4. Packer RJ, Goldwein J, Nicholson HS, et al. Treatment of children with medulloblastomas with reduced dose craniospinal radiation therapy and adjuvant chemotherapy: A Children's Cancer Group study. J Clin Oncol 1999;17:2127-36.
5. Progress of Clinical Neurosciences, Neurological Society of India 2000.
6. Subarachnoid Hemorrhage, Sen Gupta RP, McAllister VL, New York: Springer Verlag.

Non-Hodgkin's Lymphoma

34

Pamela Jayaraj
K Pavithran

The non-Hodgkin's lymphomas (NHL) are monoclonal proliferation of lymphoid tissues of either the B-cell or the T-cell varieties.

EPIDEMIOLOGY AND ETIOLOGY

Incidence

It is relatively common in developing countries. It is now considered one among the 5 top causes of cancer in young adults and there is a steady increase of incidence during the last 5 decades. NHL can occur at any age but the incidence increases with age and the male to female ratio is 1.5:1. Families have been described with high incidence among siblings and first-degree relatives. The incidence is higher in Africa and Latin America and lowest in Asia and Pacific regions. In India the incidence is 2-3 per 100,000 persons.

Etiology

a. The etiology of NHL is not clear. But it is rarely associated with inherited or acquired immune deficiency syndrome. The other rare etiological factors are:
   1. Collagen vascular disease
   2. Longstanding Sjogren's disease
   3. Klinefelter's syndrome
   4. Chediak-Higashi syndrome.
      Occupational exposure to pesticides leads to 2-5 fold increase in incidence. Workers in vinyl chloride, rubber and leather industries are at an increased risk of developing NHL.
b. Heart and kidney transplant recipients receiving immunosuppressive therapy with azathioprin or cyclosporin have a high risk of developing NHL due to altered immunity.

c. Viruses also have a role in pathogenesis of a number of lymphoma, e.g. Epstein-Barr virus (EBV) in Burkitt's lymphoma, HTLV-1 in ATLL. AIDS is associated with high incidence of NHL with frequent CNS involvement.

d. Age: The peak incidence rate is greater than that of Hodgkin's disease. About 25 percent of cases develop between 50-59 years. Maximum risk is between 60-69 years.

e. Sex: It is more common in males than females and it is 16.6 vs 11.2 per 100,000 population.

Symptoms and signs of non-Hodgkin's lymphoma (NHL) are similar to those of Hodgkin's disease (HD) except for the following:

Non-Hodgkin's lymphoma	*Hodgkin's lymphoma*
1. Lymph node presentation is noncontiguous and centrifugal.	Lymph node disease is centripetal and commonly involves axial nodes.
2. Presentation of Waldeyer's ring, epitrochlear node, GIT and testes involvement are common.	Not so common.
3. Abdominal nodal involvement is common.	Not common except in patients with B symptoms and those who are elderly.
4. Mediastinal nodal presentation is seen in less than 20 percent patients.	Mediastinal disease present in 50 percent or more.
5. Disease is rarely localized at initial presentation.	Localized nodal presentation is common.
6. Bone marrow involvement is a common occurrence.	Not common.
7. Liver involvement is a common finding in follicular lymphoma contrary to diffuse lymphoma.	Uncommon.

PATHOLOGIC CLASSIFICATION

Classification of NHL has undergone significant evolution in the last 150 years. Rappaport classification, the most popular since the 1960's is now considered inadequate. This was followed by working formulation that provides the clinicopathological types by grouping lymphomas into low, intermediate and high grade neoplasm. A few subtypes were not included in working formulation.

International Lymphoma Study Group has provided a new revised classification.

REAL classification, i.e. Revised European American classification of lymphoid diseases.

LYMPHOMA

Low Risk-indolent Lymphomas

a. B-cell lineage CLL/Small lymphocytic lymphoma with or without plasmacytoid differentiation
Lymphoplasmacytic lymphoma/Immunocytoma/Waldenstrom's hairy cell leukemia
Splenic marginal zone lymphoma
Marginal zone B-cell lymphoma
Extranodal (MALT-B-cell lymphoma)
Nodal (monocytoid)
Follicle center lymphoma/Follicular (small cell)-grade I
Follicle center lymphoma/Follicular (mixed small and large cell)-grade II.
b. T-cell lineage large granular lymphocytic leukemia, T and NK cell types
Mycosis fungoides/Sézary's syndrome
Smoldering and chronic adult T-cell leukemia/lymphoma (HTLV-1).

AGGRESSIVE LYMPHOMAS

a. B-cell lineage—prolymphocytic leukemia
Plasmacytoma/multiple myeloma
Mantle cell lymphoma
Follicle center lymphoma/Follicular, (large cell)-grade III
Diffuse large B-cell lymphoma (includes immunoblastic and diffuse large and centroblastic lymphomas)
Primary mediastinal (thymic) large B-cell lymphoma
High grade B-cell lymphoma, Burkitt-like.
b. T-cell lineage—prolymphocytic leukemia
Peripheral T-cell lymphoma, unspecified
Angioimmunoblastic lymphoma
Angiocentric lymphoma
Intestinal T-cell lymphoma
Anaplastic large cell lymphoma (T and null cell type).

Very Aggressive Lymphomas (High Risk)

a. B-cell lineage—precursor B-lymphoblastic lymphoma/leukemia
Burkitt's lymphoma/B-cell acute leukemia
Plasma cell leukemia
b. T-cell lineage—precursor T-lymphoblastic lymphoma/leukemia
Adult T-cell lymphoma/leukemia.

STAGING

The standard staging of NHL is based on Ann Arbor classification used for Hodgkin's disease. The malignant lymphomas or NHL usually occur in the elderly people and often progress early to distant nodal or extra-nodal sites and may evolve rapidly. Therefore the principle of Ann Arbor staging is not as useful a predictor of treatment outcome in malignant lymphomas as in Hodgkin's disease. Hence O'Reckly and Connors have devised a simplified staging system for clinical decision making which is based on the Ann Arbor staging, patient age and extent of tumor bulk.

In order to judge prognosis, and make appropriate therapeutic decision, the clinician must know the pathological staging (type as well as risk status) and clinical staging.

Stage I	Disease in one lymph node area only
Stage II	Disease in two or more lymph node areas on the same side of the diaphragm
Stage III	Disease in lymph node areas on both sides of the diaphragm (the spleen is considered to be nodal)
Stage III 1	Involvement of splenic, celiac or portal nodes
Stage III 2	Involvement of para-aortic, iliac or portal nodes
Stage IV	Extensive disease in liver, bone marrow or other extranodal sites
Substage E	Localized extranodal disease
Symptom status A	Absence of fevers, sweats or weight loss
Symptom status B	Unexplained fevers >38°C

Drenching night sweats

Weight loss of >10 percent in preceding 6 months.

Definition of bulk Mediastinal mass > one-third of the maximum diameter of the chest

B-CELL NEOPLASM

  I. Precursor B-cell neoplasm: Precursor B-lymphoblastic leukemia/lymphoma.

 II. Peripheral B-cell neoplasms.

    1. B-cell chronic lymphocytic leukemia/prolymphocytic leukemia/small lymphocytic lymphoma.

    2. Lymphoplasmacytoid lymphoma/immunocytoma.

    3. Mantle cell lymphoma

    4. Follicle center lymphoma. Provisional cytologic grades:

      i. small cell

     ii. mixed small and large cell

    iii. large cell

      Provisional subtype: diffuse predominantly small cell type.

    5. Marginal Zone B-cell lymphoma

6. Splenic marginal zone lymphoma
7. Hairy cell leukemia
8. Plasmocytoma/plasma cell myeloma
9. Diffuse large B-cell lymphoma
10. Burkitt's lymphoma
11. High grade B-cell lymphoma.

T-CELL AND PUTATIVE NK CELL NEOPLASMS

I. Precursor T-cell neoplasm: Precursor T-lymphoblastic lymphoma/leukemia.
II. Peripheral T-cell and NK cell neoplasms:
1. T-cell chronic lymphocytic leukemia/prolymphocytic leukemia
2. Large granular lymphocyte leukemia
3. Mycosis fungoides/Sezary syndrome
4. Peripheral T-cell lymphomas–unspecified
5. Angio-immunoblastic T-cell lymphoma (AILD)
6. Angiocentric lymphoma
7. Intestinal T-cell lymphoma
8. Adult T-cell lymphoma leukemia ATL/L
9. Anaplastic or large cell lymphoma ALCL
10. Provisional entity. Anaplastic large cell lymphoma, Hodgkin's like lymphoma.

CLINICAL FEATURES

More than 60 percent of patients present with lymph nodal disease and associated infection. The involvement of Waldeyer's ring, epitrochlear and mesenteric nodes is more suggestive of NHL than Hodgkin's disease. NHL presents with a wide spectrum from low-grade lymphoma (widely disseminated at diagnosis but follows indolent course) to high grade lymphoma (short history of localized rapidly enlarging lymphadenopathy, with or without constitution symptoms). Superficial lymphadenopathy is the most common presenting feature of NHL but may present with oropharyngeal involvement (5-10%), autoimmune cytopenias, gastrointestinal involvement (15%), CNS involvement (5-10%), seen associated with high grade NHL or skin involvement. The skin involvement is seen with T-cell lymphomas. Patients with GIT involvement have a higher frequency of oropharyngeal involvement of Waldeyer's ring (Table 34.1).

LOW GRADE

40 percent of the cases belong to this grade and are most common in middle or old age. The median age is 55 years. They are generally indolent and present with stage III or IV disease in two-thirds of patients and frequently involve bone marrow at first presentation. It can also present with painless lymphadenopathy. The effects of bone marrow infiltration or constitutional

Table 34.1: International prognostic index for NHL					
Risk factors		*Definition*	*Predictive model*		
Age		>60 yrs			
LDH		>1× normal			
ECOG		>1			
Stage		III/IV			
Extranodal sites		>1			
	No. of	*%*		*DFS*	*Overall*
Risk category	*risk factors*	*Cases*	*CR*	*of CR[a]*	*survival*
Low	0-1	35	87%	70%	73%
Low intermediate	2	27	67%	51%	51%
High intermediate	3	22	55%	49%	43%
High	4-5	16	44%	42%	26%

[a]DFS, Disease-free survival at 5 years.

symptoms are evident. The median survival is around 8 years. About 30 percent of low grade variety may transform to more aggressive histology often resistant to treatment.

Marginal zone lymphomas take 3 forms:
1. Mucosa-associated lymphoid tissue (MALT) lymphoma is associated with local invasion at site where tumor arises, e.g. stomach, small bowel, salivary gland or lung.
2. Monocytoid B-cell lymphoma is associated with Sjogren's syndrome—usually localized to head, neck and parotid gland.
3. Mycosis fungoides is a T-cell lymphoma, which presents as localized or generalized plaque or erythroderma associated with lymphadenopathy. In 50 percent median survival is 10 years but prognosis is worse with lymphadenopathy or visceral involvement.

INTERMEDIATE GRADE

The most common histology is diffuse large B-cell NHL. 50 percent of cases belong to this group. It could present with stage I or II disease in 50 percent of patients but disseminated extranodal disease is not uncommon and 1/3 patients have constitutional symptoms. Other subtypes of intermediate grade lymphoma often present with widespread disease and are more likely than the low-grade histologies to progress without treatment. Median survival is only 3 years.

The various presentations include cutaneous lesions, bone lesions, CNS disease, abdominal mass, gastrointestinal lymphoma and testicular masses. The spinal cord compression and involvement of various parenchymal and visceral sites are also seen in this grade. In view of such wide range of both lymphatic and extralymphatic disease presentations, the NHL may mimic virtually any other infectious or neoplastic condition.

AGGRESSIVE LYMPHOMA (HIGH GRADE)

These constitute 60 percent of all lymphomas. The disease-related prognostic factors are the stage, and the tumor burden, increased LDH level and the immunophenotype (whether T- or B-cell). Advanced age, poor performance status and B-symptoms are associated with poor outcome.

The majority of patients present with stage III and IV disease with a median age of 55 years. Approximately 50 percent of the patients will show relapse of the disease even after achieving complete remission with chemotherapy.

INVESTIGATIVE PROCEDURES FOR NON-HODGKIN'S LYMPHOMA

Mandatory Procedures

History and physical examination, excisional biopsy of involved node or extranodal site. Complete blood count, LDH, liver and renal function tests, and peripheral smear examination must be done.
- Chest X-ray.
- CT scan of abdomen, pelvis and thorax.
- Bilateral bone marrow study.
- ENT examination for Waldeyer's ring and nasopharynx.

Immunological markers of surface antigens to differentiate between B-cell and T-cell (This test could be done on blood, bone marrow or tissue from the lymph node).

Optional Procedures

Cytology of cerebrospinal fluid (for patients with neurologic abnormalities and small non-cleaved and lymphoblastic histology).
- X-ray and CT scan of symptomatic site.
- Bone scanning (for those with bone pain).

MANAGEMENT

In most patients with NHL, the approach to treatment is based primarily on the histological categorization into one of the 3 main groupings of clinical relevance (i.e. histologically indolent disease, low grade, intermediate risk and high risk). With the first 2 groups, the extent of the disease may also indicate the therapeutic strategy employed. In some patients with extranodal lymphoma, the specific site of disease may also influence the treatment.

The choice of therapy depends upon stage, histologic subtype, patient's age and performance status.

TREATMENT OF LOW GRADE LYMPHOMA

When the disease is localized and the patient does not have typical B symptoms, radiotherapy is the mainstay of therapy. Involved field radiotherapy is delivered to a dose of 3500-4500 cGY. The 5-year disease free survival with radiotherapy in stage I and II disease is approximately 70 percent or more. Most relapses occur outside the radiation field.

The alternative approach in limited stage disease is the "watch and wait" policy till the disease shows progression or to use chemotherapy alone. Chemotherapy regimens include cyclophosphamide, vincristine, prednisolone (CVP) or fludarabine as a single agent.

The optimum strategy for advanced stage low-grade lymphoma is controversial and meant for patients with stage III, IV and bulky stage II. The treatment approaches either of the two ranges, from the "watch and wait" policy to combination chemotherapy and chemoradiotherapy. The other systemic treatment option includes rituximab, which is an anti-CD-20 monoclonal antibody agent.

The patients who can do without initial therapy are those without B symptoms. Otherwise with bulky disease, patients are treated with radiotherapy and combination chemotherapy.

In elderly patients with intermediate or low risk, instead of multidrug CVP regimen, chlorambucil is combined with prednisolone. The dose of prednisolone is 40 mg/m^2 daily. Oral chlorambucil and prednisolone therapy are monitored by blood counts and the drugs should be stopped when there is mild myelosuppression.

Whenever urgent response is needed in an advanced low grade lymphoma the CVP regimen is given for 4-6 cycles. Radiotherapy (a dose of 30Gy) is often added to originally affected bulky nodal/extranodal sites.

Patients with advanced low grade lymphoma survive for a long period of time with periodic interventional therapy but are likely to show repeated relapses. In fact approximately 50 percent of the patients will demonstrate histological transformation from intermediate to high grade NHL.

TREATMENT OF LIMITED STAGE LARGE CELL LYMPHOMA (INTERMEDIATE GRADE)

The limited stage includes stage I or II tumor mass less than 10 gm and the absence of B-symptoms. The current treatment approach for limited stage large cell lymphoma is to deliver combination chemotherapy with or without radiotherapy to the local sites. The CHOP (cyclophosphamide + doxorubicin + vincristine + prednisolone) regimen is given for 3 cycles followed by involved field radiotherapy (IFRT). Connors et al have shown excellent cure rate of more than 80 percent with this regimen.

TREATMENT OF AGGRESSIVE LYMPHOMA (HIGH GRADE)

The initial studies showed high responses to the CHOP regimen. This regimen has remained the choice for first line chemotherapy in the majority of institutions. Unfortunately long term studies have reported a 30 percent overall 10 year survival with this regimen. Due to the limitation with CHOP schedule several other chemotherapeutic schedules were developed and studied (PROMACE/CYTA BOM, MACOP-B,M-BACOD). There was no statistical difference in survival. The fewest number of fatal toxicities was with CHOP regimen. So it seems that CHOP regimen is the most appropriate, despite its limitation (Table 34.2).

The majority of patients present with stage III and IV disease. Approximately 50 percent of the patients will show relapse of the disease even after achieving complete remission with chemotherapy.

High dose chemotherapy with stem cell transplantation is another potential modality of treatment for intermediate and high grade lymphoma.

The schedule is repeated every 21 days for 4 to 6 cycles.

ROLE OF RADIOTHERAPY IN NON-HODGKIN'S LYMPHOMA

The management of non-Hodgkin's lymphoma is primarily done with chemotherapy. The precise indications for radiotherapy are described below:

1. True stage I—II low grade NHL and stage I large cell lymphoma (intermediate grade).
   Involved field radiotherapy is curative in these patients and the dose of radiation is according to histology.
   Dose: Low grade NHL—35 Gy
   Intermediate grade NHL—40 to 45 Gy
   In stage I disease, long term cure rates range from 50 to 80 percent.
2. Involved field radiotherapy (IFRT):
   IFRT is the commonly used technique for NHL. In lymphatic and extralymphatic stage IA or stage IE disease the lymphatic region is irradiated in toto.
   In bulky stage II, stage III or stage IV disease, the patient might have residual disease after completion of chemotherapy. If there is no other

Table 34.2: Chemotherapy-CHOP regimen		
Regimen	*Dose*	*Day/Week*
C Cyclophosphamide	750 mg/m^2 IV	1
H Adriamycin	50 mg/m^2 IV	1
O Vincristine	1.4 mg/ m^2 IV	1
P Prednisolone	100 mg PO	1-5

systemic evidence of disease IFRT will improve the disease-free and long-term survival in these patients.

3. Total body irradiation (TBI):
   In advanced low grade NHL patients can be palliated by giving whole body irradiation followed by autologue bone marrow transplantation rescue. In relapsed or recurrent follicular lymphoma, cyclophosphamide and total body radiation are followed by ABMT rescue.

4. Palliative radiotherapy.
   Metastatic lymphoma to bone or spine is a common problem in NHL patients. Symptoms of pain and spinal cord compression can be palliated by radiotherapy. The usual recommended dose for bone metastasis in NHL is 30 Gy in 10 fractions over a two week period or 20 Gy in 5 fractions over a week period.

TREATMENT OF RELAPSED CASES OF NHL

A variety of regimens are used, including EPOCH, DHAP, ESHAP, etc. Some of the chemosensitive parents are considered for ABMT (Table 34.3).

a. Etoposide, cyclophosphamide, and doxorubicin dosages may be increased by 20 percent from the previous cycle's dosage if there was no evidence of absolute neutropenia (ANC, $<500/mm^3$) or thrombocytopenia (platelet count, $<25,000/mm^3$).

b. Increments in the doses of cyclophosphamide by 50 mg/m^2 and etoposide by 15 mg/m^2 during each cycle are allowed if the patient could tolerate without significant neutropenia.

FURTHER READING

1. Carbone PP, Kaplan HS, Husshoff K, et al. Report of the committee on Hodgkin's disease staging classification. Cancer Res 1970; 31:1860.
2. Connors JM, Klimo P, Fairey RN, et al. Brief chemotherapy and involved field radiation therapy for limited stage aggressive histology lymphoma. Ann Int Med 1987;107-25.
3. Fisher RI, Gaynor ER, Dahlberg S, et al. Comparison of standard regimen (CHOP) with three intensive chemotherapy regimens for advanced non-Hodgkin's lymphoma. N Eng J Med 1993;328:1002-12.
4. Harris NL, Jaffe ES, Stein H, Banks PM, Cram JKC, Cleary ML, et al. A revised European American classification of lymphoid neoplasms: A proposal from the international Lymphoid Study Group. Blood 1994; 84:1361-92.
5. Hoover RN. Lymphoma risk in populations with altered immunity: A search for mechanism. Cancer Res 1992;52:547-63.
6. Jacobson JO, Aisenberg AC, Lambarre L, et al. Mediastinal large cell lymphoma. An uncommon subset of adult lymphoma curable with combined modality. Cancer 1988;62:1893-99.
7. NCRP.National Cancer Registry Programme.Biennial Report 1988-1989. An epidemiological study. Indian Council of Medical Research, New Delhi 1992.

Table 34.3: Salvage chemotherapy regimens in aggressive NHL

Combination chemotherapy	Treatment description
EPOCH (dose adjusted)	Etoposide, 50 mg/ m^2 per day by continuous i.v. infusion for 4 days, days 1-4 (total dose/cycle, 250 mg/m^2)
	Doxorubicin, 10 mg/m^2 per day by continuous i.v. infusion for 4 days, days 1-4 (total dose/cycle, 40 mg/m^2)
	Vincristine, 10 mg/m^2 per day by continuous i.v. infusion for 4 days, days 1-4 [total dose/cycle, 1.6 mg/m^2 (no cap)]
	Prednisone, 60 mg/m^2 per dose p.o. every 12 h for 5 days, days 1-5 (total dose/cycle, 750 mg/m^2)
	Filgrastim, 5 mg/kg per day s.c. starting day 6; continuous until ANC >5,000 cells/mm^3
	Treatment is repeated every 21 days
	Cotrimoxazole (800 mg sulfamethoxazole + 160 mg trimethoprim), 1 dose p.o. 3 times weekly (e.g., Monday, Wednesday, Friday) given continuously throughout antineoplastic treatment.
DHAP	Cisplatin, 100 mg/m^2 by continuous i.v. infusion for 24 h on day 1 (total dose/cycle, 100 mg/m^2)
	Cytarabine, 2,000 mg/m^2 per dose i.v. over 3 h every 12 h for two doses on day 2 (total dose/cycle, 4,000 mg/m^2)
	Dexamethasone, 40 mg per day p.o. or i.v. for 4 days, days 1-4 (total dose/cycle, 160 mg/m^2)
	Treatment is repeated every 21-28 days
ESHAP	Etoposide, 40 mg/m^2 per day over 1 h i.v. for 4 days, days 1-4 (total dose/cycle, 160 mg/m^2)
	Methylprednisolone 250-500 mg per day i.v. for 5 days, days 1-5 (total dose/cycle, 1,250 – 2,500 mg)
	Cytarabine, 2,000 mg/m^2 i.v. over 2 h on day 5 (total dose/cycle, 2,000 mg/m^2)
	Cisplatin, 25 mg/m^2 per day by continuous i.v. infusion for 4 days, days 1-4 (total dose/cycle, 100 mg/m^2)
	Treatment is repeated every 21-28 days
CEPP(B)	Cyclophosphamide, 600 mg/m^2 per dose i.v. for two doses, 5 days 1 and 8 (total dose/cycle, 1,200 mg/m^2)
	Etoposide, 70 mg/m^2 per day i.v. for 3 days, days 1-3 (total dose/cycle, 210 mg/m^2)
	Prednisone, 60 mg/m^2 per day p.o. for 10 days, days 1-10 (total dose/cycle, 600 mg/m^2)
	Procarbazine, 60 mg/m^2 per day p.o. for 10 days, days 1-10 (total dose/cycle, 600 mg/m^2)
	Bleomycin, 15 U/m^2 i.v. on days 1 and 15 (total dose/cycle, 30 U/m^2)

8. O'Reilly SE, Conorrs JM. Non-Hodgkin's Lymphoma-Characterisation and treatment. Br Med J 1992;304:1682-87.

9. Rohatimer AZS, Johnson PW. Myeloablative therapy with autologous bone marrow transplantation as consolidation therapy for recurrent follicular lymphoma. J Clin Oncol 1994;12:1177-84.

10. Tubiana M. Prognostic factor in Non- Hodgkin's lymphomas. Int J Radiat Oncol Biol Phys 1986;12:503-14.

11. Vose JM. Classification and clinical course of low grade non-Hodgkin's lymphomas with overview of therapy. Ann Oncol 1996;7(suppl-6):513-19.

APPENDIX 12

International comparison, India and five continents—AAR (ICMR and IARC).

NON-HODGKIN'S LYMPHOMA (MALE)

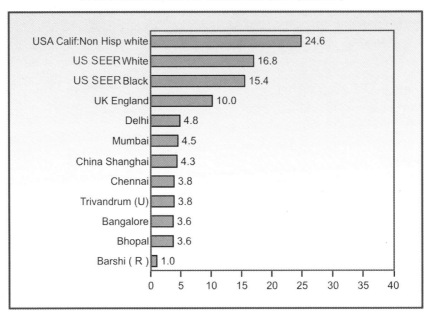

NON-HODGKIN'S LYMPHOMA (FEMALE)

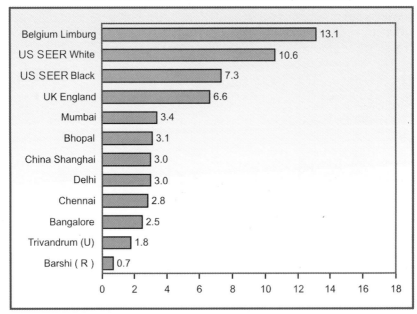

Rate per 100,000

Hodgkin's Lymphoma

35

Pamela Jayaraj
K Pavithran

Hodgkin's disease (HD), a malignancy of lymphatic systems, represents less than 2.3 percent of all new cases of cancer in India. It is a non-leukemic malignant condition arising from lymphoreticular tissues. It is one of the first tumor types that are curable at both localized and advanced stages of the disease. The first clinical and gross anatomic description of the disease was given by Thomas Hodgkin in 1832.

EPIDEMIOLOGY AND ETIOLOGY

Epidemiology

Hodgkin's disease represents 20 -25 percent of all lymphomas.

Incidence

In developing countries the overall incidence of Hodgkin's disease is lower than that in developed countries but the incidence before the age of 15 years is rising, with a modest increase throughout adolescence and young adulthood.

Sex

The disease is more common in males than in females.

Age

There is a bimodal age distribution with the first peak seen in the twenties and a second rise after the age of 50.

Etiology

The etiology of Hodgkin's disease remains undetermined. Environmental risk factors do not play a major role in Hodgkin's disease. However wood workers, farmers and workers in meat industry may be at increased risk. HIV infection is not a risk factor for the development of Hodgkin's disease.

Occasional geographic clusters of cases have suggested the possibility of a viral etiology, with perhaps a long incubation or latent period.

Recently, the Epstein-Barr virus genome has been detected by polymerase chain reaction (PCR) in Reed-Sternberg cells in about half of the Hodgkin's disease cases, most commonly in mixed cellularity type.

CLINICAL FEATURES

The onset is usually characterized by painless lymph node enlargement with or without fever, sweating, pruritus, weight loss or malaise. Cervical lymph nodes are the most commonly enlarged at the onset (60-80%) while mediastinal, axillary and inguinal nodes do so less commonly (6-20%).

Based upon Ann-Arbor symposium on staging of HD in 1970, the most important constitutional symptoms (B symptoms) are as follows:

1. Unexplained weight loss of more than 10 percent of body weight in 6 months previous to diagnosis
2. Unexplained fever with temperature above 38°C
3. Night sweats.

DIAGNOSTIC WORK-UP

1. Adequate surgical biopsy
2. Detailed history
3. A careful and detailed physical examination
4. Necessary laboratory procedures
   a. Complete blood count including an erythrocyte sedimentation rate
   b. Serum alkaline phosphatase level
   c. Evaluation of renal function
   d. Evaluation of liver function
   e. Immunological marker studies
5. Radiological studies
   a. Chest radiograph
   b. Chest and abdominal CT scan

HISTOLOGIC CLASSIFICATION OF HD-LUKES, BUTLER, HICK (1996)

Lymphocytic predominance	(15%)
Nodular sclerosis	(10%)
Mixed cellularity	(10%)
Lymphocyte depletion	(5%)

ANN ARBOR CLINICAL STAGING CLASSIFICATION, REVISED AT COTSWOLD

Stage I

Involvement of a single lymph node region or lymphoid structure (e.g. spleen, thymus, Waldeyer's ring) or involvement of a single extralymphatic site (I_E).

Stage II

It involves two or more lymph node regions on the same side of the diaphragm (hilar nodes, when involved on both sides constitute stage II disease). There is localized contiguous involvement of only one extranodal organ or site and lymph node regions on the same side of the diaphragm (II_E). The number of anatomic regions involved should be indicated by numerical subscripts.

Stage III

It involves lymph node regions on both sides of the diaphragm (III), which may also be accompanied by involvement of the spleen (IIIs) or by localized continuous involvement of only one extranodal organ site (III_E) or both (III_{ES}). Stage III may be subdivided as stage III_1, (e.g. spleen or splenic hilum, celiac or portal node involvement) or III_2 (e.g. para aortic, iliac or mesenteric node involvement).

Stage IV

There is diffuse or disseminated involvement of one or more extra nodal organs or tissues, with or without associated lymph node involvement.

RADIOTHERAPY IN HODGKIN'S DISEASE (TABLE 35.1)

Hodgkin's disease is one neoplasm where the outcome is improved due to the advancement of the radiotherapy technology. The lymphomatous cells are very radiosensitive. In fact, patients with Stage I and Stage II A may be cured by radiotherapy alone. The local control is proportionate to the total dose up to a dose of 3000 cGy. The local control attains 93 percent at a dose level of 3000 cGy. The rate of regression is a good indicator of improved local control. The recommended dose for involved site is 3600 cGy and for uninvolved site 3000 cGy. But when radiotherapy is given after chemotherapy (mechlorethamine, oncovin, procarbazine, prednisone—MOPP), the total dose for involved site is 2500 cGy.

CHEMOTHERAPY

The indications for chemotherapy in HD are:
    1. Primary treatment for advanced disease

Table 35.1: The precise indications of radiotherapy are summarized below

Stage	*Treatment technique*
Stage 1	Radiotherapy
CS –II	Extended
(Supradiaphragmatic)	Mantle field
PS IIA, IB (Supradiaphragmatic mediastinal adenopathy)	Extended Mantle field (STLI)
CS IIIA, IIIB	TLI or Combined modality (CT + IFRT)
CS IV	Combined modality
CSI –II (infradiaphragmatic)	Inverted -Y RT
PS I-II (Infradiaphragmatic)	Combined modality (CT + IFRT)
CS	— Clinical stage
PS	— Pathological stage
STLI	— Subtotal lymphoid irradiation
TLI	— Total lymphoid irradiation
IFRT	— Involved field radiotherapy
CT	— Chemotherapy

   2. Combined modality
   3. Adjuvant to radiotherapy in early stage with bulk disease
   4. Salvage therapy
   5. High dose therapy
   6. Palliative therapy

Hodgkin's disease is exquisitely sensitive to chemotherapy possibly because of a high tumor cell growth factor (>50%) as measured by immunohistochemistry. Nitrogen mustard was the first compound to be assessed for a cytotoxic effect in patients with Hodgkin's disease following the observation that mustard gas induced neutropenia. Currently, three major groups of regimens dominate the primary chemotherapy of newly diagnosed HD:

   1. MOPP and its variants
   2. ABVD (doxorubicin, bleomycin, vinblastine, dacarbazine) and
   3. various regimens combining MOPP and ABVD.

   Randomized studies have shown that ABVD is superior to MOPP.

   Various factors that adversely influence the remission and relapse are:

   1. age >40 years
   2. systemic symptoms especially fever and weight loss
   3. any prior chemotherapy
   4. stage IV disease
   5. low Hb and low lymphocyte count
   6. multiple extranodal sites and/or bulky nodal disease
   7. liver, pleura and bone marrow involvement

The other adverse factors are poor performance status, raised serum LDH and the reduced dose intensity in the chemotherapy cycles.

COMBINED MODALITY THERAPY

The combination of multidrug chemotherapy schedules and radiotherapy for advanced stage IIB, III and IV disease has been the practice in the recent times. The combined therapy is also used for bulky mediastinal disease at presentation or multiple bulky nodal and extranodal involvement.

Chemotherapy, either MOPP or ABVD should be given first to reduce the tumor bulk in involved field. In case of the initial bulky disease (LN or site) RT is included in the treatment portal to a dose of 25-30 Gy. It is preferred to reduce the radiation dose after the full course of chemotherapy in order to avoid the long term toxicities.

ABVD

Doxorubicin, 25 mg/m^2 per dose i.v. push for two doses, days 1 and 15 (total dose/cycle, 50 mg/m^2)

Bleomycin, 10 Units/m^2 per dose i.v. push for two doses, days 1 and 15 (total dose/cycle, 20 Units/m^2)

Vinblastine, 6 mg/m^2 per dose i.v. push for two doses, days 1 and 15 (total dose/cycle, 12 mg/m^2)

Dacarbazine, 375 mg/m^2 per dose i.v. infusion for two doses, days 1 and 15 (total dose/cycle, 750 mg/m^2)

MOPP

Mechlorethamine, 6 mg/m^2 per dose i.v. push for two doses, days 1 and 8 (total dose/cycle, 12 mg/m^2)

Vincristine, 1.4 mg/m^2 per dose i.v. push for two doses, days 1 and 8 (total dose/cycle, 2.8 mg/m^2)

Procarbazine, 100 mg/m^2 per dose p.o. dose for 14 doses, days 1-14 (total dose/cycle, 1,400 mg/m^2)

Prednisone, 40 mg/m^2 per dose p.o. for 14 doses, days 1-4 (cycles 1 and 14 only) (total dose/cycle, 560 mg/m^2)

Treatment cycles repeats every 28 days.

TREATMENT OF RELAPSED AND RECURRENT HODGKIN'S DISEASE

The choice of treatment of relapsed disease depends on the primary modality of treatment. If the patient was initially treated with radiation only, at the time of relapse chemotherapy regimens such as ABVD or MOPP could be initiated or *vice versa*.

If the patient was initially treated with chemotherapy and develops relapse in less than a year, non-cross resistant agents or regimens should be used.

Any patient in whom cure is not achieved with the initial course of combination chemotherapy should be considered a potential candidate for high dose chemotherapy with stem cell support. The recent clinical application of granulocyte macrophage colony stimulating factor (GM-CSF) and granulocyte colony stimulating factor (G-CSF) have been demonstrated to accelerate granulocyte recovery after ABMT (Autologous bone marrow transplantation).

FURTHER READING

1. Bigar BJ, Horm J, Goedert JJ, Melbye M. Cancer in a group at risk of acquired immunodeficiency syndrome (AIDS) through 1984. Am J Epidermiol 1987;126:578.
2. Hodgkin T. On some morbid appearances of the adsorbent glands and spleen. Med Chir Trans 1832;17:68-114.
3. Lister TA, Crowther D, Sutcliffe SB, et al. Report of a committee convened to discuss the evaluation and staging of patients with Hodgkin's disease: Cotswold's meeting. J Clin Oncol 1989;7:1630-36.
4 Lukes RJ, Butler JJ, Hicks ED. Natural history of Hodgkin's disease as related to its pathologic picture. Cancer 1966;19:317-44.
5. NCRP: National Cancer Registry Programme. Biennial Report 1988-1989. An epidemiological study. Indian Council of Medical Research, New Delhi, 1992.
6. Ultmann JE, Moran EM: Hodgkin's disease: Clinical course and complications. Arch Intern Med 1973;78:113.

Multiple Myeloma— Plasma Cell Neoplasm

36

Pamela Jayaraj
K Pavithran

Plasma cell neoplasms are a group of related disorders each of which is associated with proliferation, and accumulation of immunoglobulin-secreting cells derived from B-cell lymphocytes. They are believed to be monoclonal tumors derived from single transformed cells.

PATHOLOGICAL CLASSIFICATION

Plasma cells are found primarily in the tissues and organs of lymphoreticular system, especially the bone marrow, lymph nodes, liver, upper respiratory and gastrointestinal tract mucosa. The plasma cells are derived from the B-lymphocytes, which develop from the primitive reticular stem cells found scattered throughout all tissues, thus making it possible to find these tumors in almost any tissue or organ.

The classification of the plasma cell tumors is as follows:
Multiple plasma cell myeloma
Disseminated monosteolytic myelomatosis
Solitary plasmocytoma of the bone
Extramedullary plasmocytoma
Plasma cell leukemia
Waldenstrom's macroglobulinemia
Malignant lymphoma with M component
Myeloma is a low growth fraction tumor with only a small percentage of tumor cells in cycle at any given time. The subclinical phase can take 1-3 years; the clinical phase can last from 1 year to more than 10 years.

CLINICAL PRESENTATION

Malignant plasma cell tumors are seen at presentation in several forms, from small localized lesions to diffuse dissemination. The most common presentation is that of a disseminated disease (myeloma) with involvement of multiple skeletal sites. Common presenting complaints are bone pain (68%), infection (12%), bleeding (7%) and easy fatigability. Peripheral blood examination usually reveals anemia. Hyperglobulinemia can cause disturbances of the clotting mechanism and usually produces an elevation of the erythrocyte sedimentation rate. Hypercalcemia is present in 50 percent of the patients. Skeletal radiographs demonstrate one of the three common features: diffuse osteoporosis, well demarcated lytic lesions, or localized cystic osteolytic lesions.

Plasma cell tumors secrete measurable 'paraprotein' (either complete or incomplete immunoglobulin Ig proteins or proteins of light chains) in 95 to 99 percent of cases. These paraproteins constitute a unique 'tumor marker'.

DIAGNOSTIC WORKUP

Diagnostic Criteria for Multiple Myeloma

Major Criteria
1. Plasmacytoma on tissue biopsy
2. Bone marrow plasmacytosis with >30 percent plasma cells
3. Monoclonal globulin spikes on serum electrophoresis exceeding 3.5 g/dL for IgG or 2g/dL for IgA, greater than or equal to 1g/24 hour of kappa or lambda light chain excretion on urine electrophoresis.

Minor Criteria
a. Bone marrow plasmacytosis 10-30 percent plasma cells
b. Monoclonal globulin spikes present but < levels defined above
c. Lytic bone lesions
d. Residual normal Ig A < 100 mg/dL or IgG <600 mg/dL.

The diagnosis of myeloma requires a minimum of one major + one minor criteria or three minor criteria that should include a+ b.

ROUTINE STUDIES

General history
— Physical examination
— Bone marrow biopsy or biopsy of any mass

RADIOGRAPHIC STUDIES

— Chest film
— Skeletal survey
— MRI or CT scans of painful weight bearing areas

LABORATORY TESTS

— Complete blood cell count
— Serum B2 microglobulin (Very valuable in determining prognosis and response to therapy)

— Plasma chemistry profile
— Protein studies including immunoelectrophoresis

The diagnosis of myeloma requires a minimum of one major + one minor criteria or three minor criteria that should include a+ b. In the UK two out of three following parameters are essential for the diagnosis of multiple myeloma

1. Presence of paraproteins in the serum or urine
2. Radiological manifestations of multiple myeloma
3. Bone marrow plasmacytoma.

MYELOMA STAGING SYSTEM

Criteria measured myeloma cell mass (cells $\times 10^{12}/m^2$)

Stage I

All of the following
— Hemoglobin value >10 g/dL
— Serum calcium value normal (<12 mg/dL)
— On roentgenogram, normal bone structure
— Solitary bone plasmacytoma only <0.6 (low)
— Low M component production rate
— IgG value <5 g/dL
— Ig A value <3 g/dL
— Urine light chain component on
— Electrophoresis <4 g/24 hr

Stage II Overall data does not fit either Stage 1 or Stage 111 Stage III
— One or more of the following hemoglobin values <8.5 g/dL
— Serum calcium value >12 mg/dL
— Advanced lytic bone lesions (scale 3) Radiograph shows multiple lytic lesions

High M component production rates   >1.2 (high)
Ig G value   > 7 g/dL
IgA value   > 5 g/dL
Urine light chain M component on
Electrophoresis >12 g/24 hr
Subclassification
A = relatively normal renal function (serum creatinine value >2 mg/dl)
B = abnormal renal function (serum creatinine value <2 mg/dl)

PROGNOSTIC FACTORS

Multiple prognostic factors in myeloma include degree of bone marrow involvement, tumor mass, renal status, chromosome ploidy, intrinsic drug sensitivity and kinetic parameters. However, the most easily measurable and quantifiable and highly predictive parameters are the serum b2-microglobulin level and the serum albumin level.

GENERAL MANAGEMENT

Both chemotherapy and radiation therapy are effective in the palliation of myeloma.

CHEMOTHERAPY

The mainstay of chemotherapy in myeloma for the past two decades has been melphalan frequently in combination with prednisone. The reported response rates range from 45 to 70 percent of patients. The median duration of response is approximately 24 months, with a median survival time of 30 months. Additional agents with demonstrated efficacy are cyclophosphamide, BCNU (carmustine), doxorubicin and lumestine.

Multiple myeloma is not a curable disease. More recent combination therapy may reduce the paraprotein levels quicker than melphalan and prednisone. However there is no survival advantage unless followed by stem cell transplantation of bone marrow.

The duration of chemotherapy is controversial. The cessation of therapy may result in relapse and response to retreatment may be more difficult. Continued chemotherapy may lead to refractory anemia or development of secondary acute leukemia.

Allogenic bone marrow transplantation has been tried in patients with myeloma with variable response depending on the prognostic factors of extended prior treatment stage of disease and age of the patient.

Supportive care is extremely important and includes treatment of anemia, hypercalcemia, hyperuricemia, azotemia and frequent infections.

RADIATION THERAPY

Radiation therapy plays an essential role in the management of plasma cell tumors and is used primarily as an adjuvant in myeloma. The indications of radiotherapy are as follows:
   a. As primary treatment in localized presentations (Solitary plasmacytoma of bone and extramedullary plasmacytoma).
   b. For palliation of pain not controlled by chemotherapy from bone lesions of disseminated disease.
   c. For prevention of pathologic fractures in weight bearing bones.
   d. For relief of spinal cord compression and nerve root compression.

Large field irradiation, such as hemibody irradiation (HBI), sequential HBI, or total-body irradiation can also relieve pain in multiple sites and is a more cost-effective approach. However the role of HBI or TBI is controversial. It appears that chemotherapy is superior as part of the initial treatment. However, large field irradiation is used in patients who have become radioresistant.

FURTHER READING

1. Alexanian R. Localized and indolent myeloma. Blood 1980;56:521.
2. Bataille R, Harousseau JL. Multiple myeloma. N Engl J Med 1997;336:1657-63.
3. Bergsagel DE. Chemotherapy of myeloma. In Malpas JS, Bergsagel DE, Kyle RA (Eds): Myeloma: Biology and Management. Oxford University Press, 1994;273-306.
4. Bergsagel PL, Kuehl WM. Chromosome translocations in multiple myeloma. Oncogene 2001;20(40):5611-22.
5. Dalton WS, Bergsagel PL, Kuehl WM, Anderson KC, Harousseau JL. Multiple Myeloma: Hematology 2001;157-77.
6. Kovacsovics TJ, Delaly A. Intensive treatment strategies in multiple myeloma. Semin Hematol 1997;34:49.

Acute Leukemias

37

K Pavithran
Paul Puthuran

Acute leukemias are a heterogeneous group of neoplasms arising from clonal, neoplastic proliferations of immature cells of the hematopoietic system, which are characterized by aberrant or arrested differentiation. It was in 1845 that Virchow recognized and identified leukemia although Velpeau (1827) had earlier provided the first accurate description of a case of leukemia. It was Ebstein who introduced the term acute leukemia in 1889. Acute leukemias are broadly divided into nonlymphocytic (commonly referred to as myeloid) and lymphoid categories based on the cell of origin.

EPIDEMIOLOGY

Acute leukemias account for less than 3 percent of all cancers. Leukemia is the most common of all childhood malignancies accounting for nearly one-third of all cases occurring before the age of 15 years. Acute lymphocytic leukemia (ALL) accounts for 80 percent of childhood leukemias, acute myeloid leukemia (AML) for 15-18 percent and chronic myeloid and myelomonocytic leukemia accounts for the remainder. In adults acute myeloid leukemia is three to four times more common than acute lymphatic leukemia. It is commoner in patients above 50 years of age. Acute lymphatic leukemia in adults can occur at any age. Published data from India indicate an AAR of 1.4 to 2.3/100,000. The incidence of myeloid in comparison to lymphoid leukaemias is slightly higher in males but distinctly higher in females. Consequently the male-female ratio is less than that of lymphoid leukemias. In both males and females in Barshi, Bhopal and Delhi, myeloid leukaemias are one of the ten leading sites of cancer. The AAR seen in the West is 2-3 times higher than in India.

ETIOLOGY

The cause of most acute leukemias is unknown. Clustering of leukemias in several families has been reported. Consanguinity of parents has also been noted. In Down's syndrome there is a twenty-fold increased risk of leukemia. Higher risk is also noted in patients with Fanconi's anemia, Klinefelter's syndrome, Bloom's syndrome and ataxia telangiectasia. As much as 20 percent of AML may be attributable to smoking. Markedly increased incidence of AML was observed among atomic bomb survivors in Japan. The incidence peaked at 5-6 years and has come back to base line levels in 15 years.

The following factors are incriminated in the etiology of acute leukemia:
1. Ionizing radiation
2. Chemotherapeutic agents. These include alkylating agents such as cyclophosphamide, nitrogen mustard, chlorambucil, etc.
3. Chemicals-Benzene
4. Smoking
5. Congenital abnormalities
   a. Down's syndrome
   b. Bloom's syndrome
   c. Neurofibromatosis
   d. Ataxia telangiectasia
   e. Klinefelter's syndrome
6. Bone marrow failure syndromes
   a. Fanconi's anemia
   b. Dyskeratosis congenita
   c. Kostmann agranulocytosis
7. Retrovirus: HTLV-1 (Adult T-cell leukemia virus).

CLINICAL PRESENTATION

Patients with acute leukemia typically present with a 1 to 3 months history of fatigue (due to anemia), fever and bleeding tendencies. These are the three commonest signs at the time of presentation of a patient with leukemia. The physical examination typically shows pallor and hemorrhage (in the gums, as epistaxis, in the stool, in the skin as petechiae or ecchymoses, or as fundal hemorrhage). Hepatomegaly, splenomegaly and lymphadenopathy are more common in ALL and in monocytic subtypes of AML. Mediastinal lymph node enlargement is found in more than 50 percent cases with T-cell ALL. Gum hypertrophy is common with acute myelomonocytic and monocytic leukemias. Rarely patients can present with isolated tumors of myeloblasts (chloromas/granulocytic sarcomas).

In childhood leukemias, bone pain is not uncommon. Features of meningeal involvement develop in less than 10 percent, at the time of diagnosis. CNS involvement is seen in 10-15 percent of ALL at presentation. 1 percent of patients present with painless enlargement of the testes due to leukemic infiltration.

DIAGNOSIS

Anemia, thrombocytopenia and elevated leukocyte count with blasts are pathognomonic of acute leukemia. Anemia is found in most patients and more than 50 percent will have associated thrombocytopenia. The white blood cell (WBC) count can be normal, reduced or elevated; less than 20 percent of patients have greater than 100,000 cells/μL, and an equal number of patients have less than 5000 cells/μL. Acute monocytic leukemias and T-cell leukemias may have the highest WBC counts. Acute promyelocytic leukemia (APML) is often associated with disseminated intravascular coagulation (DIC). The clinical presentation of AML cannot usually be distinguished from ALL without examination of the blasts for immunophenotype and morphology. A bone marrow aspirate and biopsy, with appropriate cytochemical, immunochemical, and genetic evaluations, must be done in all cases. Even in the severely neutropenic and thrombocytopenic patient a bone marrow aspiration and biopsy can be safely performed and posterior iliac crest is the preferred site for bone marrow examination.

When blasts are more than 20 percent, a diagnosis of AML is confirmed. 'Auer rods' are present in 50 percent of newly diagnosed cases of AML. In ALL the blasts are small or large which are either homogeneous or heterogeneous. These are classified as L1 to L3 based on the size of the cell, degree of basophilia in the cytoplasm and the characteristics of the nucleoli. However in 15 percent of cases, any definite morphological distinction between an immature AML-variant and ALL cannot be made morphologically. The use of monoclonal antibodies that identify myeloid and lymphoid-associated antigens is very useful in these cases.

CLASSIFICATION

Any classification system of leukemia must answer the following three questions:

1. What is the lineage?
2. What is the maturational stage?
3. What is the genotype?

Because the treatments of ALL and AML may differ significantly, the most important first step in the diagnostic assignment is to distinguish the lymphoid and myeloid lineages to assign therapy. If myeloid, the next step is to see whether it is APML or non-APML and study the cytogenetic features. Identification of APML is important because retinoic acid is used as a differentiating agent along with chemotherapy and has the best prognosis among all types of AML (70% 5 yr survival). Among the lymphoid neoplasms, the distinction of FAB L3-ALL (Burkitt's type; mature B cell) is the second important step, as treatment strategies and prognosis differ with this subgroup (Figs 37.1 and 37.2, Plate 3; 37.3 and 37.4, Plate 4; 37.5 and 37.6, Plate 5; 37.7 and 37.8, Plate 6; 37.9 and 37.10, Plate 7 and 37.11, Plate 8).

Plate 3

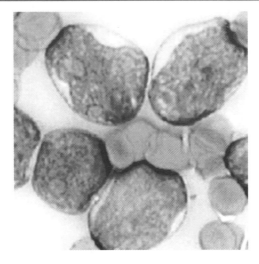

Figure 37.1: AML-MO Poorly differentiated blast cells with granulocytes. Definitive diagnosis of AML-MO requires demonstration of MPO by transmission electron microscope and the absence of antigen from the lymphoid series. No morphological or cytochemical evidence of granulocytic lineage is observed

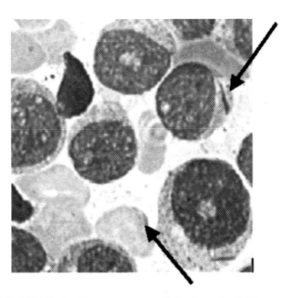

Figure 37.2: AML-M1 Blast with one or more distinct nucleoli. Fine azurophilic granules and occasional Auer rods (closed arrows) are seen

Plate 4

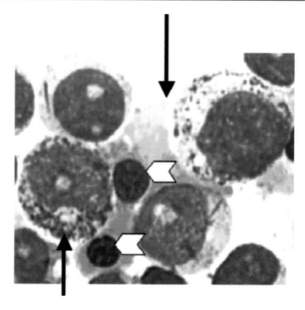

Figure 37.3: AML-M2 Blast with significant maturation characterized by presence of prominent granules (closed arrow) and presence of Auer rods.Two late stages of immature RBCs (open arrow) are also seen

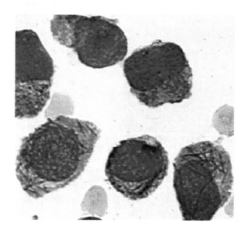

Figure 37.4: AML-M3 Promyelocytic with heavy granulation and presence of Auer rods, in bundles forming faggots

Plate 5

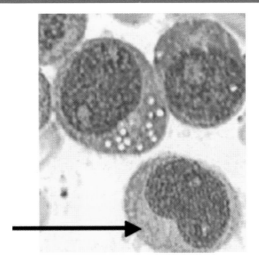

Figure 37.5: AML-M4 Myeloid cells with granulation of monocytic precursors with abundant cytoplasm and reniform nucleus (closed arrow)

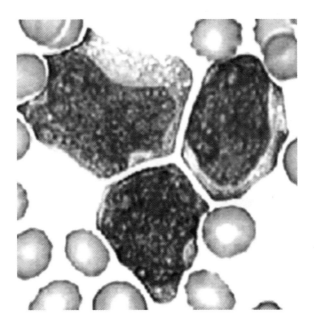

Figure 37.6: AML-M5 Immature monoblasts with round to oval nuclei with delicate chromatin and abundant rim of cytoplasm

Plate 6

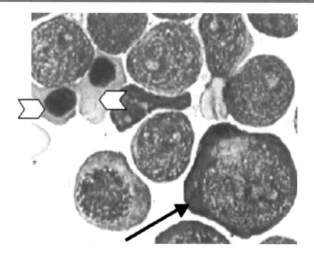

Figure 37.7: AML-M6 Erythroid precursor in different stages of maturation. Early stage (closed arrow), late stage (open arrow) and immature blasts

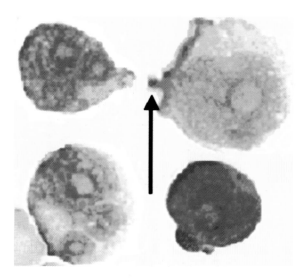

Figure 37.8: AML-M7 Acute megakaryocytic leukemia. Megakaryoblasts with single to multiple nuclei, having fine reticulated chromatin pattern and abundant cytoplasm. Cytoplasmic blebs formation (closed arrow) as of platelet budding is evident

Plate 7

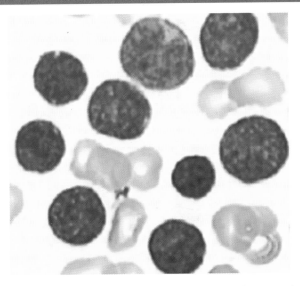

Figure 37.9: ALL-L1 Uniformly small blasts with regular large nucleus having coarse chromatin. Moderately basophilic scanty cytoplasm

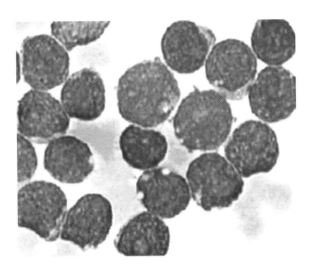

Figure 37.10: ALL-L2 Larger and heterogeneous blasts with irregular nucleus with greater number of nucleoli and abundant basophilic cytoplasm

Plate 8

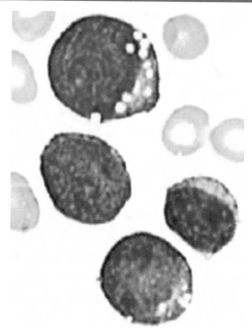

Figure 37.11: ALL-L3 Large homogeneous blasts. Nuclear chromatin freely stippled with prominent nucleoli and deep basophilic vacuolated cytoplasm

Previously used French-American-British (FAB) classification (Table 37.1) relied primarily on morphology and cytochemistry. The FAB criteria are based on a Wright-stained peripheral blood smear and bone marrow aspirate. Four basic histological stains are required and these are PAS (Periodic Acid Schiff) reagent, Sudan black, Peroxidase and Esterase. Most lymphoblasts are PAS positive whereas myeloblasts are PAS negative. Sudan black staining pattern is similar to the peroxidase reactivity. Myeloblasts are generally positive and lymphoid precursors are negative. In general it is a sensitive marker of myeloblasts and is helpful in differentiating immature cells that appear undifferentiated on smear examination.

Knowledge of the exact immunophenotype and the genotype is very important before commencing the most appropriate definitive treatment, such as high-dose consolidation chemotherapy, BMT, or prolonged maintenance therapy in these patients. The WHO classification was developed integrating all these features (Table 37.2).

IMMUNOPHENOTYPING OF ACUTE LEUKEMIAS

The lineage and state of maturation of normal hematopoietic cells may be identified by the use of a flow cytometer to determine the cell size, granularity, and the presence or absence of a panel of cell surface or cytoplasmic differentiation antigens. Acute lymphoid leukemias of T-cell lineage are characterized by expression of the T-cell markers CD2, CD5, CD7, and sometimes CD1. Acute lymphoid leukemias of B-cell lineage express CD 10, CD19, CD22, and, depending on maturational stage, CD20, and surface immunoglobulin. Acute myeloid leukemias express CD13, CD15, CD33, and, more often if monocytoid, CD14. Terminal deoxyribonucleotidyl transferase (Tdt) is expressed by most lymphoid blasts and approximately 20 percent of myeloid blasts. HLA-DR is found on virtually all B-lineage leukemias, most myeloid and monocytic leukemias (except FAB M3).

Based on the immunophenotype ALL can be:
1. Pre-B-cell ALL: This represents approximately 70 percent of patients. The term pre-B refers to the fact that these cells are committed to the B-cell lineage and expression of typical early B-cell markers such as CD19 and terminal deoxyribonucleotidyl transferase, but do not express surface immunoglobulin. In addition the lymphoblasts of

Table 37.1: FAB classification of ALL
1. L1—Uniformly small blasts with regular nuclear shape. Moderately basophilic scanty cytoplasm with inconspicuous nucleolus.
2. L2—Larger and heterogeneous blasts with irregular nucleolus. Abundant basophilic cytoplasm with greater number of nucleoli.
3. L3—Large homogeneous blasts. Nuclear chromatin is freely stippled. Deep basophilic vacuolated cytoplasm is observed with prominent nucleoli.

Table 37.2: WHO classification of acute myeloid leukemia

I. Acute myeloid leukemias with recurrent cytogenetic translocations
    - AML with t(8;21)(q22;q22),AML1(CBFa)/ETO
    - Acute promyelocytic leukemia (AML with t(15;17)(q22;q11-12) and variants, PML/RARa)
    - AML with abnormal bone marrow eosinophils (inv(16)(p13q22) or t(16;16)(p13;q11), CBFb/MYH11X)
    - AML with 11q23 (MLL) abnormalities
II. Acute myeloid leukemia with multilineage dysplasia
    - with prior myelodysplastic syndrome
    - without prior myelodysplastic syndrome
III. Acute myeloid leukemia and myelodysplastic syndrome, therapy related
    - Alkylating agent related
    - Epipodophyllotoxin related (some may be lymphoid)
    - Other types
IV. Acute myeloid leukemia not otherwise categorized
    - AML minimally differentiated
    - AML without maturation
    - AML with maturation
    - Acute myelomonocytic leukemia
    - Acute monocytic leukemia
    - Acute erythroid leukemia
    - Acute megakaryocytic leukemia
    - Acute basophilic leukemia
    - Acute panmyelosis with myelofibrosis

ALL was divided into three subtypes (L1, L2, L3) according to the FAB classification (Table 37.1). However, except for L3, L1 and L2 morphology does not predict immunophenotype, genetic abnormalities or clinical behavior. So these terms are no longer retained in the WHO classification (Table 37.3).

patients with pre-B-cell ALL typically express CD10, which was previously known as common ALL antigen (CALLA).

2. T-cell disease: T-cell ALL and lymphoblastic lymphoma are essentially the same disease.

3. The third and least common subtype (approximately 5% of adult ALL) is mature B-cell ALL. These leukemic cells are express surface immunoglobulin.

More than 70 percent of adult ALL are of B-cell origin and the rest belong to T-cell lineage. In childhood ALL 20 percent of cases are of T-cell origin and the remainder is of precursor B-cell origin (Table 37.3).

CYTOGENETICS AND MOLECULAR GENETICS OF ACUTE LEUKEMIAS

Karyotype is rapidly becoming the gold standard for diagnosis and prognosis in many subtypes of acute leukemia. However, this facility is available only in major institutions. In ALL, the presence of t(9;22) is found

Table 37.3: WHO classification of acute lymphoid leukemias
Precursor B-cell acute lymphoblastic leukemia (cytogenetic subgroups)
t(9;22)(q34;q11); BCR/ABL
t(v;11q23); MLL rearranged
t(1;19)(q23;p13) E2A/PBX1
t(12;21)(p12;q22) ETV/CBF α
Precursor T-cell acute lymphoblastic leukemia
Burkitt cell leukemia

in up to 30 percent of adults: t(4;11), −7 or +8, which are infrequently seen, are poor prognostic signs. Abnormal karyotypes are seen in approximately 80 percent of patients with AML. Based on the karyotype and its clinical significance AML is divided into three subtypes.

Cytogenetic classification of AML:

Favorable: t(8;21), t(15;17), inv(16)/t(16;16)/del(16q)
Intermediate: +8, −Y, +6, del(12p); normal karyotype
Unfavorable: −5, del(5q), −7/del(7q), complex karyotype

SECONDARY LEUKEMIA

Leukemia occurring after treatment of another malignancy is called secondary leukemia. It is seen after chemotherapy for primary childhood cancer, breast cancer and Hodgkin's disease or following myelodysplasia. Several factors such as radiation therapy and chemotherapeutic agents, which are leukemogenic, can cause chromosomal damage. In Hodgkin's disease, those who have received MOPP therapy have greater tendency to develop AML than those with ABVD treatment. The risk is greater when chemotherapy combined with radiotherapy is given. Secondary leukemia generally carries a poor prognosis and the response to treatment is often unsatisfactory.

PROGNOSTIC FACTORS IN AML

	Favorable	*Unfavorable*
Age	< 40	> 60
WBC count	< 10,000/mm³	> 100,000/mm³
Cytognetics	t(8;21), t(15;17), inv 16	−5,del(5q), −7/del(7q)
Origin	de novo	secondary

TREATMENT OF ACUTE LEUKEMIA

The goal of therapy in acute leukemia is the eradication of the leukemic clone with the restoration of normal hematopoiesis. The basic treatment is aimed at 'remission-induction', 'consolidation of remission' and 'remission-maintenance'. Remission induction is achieved by inflicting severe marrow hypoplasia with chemotherapy and allowing the normal residual stem cells to regroup faster than leukemic cells.

MANAGEMENT OF AML

Appropriate treatment of AML requires aggressive chemotherapy resulting in severe and prolonged pancytopenia. Patients with AML are more susceptible to infections with gram negative enteric organisms, staphylococci and fungi and need appropriate and intense antimicrobial therapy. Supportive treatment includes proper hydration, packed cell transfusion and platelet transfusion (when platelet count is less than $20,000/mm^3$).

DRUG TREATMENT OF AML

Previously all types of AML were treated as one disease. Now with the better understanding of the biology of disease, it is treated depending upon the risk subtypes. Of these the most important determinant is karyotype. For the purpose of treatment AML can be divided into:
1. APML, and AML other than APML
2. AML in the young vs AML among the elderly.

INDUCTION OF REMISSION

Standard induction regimen consists of cytosine arabinocide (Ara-C) and daunorubicin. The induction treatment is the same irrespective of the risk groups. Instead of daunorubicin, idarubicin or mitoxantrone can also be used with equally good response rates. The other agents, which are effective are thioguanine, etoposide and amsacrine and are used in various combinations.

Ara-C is usually given as a 7 day continuous infusion at the rate of 100 $mg/m^2/day$ or $100 mg/m^2$ twice daily as a 3 hr infusion and daunorubicin at a dose of 45 mg/m^2 per day for 3 days. This is referred to as the 3/7 regime. With this regimen a complete remission is achieved in 60-70 percent of AML. Complete response (CR) is defined as circulating neutrophils of more than $1500/mm^3$, platelets over $100,000/mm^3$ and a bone marrow aspirate containing less than 5 percent blasts along with 20 percent cellularity showing normal maturation of all lineages. Peripheral blood smear should not contain circulating blasts and there should be no evidence of extramedullary disease. These criteria must be sustained for a period of at least 4 weeks.

A repeat bone marrow is done once the count starts recovering (usually 3 weeks) and second chemotherapy is planned depending on the result (whether in remission or not). In some centers, bone marrow is done on day 14, to assess remission status; if remission is not achieved, a second chemotherapy is started. If 2 courses fail, one has to look for alternative treatment. Remissions obtained after more than 2 courses of chemotherapy are short-lived. Approximately one half of patients who fail to enter into remission die during induction due to infections or hemorrhagic complications. The other half is also expected to have a short life expectancy (1-1.5 years).

POST-REMISSION THERAPY

Currently, the options for post-remission therapy in younger patients with AML involve three forms of dose-intensive treatments: high-dose chemotherapy, allogenic and autologous transplantation. The choice of post-remission therapy is determined by the prognostic group, based on the cytogenetics at presentation.

AML WITH FAVORABLE CYTOGENETICS

They do well following high dose cytosine arabinoside based (3 g/m^2 iv bid × 3 days) consolidation therapy. The optimal number of cycles is controversial, but it varies from 2 to 4. Whether autologous stem cell transplantation should be offered as a part of post-remission strategy to patients with favorable cytogenetics remains controversial. Autologous transplantation provides about 10 percent benefit over high dose cytosine arabinoside, provided it is done in an experienced center, where transplant related mortality is very low. Allogenic transplantation is not needed in this group of patients as none of the randomized studies demonstrated any advantage in this subset of patients.

AML WITH INTERMEDIATE RISK CYTOGENETICS

If an HLA matched sibling donor is available, allogenic BMT is the most appropriate form of therapy for these patients. Once the patient is in remission, it is better to go for transplant immediately as there is no additional benefit with further post-remission chemotherapy. However, for those who are going for an autotransplant, it is better to give further high dose cytosar based chemotherapy before the transplant.

AML WITH UNFAVORABLE CYTOGENETICS

This group has long been recognized to have the poorest prognosis among patients with AML. While the initial response rates may exceed 50 percent, the overall long-term survival remains poor, whatever mode of post-remission therapy is employed. If an HLA identical donor is available patients should be referred for this procedure after induction therapy. Because of the extremely high risk of relapse and poor long term outcome, if an HLA matched sibling donor is not available, matched unrelated donor, or haploidentical family donor can be used, with good long term survival rates.

AML IN THE ELDERLY

The prognosis is generally poor in this group of patients despite all forms of treatment. This is because AML in the elderly differs from AML in the young by many features.

1. Increased incidence of drug resistance-MDR gene expression 71 percent vs 35 percent
2. Less occurrence of favourable cytogenetics
3. Poor tolerance to chemotherapy
4. Co-morbid illnesses, e.g. diabetes, hypertension, coronary artery disease
5. Greater incidence of AML arising from prior myelodysplasia.

With the standard induction treatment, the response rate is only 45-50 percent with a median survival of 6 months and 5 year survival of 7.6 percent. The ideal induction regimen for older patients has not yet been defined. High dose cytosine arabinoside has not been able to confer any benefit in the elderly patients. As resistance is one of the major reasons for failure of treatment, cyclosporine and PSC833 have been evaluated in randomized studies to reverse drug resistance, however, so far the results are not encouraging.

ACUTE PROMYELOCYTIC LEUKEMIA

Acute Promyelocytic Leukemia (APML) is treated with oral administration of all-transretinoic acid (ATRA); 45 milligrams per square meter per day in two divided doses along with chemotherapy (daunorubicin). This can induce remission in >90 percent of patients with APML. ATRA is not a cytotoxic agent, but instead, causes a proliferation of the abnormal clone coincident with maturation, eventual terminal differentiation, and ultimately, apoptotic cell death. Administration of ATRA leads to rapid resolution of coagulopathy in the majority of patients. Administration of ATRA can lead to hyperleukocytosis, as well as a syndrome of respiratory distress known as the "retinoic acid syndrome" (RAS). RAS is characterized by fever, dyspnea, peripheral edema with resultant weight gain, pleural and pericardial effusions and hypotension. The treatment consists of administration of high doses of steroids (dexamethasone). There is no role for high dose cytosine arabinoside in post remission therapy. Once in remission they have to be on maintenance therapy with pulse doses of ATRA with or without 6-mercaptopurine and methotrexate for 1 year. Bone marrow transplantation is indicated in patients with minimal residual disease (PML-Ra positive by RT-PCR) or in relapse. Arsenic trioxide is very useful in relapsed cases.

RELAPSED AND REFRACTORY AML

Several factors like age, duration of first remission and cytogenetic findings have to be taken into consideration before planning treatment of relapsed

AML. The most important of these is duration of first remission. Those patients whose remission lasted for 2 years or more will achieve a second remission in 50-60 percent of cases, when the same initial chemotherapy is repeated. For those patients whose remissions were less than 1 year in duration or who failed to achieve a first remission (primary refractory disease) only 10 percent to 20 percent attain complete remission. Long-term survival at 3 years in the long remission group is approximately 20-25 percent, while shorter duration remission groups have virtually no 3 years survivals. Therefore, treatment decisions must be based, in large part, upon individual, potential for obtaining and maintaining a second remission. After inducing remission these patients should undergo allogenic BMT. In elderly patients who are not candidates for BMT, gemtuzumab ozogamicin can be considered.

ROLE OF GROWTH FACTORS IN AML TREATMENT

Hematopoietic growth factors (G-CSF, GM-CSF) have been used during the induction and post-remission treatment of AML. In many of these trials the duration of neutropenia could be reduced by 2-3 days. Other than that there is no significant benefit on infection rates or survival.

MONOCLONAL ANTIBODY THERAPY IN AML

By targeting features unique to malignant cells, these treatments conceptually allow for eradication of malignant clones while sparing normal tissue. The CD33 antigen is expressed on committed myeloid precursor cells but not in hematopoietic stem cells. The CD33 antigen is also expressed by leukemic blast in at least 90 percent of patients with AML. Gemtuzumab ozogamicin (Mylotarg) is composed of an anti CD33 antibody, complexed to clicheamicin, an antitumor antibiotic that generates double-stranded DNA breaks, resulting in cellular death. It produces 20-30 percent complete response. Currently it is approved for use in relapsed or refractory AML in patients older than 60 years.

MANAGEMENT OF ACUTE LYMPHATIC LEUKEMIA

The cure rate in children with ALL is as high as 80 percent. Unfortunately the adult response is rather poor with only 20-30 percent surviving for 5 years. This difference is due to differences in the biology of the disease in adults.
1. Poor tolerance of intensive therapy.
2. Increased incidence of unfavorable cytogenetic subgroups [particularly t(9;22) and t(4;11)] and a decreased incidence of favorable cytogenetic subgroups such as hyperdiploidy or t(12;21).
3. Comorbid illnesses.

PROGNOSTIC FEATURES

1. Age-<1year and >9 years: poor prognosis.
2. White blood cell count: High count associated with poor prognosis.
3. Leukemic cell immunophenotype: T cell has a favorable prognosis, pre-B cell has an intermediate prognosis, whereas mature B-cell disease has a poor prognosis with standard regimens.
4. Cytogenetics: Philadelphia chromosome-positive disease has a worse prognosis; hyperdiploidy: good prognosis.

The different phases of treatment are:
— Induction
— Consolidation
— CNS prophylaxis
— Remission maintenance

DRUG TREATMENT OF ALL

The mainstay of induction therapy for ALL has been the combination of vincristine and prednisone. Addition of an anthracycline to induction therapy was found to increase the likelihood of achieving a complete remission CR. Current standard induction therapy consists of prednisone and vincristine, daunorubicin and L-asparaginase. In adult ALL, the role of L-asparaginase is not clear.

POST-REMISSION THERAPY-ALL

There are various protocols available for consolidation and maintenance therapy. The drug most prominently used in consolidation of ALL are Ara-C along with epidophyllotoxins, or antimetabolites (such as methotrexate or 6-mercaptopurine).

The CNS directed therapy has become an integral component of the management of ALL. The two commonest extramedullary sites are the CNS and the testes. There are three ways of CNS directed therapy.

Cranial irradiation and intrathecal methotrexate.

Intrathecal multiple drug therapy consisting of methotrexate, cytosine arabinoside and hydrocortisone.

Intermediate or high dose systemic methotrexate plus intrathecal methotrexate.

The combination of intrathecal methotrexate and cranial irradiation remains the preferred approach. In children with low risk disease CNS radiation is not necessary.

Most maintenance regimens however rely on a combination of 6-MP (6-mercaptopurine) and methotrexate. 6-MP is given daily along with weekly methotrexate for 24 months. Other drugs used in remission maintenance include L-asparaginase and anthracycline. The cancer and leukemia group B (CALGB) study clearly demonstrated that remission was better for patients who received consolidation and maintenance therapy. Maintenance therapy is advised for a period of 2 years since maximal relapse is seen within 12-18 months after remission-induction.

Two subtypes of adult ALL require special consideration. B-cell ALL (Burkitts type) is not usually cured with typical ALL regimens. Aggressive brief duration high-intensity regimens similar to those used in aggressive non-Hodgkin's lymphoma have shown high response rates and cure rates (75% complete remission; 40% failure-free survival). T-cell ALL, including lymphoblastic lymphoma, has shown high cure rates when treated with cyclophosphamide-containing regimens.

RELAPSED OR REFRACTORY ACUTE LYMPHOBLASTIC LEUKEMIA

10 percent to 25 percent of patients have diseases resistant to vincristine/ prednisone-based regimens and 60 percent to 70 percent of patients achieve a complete relapse (CR) later. Mainly two types of regimens are used in these patients:

1. regimens used for newly diagnosed patients, e.g. for patients with late relapse
2. those that involve high-dose chemotherapy. High-dose cytarabine-based regimens in combination with other agents have the greatest likelihood of inducing a second CR. However, second CRs are short-lived. So these patients should be offered allogenic transplant.

CENTRAL NERVOUS SYSTEM RELAPSE IN ACUTE LYMPHOBLASTIC LEUKEMIA

CNS relapse occurs in approximately 10 percent of patients who have received appropriate prophylaxis. In the majority of patients, bone marrow relapse occurs simultaneously or later. Patients with isolated CNS relapse should receive reinduction chemotherapy as well. Treatment of established CNS disease requires a combination of radiotherapy and intrathecal chemotherapy. Radiotherapy should consist of 1800 to 2400 cGy administered to the whole brain.

ROLE OF ALLOGENIC BMT IN ALL

The only group for whom allogenic transplant in the first CR can be routinely recommended is patients with t(9;22) and t(4;11) disease. For all other patients, allogenic transplant should be reserved for the second CR.

FURTHER READING

1. Bandini G, Zuffa E, Rosti G, et al. Long term outcome of adults with acute myelogenous leukemia. Br J Hematol 1991;7:486.
2. Bleyer WA. Central nervous system leukemia. In: Henderson ES, Lister TA (Eds): Leukemia (5th ed). Philadelphia: WB Saunders, 1990.

3. Conde E, Iriondo A, Rayon C, et al. Sclogenic bone marrow transplant versus intensification chemotherapy for acute myelogenous leukemia in first remission. A prospective controlled trial. Br J Hematol 1988;68:219.

4. Estey EH, Smith TL, Keating MJ, et al. Prediction of survival during induction therapy in patients with newly diagnosed acute myeloblastic leukemia. Leukemia 1989;3:257.

5. Giles FJ, Keating A, Goldstone AH, et al. Acute myeloid leukemia. Hematology (Am Soc Hematol Educ Program) 2002;73-110.

6. Giles FJ. Gemtuzumab ozogamicin: promise and challenge in patients with acute myeloid leukemia. Expert Rev Anticancer Ther 2002;2:630-40.

7. Harris NL, Jaffe ES, Diebold J, et al. The World Health Organization Classification of Neoplasms of the Hematopoietic and Lymphoid Tissues: Report of the Clinical Advisory Committee Meeting - Airlie House, Virginia, November, 1997. Hematol J 2000;1:53-66.

8. Hoelzer D, Ludwig WD, Thiel E, et al. Improved outcome in adult B-cell acute lymphoblastic leukemia. Blood 1996;87:495-508.

9. Hoelzer D, Thiel E, Loffler H, et al. Prognostic factors in a multicenter study for treatment of acute lymphoblastic leukemia in adults. Blood 1988; 71: 123-31.

10. Leopold LH, Willemze R. The treatment of acute myeloid leukemia in first relapse: A comprehensive review of the literature. Leuk Lymphoma. 2002;43:1715-27.

11. Morra E, Lazzarino M, Inverdadi D, et al. Systemic high dose ara-c for the treatment of meningeal leukemia in adult acute lymphoblastic leukemia and Non-Hodgkin's lymphoma. J Clin Oncol 1986;4:1207.

12. Popat U, Carrum G, Heslop HE. Haemopoietic stem cell transplantation for acute lymphoblastic leukaemia. Cancer Treat Rev 2003;29:3-10.

13. Preisler HD, Anderson K, Rai K, et al. The frequency of long term remission in patients with acute myelogenous leukemia treated with conventional chemotherapy. Br J Hematol 1989;71:189.

14. Rubnitz JE, Pui CH. Recent advances in the treatment and understanding of childhood acute lymphoblastic leukaemia. Cancer Treat Rev 2003;29:31-44.

15. Schiffer CA, Larson RA, Bloonefield C. Cancer and leukemia group B (CALGB) studies in adult acute lymphocytic leukemia. Leukemia 1992;6(Suppl 2):171.

16. Stone RM. The difficult problem of acute myeloid leukemia in the older adult. Cancer J Clin 2002;52:363-71.

17. Wetzler M, Dodge RK, Mrozek K, et al. Prospective karyotype analysis in adult acute lymphoblastic leukemia: the Cancer and Leukemia Group B experience. Blood 1999;93:3983-93.

18. Wolf SN, Herzig RH, Fay JW, et al: High dose cytarabine and daunorubicin as consolidation therapy for acute myeloid leukemia in first remission. Long term follow up and results. J Clin Oncol 1989;7:1260.

APPENDIX 13

International comparison, India and five continents—AAR (ICMR and IARC).

LYMPHOID LEUKEMIA (MALE)

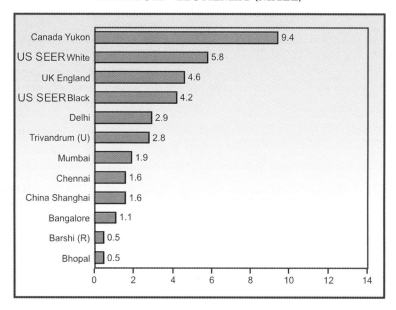

MYELOID LEUKEMIA (MALE)

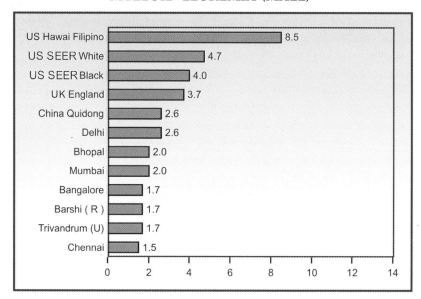

Rate per 100,000

Chronic Leukemias

38

K Pavithran, Paul Puthuran

The chronic leukemias are a group of heterogeneous proliferative disorders derived from lymphoid or myeloid precursor cells that retain some capacity for differentiation to recognizable mature elements. The natural history of the chronic leukemias tends to be longer than that of acute leukemias. Broadly there are two types: chronic myeloid leukemia and chronic lymphatic leukemia.

CHRONIC MYELOID LEUKEMIA

Chronic myeloid leukemia (CML) is a myeloproliferative disorder characterized by clonal expansion of a transformed primitive hematopoietic progenitor cell. It is the commonest type of leukemia seen in India, accounting for 30 percent of all leukemia cases.

EPIDEMIOLOGY

The incidence of CML is 1 to 2 per 100,000 population with a male to female ratio of 1.4 to 2.2:1.0. The median age at presentation is between 45 and 55 years. One-third of the patients are above sixty. CML is uncommon in children and adolescents in whom it accounts for less than 5 percent of the leukemias.

The etiology of CML is unknown. Studies from the atomic bomb survivors in Hiroshima and Nagasaki revealed that there was a higher incidence of leukemia appearing after 3 years and reaching a peak frequency between 5 and 10 years.

PATHOGENESIS

CML is classically associated with the presence of Philadelphia (Ph) chromosome. First described by Nowell and Hungerford in 1960, it results from reciprocal translocation of genetic material (containing proto-oncogene c-abl) from chromosome 9 to chromosome 22 (at the breakpoint of the bcr locus). The resultant chromosome 22 containing bcr-abl fusion gene is called the Ph chromosome. It is the hallmark of CML and is found in 95 percent of patients. The remainder has complex or variant translocations involving additional chromosomes that have the same end result, which is the fusion of the *bcr* gene on chromosome 22 to the *abl* gene on chromosome 9. Ph chromosome is also found in 5 percent of children and 25 percent of adults with acute lymphatic leukemia and in 20 percent of patients with acute myeloid leukemia. Abl proteins are non-receptor tyrosine kinases that have important roles in signal transduction and the regulation of cell growth. Depending on the site of the breakpoint in the *bcr* gene, three main types of bcr-abl genes can be formed. The fusion protein can vary in size from 185 to 230 kd. Nearly all patients with typical chronic phase CML express a 210 kd bcr-abl protein, whereas patients with Ph chromosome-positive acute lymphoblastic leukemia express either a 210 or 185/190 kd bcr-abl protein. In a subset of patients with CML a larger 230 kd bcr-abl fusion protein was found and it was associated with a lower white blood count and slower progression to blast crisis. The 185/190 kd bcr-abl protein has higher specific activity as a tyrosine kinase and is a more potent oncogene than the 210 kd protein, suggesting that the magnitude of the tyrosine kinase signal affects the disease phenotype.

The resultant fusion product bcr/abl, encodes a fusion protein with elevated and dysregulated tyrosine kinase activity. The normal P145^{ABL} exchange between the cytoplasm and the nucleus. The activity and intra-cellular localization of P145 abl is regulated by integrins.

1. Bcr/abl acts as a mitogen by activating Ras (oncogene) signal transduction pathway leading to increase in C-myc and C-fos and subsequent increase in gene transcription and activation of Cyclin-D complexes. Cyclin dependent kinases allow the cells to move from G1 phase of the cell cycle to S phase.

2. Bcr/abl inhibits apoptosis thus leading to accumulation of cells.

3. 4β integrins are important for the adhesion of normal progenitors to the marrow microenvironment; this effects the progenitor proliferation and differentiation. Bcr/abl blocks normal integrin function and thereby reduces adhesion of progenitor cell to stromal elements, so that the stem cells escape physiological inhibitory regulation. During evolution to blast crisis, a range of nonrandom secondary chromosome change occurs, including duplication of the Ph chromosome, trisomy 8 and isochromosome 17q. Molecular abnormalities include abnormalities in p53, RB1, c-MYC, RAS and AML-EVI-I. Alterations in p53 are associated exclusively with myeloid transformation whereas abnormalities of RB1 are associated with lymphoid transformation.

CLINICAL FEATURES

The median age at diagnosis is 50 years, but people of all age groups are affected, including children. The age of presentation is one decade earlier in Indian patients. In some the detection of the disease is accidental. The common symptoms include fatigue, weight loss, weakness, pallor and upper abdominal discomfort due to organomegaly (due to massive spleno-megaly). The most common abnormality on physical examination is splenomegaly, which is present in up to half of patients.

The disease has three stages:
— Initial chronic phase
— An accelerated phase
— Blast crisis.

The natural history of CML is progression from a benign chronic phase to a rapidly fatal blast crisis, generally over 3 to 5 years. The initial chronic phase may last for a few years and the diagnosis is sometimes arrived at on routine examination by detecting abnormal leukocyte count in an otherwise asymptomatic individual. Less commonly the terminal event is characterized by a transformation to myelofibrosis and osteosclerosis leading to marrow failure.

Transformation from the chronic phase to an accelerated phase occurs in about 2-6 years, following which it rapidly progresses to the blastic phase. The chronic phase of CML is usually benign and with appropriate medication the patient can lead a normal life. Once transformation to an accelerated phase occurs, treatment is difficult and therefore carries a grave prognosis.

DIAGNOSIS

The peripheral smear reveals an admixture of mature and immature granulocytes, circulating myeloblasts and prominent basophilia. In the chronic phase 5-15 percent myeloblasts can be seen in the peripheral blood. The accelerated phase is characterized by basophilia (>20%), thrombo-cytopenia, peripheral blood blasts between 15-30 percent or myeloblast plus promyelocytes more than 30 percent and additional cytogenetic abnormalities like double Philadelphia chromosome, trisomy 8 or isochromosome 17. Blast crisis or transformation to acute leukemia is defined as more than 30 percent myeloblasts in the peripheral blood or bone marrow. Leukocyte alkaline phosphatase activity is low or absent in uncomplicated patients. It is elevated in leukemoid reactions and normal or elevated in most other myeloproliferative disorders such as poly-cythemia vera and myelofibrosis.

The bone marrow is hypercellular—primarily because of an expanded, immature (but not blastic) granulocyte compartment—and the numbers of megakaryocytes and red cell precursors are often increased.

Marrow or blood karyotypes demonstrate the Ph chromosome in 90 percent of patients, although it may not be present in every metaphase examined. In up to one-third of those patients who are Ph negative by conventional cytogenetics, molecular studies (PCR and FISH-fluorescent *in situ* hybridisation) will be able to detect bcr-abl rearrangements. The remaining patients are Ph and bcr-abl negative. The prognosis is poor in these patients.

TREATMENT

Over the years the treatment of CML has evolved through many phases-arsenicals, radiotherapy and in the 1950's chemotherapy. In the 1980's interferon (IFN) and bone marrow transplantation were added to the treatment of CML and in 2000's imatinib mesylate.

CONVENTIONAL CHEMOTHERAPY

Busulfan and hydroxyurea control the signs and symptoms of CML but they do not have any effect on the progression of the disease. Busulfan (4-8 mg/day) controls cell count by acting on the stem cells. So it takes about 3 weeks before the count starts falling. Side effects are also many. It is best to avoid in patients who are being prepared for bone marrow transplantation (BMT) as the incidence of veno-occlusive disease is high. Hydroxyurea (1-3 g/day) is useful in bringing down the counts rapidly as it acts on the proliferating cells and is usually well tolerated. Hydroxyurea is preferred to busulfan because of the better toxicity profile and the effect on the prolongation of survival.

INTERFERON (IFN)

Because the majority of patients with CML are not candidates for allogenic transplantation, alternative therapies have been studied extensively. One such therapy is interferon. Both IFN α2a and α2b, are used in the treatment of CML. IFNα acts by
  i. induction of FAS and its ligand on CML progenitors, facilitating cell death of early stem cell population.
 ii. restoring integrin-dependent adhesion and adhesion-mediated proliferation inhibitor signalings.
iii. augmentation of cellular antigen presentation leading to increased recognition of CML cells by cellular immune system. IFNα induces hematologic remission in 70-80 percent of previously untreated patients and major complete remission in between 5-25 percent. IFNα has only modest activity in the late chronic phase (defined as CML diagnosed for more than one year) of CML in patients. Data on the efficacy of interferon is derived from the major randomized controlled clinical trials. The individual patient data from these trials were

pooled and analyzed by the CML trialists collaborative group. The 5-year survival rates for patients on chemotherapy were found to be 42 percent and 57 percent for patients on IFNα. In those who achieve major or complete cytogenetic remission median survival is prolonged by 20 months. IFNα prolongs survival by delaying blast crisis. Only 5 to 10 percent of patients have sustained complete disappearance of the Ph chromosome, and they survive the longest.

THERAPY INITIATION

Initially the tumor load has to be reduced below $20 \times 10^9/L$ with hydroxyurea. Side effects with IFNa are related to tumor load. The CML cells contain high levels of cytokines (leukotriene 4) that may induce an inflammatory response on release following cell kill. Initiate treatment with IFN 3 MU daily and then increase the dose gradually. Tachyphylaxis develops in 1-2 weeks. Initial side effects are mainly flu like symptoms (fever, myalgia, rhinitis). This can be prevented by premeditation—with paracetamol and taking the dose at bedtime. Delayed side effects (persistent fatigue, weight loss, neurotoxicity, insomnia and autoimmune phenomena) are dose limiting and occur in about 10 percent of patients. Tricycle antidepressants are useful for the neurologic side effects. The actual dose of IFNα is important for achieving cytogenetic remission. However, the best dose at which to start IFNa therapy in newly diagnosed patients is still not certain. At present it varies from $3-5 \text{ MU}/m^2$ daily to 3 times per week. Medical research council (MRC) study showed a survival advantage for patients receiving IFNα even without achieving a cytogenetic response.

IFNα WITH CYTOSINE ARABINOSIDE (ARA-C)

The rationale behind the use of combination treatment is that Ara-C selectively suppresses the growth of CML cells compared to that of normal hematopoietic cells *in vitro*. So combination of daily IFNa and low dose Ara-C (10-20 mg/day for 10 days a month) was preferred to IFN alone. The WBC count should be maintained between $3-5 \times 10^9/L$. The dose should be reduced only if the WBC count is less than $2 \times 10^9/L$ or the platelet count is less than $50 \times 10^9/L$ or in the presence of grade 2-4 toxicity.

IMATINIB MESYLATE

Imatinib mesylate is an orally active tyrosine kinase inhibitor. It selectively suppresses the growth of CML cells. The half life of this compound is 13-19 hrs, making single daily doses possible. It is well tolerated. Randomised studies have shown Imatinib mesylate to be much superior to IFNα plus cytarabine in newly diagnosed patients in regard to improved complete cytogenetic response and overall survival. Imatinib therapy may be instituted as soon as the diagnosis of Ph-positive CML has been established, even if the white blood count (WBC) is very high. For patients with elevated WBCs who begin imatinib while on hydroxyurea, the hydroxyurea may need to be continued for 1 to 3 weeks, closely monitoring the WBC. For patients with a WBC over 20,000/mm^3, concomitant therapy with allopurinol is recommended until the WBC is consistently less than 20,000/mm^3. The dose is 400 mg/day for patients in chronic phase and 600 mg/day for patients in accelerated phase or blast crisis. Currently imatinib mesylate is the preferred agent for the treatment of CML in chronic phase. If there is no major cytogenetic response at the end of 6 months they should be offered allogenic BMT or other forms of therapies.

EFFICACY ASSESSMENT

Patients should be monitored with blood counts and cytogenetic studies in all cases and molecular studies especially in the post-transplant setting.

CRITERIA FOR RESPONSE ASSESSMENT

Complete hematologic remission: normalization of WBC count to $<9 \times 10^9$/L with normal differential, normal platelet count and disappearance of all symptoms and signs of disease.

Partial hematologic remission: Normalization of WBC with persistent immature peripheral cells or splenomegaly or thrombocytosis at 50 percent pre-treatment level.

Cytogenetic remission: Complete; no evidence of Ph+ve cells; partial 1-34 percent of metaphases Ph+ve; a minor 35-90 percent metaphases Ph+ve.

MINIMAL RESIDUAL DISEASE (MRD)

MRD means the disease that cannot be detected by conventional investigations. The methods available for detection of MRD are cytogenetics, fluorescence *in situ* hybridisation (FISH), hypermetaphase FISH and reverse transcriptase PCR (RT-PCR). Cytogenetic study has to be done every 3-6 months. The relapse can be molecular relapse (increasing numbers of bcr/abl transcripts while the marrow is still entirely Ph negative), cytogenetic relapse (Ph+ve) or hematological relapse. Molecular relapse is defined as bcr/abl transcripts >1000 transcripts/mg RNA.

ALLOGENIC BONE MARROW TRANSPLANTATION (ALLOBMT)

This is the only curative treatment for CML. Unfortunately it is available to only 15-25 percent of these patients because of advanced age, non-availability of an HLA identical donor and lack of resources. AlloBMT is associated with significant morbidity and mortality. Even today the transplant related mortality is about 30 percent. The antileukemia effect is due to the myeloablative effect of chemotherapy and graft-versus-leukemia (GVL) effect. The GVL effect is mediated through:

1. CD_4+ve T lymphocytes exert cytotoxicity to CML cells and inhibits CFU-GM and BFUE Cytotoxicity is mediated through the Fas/Fas ligand pathway.
2. cytokines and IFN inhibit CML progenitor cells.

The commonly used conditioning regimens are busulfan/cyclophosphamide (BU/CY) and busulfan/total body irradiation (BU/TBI). Of these BU/CY regimen is better tolerated than CY/TBI and has fewer complications. In patients who have an HLA-identical sibling donor and who are below forty, the success rate is about 60 to 70 percent when measured by 10-year survival. Adverse pre-transplant prognostic factors are advanced age (>55 yrs), prior therapy with busulfan, male recipient-female donor, and transplant during the late chronic phase and donor T lymphocyte depletion. Prior therapy with interferon was found to have an adverse effect in earlier studies but a recent study indicated that IFNα does not influence the outcome of allogenic stem cell transplantation unless it is given within 3 months prior to transplantation. Causes of death following allogenic BMT are GVHD, infections, lung toxicity and relapse in decreasing order of frequency. BMT done during the accelerated phase and blast crisis generally does very poorly and has a very high risk of relapse after BMT.

MATCHED UNRELATED OR MISMATCHED RELATED DONORS

Unrelated alloBMTs carry a higher incidence of moderate to severe acute GvHD and a higher morbidity in patients receiving transplants from matched unrelated donors. However, data from the National Marrow Donor Program (NMDP) shows that unrelated alloBMT is effective and feasible. Extended family typing will identify one HLA antigen mismatched related donor in about 5-10 percent of patients; without an HLA identical sibling donor. Transplant with one antigen mismatched related donor results in survival similar to that using matched unrelated donors. Suitable candidates for matched unrelated donor BMT are young patients (<30 yrs) in chronic phase who have a matched donor and have exhibited resistance to IFNα therapy.

RELAPSE FOLLOWING BMT

Treatment options available are supportive care, chemotherapy (hydroxyurea), IFNα, second allogenic BMT and adoptive immunotherapy with donor lymphocyte infusion (DLI). Donor lymphocyte infusion induces remission in more than 70 percent of patients with relapsed CML, following allogenic BMT. Induction of GVL with DLI is very useful for patients who relapse with chronic phase CML. The effectors of this GVL effect are thought to be donor T cells. Treatment related mortality is about 20 percent. The major toxicities are bone marrow aplasia and GVHD.

INVESTIGATIONAL APPROACHES

These include autologous BMT, chemotherapy with newer agents-pegylated IFNα, ocfosfate, homoharringtonine, decitabine, farnesyl transferase inhibitors, inhibition of bcr/abl gene products [antisense oligonucleotide (AS-ODN) therapy] and vaccination strategies.

FURTHER READING

1. Allan NC, Richards SM, Shepherd PCA. UK Medical research council randomised multicenter trial of interferon alpha for chronic myeloid leukemia improved survival irrespective of cytogenetic response. Lancet 1995;345:1392-97.
2. Bernstein R. Cytogenetics of chronic myelogenous leukemia. Semin Hematol 1988;25:20-34.
3. Bhatia R, Forman SJ. Autologous transplantation for the treatment of chronic myelogenous leukemia. Hematol/Oncol Cli North Am 1998;12:151-71.
4. Clift RA, Radich J, Appelbaum FR, et al. Long-term follow-up of a randomized study comparing cyclophosphamide and total body irradiation with busulfan and cyclophosphamide for patients receiving allogenic marrow transplants during chronic phase of chronic myeloid leukemia. Blood 1999;94:3960-62.
5. Faderl S, Talpaz M, Estrov Z, et al. The biology of chronic myeloid leukemia. N Engl J Med 1999;341:164-72.
6. Goldman JM, Druker BJ. Chronic myeloid leukemia: Current treatment options. Blood 2001;98:2039-42.
7. Guilhot F, Chastang C, Michallet M, et al. Interferon α-2b combined with cytarabine versus interferon alone in chronic myelogenous leukemia. French chronic myeloid leukemia study group. New Engl J Med 1997;337:223-29.
8. Hansen JA, Gooley TA, Martin PJ, et al. Bone marrow transplants from unrelated donors for patients with chronic myeloid leukemia. New Engl J Med 1998;338:962-68.
9. Kantarjian HM, O'Brien SM, Anderlini P, Talpaz M. Treatment of chronic myeloid leukemia current status and investigational options. Blood 1996;87:3069-81.
10. Kantarjian HM, Smith TL, O'Brien, et al. Prolonged survival in CML after cytogenetic response to interferon therapy. Ann Intern Med 1995;122:254-61.
11. Mackinnon S. Donor leukocyte infusion. Baillieres Clin Hematol 1997;10:357-67.
12. Pavithran K, Thomas M. Chronic myeloid leukemia. Recent advances. Journal of Internal Medicine of India 2000;3:91-97.
13. Popplewell L, Forman SJ. Allogenic hematopoietic stem cell transplantation for acute leukemia, chronic leukemia and myelodysplasia. Hematol/Oncol Clin Nor Am 1999;13:987-1015.
14. Rushing D, Goldman A, Gibbs G, et al. Hydrea vs Busulfan in the treatment of Chronic myelogenous leukemia. Am J Clin Oncol 1982;5:307-13.
15. Talpaz M, Kantarjan H, Kurzrock R, et al. Interferon α-produces sustained cytogenetic response in chronic myeloid leukemia. Philadelphia chromosome patients. Ann Intern Med 1991;114:532-38.
16. The chronic myeloid leukemia Trialists' Collaborative group. Interferon alpha vs Chemotherapy for CML: A meta-analysis of seven randomised trials. J Natl Cancer Inst 1997;89:1616-20.

17. Tura, on behalf of the Italian Cooperative Study group on CML (ICSG on CML): Cytarabine increases karyotypic response in alpha interferon treated CML patients: Results of a national prospective randomized trial. Blood 1998;92(suppl):317.
18. Verfaillie CM. Biology of chronic myelogenous leukemia. Hematol/Oncol Clin North Am 1998;12:1-29.

CHRONIC LYMPHOCYTIC LEUKEMIA

Chronic lymphocytic leukemia (CLL) is a disease characterized by the accumulation of resting neoplastic B-lymphocytes in bone marrow, lymphoid tissues, and peripheral blood. This accumulation is considered to result from the prolonged survival of B-CLL cells arrested in the G0 stage of the cell cycle. CLL is the most frequent form of leukemia in adults in western countries, accounting for 25 percent of all leukemias, but is rare in India. The etiology of CLL is unknown.

CLINICAL FEATURES

CLL is a disease of the elderly. Median age of patients at diagnosis is 60-65 years. The most common presenting features are lymphadenopathy (20-30%), splenomegaly (15-25%), anemia and/or thrombocytopenia (10-15%). B symptoms (i.e. fever, night sweats, weight loss) are infrequent in CLL patients and should raise the possibility of disease transformation. Physical examination will reveal lymphadenopathy often associated with hepatosplenomegaly. Frequently, the presence of lymphadenopathy or an abnormal CBC performed during a routine medical examination is the only reason to consider the diagnosis. In a small proportion of CLL, usually less than 5 percent of the cases evolve into a more aggressive lymphoproliferative disorder known as Richter's syndrome. It is characterized by increase in lymphadenopathy, fever, abdominal pain, weight loss, progressive anemia and thrombocytopenia with a rapid rise in peripheral lymphocyte count. The lymph node biopsy reveals a large cell or immunoblastic lymphoma. Hypogammaglobulinemia is observed in 20-30 percent of the cases and is considered to be the main cause of recurrent infections. 15-30 percent of the patients develop either a positive Coombs' test or clinically overt autoimmune hemolytic anemia.

DIAGNOSIS

The National Cancer Institute-Sponsored Working Group (NCI-WG) criteria are used for the diagnosis. Lymphocytosis >5 × 10^9/l) =1 B-cell marker (CD19, CD20, CD23) + CD5, atypical cells (e.g. prolymphocytes) <55 percent, bone marrow lymphocytes >30 percent. CLL has to be differentiated from other disorders with increased numbers of circulating atypical lymphoid cells e.g. prolymphocytic leukemia (PLL), hairy cell leukemia (HCL) and from non-Hodgkin's lymphoma (NHL) in a leukemic phase (e.g. mantle cell NHL).

STAGING

Staging system of CLL has been developed to predict prognosis and for the purpose of treatment. Rai and Binet staging systems are the most commonly used staging systems in CLL (Table 38.1).

BINET CLASSIFICATION

Clinical stage A: no anemia or thrombocytopenia and fewer than three areas of lymphoid involvement*.

Clinical stage B: no anemia or thrombocytopenia with three or more areas of lymphoid involvement.

Clinical stage C: anemia and/or thrombocytopenia regardless of the number of areas of lymphoid enlargement.

PROGNOSTIC FACTORS

Unfavorable prognostic factors, independent of clinical stage, are age (>55 years), male sex, black race, and poor performance status. There are no differences between older and younger CLL patients in presenting features, response rates, or duration of response. Laboratory prognostic factors which may predict the outcome include lymphocyte doubling time, with a 12-month cut-off, B2-microglobulin, soluble CD23, and LDH.

TREATMENT

Since no therapy has markedly altered the natural course of the early stage disease many follow the policy of observing the patient for a period

Table 38.1: Rai staging. According to modified Rai staging system the disease is staged as follows		
Rai Stage	*Three-stage system*	*Median survival*
0	Low risk group: lymphocytosis in the blood and bone marrow.	More than 10 years
I/II	Intermediate risk lymphocytosis+ Lymphadenopathy+ Splenomegaly ± hepatomegaly.	7 yrs
IV/V	High risk group: lymphocytosis + anemia thrombocytopenia	2-4 yrs

*Lymphoid areas include cervical, axillary, inguinal, and spleen.

of 3-6 months. The decision for therapeutic intervention is made under the following conditions:

- Progressive symptoms due to the disease
- Worsening of bone marrow failure with anemia and thrombocytopenia
- Massive splenomegaly
- Bulky lymphadenopathy
- Lymphocyte doubling time of less than 6 months

Active drugs include alkylating agents especially chlorambucil, cyclophosphamide and nucleoside analogues, fludarabine, 2-chlorodeoxyadenosine and pentostatin. Chlorambucil is the first line drug either given as a daily oral dose of 4-8 mg/m^2 for 2 weeks or as pulses of 15 to 30 mg/m^2 every 2 to 4 weeks. The cycles are repeated every month. The intermittent therapy seems to be better tolerated. There is no indication for maintenance therapy following maximal response.

Combination therapy is only advocated when the patient fails to respond to single agent chlorambucil therapy. Fludarabine is the most active agent for the treatment of CLL. The recommended dose is 25 mg/m^2/day by intravenous route for 5 consecutive days. This drug is given 40 mg/m^2 orally for 5 days; this is repeated every 4 weeks for 4-6 cycles. Fludarabine induces complete remissions in approximately 30 percent of previously untreated patients, with an overall response rate higher than 70 percent. The major toxicity associated with fludarabine therapy is severe immunosuppression. Currently fludarabine is the preferred agent for initial treatment for most patients with CLL. This is based on the results from four randomized controlled trials which showed significant improvement in DFS.

Combination regimens have not been found to be superior to single-agent therapy for CLL. The most commonly used multiagent regimen are chlorambucil, prednisone (CP) or cyclophosphamide, vincristine, and prednisone (CVP).

Campath I is clearly an extremely effective therapy in refractory chronic lymphocytic leukemia (CLL). Campath is a humanized monoclonal antibody directed against CD52, an antigen expressed on all lymphocytes. Dose is 30 mg by a 2-hour infusion three times a week for up to 12 weeks. Responses occur in approximately one-third of the patients who have been unsuccessful with other treatments, including fludarabine.

BONE MARROW TRANSPLANTATION

When donors are available myeloablative allogenic bone marrow transplant may be considered as a treatment option for young patients but the results are not encouraging. Nonmyeloablative allotransplant may be considered for older patients or young patients with poor prognostic features who are not eligible for myeloablative protocols.

PROLYMPHOCYTIC LEUKEMIA (PLL)

PLL can occur either de novo or, less often, as a transformation from CLL. PLL cells are large, with a round nucleus and a prominent nucleolus. Patients with de novo PLL tend to be older than those with transformed PLL. They are usually symptomatic and generally present with marked splenomegaly and a higher white blood cell count but less lymphadeno-pathy. The clinical course is usually aggressive. PLL patients are usually refractory to therapy. Transient clinical responses lasting six to nine months have been reported with fludarabine and pentostatin (Table 38.2).

HAIRY CELL LEUKEMIA

Hairy cell leukemia is an indolent lymphoproliferative malignancy characterized by infiltration of the bone marrow, liver, spleen, and occasio-nally lymph nodes with a malignant B-cell with hair-like cytoplasmic projections. HCL was initially described by Bouroncle et al in 1958.

Most patients present with splenomegaly and pancytopenia, and occasionally, lymphadenopathy. Splenomegaly can be massive. Infections are common and are attributed to immunosuppression due to neutropenia, monocytopenia, and a deficiency of natural killer cells and dendritic cells. There is an increased incidence of second malignancies. Diagnosis is based on morphology, cytochemistry and flow cytometric analysis. The neoplastic cell in HCL is an abnormal lymphocyte with morphological features that permit distinction from other lymphoproliferative disorders. The cells are small with round, oval and reniform nuclei that have smooth nuclear margins, granular chromatin and a single small nucleolus. The ample cytoplasm is grey-blue and textured with margins that are often frayed with fine projections imparting a 'hairy' appearance. Because HCL induces bone marrow fibrosis, bone marrow aspirates are usually dry tap. Tartrate-resistant acid phosphatase (TRAP) stain is helpful in identifying HCL cells. The immunophenotypic profile of typical HCL is remarkably consistent. Pan B-cell antigens are expressed, with high intensity of CD20 and CD22. In addition, the cells express CD11c, CD25 and CD103. Surface immunoglobulin is usually brightly positive. This

Table 38.2: Differences between de novo PLL and CLL/PLL		
	CLL transformation de novo PLL	*CLL/PLL*
Age	60s	70s
Lymphocytosis	Moderate	Marked
Splenomegaly	Moderate	Marked
Lymphadenopathy	Moderate	Rare
Cytogenetics	Trisomy 12, 11q	t(6;12)
Response to therapy	Fair	Poor

characteristic phenotype will be expressed in greater than 90 percent of cases of HCL.

HCL may be an indolent disorder, and 10 percent of patients may never require treatment. In most patients, however, treatment is eventually warranted because of massive or progressive splenomegaly, worsening blood counts and recurrent infections. Previously splenectomy was the standard treatment for HCL. In most patients, this procedure improves symptoms, however it does not affect the disease itself. Interferon produces responses in 80 percent of patients; however, only 10 percent of these are complete responses and recur when the therapy is discontinued. Currently cladribine is the preferred agent for HCL. Cladribine is administered by a continuous intravenous infusion at a dose of 0.09 mg/kg in 500 ml 0.9 percent sodium chloride daily over a 7-day period. Single course of cladribine produces responses in more than 90 percent of patients, including 65 to 80 percent complete remissions. The majority of hairy cell leukemia patients treated with cladribine enjoy long-lasting complete remissions, and those patients who relapse can frequently be retreated successfully with cladribine. Additional salvage therapies include pentostatin, splenectomy, rituximab (mabthera) and BL-22 immunotoxin.

FURTHER READING

1. Andritsos L, Khoury H. Chronic lymphocytic leukemia. Curr Treat Options Oncol 2002;3:225-31.
2. French Cooperative Group on CLL, Johnson S, Smith AG, et al. Multicentre prospective randomised trial of fludarabine versus cyclophosphamide, doxorubicin, and prednisone (CAP) for treatment of advanced-stage chronic lymphocytic leukemia. Lancet 1996;347:1432.
3. Goodman GR. Cladribine in the treatment of hairy-cell leukaemia. Best Pract Res Clin Haematol 2003;16:101–16.
4. Jacobs P, Wood L. Chronic lymphocytic leukaemia—The haematologic basis for diagnosis and treatment. Hematology 2002;7:33-41.
5. Leporrier S, Chevret B, Cazin B, et al. Randomized comparison of fludarabine, CAP and ChOP, in 695 previously untreated stage B and C chronic lymphocytic leukemia (CLL). Early stopping of the CAP accrual. Blood 1997;90 [Suppl 1]:529(abst 2357).
6. Montserrat E. Current and developing chemotherapy for CLL. Med Oncol 2002;19: Suppl:11-9.
7. Osterborg A, Mellstedt H, Keating M. Clinical effects of alemtuzumab (Campath-1H) in B-cell chronic lymphocytic leukemia. Med Oncol 2002;19: Suppl:21-26.
8. Pangalis GA, Vassilakopoulos TP, Dimopoulou MN, et al. B-chronic lymphocytic leukemia: Practical aspects. Hematol Oncol 2002 ;20:103-46.
9. Rai KR, Peterson B, Elias L, et al. A randomized comparison of fludarabine and chlorambucil for patients with previously untreated chronic lymphocytic leukemia. A CALGB, SWOG, CTC/NCI-C and ECOG inter-group study. Blood 1996;88[Suppl 1]:141(abst 552).
10. Spriano M, Chiurazzi F, Liso V, et al. Multicentre prospective randomized trial of fludarabine versus chlorambucil and prednisone in previously untreated patients with active B-CLL. Proceedings of the Eighth International Workshop on CLL. 1999:52 (abst P086).

Myelodysplastic Syndromes

39

Antony Thomas

Myelodysplastic syndromes (MDS) are a group of acquired disorders involving bone marrow stem cells, and are characterized by irreversible ineffective hematopoiesis. This results in cellular or hypercellular bone marrow with peripheral cytopenia (hence ineffective hematopoiesis) and morphologic abnormalities involving one or more of myeloid cell lineages.

MDS has been introduced as a set of disorders that fall into "no man's land" between normalcy and acute leukemia. The clinical and morphologic distinction of MDS from AML is frequently difficult, and the number of blast cells in the marrow is a requisite for the diagnosis. A blast count of 20 percent or more is seen in AML and 19 percent or less is noted in MDS. MDS predominantly occurs in older adults with a median age of 70 years. MDS that occurs insidiously is termed primary MDS and that occurs as a result of exposure to previous alkylating agent therapy and/or radiotherapy is termed secondary or therapy-related MDS. MDS may remain indolent, or may progress to bone marrow failure or to leukemia.

The commonest clinical features of MDS are anemia, intercurrent infections and bleeding episodes.

CLASSIFICATION OF MYELODYSPLASTIC SYNDROMES

Classifications by FAB group (1976 and 1982) describe MDS with bone marrow blast count as 29 percent or less and also include chronic myelomonocytic leukemia (CMML). However recent studies limits the bone marrow blast cell count to 19 percent and removes CMML from MDS, as it shows both myelodysplastic and myeloproliferative features. CMML is now placed in myelodysplastic/myeloproliferative disorders. The scheme of WHO classification of MDS (2001) is given below:

— Refractory anemia

— Refractory anemia with ringed sideroblasts

— Refractory cytopenia with multilineage dysplasia

— Refractory anemia with excess blasts

— Myelodysplastic syndrome, unclassifiable

— Myelodysplastic syndrome associated with del (5q) chromosome abnormality.

The salient morphologic and prognostic features of MDS are mentioned in Table 39.1. Progression of MDS depends on cytopenia, percent of marrow blasts, and type of cytogenetic abnormalities. Isolated del(5q) is associated with good prognosis, however presence of complex genetic abnormalities or abnormalities of chromosome 7 indicate poor prognosis. Age is also important in predicting prognosis; patients below 60 years has better survival compared to older patients (Table 39.1).

At this point it is important to consider the general differentiating / diagnostic features in myelodysplastic syndromes, acute myeloid leukemia and chronic myeloid leukemia, depicted in Table 39.2.

TREATMENT ASPECT IN MDS

The management of patients with MDS depends on the age, clinical features, and evaluation of the prognostic features and evolution of the disease process. Blood transfusion, intensive chemotherapy and allogenic stem cell transplantation will help in a small percent of cases.

Table 39.1: Morphologic and prognostic features in MDS	
MDS–Low risk group	*Good survival*
Refractory anemia (RA)	Anemia, <5 percent , bone marrow blasts, <15 percent
	Ringed sideroblasts, dysplasia involving erythroid series only.
Refractory anemia with ringed sideroblasts (RARS)	Anemia, <5 percent bone marrow blasts, 15 percent or More ringed sideroblasts, dysplasia involving erythroid series only.
MD-High risk group Refractory cytopenia with multilineage dysplasia (RCMD)-with or without ringed sideroblasts	High chance for evolution to leukemia Peripheral cytopenias (bicytopenia or pancytopenia), <5 percent bone marrow blasts, dysplasia of two or more myeloid cell lines.
Refractory anemia with excess blasts-1 (RAEB-1)	Peripheral cytopenias, 5-9 percent bone marrow blasts, unilineage or multilineage

Table 39.2: Diagnostic features in MDS, AML and CML			
	MDS	*AML*	*CML*
Bone marrow	Cellular/hypercellular Blasts 19% or less Dysplasia of one or more myeloid lineage	Usually hypercellular Blasts 20% or more Dysplasia may be present	Hypercellular Blasts <10% Relatively normal Morphology
Peripheral blood	Cytopenia	Variable count	Increased count
Hematopoiesis	Ineffective	Ineffective or effective	Effective

FURTHER READING

1. Benett JM, Catovsky D, Daniel MJ, et al. Proposals for the classification of myelodysplastic syndromes. British Journal of Haematology 1982; 33:451.
2. Brunning RD, Bennet JM, Flandrin G, Matutes E. Myelodysplastic syndromes: WHO classification of tumors of haematopoietic and lymphoid tissues: Lyon: IARC Press 2001;62-73.
3. Delacretaz F, Schmidt P, Piguet D, et al. Histopathology of myelodysplastic syndromes: The Fab classification (proposals) applied to bone marrow biopsy. Am J Clin Path 1987;87:180-91.
4. Robert WM, Paul MA. Diagnosis, classification and course of myelodysplastic syndromes. Clinics in Laboratory Medicine 1990;10(4):683-706.

Thyroid Carcinoma

40

AR Rama Subbu

EPIDEMIOLOGY

Thyroid carcinoma is not a very common tumor. The incidence varies between 6 and 25 per million populations in various countries.

INCIDENCE

Sex: Male:female ratio is 1: 1.25.

Age: The age incidence is uniformly spread out between 20-70 years. Peak incidence is in the third and fourth decades.

Thyroid carcinoma is usually derived from follicular cells but the uncommon medullary carcinoma arises from parafollicular or C cells.

Four distinct histologic types of follicular cell-derived cancer FCDC are recognized. The substantial majority are papillary; the other histological types are follicular, oxyphilic or Hurthle cell and anaplastic.

CLASSIFICATION

A. American Thyroid Association Classification
   Differentiated Carcinomas:
   a. Papillary
      i. Pure papillary
      ii. Mixed follicular and papillary
   b. Follicular
      i. Invasive
      ii. Non-invasive
   c. Medullary
B. WHO classification
   Differentiated:
   a. Follicular
   b. Papillary
   c. Squamous cell
   d. Medullary

Undifferentiated:
a. Spindle cell
b. Giant cell
c. Small cell

Probably the most useful classification:

Well-differentiated:
a. *Papillary*: Papillary and follicular variant 80-90%
b. *Follicular*: With microscopic and macroscopic invasion, Hurthle 10-20%
c. *Medullary*: Sporadic and familial 6-8%

Undifferentiated:
a. *Anaplastic*: Spindle cell, giant cell, and small cell 2-4%
b. Lymphoma 4-5%
c. Metastatic < 1%

Clinically recognized thyroid carcinomas constitute less than 1 percent of malignant tumors and it is the commonest endocrine malignant condition. It has been noted that this type of cancer is responsible for more deaths than all other endocrine cancers combined. Slow growth, delayed symptoms, low morbidity and mortality generally characterize thyroid cancers. At initial assessment, most patients with thyroid cancer have a palpable neck mass, which may represent either the primary intrathyroidal tumor or metastatic regional lymphadenopathy.

ETIOLOGIC FACTORS

Prolonged TSH stimulus:
a. Thyroid cancer is experimentally produced in animals by severe iodine restriction, goitrogens (such as cabbage and rapeseed), subtotal gland resection, and RAI singly or in various combinations.
b. There are case reports of thyroid cancer developing in the untreated hyperplastic glands of congenital cretins.

PATHOGENESIS

1. *Oncogenes* Rearrangements of the tyrosine kinase domains of the RET and TRK genes with the amino terminal sequence of an unlinked gene are found in some papillary carcinomas. RET rearrangements are found in 3 to 33 percent of the papillary carcinomas unassociated with irradiation and in 60 to 80 percent of those occurring after radiation.
2. *Radiation* External radiation administered in childhood for benign conditions of the head and neck regions increases the risk for papillary carcinoma.

Latency period is at least 5 years and the risk is maximal at about 20 years and then decreases gradually. High incidence of malignancy is reported at a dose of 200 to 1000 rads and at greater than 2000 rads, the risk is low. The risk is not increased in patients given Iodine[131] for diagnostic or therapeutic purposes. A significant number of adults exposed to the intensive radiation of the Hiroshima explosion have developed thyroid cancer.

3. Less well-defined etiologic factors:
   a. The relationship of longstanding non-toxic colloid goiter to papillary and anaplastic carcinoma.
   b. The relationship of follicular adenoma as a pre-malignant lesion to follicular carcinoma.
   c. The role of genetics and neural crest analogue to medullary carcinoma.

PATHOLOGY

Thyroid tumor usually presents as an asymptomatic thyroid nodule.

It can also present as a dominant nodule in a multinodular goiter. Bilateral discrete nodules suggest familial medullary thyroid carcinoma. Anaplastic carcinoma may present as a fixed or rapidly enlarging tumor with symptoms of hoarseness, dysphagia, stridor, or neck pain.15-20 percent of all solitary thyroid nodules are malignant.

6-10 percent of all multi-nodular goiters (non-toxic) are malignant.

0.01- 0.10 percent of all thyrotoxic glands are malignant.

Metastatic disease: It occurs in 4 percent of all papillary carcinomas. Pregnancy has no apparent effect on the course of thyroid cancer.

Blood spread is common in follicular carcinomas (16%-33%) but may occur with any variety of tumor. Metastases are commonest in the lungs but also are seen in bone, contralateral thyroid lobe and adjacent cervical structures. The thyroid carcinoma has an unusual predilection to bones and occurs in 8 percent of cases. The lymphatic spread is in the first instance to the jugular group of deep cervical nodes.

PATHOLOGY OF THYROID CANCER

Well differentiated
— Papillary
— Follicular
Moderately differentiated
— Papillary variants
— Tall cell
— Columnar
— Diffuse sclerosis
Hurthle cell carcinoma
— Poorly differentiated/undifferentiated
Anaplastic thyroid carcinoma
Medullary thyroid carcinoma

Lymphoma

Sarcoma and others

Diagnostic work-up

History and physical examination:

History: 20 percent have a family history of goiter.

Women develop nodules more frequently than men.

Risk of malignancy:

— Men have a higher risk of malignancy.

— Overall risk for malignancy is 5 to 10 percent.

— Risk with history of thyroid radiation is 35 percent.

High risk lesions:

— Solitary nodule/dominant nodule/change in nodule.

— Rapid increase in size, pain and pressure on trachea causing hoarseness, dyspnea, dysphagia and in a few cases Horner's syndrome may be present.

DIAGNOSTIC PROCEDURES

Fine Needle Aspiration Cytology (FNAC)

Fine needle aspiration cytology is the best method available to differentiate between benign and malignant nodules. It is often the first and the only test performed to decide whether the patient is a candidate for surgical or nonsurgical treatment. Accuracy of cytologic diagnosis from FNAC is between 70-97 percent. Any thyroid nodule more than 1.5 cm should be evaluated with an FNAC. Needle aspiration of fluid-filled cyst may be useful and avoids unnecessary surgery.

When there is a high index of suspicion for thyroid malignancy based on history or physical examination, surgical exploration is undertaken without prior FNAC, as in the following situations:

1. Presence of hard, irregular or fixed thyroid mass:
2. Recurrent laryngeal nerve paralysis
3. Thyroid mass with history of prior radiation to the head and neck
4. Enlarged lateral cervical lymph nodes
5. Patients under 20 or over 70 years of age

When the thyroid stimulating hormone (TSH) assay is low (hyperthyroidism) or high (hypothyroidism) and the findings are confirmed by abnormal thyroxine and triiodothyronine levels, FNAC need not be performed. When the TSH is high, antibodies may be tested for and if the levels are elevated, the diagnosis is probably Hashimoto's thyroiditis and surgery is not indicated.

Radioactive Iodine (RAI ^{131}) Scintiscan

The most commonly used isotopes for thyroid imaging are technetium (99 m Tc) and radioiodine (I^{123}, I^{131}). Most thyroid cancers concentrate

RAI poorly; therefore, presenting a "cold" area in contrast to the normal surrounding gland. Thus cold nodules are suspicious for cancer, however they are also seen in colloid nodules, cysts, calcifications, hemorrhages and benign adenomas. Of the cold nodules, 10 to 15 percent are malignant. It is not necessary to operate on all cold nodules. Hot nodules essentially exclude malignancy.

Many nodules discovered on palpation or visualized on ultrasound are not delineated on isotope scanning; these nodules concentrate tracer in a manner similar to that of normal tissue and are designated as "warm" nodules and are rarely malignant; they are not operated upon. They will often shrink or disappear with thyroid hormone administration. Iridium[111] octreotide scintigraphy is useful in the detection of medullary carcinoma with sensitivity of around 70 percent.

In patients who have been operated upon for medullary thyroid cancer and who have persistent or recurrent calcitonin elevation, Iridium[111] octreotide may indicate the location of recurrence. Metastatic foci of tumor are not demonstrable by other imaging modalities.

Ultrasonography of thyroid gland: Ultrasound will detect nodules as small as 2-3 mm and will distinguish solid masses from cysts. Malignant changes may be suspected if the margins of the nodule are irregular. Ultrasound may be used to guide FNAC and to diagnose the multinodular goiter and to identify the dominant lesion. It is most useful in the follow up of non-operated nodules and to determine whether the nodule is decreasing or increasing in size while being observed or treated with thyroid hormone. It is also useful in the follow-up of patients treated for thyroid carcinoma to detect small or inaccessible nodules that may represent recurrence of the thyroid cancer.

METASTATIC SURVEY

The presence of osteolytic bone lesions, mediastinal node enlargements or soft metastatic infiltrates in the lung of a patient with a solitary thyroid nodule or multinodular goiter should lead one to suspect thyroid carcinoma. In the rare instances when these metastases are functioning, the localization with RAI scanning technique is diagnostic.

RADIOLOGICAL EXAMINATION OF NECK

Barium swallow showing displacement and fixation of the trachea by a goiter may add to one's suspicion of malignancy. Tracheal stenosis is readily seen in regular chest film. Uniform hazy calcifications in streaked or nebular formation are seen in soft tissue X-rays in the papillary and follicular carcinomas.

INDIRECT LARYNGOSCOPY

This should be performed routinely.

Unilateral or bilateral vocal cord paralysis is often an ominous sign of invasive thyroid carcinoma.

TRANSILLUMINATION

This may be positive in a simple fluid filled colloid cyst if it is very superficial.

LABORATORY STUDIES

TSH assay should be done in all patients with thyroid nodules to detect hyper-or hypothyroidism. In nodular thyroid masses, especially those with hypothyroidism, levels of serum antibodies are helpful to diagnose Hashimoto's thyroiditis. Serum thyroglobulin level is not useful in the evaluation of a thyroid nodule but is of great value in the follow up of thyroid cancer patients who are treated with thyroidectomy. In patients with the family history of medullary cancer, calcitonin levels and genetic testing for the RET oncogene are of value in the diagnosis of MEN-2 syndrome. If FNAC cytology reveals medullary carcinoma, calcitonin levels should be obtained preoperatively. Serial calcitonin levels should be obtained postoperatively in all patients operated upon for medullary carcinoma. Rare cases of hyperthyroidism with carcinoma *in situ* and functioning follicular carcinoma with extensive metastases will elevate all the thyroid function tests. Carcino embryonic antigen or CEA is elevated in medullry and anaplastic thyroid carcinoma. DNA analysis of peripheral blood is a highly reliable method for identifying the presence of RET mutation.

Thyroid angiography: This technique is cumbersome and requires a skilled team.

TNM classification of malignant tumors of the thyroid (Table 40.1):

Anatomic staging: Scheme for categorizing patients with well-differentiated thyroid cancer; prognostic risk categories.

AMES: Age, metastases, extent of primary cancer, tumor size (Table 40.2).
Low risk/High risk
Age: Males <40 years, females < 50 yrs/males >40 yrs, females>50 yrs
Metastases: no distant metastases/distant metastases.
Extent: Intrathyroidal papillary or follicular with minor capsular invasion/extrathyroidal papillary or follicular with major invasion.
Size: < 5 cm/> 5 cm.

Low-risk patients are (1) any low-risk age group without metastases or (2) high-risk age group without metastases and with low-risk extent and size.

High-risk patients are (1) any patient with metastases or (2) high-risk age group with either high-risk extent or size.
DAMES: AMES system modified by tumor cell DNA content measured by flow-cytometry.

Table 40.1: Primary tumor (T stage)

Tx	—	Tumor cannot be assessed
T0	—	No clinical evidence of tumor
T1	—	Tumor < 1 cm
T2	—	Tumor > 1 cm and < 4 cm
T3	—	Tumor > 4 cm
T4	—	Tumor extending beyond thyroid capsule

Regional lymph nodes (N Stage)

N0	—	No palpable nodes
N1	—	Regional nodal metastases
N1a	—	Ipsilateral nodes
N1b	—	Contralateral, bilateral, or mediastinal nodes

Distant metastases (M stage)

Mx	—	Metastases cannot be assessed
M0	—	No evidence of distant metastases
M1	—	Distant metastases present

Table 40.2: Clinical staging of thyroid cancer

Medullary:

Stage I	T1	N0	M0
Stage II	T2	N0	M0
Stage III	Any T	N1	M0
Stage IV	Any T	Any N	M1

Undifferentiated: All cases stage IV

Papillary or follicular:

	Cases < 45 years of age			Cases >45 years of age.		
Stage I	Any T	Any N	M0	T1	N0	M0
Stage II	Any T	Any N	M1	T2	N0	M0
Stage III				T3,T4	N0	M0
Stage IV				Any T	Any N	M1

Low risk AMES + euploid = low risk.

High risk AMES + aneuploidy = high risk.

Age: age, tumor grade, tumor extent, tumor size.

Prognostic Score (PS) = 0.05 × age in years (except patients < 40 yrs = 0) +1 (grade 2) or +3 (grade 3 or 4), + 1 (if extrathyroidal) or + 3 (if distant metastases),+ 0.2 × tumor size in cm (maximum diameter)

PS range: 0-11.65, median 2.6.

Risk categories: 0-3.99, 4-4.99, 5-5.99, >6.

MACIS: metastasis, age, completeness of resection, invasion, size.

PS= 3.1(age < 39 yrs) or 0.08 × age (if age >40), + 0.3 × tumor size in cm, +1 (if incompletely resected) +1 (if locally invasive) + 3 (if distant metastases).

PS risk categories: 0-5.99,6-6.99, 7-7.99, >8

Thyroid carcinoma may spread in the following ways:
a. Intraglandular:
   1. Direct extension through true or pseudo-capsule to invade normal parenchyma.
   2. Multifocal seeding progressing to bilateral involvement via thyroidal lymphatics.
b. Extraglandular:
   1. Direct invasion of lobe capsule and isthmus into neighbouring muscle, connective tissue, nerves or trachea.
   2. Lymphatic spread to regional, mediastinal or more distant nodes.
   3. Blood vessel invasion and metastases to distant sites.

PATHOLOGIC STAGING

a. Histologic classification: Papillary carcinoma of the thyroid is:
   1. Papillary
   2. Papillary with follicular elements
b. Follicular or Hurthle cell carcinoma of the thyroid is:
   1. Type 1 follicular variant of papillary carcinoma
   2. Type 2 localized follicular carcinoma
   3. Type 3 invasive follicular carcinoma.
c. Medullary carcinoma
d. Anaplastic carcinoma.

GRADING

Grade I: Encapsulated circumscribed neoplasms with only minimal invasion of adjacent gland or vessels.

Grade II: More extensive infiltration of surrounding gland, less differentiated, greater cellular pleomorphism and mitosis.

Grade III: Extensive growth in gland often with extraglandular invasion, dedifferentiated, pleomorphic with multinucleated cells and are very mitotic.

PATHOLOGIC BEHAVIOR

Carcinoma thyroid is usually derived from follicular cells but the uncommon medullary carcinoma arises from the parafollicular or C- cells. Four distinct histologic types of FCDC -Follicular cell-derived cancers are recognized.

WELL-DIFFERENTIATED THYROID CARCINOMA

Papillary Carcinoma

This is the most common type of thyroid carcinoma. Since iodine supplementation started in endemic areas, the incidence of papillary carcinoma has increased compared with that of follicular thyroid carcinoma. More than 50 percent of all adult and 70 percent of all childhood thyroid cancers are papillary carcinomas.

Papillary carcinoma is one of the least aggressive human cancers and has the best prognosis. It invades the lymphatics and causes metastatic spread to the regional lymph nodes and microscopic metastatic lesions in the gland. Some rare variants of papillary carcinoma are more aggressive:

1. Tall-cell variant
2. Columnar variant
3. Diffuse sclerosis variant

Most papillary tumors contain a mixture of papillary and colloid filled follicles and in some, the follicular structure predominates. Histologically the tumor shows papillary projections with characteristic pale, empty nuclei (Orphan Annie-eyed nuclei).

Colloid goiter associated with papillary cancer has a dense appearance and is referred to as "bubble gum" colloid. Psammoma bodies may also be present. Multiple foci may occur in the same lobe as the primary tumor or less commonly in both lobes. They may be due to lymphatic spread in the rich intrathyroidal lymph plexus or to multicentric growth.

Spread to the lymph nodes is common but blood-borne metastases are unusual unless the tumor is extrathyroidal. The term extrathyroidal indicates that the primary tumor has infiltrated through the capsule of the thyroid gland.

Occult Carcinoma

Papillary carcinoma may present as an enlarged lymph node in the jugular chain with no palpable abnormality of thyroid. The primary tumor may be no more than a few millimeters in size and is termed 'occult' (The term is now applied to all papillary carcinomas less than 1.5 cm in diameter).

Follicular or Hurthle Cell Carcinoma

Follicular carcinoma constitutes about 30 percent of all thyroid cancer. Since the initiation of Iodine-prophylaxis, follicular carcinoma is diagnosed less frequently. Metastatic spread is through vascular invasion rather than lymphatic spread and lymph node involvement is very rare. Malignant cells readily invade blood vessels and cause distant metastases especially to bone. One variety of follicular cancer is more aggressive, often bilateral, tends to recur and has a grave prognosis.

In contrast to papillary thyroid cancer, neck nodal metastases are the exception in FTC, but they are somewhat more commonly seen in those patients with the oxyphilic or Hurthle cell variant of FTC. Hurthle cell tumors are a variant of follicular neoplasm in which oxyphil (Hurthle, Askanazy) cells predominate histologically. It is doubtful if Hurthle cell neoplasms are ever benign and they may be associated with a poorer prognosis.

Medullary Thyroid Carcinoma (MTC)

MTC may be sporadic, familial or hereditary. Traditionally more than 70 percent MTC, are thought to be sporadic and these tumors tend to be unicentric and confined to one lobe. In contrast, the familial MTC occurring in the kindred with multiple endocrine neoplasia type II A and B tends to be bilateral and multicentric. Incidence of MTC is 5-9 percent. It arises from Parafollicular 'C' cells which produce calcitonin (which lowers serum calcium). Serum calcitonin is one of the most sensitive tumor markers in oncology. Because MTC can occur in association with familial cancer syndromes (MEN 2A, MEN 2B and familial MTC), members of the family should be screened for the presence of Ret mutations if one among them has MTC of any variety. Surgical treatment at a younger age, before the development of metastases, can be performed safely and will likely cure patients of an otherwise incurable disease. Bony metastases, particularly at the base of the skull have a bad prognosis and can be detected only by Technetium 99 scan. Patients with MTC should also be screened for pheochromocytoma because this tumor occurs in approximately 40 percent of MEN 2 patients. MTC appears as solid and anaplastic, but is actually somewhat indolent.

Nodal involvement is common, as are metastases. Its hallmark is its association with extensive amyloid deposits throughout the tumor.

It appears often in association with genetic disorders of neural crest analouge, i.e. pheochromocytoma, neurofibromatosis. At times, the tumor may elaborate ACTH and cause Cushing's syndrome. Diarrhea is a feature in 30 percent of cases and may be due to 5-hydroxytryptamine or prostaglandins produced by the tumor cells. MTC may occur in combination with adrenal pheochromocytoma and hyperparathyroidism (usually due to hyperplasia) in the syndrome MEN 2A.

When the familial form is associated with prominent mucosal neuromas involving the lips, tongue and inner aspect of the eyelids with occasionally a Marfanoid habitus, the syndrome is referred to as MEN 2B. Involvement of lymph nodes occurs in 50-60 percent of cases of MTC and blood-borne metastases are common. Tumors are not hormone dependent and do not take up Radioiodine. The course of the tumor is unpredictable, in general, life expectancy is good.

The treatment for MTC is total thyroidectomy and paratracheal lymph node resection. In 1993, MEN 2A and familial MTC were shown to be associated with mutations in exon 10 or 11 of the Ret protooncogene located on chromosome 10. The gene mutation can be detected by the use of polymerase chain reaction (PCR) followed by restriction analysis.

The immediate family members of all patients with MTC should be evaluated for a possible gene mutation. This is particularly important in case of MEN 2B syndrome where the MTC tends to be aggressive and may appear by two years of age. Total thyroidectomy is recommended as soon as the syndrome is recognized, preferably before the age of two. The MTC in MEN 2A syndrome is less aggressive and tends to appear after the age of 12.There is less urgency to proceed with the total thyroidectomy, however, it should be accomplished by the age of six.

Anaplastic Carcinoma

This occurs mainly in elderly women. It is a very aggressive tumor and appears as small, giant or spindle cell cancers, which grow rapidly, produce several local symptoms and signs by extensive invasion, metastasize widely and unless diagnosed at the early nodular stage, are fatal within 1-2 years. The tumor presents with rapidly growing mass, with invasion of trachea, larynx (stridor), recurrent laryngeal nerve (hoarseness) and esophagus (dysphagia). Most patients die of aggressive locoregional disease with upper airway obstruction or respiratory failure. An attempt at curative resection is only justified if there is no infiltration through the thyroid capsule and no evidence of metastases.

Rare Cancers: Malignant Lymphoma

In the past many malignant lymphomas were diagnosed as small round cell anaplastic carcinomas. Although the diagnosis may be made or suspected on FNAC, sufficient material is seldom available for immuno-cytochemical classification. Large needle (tru-cut) or open biopsy is usually necessary. In patients with tracheal compression, isthmusectomy is the most appropriate form of biopsy. Rarely the tumor is part of widespread malignant lymphoma disease, and the prognosis in these cases is poor.

Metastatic Thyroid Cancer

It does not always follow the histologic pattern of the primary thyroid tumor. Thus one may find a bone metastasis with a differentiated follicular pattern from a pure papillary primary carcinoma, etc. Cancer metastatic to the thyroid is a rare thyroid lesion. Thyroid resection is rarely performed for a secondary malignant lesion. Greater attention is concentrated on treating the primary tumor, usually by systemic chemotherapy or palliative irradiation.

Principles of treatment of well-differentiated thyroid carcinoma:
1. Surgery
2. Iodine[131]
3. Chemotherapy
4. External radiation
5. Thyroxine treatment (thyroid-suppressive)

Early diagnosis and extirpation are essential before intraglandular or extraglandular invasion occurs or metastases develop in distant sites. Because recurrence, morbidity and death may be long delayed, all forms of treatment are difficult to evaluate. Host factors and biological behavior of the tumor may be more important than the procedures.

SURGERY: EXTENT OF THYROIDECTOMY

Determining the extent of thyroidectomy in the management of differentiated thyroid cancer is controversial. The principal reason for this controversy is the fact that the majority of patients with differentiated thyroid cancer do extremely well; patients survive for decades. If the lesion is <1.5 cm, lobectomy is appropriate.

1. *For papillary cancer*
   Total thyroidectomy and modified node resection on homolateral side. Bilateral node resection. In 20 percent of cases, the nodes are positive is the contralateral lobe.
2. *For follicular cancer*
   Type I and II lobectomy and isthmectomy with local node excision when indicated. Type III-as above for papillary cancer.
3. *For medullary cancer*
   Total thyroidectomy and local node excision.
4. *For anaplastic cancer*
   Total thyroidectomy only in rare situation when process is localized. Most patients are inoperable and require tracheotomy when the airway is involved.

INDICATIONS FOR TOTAL THYROIDECTOMY

1. High risk patients with high-risk tumor.
2. Young patients with bulky nodal disease requiring RAI ablation.
3. Patients with
   — Gross disease in both lobes of the thyroid.
   — Gross extrathyroidal tumor requiring RAI ablation.
   — Preoperative diagnosis of poorly differentiated tumor.
   — Medullary thyroid carcinoma.
   — Thyroid cancer and a history of radiation.
   — Operable anaplastic thyroid carcinoma.
   — Distant metastasis requiring RAI ablation.

The optimal treatment for nearly all cases of thyroid cancer is total thyroidectomy with resection of paratracheal lymph nodes. Papillary carcinoma is frequently multicentric and bilateral. Examination of grossly uninvolved lobes shows that 25-30 percent of them contains additional foci of carcinoma. Recurrence rate of 7-20 percent has been reported following less than total thyroidectomy. For small occult papillary or follicular cancers found incidentally during operations for Graves' disease or multinodular goiter, sub-total thyroidectomy is adequate treatment.

Anaplastic or giant-cell thyroid carcinoma is usually far advanced when first seen; the prognosis following thyroidectomy is poor; optimal treatment is combined radiation and chemotherapy. If a diagnosis of lymphoma is made, treatment is non-surgical; radiation and/or chemotherapy is indicated. About 90 percent of patients with well- differentiated carcinoma of the thyroid can be classified as low risk and about 95 percent of these patients who have had a thyroid lobectomy or a sub-total thyroidectomy have been found to be disease-free at 20 years. The fact that total thyroidectomy can be accomplished with minimal morbidity is not an indication to perform the operation on a patient who will not benefit from the procedure.

PARATHYROIDS

To avoid the problem of permanent hypoparathyroidism following a total thyroidectomy, routine removal and transplantation of a normal parathyroid gland into ipsilateral sternomastoid muscle has been recommended. If the main arterial blood supply to a parathyroid is ligated or divided, and the parathyroid is left attached to a thyroid remnant, sufficient collateral blood supply to the parathyroid may preserve its function.

LARYNGEAL NERVES

It is essential that the laryngeal nerves be protected from injury during the performance of a thyroidectomy. Injury to recurrent laryngeal nerve is best avoided by gentle exposure and visualization of the RLN through its course in the operative field. This approach is essential in preoperative thyroid surgery where the recurrent nerves are at high risk. Invasion of the RLN by cancer does not always result in vocal cord paralysis. If one cord is paralyzed changes in the voice may be subtle or absent. It is mandatory to visualize the vocal cords by indirect or fiberoptic laryngoscopy preoperatively and postoperatively. In patients with papillary carcinoma, if the RLN is adherent to the cancer or to paratracheal lymph nodes, every effort should be made to preserve part or all of the RLN even if one must shave it off the tumor. If the nerve is encased in the tumor and a portion of the RLN is sacrificed, nerve reanastomosis or insertion of a nerve graft should be done—the success rate is about 50 percent. Injury or involvement of both RLN by cancer will result in bilateral vocal cord paralysis; the cords may be in the adductor position with marked narrowing of the glottis, requiring tracheostomy or they may be in the cadaveric position (midway between adduction and abduction) in which case tracheostomy may be deferred.

EXTRATHYROIDAL EXTENSION OF THYROID CARCINOMA

Well-differentiated thyroid carcinoma is slow growing and if untreated, eventually invades adjacent tissues. The most frequently involved structure is the sternothyroid muscle, which is often resected with the thyroid gland with no significant effect on survival. If the tumor can be completely resected portions of trachea, esophageal wall and/or laryngeal cartilage involved by cancer should be removed with the thyroid gland. Portions of trachea up to 5-6 tracheal rings can be resected with immediate reconstruction. In case the muscular layer of esophagus is invaded, excision without entering the mucosa can often be performed. Attempts to treat small areas of carcinoma, left behind after surgery by external radiation or with radioactive iodine have not often been successful.

LYMPH NODE INVOLVEMENT

Papillary carcinoma of thyroid metastasizes to lymph nodes early, especially in children and young adults. When pre- and para-tracheal nodes are encountered during thyroidectomy they are resected with the thyroid gland. Removal of the enlarged node or nodes "cherry picking" is not adequate since other nodes will usually appear later. The optimal treatment for metastatic lymph nodes in the lateral neck is a modified radical neck dissection.

THYROID HORMONE—THERAPY IN THYROID CARCINOMA

Most or all patients who have had differentiated thyroid cancer should receive thyroid hormone. The dosage of thyroid hormone to be administered should not only be sufficient to prevent hypothyroidism but a dose high enough to lower serum TSH levels. The ideal dosage is that which results in normal serum thyroxine levels and low serum levels of TSH as determined by sensitive radio-immuno assay measurement. TSH suppression is not only warranted in patients with thyroid carcinoma but also in patients with recurrent or metastatic disease.

RADIOIODINE IN THE MANAGEMENT OF THYROID CARCINOMA

The second most frequently used postoperative adjuvant therapy for patients with FCDC is remnant ablation with radioiodine.

Areas of differentiated thyroid carcinoma often take up radioactive iodine offering the opportunity to detect such foci and in many cases to treat and destroy them. In order for radioactive iodine to be effective, all the normal thyroid tissue must be removed or ablated since normal thyroid tissue has a much greater avidity for radioiodine than differentiated thyroid cancer. For this reason, a total thyroidectomy is the optimal treatment of thyroid carcinoma. All the patients with differentiated thyroid cancer following total thyroidectomy are evaluated at regular intervals of 3 months for the first year, and six months in the second year. No thyroid hormone replacement is given for a period of 3 to 4 weeks at which time serum TSH and serum thyroglobulin levels are obtained. If the TSH level is 30 u/ml or higher, 2.5 mCi of I^{131} is administered; radioiodine uptake in the neck is measured in 24-48 hours and whole body scans are obtained usually after 48-72 hours. When the uptake is below 1 percent and there are no foci seen in the scan, the patient is started on thyroid hormone replacement. Levothyroxine (T4) is given in 100-150 ug/day dosage and thyroid function tests performed after 3-4 weeks; the dose is adjusted to maintain normal T4 levels with suppressed TSH. If foci of uptake in the thyroid bed are found with the uptake of 1 percent or lower and a negative body scans, an outpatient dose of radioiodine 29 millicuries is given. If the uptake is above 1 percent or metastatic foci are found in the lateral neck, lungs or bone, a larger therapeutic dose, 100-300 millicuries is administered; this requires isolation in a hospital for 2-3 days.

Not all foci of differentiated thyroid cancer take up radioactive iodine. The uptake is generally better in younger patients and may be poor or absent in poorly differentiated tumors.

Metastases from Hurthle cell carcinoma occasionally pick up radioiodine after resection of the entire thyroid gland. Sestamibi 99mTc concentrates well in Hurthle cell tumors and may be the agent of choice for imaging patients suspected of metastasis from Hurthle cell carcinoma.

EXTERNAL IRRADIATION

External irradiation is rarely used as adjunctive therapy in the initial management of patients with follicular cell derived cancer (FCDC). It may be beneficial, however, in patients with poorly differentiated (higher histologic grade) tumors that do not concentrate RAI. It also may be considered in the postoperative management of patients with FCDC who have gross evidence of local invasion and who are presumed to have microscopic residual disease after primary surgical treatment. A similar argument can be made for patients with medullary thyroid cancer (MTC) who have locally invasive disease. No convincing efficacy has been found, however, in irradiating the neck of patients with MTC who have post-operative hypercalcitoninemia. They may not give imaging or clinical evidence of persistent disease. The situation differs considerably with respect to less well-differentiated thyroid malignant lesions. Radiation therapy is almost routinely performed after biopsy or subtotal tumor resection for anaplastic thyroid cancers. Care is taken to subject the involved field for radiation after chemotherapy. Similarly, in patients with primary non-Hodgkins lymphoma of the thyroid, it is routinely used. Treat the thyroid after accurate disease staging.

CHEMOTHERAPY

In patients with differentiated FCDC, chemotherapy is restricted to those tumors that are surgically unresectable, are unresponsive to RAI, have been treated with, or are not amenable to external irradiation. In this unusual circumstance, combination chemotherapy does not seem to be clearly superior to doxorubicin monotherapy. Neither program, unfortunately, has resulted in frequent examples of tumor regression. Adjuvant chemotherapy has rarely been administered in the primary management of MTC and is probably not justified. In contrast, in disseminated thyroid lymphoma, the treatment of choice after initial surgical intervention would routinely include an anthracycline-based chemotherapy, usually a CHOP regimen-cyclophosphamide, hydroxydaunomycin (doxorubicin), oncovin (vincristine), and prednisone. In patients with anaplastic thyroid cancer, survival has not been altered by surgical treatment, radiation therapy or chemotherapy alone.

LONG TERM FOLLOW-UP

Tumor Markers

After the elimination of thyroid tissue by total thyroidectomy, or by combined surgical treatment and RAI, increased thyroglobulin (Tg) levels may be useful indicators of the presence of metastatic FCDC, whereas subnormal or undetectable Tg levels fairly reliably indicate the absence of metastatic involvement. For patients with MTC, the classic tumor marker, used both in diagnosis and follow-up, has been the immunoreactive calcitonin (IRC) level basal and stimulated. A second major tumor marker for MTC is Carrion embryonic antigen (CEA). In general the CEA level is higher in more malignant MTC, whereas the IRC level is higher in the more differentiated MTC.

Imaging Studies

Whole body scans are performed within 6-8 weeks after an attempted total thyroidectomy or 3-6 months after RRA. In those patients with FCDC, negative whole body scans but elevated serum Tg levels or a strong clinical suggestion of a recurrence, additional imaging is necessary. Pulmonary metastatic lesions are common in this circumstance and occasionally they may be visible on a chest roentgenogram. More often the metastatic growths are micronodular and may be visualized only by high-resolution computed tomographic scanning. Similarly occult non-iodophilic osseous metastatic lesions can often be localized by isotope bone scanning.

Imaging with radioiodine II31TBS (Total body scanning) may identify residual tumor as well as metastatic lesions in the other parts of the body.

PERSISTENT OR RECURRENT DISEASE

SECONDARY SURGICAL INTERVENTION

If clinically significant, often palpable, disease recurs because of either FCDC or MTC in the neck (bed or nodes); it should be considered for surgical excision along with excision of any infiltrated local tissues. It should include section of airway. If in FCDC, bulky metastatic lesions should develop in the mediastinum and do not actively take up I^{131} they should also be considered for surgical intervention. Occasionally thoracotomy may be considered in a patient with metastatic FCDC localized to a focal area of the lung. Lesions in long bones may sometimes be excised especially when a risk of pathologic fracture exists. Neurosurgical intervention may be necessary, as spinal stabilization. If there is a danger of cord compression due to vertebral metastasis, or an apparently solitary cerebral tumor metastatic from FCDC surgical resection could be considered in selected cases.

RADIOACTIVE IODINE

If metastatic disease is discovered on a whole body scan with I^{131} in a patient with FCDC, RAI therapy would generally be administered. Before treatment with $I^{131,}$ a 10-day low iodine diet may enhance the uptake of the isotope by iodine-concentrating cells. A post-treatment whole body scan should be performed 4 to 10 days after RAI therapy to document the extent of I^{131} uptake by the FCDC.

RADIATION THERAPY

If surgical removal of local neck recurrence of FCDC or MTC is deemed either too difficult or unacceptable to the patient, radiation therapy may provide alleviation in a high percentage of cases.

CHEMOTHERAPY

Various combinations of chemotherapy for recurrent progressive MTC, such as dacarbazine alone or with combination with 5-fluorouracil, streptozocin, cyclophosphamide or vincristine. Survival for more than 2 years after initiation of chemotherapy is however rare.

FUTURE OPTIONS

Several evidence based reviews of management of thyroid cancer are available which discuss various controversial aspects of treatment. The balance of evidence favors an approach in which most patients with differentiated thyroid cancer will have FNAC for diagnosis and treatment planning. Those with tumors of more than 1 cm diameter will generally undergo total or near-total thyroidectomy with central node dissection usually followed by I^{131} therapy and TSH suppression. Serum thyroglobulin is used to monitor for recurrence, with isotope scans when indicated. External beam radiotherapy is rarely required. Recombinant human TSH is now available and has an evolving role in managing selected cases. Follow up should be life-long because thyroid cancer has a long natural history; late recurrences do occur and can be successfully treated.

Employing a single aggressive therapeutic approach for all patients with well-differentiated carcinoma of thyroid will prevent recurrent disease from developing in all but 7 percent of patients.

These conceptual guidelines set forth by the American Association of Clinical Endocrinologists (AACE) and British Thyroid Association present a consensus of approaches to the management of patients with thyroid carcinoma. The field is highly complex and a considerable diversity of opinion prevails. Adherence to these guidelines should eliminate the possibility of either overaggressive treatment in a patient with an excellent prognosis or inadequate therapy for the unusual patient with a high risk of tumor recurrence and possible death from cancer.

FURTHER READING

1. Agrawal S. Diagnostic accuracy and role of fine needle aspiration cytology in management of thyroid nodules. J Surg Oncol 1995;58:168-72.
2. Andersen PE, Kinsella J, Loree TR, Shaha AR, Shah JP. Differentiated carcinoma of the thyroid with extra-thyroidal extension. Am J Surg 1995;170:467-70.
3. Arad E, O'Mara RE, Wilson GA. Ablation of remaining functioning thyroid lobe with radioiodine after hemithyroidectomy for carcinoma. Clin Nucl Med 1993;18:662-63.
4. Attie JN. Modified neck dissection in the treatment of thyroid cancer. A safe procedure. Eur Cancer Clin Oncol 1988;24:325-24.
5. Cady B, Cohn K, Rossi RL, et al. The effect of thyroid hormone administration upon survival in patients with differentiated thyroid carcinoma. Surgery 1985;98:1171-78.
6. Carmeci C, Jeffrey RB, McDougall IR, Nowels KW, Weigel RJ. Ultrasound-guided fine-needle aspiration biopsy in the diagnosis of thyroid nodules. Br J Surg 1994;81:1151-54.
7. Cavalieri RR. Nuclear imaging in the management of thyroid carcinoma. Thyroid 1996;6:485-92.
8. Chen H, Zeiger MA, Clark DP, Westra WH, Udelsman R. Papillary carcinoma of the thyroid: Can operative management be based solely on the fine-needle aspiration? J Am Coll Surg 1997;184:605-10.
9. Chen H, Nicol TL, Zeiger MA, et al. Hurthle cell neoplasms of the thyroid. Ann Surg 1998;227:542-46.
10. Donis-Keller H, Dou S, Chi D, et al. Mutations in the RET proto-oncogene are associated with MEN 2A and FMTC. Hum Mol Genet 1993; 2:851-56.
11. Fraker DL. Radiation exposure and other factors that predispose to human thyroid neoplasia. Endocr Surg 1995;75:365-75.

12. Grossman RF,Tu S-H, Duh Q-Y, Siperstein AE, Novosolov F, Clark OH. Familial nonmedullary thyroid cancer. Arch Surg 1995;130:892-97.

13. Harness JK, Fung L, Thompson NW, et al. Total thyroidectomy: Complications and technique. World J Surg 1986;10:781-86.

14. La Quaglia MP, Corbally MT, Heller G, et al. Recurrence and morbidity in differentiated thyroid carcinoma in children. Surgery 1988;104:1149-56.

15. Lin J-D, Kao P-F, Chao T-C. The effects of radioactive iodine in thyroid remnant ablation and treatment of well differentiated thyroid carcinoma. Br J Radiol 1998;71:307-13.

16. Maxon HR, Smith HS. Radioiodine-131 in the diagnosis and treatment of metastatic well differentiated thyroid cancer. Endocrinol Metab Clin North Am 1990;19:685-718.

17. Moley JF. Medullary thyroid cancer. Surg Clin NA 1995;75:405-20.

18. Patwardhan N, Cataldo T, Braverman LE. Surgical management of the patient with papillary cancer. Surg Clin North Am 1995;75:449-64.

19. Sabel MS, Staren ED, Gianakakis LM, Dwarakanathan S, Prinz RA. Effectiveness of the thyroid scan in evaluation of the solitary thyroid nodule. Am Surg 1997;63:660-64.

20. Schlumberger MJ. Papillary and follicular thyroid carcinoma. N Engl J Med 1998; 338:297-305.

21. Singer PA, Cooper DS, Daniels GH, et al. Treatment guidelines for patients with thyroid nodules and well-differentiated thyroid cancer. Arch Intern Med 1996;156:2165-72.

22. Soh EY, Clark OH. Surgical considerations and approach to thyroid cancer. Endocrinol Metab Clin North Am 1996;25:115-39.

23. Tallroth E, Backdahl M, Einhorn J, et al. Thyroid carcinoma in children and adolescents. Cancer 1986;58:2329.

24. Weigal RJ. Advances in the diagnosis and management of well-differentiated thyroid cancers. Curr Opin Oncol 1996;8:37-43.

APPENDIX 14

International comparison; India and five continents—AAR (ICMR and IARC).

THYROID CANCER (FEMALE)

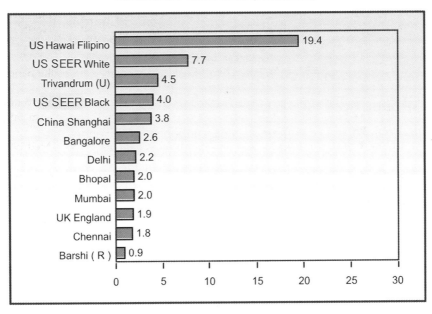

Rate per 100,000

Adrenal and Retroperitoneal Tumors

41

Abraham Kurian
Iqbal S Shergill
Kim Mammen

INTRODUCTION

The adrenal glands are an important component of the endocrine system, involved in the biochemical homeostasis of the human body. Malignant and benign tumors of the adrenal gland are an extremely rare entity, however, they are clinically important as they often present with endocrine disorders and occasionally as a life threatening acute emergency.

SURGICAL ANATOMY AND PATHOLOGY

The adrenal glands are paired organs weighing approximately 4 g and situated in the retroperitoneum in close relationship with the kidneys. As a result of their anatomical location they are also referred to as suprarenal glands. For consistency, the term adrenal gland will be used throughout this text. The left adrenal gland is crescentic in shape and extends along the medial border of the left kidney, whereas the right is pyramidal and overlies the upper pole of the right kidney. The left gland lies on the left crus of the diaphragm, behind the pancreas, lesser sac and the stomach. The right adrenal lies behind the right lobe of the liver and extends medially behind the inferior vena cava. It rests posteriorly on the diaphragm. Three arteries supply each adrenal gland, namely: (1) adrenal branch of the inferior phrenic artery, (2) adrenal branch of the aorta, and (3) adrenal branch of the renal artery. The venous drainage is via one vein, which drains into the renal vein on the left and the inferior vena cava on the right. Despite the difference in their anatomical relationships, both adrenals are structurally identical, with each one consisting of two distinct parts. There is a yellow colored outer cortex, derived from the primitive mesoderm, and an inner medulla, which is dark brown originating from the neuroectoderm. The adrenal cortex contains cords of epithelial cells in zones, which secrete different hormones. From the outside inward, these zones are the zona glomerulosa, zona fasciculata and zona reticularis. The importance of these zones is that each one secretes different hormones with differing effects on the endocrine system. The cells of the zona glomerulosa secrete mineralocorticoids (aldosterone), the zona fasciculata produce glucocorticoids (cortisol) and the zona reticularis is where androgenic steroids are released. The adrenal medulla is distinct from the adrenal cortex and consists of cells similar to sympathetic neurons. These cells secrete catecholamines (epinephrine and norepinephrine).

CLASSIFICATION

A classification based on the anatomical location, and the histological origin, allows the most convenient discussion of the different adrenal tumors, which exist (Figure 41.1).

Adrenal cortex-primary tumors arising from epithelial cells.

ADRENAL ADENOMA

An adrenal adenoma is by definition a benign tumor derived from the adrenal cortex. The underlying etiology for the development of an adenoma is not known. Adenomas present mainly in adults, but cases have been reported in patients of all ages. Some evidence suggests that the incidence in teenage girls is slightly higher than that of teenage boys,

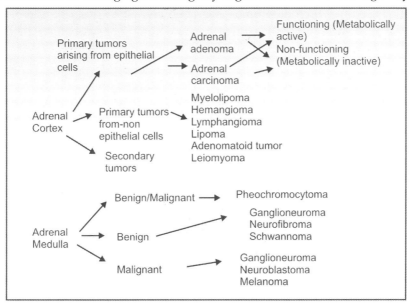

Figure 41.1: Classification of adrenal tumors

but no satisfactory explanation for this finding has been given. Indeed, there is no sex-related predilection in adults. Macroscopically, an adrenal adenoma is composed of firm yellow colored tissue, similar to normal adrenal cortex. This type of neoplasm is well circumscribed with a visible capsule and any remaining adrenal tissue is usually compressed to the edge. Most adrenal adenomas weigh between 20 and 50 gm, whereas most adrenocortical carcinomas are much bigger with the critical cut off weight being 100 gm. During microscopic examination well-differentiated cells resembling the zona fasciculata of the adrenal cortex are commonly seen. Occasionally, some cellular pleomorphism may also be present.

The diagnosis of an adrenal adenoma may be made with a thorough history, physical examination and appropriate investigations. In the majority of cases, clinical presentation occurs as the adenoma is "functioning". This describes an adenoma that is metabolically active and producing excessive amounts of adrenal cortical hormones. Adenomas, which are not producing endocrine hormones, are called "non-functioning". The hormones commonly secreted in a functioning adenoma are aldosterone and cortisol, and therefore patients present with clinical features of primary hyperaldosteronism (Conn's syndrome) or hypercorticism (Cushing's syndrome). These clinical syndromes and their investigations are described separately below. Occasionally, functioning adenomas produce sex hormones and patients may present with virilization, but these cases are extremely uncommon. Interestingly, with the increased reliance on investigations for diagnosing non-specific symptoms, many adrenal adenomas are now being detected incidentally and the name "incidentaloma" has been coined to describe them. The majority of these adenomas are non-functioning. The investigations of an adenoma include a CT scan of the abdomen in all patients to elucidate the size of the adenoma and its anatomical relations to the surroundings. MRI scanning has also been advocated in the investigation of these tumors to delineate the anatomy further. In cases where there is doubt, percutaneous adrenal core needle biopsy may be attempted to obtain an adequate specimen for analysis. However, this procedure is not without its complications, with pneumothorax, hemorrhage and pancreatitis occurring in 3 percent of cases. In addition, although the histological results obtained from the needle biopsy may be reliable in differentiating metastatic lesions from adenomas: they are less useful in distinguishing between adrenal adenoma and adrenocortical carcinoma.

Surgery is the preferred treatment for adrenal adenomas. Open adrenalectomy for large tumors is recommended whereas smaller tumors may be treated with a laparoscopic approach. Importantly, in functioning adenomas secreting cortisol, preoperative steroid cover is necessary because of the prolonged suppression of the contralateral adrenal gland. Further steroidal treatment may be required in the postoperative period, as recovery may sometimes take up to two years. In around 25 percent of cases, patients may never become steroid-free.

ADRENOCORTICAL CARCINOMA

A malignant cancer of the adrenal cortex arises from epithelial cells and is therefore called an adrenocortical carcinoma. Adrenocortical carcinoma is an extremely rare tumor, with an incidence of around 1 to 2 persons per million population. It usually occurs in adults, with a median age of 44 years at the time of diagnosis. In the early stages of the disease adrenocortical carcinomas may be curable, but only one-third of malignancies are pathologically localized at the first presentation. Following adrenalectomy, most carcinomas weigh more than 100 gm, differentiating them from their benign counterparts. Microscopically, adrenocortical carcinomas are mostly composed of diffusely arranged cells with varying degrees of pleomorphism. Nuclear atypia and hyperchromasia are usually present and many areas of necrosis are found. The fibrous capsule and venous and sinusoidal blood vessel walls are mostly infiltrated with cancer cells.

Clinically, the majority of patients (60%) have functioning tumors and present with symptoms related to excessive hormone secretion from the carcinoma such as Cushing's syndrome, Conn's syndrome, hyperandrogenism and hyperestrogenism. Conversely, non-functioning carcinomas present with non-specific symptoms such as vague abdominal pain, abdominal masses, fatigue and weight loss, and in fact may only be detected following symptoms of local invasion by tumor or by metastases to the peritoneum, lung, liver and bone. Investigations aim to confirm the diagnosis biochemically and radiologically, followed by staging of the tumor radiologically. The stage of adrenocortical carcinoma is determined by the size of the primary tumor, the degree of local invasion, and whether it has spread to regional lymph nodes or distant sites (Table 41.1).

Staging investigations should include CT of the abdomen. MRI scans (T1 weighted images) are an alternative non-invasive method to CT in distinguishing between benign and malignant adrenal masses. In addition, MRI can also often clearly demonstrate any evidence of extracapsular

Table 41.1: TNM classification

T1:	Primary tumor no more than 5 cm in size; no local invasion
T2:	Primary tumor greater than 5 cm in size; no invasion
T3:	Primary tumor of any size, locally invading but not involving adjacent organs
T4:	Tumor of any size, locally invading adjacent organs
N0:	No regional positive nodes
N1:	Positive regional nodes
M0:	No (known) distant metastasis
M1:	Distant metastasis present

tumor invasion, extension into the vena cava or distant metastasis. Adrenal venography and selective angiography may provide additional staging information in smaller lesions and for distinguishing tumors of the adrenal gland from tumors of the upper pole of the kidney. The presence of metastatic lesions can be detected using chest radiograph, ultrasound scan of the liver and bone scans. These investigations allow effective palliation of both functioning and non-functioning lesions, according to stage. Radical surgical excision is the treatment of choice for localized malignancies and remains the only method by which long-term disease-free survival may be achieved. The overall 5-year survival for tumors resected for cure is approximately 40 percent. Survival for patients with late stage tumors is depressingly poor. In some cases, palliation of metastatic functioning tumors can be achieved by resection of both the primary tumor and metastatic lesions. Clinical trials are currently in progress addressing the use of palliative antihormonal therapy, systemic chemotherapy and radiation therapy in unresectable or widely disseminated tumors.

PRIMARY HYPERALDOSTERONISM (CONN'S SYNDROME)

Dr JW Conn, an American endocrinologist, first discovered primary hyperaldosteronism in 1955 in a patient who had symptoms attributable to an aldosterone producing adenoma. The name Conn's syndrome was subsequently used to describe cases of primary hyperaldosteronism. In this syndrome, there is excessive and unregulated secretion of aldosterone from the zona glomerulosa of the adrenal cortex and in up to 80 percent of cases the etiology is a benign cortical adrenal adenoma. The majority of the remaining cases are due to bilateral adrenal hyperplasia, with adrenal carcinoma only accounting for <1 percent of patients. Overall, Conn's syndrome remains extremely rare, with reports of only one new case in a million people each year.

Clinical presentation is usually with hypertension, however, many patients will also have non-specific symptoms such as polyuria, nocturia, muscle weakness and headaches. The diagnosis is confirmed biochemically, based on the physiological effects of aldosterone.

Patients with Conn's syndrome have high plasma aldosterone with concomitant low plasma renin activity, hypokalemia and a metabolic alkalosis. Interestingly, traditional teaching was to limit investigation for Conn's syndrome to patients who have hypokalemia, or in whom blood pressure was difficult to control with medication. Using these criteria, it was found that many patients with Conn's syndrome were missed. The current trend is to investigate all patients with clinical suspicion of primary hyperaldosteronism. In addition to biochemical analysis, CT scan of the abdomen is sensitive enough to identify an adenoma in 90 percent of patients and the main differential diagnosis of adrenal hyperplasia can be excluded in the absence of bilaterally enlarged adrenal glands. In cases where localization is in doubt (e.g., which adrenal gland is oversecreting aldosterone?), adrenal vein sampling for aldosterone and renin may be performed radiologically. This is an invasive procedure and carries with it some morbidity.

The treatment for Conn's syndrome depends on the underlying cause, but it is generally considered that medical treatment is indicated for bilateral adrenal hyperplasia, and surgical intervention for an adrenal adenoma and rare cases of adrenocortical carcinoma. Without an effective drug therapy, or operative treatment, hypertension in these patients with Conn's syndrome is extremely difficult to control. Poorly controlled high blood pressure is associated with increased rates of stroke, heart disease and kidney failure. Drugs such as spironolactone, triamterene and amiloride are used for bilateral adrenal hyperplasia with good outcomes.

Whenever surgical removal of an adenoma is contemplated, it can be done using a traditional open procedure or laparoscopically for smaller tumors. While awaiting operation, patients may require potassium supplementation for hypokalemia. Very rarely, emergency in-patient treatment with intravenous potassium is necessary, if life threatening hypokalemia is present.

CUSHING'S SYNDROME

In 1932, Dr Harvey Cushing described eight patients with symptoms attributable to a syndrome caused by excessive secretion of cortisol. Cushing's syndrome as it is now known to occur either as a result of endogenous overproduction of glucocorticoids (cortisol) or due to excess levels of exogenously administered glucocorticoids.

There is either excess production occurring primarily from the adrenal gland or secondary to excess adrenocorticotropic hormone (ACTH) production. The causes of primary, or ACTH independent, Cushing's syndrome are an adrenal adenoma (10%), adrenocortical carcinoma (5%) or adrenal hyperplasia (3%). ACTH dependent Cushing's syndrome occurs when ACTH is secreted by the pituitary (70%)-called Cushing's disease, or because of an ectopic nonpituitary tumor (10%) such as oat cell lung carcinoma, small cell lung carcinoma and carcinoid tumors. Ectopic corticotropin-releasing hormone (CRH) secretion is a very rare cause of Cushing's syndrome (2%). In the majority of cases of exogenous Cushing's syndrome, steroids are the etiological factor. Overall, Cushing's syndrome is more common in females than males, with an incidence ratio of approximately 5:1. There is no satisfactory explanation for this sex difference. Cushing's syndrome caused by an adrenal or pituitary adenoma commonly occurs in patients aged 25-40 years, although specific etiological factors are unknown. Ectopic ACTH production usually occurs later in life and is found to be more common in males, as a result of the increased incidence of lung tumors in this population.

The diagnosis of Cushing's syndrome can be made clinically with the well-described classical features of this condition. Typically patients have a rounded face, truncal obesity, buffalo hump, virilization (females), impotence or gynecomastia (males), increased bruising and striae, peripheral extremity muscle wasting and variable mental aberrations, accompanied by a history of hypertension, osteoporosis and diabetes. However, in all cases the diagnosis should be confirmed biochemically and the underlying etiology must be detected and corrected, as this is a potentially reversible condition. Biochemical investigations begin by detecting a loss of the normal diurnal variation in cortisol levels in serum. In normal individuals, cortisol levels are highest in the morning and lowest at night. In Cushing's syndrome the levels remain high throughout the day. To distinguish between the commonest causes of Cushing's syndrome, that is adrenal adenoma, adrenocortical carcinoma and Cushing's disease, the overnight dexamethasone suppression test is performed. At 11pm of Day 1 of the test, dexamethasone is administered and measuring the serum cortisol at 8 am on Day 2 follows this up. In Cushing's disease cortisol levels are suppressed to normal levels (<50 nmol/L), whereas there is no suppression in cases of adrenal adenoma and adrenocortical carcinoma. Furthermore, ACTH measurements can be carried out to detect cases of ectopic ACTH production, where high levels of ACTH would be expected. If the adrenal glands are suspected to be the cause of hypercorticolism, a CT scan of the abdomen is mandatory to distinguish between adenoma and carcinoma. If there is doubt, T2 weighted images on MRI may distinguish adenoma (low signal intensity and usually <6 cm) from a carcinoma (high signal intensity and >6 cm). Treatment in both cases is surgical adrenalectomy, which may be carried out laparoscopically in cases of small adenoma.

ADRENAL CORTEX–PRIMARY TUMORS ARISING FROM NON-EPITHELIAL CELLS ADRENAL MYELOLIPOMA

This is a rare benign tumor of the adrenal composed of mature adipose tissue and a variable amount of hematopoietic elements. The incidence is around 0.2 percent. Most lesions are small and asymptomatic, only being discovered incidentally at autopsy or on imaging studies performed for other reasons. CT scan readily identifies the fatty component within the myelolipoma. In addition, osseous metaplasia may be detected within the mass. The main clinical importance is the risk of rupture of the mass, either spontaneously or by trauma, with resultant retroperitoneal hemorrhage. Patients with small asymptomatic myelolipomas are monitored clinically for symptoms, whereas symptomatic tumors are treated by adrenalectomy.

ADRENAL HEMANGIOMA

Adrenal hemangiomas are rare benign tumors. They are well circumscribed and comprise closely adjacent vascular channels of varying sizes that are lined with a single layer of endothelium. Most adrenal hemangiomas are small and asymptomatic, and will only become symptomatic when they reach a size large enough to exert pressure. Occasionally they may be the cause of an intra-adrenal or retroperitoneal bleeding following spontaneous or traumatic rupture. Radiological findings on abdominal x-rays and CT scan of the abdomen show the pathognomonic feature of an adrenal gland hemangioma-round calcifications with translucent centers, typical of phleboliths. Despite this feature, diagnosis is usually made postoperatively following surgical removal.

ADRENAL CORTEX—SECONDARY TUMORS

Adrenal Metastases

Adrenal metastases are detected in approximately 30 percent of patients dying of cancer, with half of these cases having bilateral adrenal gland involvement. The commonest sites of their primaries, in order, are lung, colorectal, breast, prostate and melanoma. On an average, adrenal metastases are about 5 mm in size macroscopically and microscopically located in the zona fasciculata and zona reticularis. They may present with non-specific symptoms or may be quiescent, with symptoms only from the primary tumor. Detailed biochemical and radiological investigations to rule out adrenal adenomas and adrenal carcinomas are mandatory. Interestingly, confirmation of the diagnosis can only be achieved histologically following surgical resection.

ADRENAL MEDULLA—BENIGN/MALIGNANT

Pheochromocytoma

Pheochromocytoma is a tumor derived from the chromaffin cells of the adrenal medulla and is associated with pathologic secretion of catecholamines (epinephrine and norepinephrine). Its name originates from the Greek word *phaios,* meaning dark or dusky, and *chrome,* meaning color, describing the chromaffin reaction seen in these tumors. The true incidence and prevalence of this tumor are unknown. However, tumors are believed to be responsible for approximately 0.1-0.5 percent of patients with newly diagnosed hypertension. Pheochromocytomas are mainly found in adults aged 20 to 40 years with an equal male to female ratio. In children, the disease is almost always inherited. The underlying etiology is not known. Pheochromocytoma is sometimes called the "10 percent" tumor, as 10 percent occur in children, 10 percent in patients with multiple endocrine neoplasia (MEN) syndrome and 10 percent of tumors are extra-adrenal, because chromaffin tissue is also present at other anatomical locations such as the pelvis and mediastinum.

Clinical symptoms of pheochromocytoma are those of excessive catecholamine secretion including headaches, sweating and palpitations. In the absence of this classic triad, symptoms are usually non-specific symptoms such as tremor, nausea, dyspnea, fatigue, dizziness and chest or abdominal pain. Interestingly, with increasing radiological evaluation in the form of ultrasound scans for non-specific symptoms, pheochromocytoma may present as an incidentaloma. Physical examination findings include hypertension, which may be sustained or paroxysmal. Orthostatic hypotension may also be present. Patients commonly have tachycardia, arrhythmias, tremor and lean body habitus. In advanced cases, an intra-abdominal mass may be noted. If it is part of the MEN syndrome, clinical signs of these syndromes may also be present. As with the other adrenal tumors, the diagnosis is confirmed biochemically and radiologically. Excessive catecholamines or their metabolites may be measured in serum or urine. In practice, 24-hour urine collection is taken for vanillylmandelic acid and urinary free catecholamines, metanephrine and normetanephrine.

Once an adrenal or extra-adrenal tumor is detected biochemically, CT or MRI of the region is performed for anatomic localization prior to surgical removal. CT scan is an excellent initial investigation because 97 percent of tumors are infradiaphragmatic and 90 percent are intra-adrenal. MRI has the advantage of improved soft tissue characterization with a characteristic high signal intensity on T2 weighted images. Some clinicians use Metaiodobenzylguanidine (MIBG) uptake scanning as the initial screening modality because it enables whole-body imaging, which makes it useful for detection of extra-adrenal tumors and metastatic deposits.

Optimal treatment for pheochromocytoma includes prompt surgical referral for excision because patients are at significant risk for lethal complications such as hypertensive crisis and adrenal hemorrhage. A preoperative biopsy is seldom performed, and in fact may be dangerous because hypertension is triggered by direct manipulation of the adrenal gland. Open surgical excision of the tumor is usually carried out, although there has been a recent trend to carry out laparoscopic adrenalectomy, in tumors less than 5 cm. It is Important that the patients with pheochromocytoma require preoperative medical treatment to prevent cardiovascular morbidity due to severe hypertension. Previously, antihypertensive drugs, such as the non-competitive alpha-blocker phenoxybenzamine were used for 4 weeks prior to surgery to normalize the blood pressure. Recently, newer agents such as prazosin, terazosin and doxazosin are used. Very rarely beta-blockers may be required to treat coexisting arrhythmias. During the perioperative period, meticulous fluid management is necessary and handling of the tumor is kept to a minimum to avoid fluctuations in blood pressure. Careful communication between surgeon and anesthetist is mandatory for a successful outcome. Postoperative follow up following recovery is essential because of the risk of recurrence and further metastatic disease. Routine monitoring of the blood pressure and repeat biochemical evaluation are indicated if hypertension recurs.

FURTHER READING

1. Bernini GP, Moretti A, Bonadio AG, Menicagli M, Viacava P, Naccarato AG, Iacconi P, Miccoli P, Salvetti A. Angiogenesis in human normal and pathologic adrenal cortex. J Clin Endocrinol Metab 2002;87(11):4961-65.
2. Danilowicz K, Albiger N, Vanegas M, Gomez RM, Cross G, Bruno OD. Androgen-secreting adrenal adenomas. Obstet Gynecol. 2002;100(5 Pt 2):1099-1110.
3. Grant CS, Hay ID, Gough IR, et al. Local recurrence in papillary thyroid carcinoma: Is extent of surgical resection important? Surgery 1998;104:954-62.
4. Hase T, Ohta S, Bertherat J, Billaud L, Guilhaume B. Cushing's syndrome and adrenal insufficiency in pregnancy. Ann Endocrinol (Paris) 2002;63(5):452-56. French.
5. Hundahl SA, Fleming ID, Fremgen AM, et al. A National Cancer Data Base report on 53,856 cases of thyroid carcinoma treated in the U.S., 1985-1995. Cancer 1998;83:2638-48.
6. Icard P, Chapuis Y, Andreassian B, et al. Adrenocortical carcinoma in surgically treated patients: A retrospective study on 156 cases by the French Association of Endocrine Surgery. Surgery 1992;112:972-79.
7. Lutton JP, Cerdas S, Billaud L, et al. Clinical features of adrenocortical carcinoma, prognostic factors, and the effect of mitotane therapy. N Engl J Med 1990;322:1195-1201.
8. Mukherjee S, Ghosh AK, Mullick RN. Left sided cervical and thoracic malignant extra-adrenal pheochromocytoma. J Assoc Physicians India 2002;50:1079-81.
9. Norton JA. Adrenal tumors. De Vita VT Jr, Hellman S, Rosenberg SA (Eds). Cancer: Principles and Practice of Oncology (5th ed). Philadelphia: Lippincott-Raven, 1997;1659-77.
10. Schocket LS, Syed NA, Fine SL. Primary adrenal lymphoma with choroidal metastases. Am J Ophthalmol 2002;134(5):775-76.
11. Zielasek J, Bender G, Schlesinger S, Friedl P, Kenn W. A woman who gained weight and became schizophrenic. Lancet. 2002;360(9343):1392.

Pediatric Solid Tumors

42

Mohan Abraham

LIVER TUMORS

Liver tumors are not common in the pediatric age group. About 75 percent are malignant. Hepatoblastoma (HB) and hepatocellular carcinoma account for 90 percent of these tumors. Infantile hemangioendothelioma, mesenchymal hamartoma and undifferentiated embryonal sarcoma contribute the remaining 10 percent.

HEPATOBLASTOMA AND HEPATOCELLULAR CARCINOMA

Hepatoblastoma is the most common hepatic tumor. 90 percent occur in the first 5 years;68 percent in the first 2 years and 4 percent occur at birth. With increasing survival of low birth weight babies, an increase in the incidence of hepatoblastoma in the low birth weight group has been noted. A 0.7 percent incidence in 1985 to 1989 increased to 8.6 percent in 1990 to 1993. Prolonged use of oxygen, assisted ventilation and frusemide have been found associated with higher stages of tumor.

SIGNS AND SYMPTOMS

An abdominal mass occurs in 68 percent of cases, abdominal distension occurs in 28 percent, anorexia and weight loss occur in 23 percent of cases. 19 percent of children come with abdominal pain and 11 percent come with vomiting. Male to female ratio is 3:1. Fever and thrombocytosis have also been noted. Human chorionic gonadotropin produced by hepatoblasts can give rise to precocious puberty.

LABORATORY FINDINGS

Anemia occurs in 65 percent of cases. Thrombocytosis exceeding 500,000/mm^3 occurs in 35 percent of cases. Alpha-fetoprotein (AFP) is the most important laboratory investigation. It is raised in almost 90 percent of cases and AFP can predict the outcome and also monitor the recurrence.

AFP may be low in undifferentiated tumors or may be high in highly invasive tumors. Both extremes have poor prognosis. Patients in whom AFP fails to fall significantly after surgery and chemotherapy have a poorer outcome than those who show a significant decrease in the AFP levels. It is important to remember that in the newborn period, AFP levels are normally high, ranging from 25,000 ng/ml to 50,000 ng/ml. Only by 6 months of age this falls to 25 ng/ml. So AFP may remain appropriately high for the age in children below 6 months of age even after complete excision of the tumor. High levels of AFP initially means poor prognosis in HCC.

IMAGING

Ultrasound is the initial modality of imaging. It will help to differentiate between solid and cystic lesions and also the extent of involvement.

Chest radiographs should be obtained as routine to rule out pulmonary metastasis.

CT scan and MRI are of great help in differentiating between hepato-blastoma, hepatocellular carcinoma, focal nodular hyperplasia, mesen-chymal hamartoma and abscesses. Speckled or amorphous calcification can be seen in 50 percent of cases of hepatoblastoma. MRI has more diagnostic accuracy especially in cases of recurrence. Hepatic vasculature is also seen better with MRI. Angiograms have only therapeutic indication now for the purpose of chemoembolisation.

PATHOLOGY (Figs 42.1 and 42.2, Plate 9)

Hepatoblastoma usually presents as a large solitary intrahepatic tumor, surrounded by a pseudo capsule in 80 percent of cases. Right lobe is involved in 58 percent and left in 15 percent of cases. Bilobar disease can occur in 27 percent either as multicentric disease or by exstension. Most of the time the tumor is resectable. Hepatoblastoma has six histological subtypes based on the predominant cell type.

EPITHELIAL

1. Fetal
2. Embryonal
3. Macrotrabecular
4. Small cell
5. Teratoid
6. Nonteratoid

Table 42.1: Children's Cancer Study Group staging of HB and HCC	
Stage I	Complete resection
Stage II	Microscopic residual tumor
	Intrahepatic
	Extrahepatic
Stage III	Gross residual tumor
	Primary completely resected, nodes positive, or tumor spill
	Primary not completely resected, or nodes positive, or tumor spill
Stage IV	Metastatic disease
	Primary completely resected
	Primary not completely resected

MIXED EPITHELIAL/MESENCHYMAL

Haas et al reported 92 percent 2 years survival in stage 1 patients with pure fetal histology; while only 57 percent of stage 1 patients with all other histological types were alive at the end of two years.

Hepatocellular carcinoma presents with multicentric or extensive involvement of both lobes and usually is unresectable. However fibrolamellar variant of HCC has more resectable lesions.

TREATMENT

About 40 to 60 percent of patients with HB are inoperable when first diagnosed and 10 to 20 percent have pulmonary metastasis. However 85 percent of these tumors can be made resectable and converted to stage 1 or 2 categories by chemotherapy. Routine administration of chemotherapy including transarterial chemoembolisation is part of many protocols now. Ifosfamide, cisplatin, and doxorubicin (IPA) are the standard chemotherapeutic agents used. Carboplatin and etoposide (CARBO/VP 16) have also been used in patients with advanced or recurrent disease.

SURGERY

Surgery remains the mainstay of treatment. Survival is directly proportional to the amount of tumor removed. Except the small tumors, most cases need preoperative chemotherapy. Preoperative chemotherapy has increased resectability from 40 to 90 percent. In extensive tumors liver transplantation has been tried with good results. However in the Indian situation, the high cost for the procedure and the immunosuppressive therapy, after surgery, make transplantation inaccessible for most. Incomplete resection, extensive involvement—multifocal or bilobar and vascular invasion—predict poor outcome. The actual size of the tumor does not have that much of significance as far as prognosis is concerned (Table 42.1).

LIVER TRANSPLANTATION

Orthotopic liver transplantation has proved to be of great help in extensive tumors. For HBL, 1-year, 3-year, and 5-year post-transplantation survival rates were 92 percent, 92 percent, and 83 percent, respectively. Intravenous invasion, positive hilar lymph nodes and contiguous spread did not have a significant adverse effect on the outcome. For HCC, the overall 1-year, 3-year, and 5-year disease-free survival rates were 79 percent, 68 percent, and 63 percent respectively. Vascular invasion, distant metastasis, lymph node involvement, tumor size, and gender were significant risk factors for recurrence.

RADIATION THERAPY

The role for radiation therapy is limited. Radiotherapy is ineffective in HCC, but can control local tumor if incompletely resected.

PROGNOSIS

Survival rates vary with stage. Overall survival rates vary from 65 to 70 percent. For stage 1 it approaches 100 percent. For stage 2 lesions it is 75 to 80 percent, for stage 3 it is 65 to 68 percent and for stage 4 it is 0 to 27 percent.

UNDIFFERENTIATED EMBRYONAL SARCOMA

It occurs in children 6 to 10 years of age. It is a highly malignant tumor. There is no racial or sexual predilection. The majority present with abdominal mass or abdominal pain. Abdominal pain due to tumor rupture has been reported in 3 patients.

AFP is usually negative. Serum bilirubin is rarely elevated. MRI and CT scans may show a misleading cyst-like lesion. Ultrasound will show that it is predominantly solid.

The tumor occurs mostly in the right lobe of the liver and can vary greatly in size. Cut section shows a soft fluctuant lesion with solid, cystic or gelatinous areas. It may have large areas of hemorrhage and necrosis.

Surgical resection is recommended when possible. Multiagent chemotherapy and radiotherapy have been employed with varying results. 67 cases reported over a period of 15 years showed a 2-year survival of 9 percent. 73 percent of patients were either dead or had demonstrable tumor at the end of 36 months.

HEMANGIOENDOTHELIOMA

Infantile hemangioendothelioma usually presents before six months of age;one-third of the cases, presents in the first one month. Only rarely it is seen over 3 years of age. Girls are affected more than boys in a ratio of 2:1.

Enlarging abdomen is the usual clinical complaint;10 to 15 percent can present with complications like congestive cardiac failure, Kasabach-Merritt syndrome or hemorrhage. Occasionally they can present with jaundice, liver failure or rupture. Hemangiomas in other sites will be an indicator of the possibility of hemangioendothelioma of liver when there is hepatomegaly. Angiosarcoma of the liver following resection of hemangioendothelioma has been reported in one child.

LABORATORY FINDINGS

Anemia occurs in 50 percent of cases with hemoglobin level below 10 gm/dl;in 32 percent aspartate aminotransferase is elevated above 100 U/L, in 20 percent bilirubin is elevated. Alpha-fetoprotein is not elevated when adjusted for the age.

IMAGING

Contrast enhanced CT confirms the diagnosis. Hypodense lesion in non-contrast phase, which shows peripheral enhancement during the dynamic bolus CT, and becomes isodense to parenchyma during delayed phase confirms the diagnosis.

Ultrasound may show multiple hypoechoic lesions. Angiography is indicated if therapeutic immobilization is considered.

MANAGEMENT

In the presence of congestive cardiac failure, the child is initially managed with diuretics and digitalis. Steroids produce accelerated regression of the tumor. Prednisolone is given 4 to 5 mg/kg/day for 28 days. Alpha interferon has also been used with success. Experience in treating peripheral hemangiomas indicates a greater success rate with alpha 2a interferon compared to steroids in inducing accelerated regression. If the lesions are localized resection can be attempted. Transarterial embolisation is another option worth considering.

MESENCHYMAL HAMARTOMA

Mesenchymal hamartomas usually present as painless abdominal swellings. 85 percent of lesions occur in children below 2 years of age. Only 5 percent occur above 5 years of age. The lesions are usually small at the time of birth and enlarge gradually as fluid accumulates in the cysts. Rupture of the cysts can give rise to neonatal ascites.

PATHOLOGY

Mesenchymal hamartoma arises from a mesenchymal rest that becomes isolated from the normal portal triad structure and develops independently. The tumor grows along bile ducts and may incorporate normal liver tissue. Mesenchymal rest contains blood vessels and bile ducts;the biological behavior depends on the amount of these tissues present in the tumor. It may be cystic or predominantly vascular.

LABORATORY PARAMETERS

They are nonspecific.

Alpha fetoprotein is usually normal when adjusted for the age.

IMAGING

Ultrasonography will show a predominantly cystic tumor, which may be pedunculated. Cysts may be septate. These features distinguish it from hepatoblastoma and hemangioendothelioma. MRI and CT will show the same findings.

TREATMENT

Since this is a benign tumor extensiveness of surgery should be weighed against the possible risk to life and benefit to the patient. If resection is possible without imparting high morbidity, it is recommended. Marsupialization is known to have recurrences. Spontaneous involution has been reported.

HEPATOCELLULAR ADENOMA

Hepatocellular adenoma (HCA) is mostly an adult tumor. It occurs in children who are on anabolic steroids or who had multiple blood transfusions for chronic anemia. It also occurs in children with type 1 glycogen storage disease;probably because of regional imbalance in insulin and glucagon metabolism.

They usually present as asymptomatic mass. Liver enzymes and alpha-fetoprotein levels are normal. It has a high propensity for intraperitoneal hemorrhage from spontaneous rupture. Tumor can regress with correction of glycogen storage disease. Resection of tumor is recommended in children without any metabolic problem and not on steroids because of the known association of HCA and HCC. If resection is difficult, careful monitoring of the lesion and alpha fetoprotein is mandatory.

FOCAL NODULAR HYPERPLASIA

Focal nodular hyperplasia is usually found incidentally while investigating for other reasons. They are irregular non-tender masses. They may be found along with vascular malformations or hemangiomas. Ultrasonography may show an iso, hypo- or hyperechoic mass. CT will show a hypervascular tumor with a stellate central scar. Since malignancy or hemorrhage does not occur in these lesions conservative management is recommended.

FURTHER READING

1. Achilleos OA, Buis LJ, Kelly DA, et al. Unresectable hepatic tumors in childhood and the role of liver transplantation. J Pediatr Surg 1996;31:1563–67.
2. Awan S, Davenport M, Portmann B, et al. Angiosarcoma of the liver in children. J Pediatr Surg 1996;31:1729–32.
3. Barnhart DC, Hirschl RB, Garver KA, et al. Conservative management of mesenchymal hamartoma of the liver. J Pediatr Surg 1997;32:1495.
4. Becker JM, Heitler MS. Hepatic hemangioendotheliomas in infancy. Surg Gynecol Obstet 1989;168:189–200.
5. Conran RM, Hitchcock CL, Waclawiw MA, et al. Hepatoblastoma: The prognostic significance of histologic type. Pediatr Pathol 1991;12:167–83.
6. Ehrlich PF, Greenberg ML, Filler RM. Improved long-term survival with preoperative chemotherapy for hepatoblastoma. J Pediatr Surg1997;32:999–1002.
7. Filler RP, Ehrlich P, Greenberg M, et al. Preoperative chemotherapy in hepatoblastoma. Surgery 1991;110:591–97.
8. Fuchs J, Bode U, von Schweinitz D, et al. Analysis of treatment efficiency of carboplatin and etoposide in combination with radical surgery in advanced and recurrent childhood hepatoblastoma: A report of the German Cooperative Pediatric Liver Tumor Study HB 89 and HB 94. Klin Padiatr 1999;211:305–09.
9. Geiger JD. Surgery for hepatoblastoma in children. Curr Opin Pediatr 1996;8:276–82.
10. George J, Cohen M, Tarver R, et al. Ruptured cystic mesenchymal hamartoma: An unusual cause of neonatal ascites. Pediatr Radiol 1994;24:304–05.
11. Haas JE, Muczynski KA, Krailo M, et al. Histopathology and prognosis in childhood hepatoblastoma and hepatocarcinoma. Cancer 1989;64:1082–95.
12. Haas T, Kodama M, Kishida A, et al. Successful management of infantile hepatic hilar hemangioendothelioma with obstructive jaundice and consumption coagulopathy. J Pediatr Surg 1995;30:1485–87.
13. Habrand JL. Is there a place for radiation therapy in management of hepatoblastomas and hepatocellular carcinomas in children? J Radiat Oncol Biol Phys 1992;23:525.
14. Heimann A, White PF, Riely CA, et al. Hepatoblastoma presenting as isosexual precocity. The clinical importance of histologic and serologic parameters. J Clin Gastroenterol 1987;9:105–10.
15. Ikeda H, Matsuyama S, Tanimura M. Association between hepatoblastoma and very low birth weight: A trend or a chance? J Pediatric 1997;130:557–60.
16. Lack EE, Schloo BL, Azumi N, et al. Undifferentiated (embryonal) sarcoma of the liver. Clinical and pathologic study of 16 cases with emphasis on immunohistochemical features. Am J Surg Pathol 1991;15:1-16.
17. Maruyama K, Ikeda H, Koizumi T, et al. Prenatal and postnatal histories of very low birthweight infants who developed hepatoblastoma. Pediatr Int 1999;41:82–89.

18. Reynolds M. Conversion of unresectable to resectable hepatoblastoma and long-term follow-up study. World J Surg 1995;19:814–16.
19. Samuel M, Spitz L. Infantile hepatic hemangioendothelioma: The role of surgery. J Pediatr Surg 1995;30:1425.
20. Selby DM, Stocker JT, Waclawiw MA, et al. Infantile hemangioendothelioma of the liver. Hepatology 1994;20:39–45.
21. Stocker J, Conran R, Selby D. Tumor and pseudotumors of the liver. In: Stocker J, Askin F (Eds): Pathology of Solid Tumors in Children. London: Chapman and Hall, 1998;83–110.
22. Stocker J, Conran R. Hepatoblastoma. In Okuda K, Tabor E (Eds): Liver Cancer. New York: Churchill Livingstone, 1997;263–78.
23. Tagge D. Hepatocellular carcinoma: Impact on survival. J Pediatr Surg 1992;27:292–97.
24. Thomas MD, Stocker J. Hepatic tumors in Children, Clinics in Liver Disease,Volume 5 Number 2001.
25. Van Tornout JM, Buckley JD, Quinn JJ, et al. Timing and magnitude of decline in alpha-fetoprotein levels in treated children with unresectable or metastatic hepatoblastoma are predictors of outcome: A report from the Children's Cancer Group. J Clin Oncol 1997;15:1190–97.
26. Von Schweinitz D, Hecker H, Schmidt-von-Arndt G, et al. Prognostic factors and staging systems in childhood hepatoblastoma. Int J Cancer 1997;74:593–99.
27. Von Schweinitz D, Wischmeyer P, Leuschner I, et al. Clinico-pathologic criteria with prognostic relevaance in hepatoblastoma. Eur J Clinid 1994;30A:1052–58.
28. Vos A. Primary liver tumors in children. Eur J Surg Oncol 1995;21:101–05.

NEPHROBLASTOMA

CLINICAL PRESENTATION

Most of the children with nephroblastoma (Wilms' tumor) present with an asymptomatic abdominal mass. Median age for presentation is 36.5 months for boys and 42.5 months for girls. Median age for presentation in case of bilateral tumors is 29.5 months for boys and 32.6 months for girls. Incidence is equal in boys and girls. Incidence is higher in African children.

ASSOCIATED ANOMALIES

Genitourinary anomalies like hypospadias, cryptorchidism and renal fusion anomalies occur in 4.5 percent of patients with Wilms' tumor. Associated syndromes include: Denys-Drash syndrome (male pseudo-hermaphroditism, renal mesangial sclerosis, and nephroblastoma), Beckwith-Wiedemann syndrome (exomphalos, visceromegaly, macro-glossia, hepatomegaly, hemihypertrophy and hyperinsulinemic hypoglycemia) and WAGR syndrome (Wilms' tumor, aniridia, genital anomalies, and mental retardation).

MOLECULAR GENETICS

Tumor Suppressor Genes

They occur in two copies and both of them have to be activated for the tumor to manifest. In many cases one allele is inactivated by mutation and the second allele is inactivated by loss of chromosomal material by loss of heterozygocity.

WT1

This is a complex gene and is encoded by 10 exons. It is found on chromosome 11p13. A mutation of the WT1 gene is present in patients with the Denys-Drash syndrome. It acts to regulate the transcription of other genes.

WT2

A second suppressor gene called WT2 is found on chromosome 11p15. This has been linked to Beckwith-Wiedemann syndrome.

PATHOLOGY (Fig. 42.3, Plate 9)

The tumor is composed of blastema, tubules and stroma. Classic Wilms' tumors are heterogeneous and may contain adipose tissue, skeletal muscle cartilage and bone. If only one component is present, they are called monophasic tumors.

Presence of anaplasia indicates poorer prognosis. Anaplasia is rarely found below two years of age. Incidence increases to 13 percent by 5 years of age. Tumors with anaplasia are also called tumors with unfavorable histology.

IMAGING

Ultrasound is the initial mode of imaging. CT or MRI can follow this. MRI has the additional advantage of assessing the vascular invasion more accurately. If the patient cannot afford MRI, as it occurs with many poor patients in India, an intravenous urogram can be done by injecting the dye in a leg vein as a bolus and taking the pictures while injecting. This will visualize the inferior vena cava and any thrombus if present. X-ray of the chest is mandatory to look for metastasis. CT will show metastasis not seen in X-rays, but the management of these patients is controversial.

MANAGEMENT

National Wilms' Tumor Study (NWTS) does not recommend preoperative chemotherapy in resectable lesions. Chemotherapy regresses the tumor and during surgery accurate staging becomes impossible leading to recurrences. However International Society of Pediatric Oncology (SIOP) recommends preoperative chemotherapy with a view to decrease

Plate   9

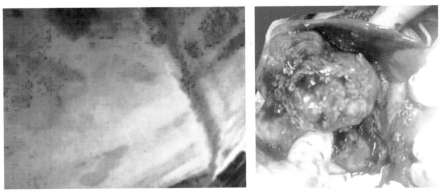

Figure 42.1: Teratoid type of hepatoblastoma. Note the extensive calcification

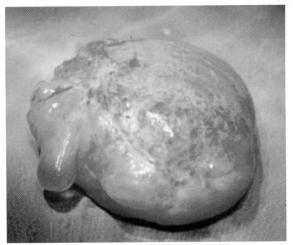

Figure 42.2: Mesenchymal hamartoma-resected specimen.
Note the succulent nature

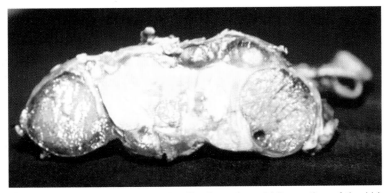

Figure 42.3: Nephroblastoma originating from the middle portion of the kidney

Plate   10

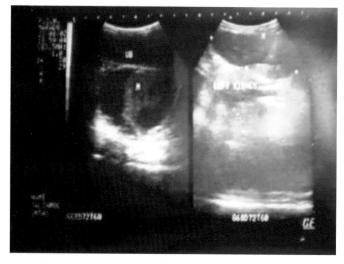

Figure 42.4: Ultrasound picture showing cystic and solid components in Type 4 teratoma and obstruction to left ureter

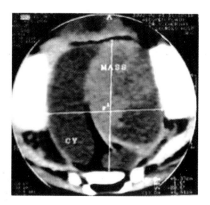

Figure 42.5: CT scan of Type 4 lesion

intraoperative tumor rupture, surgical morbidity and maintain or improve the outcome as compared to postoperative adjuvant chemotherapy (Table 42.2).

SURGICAL MANAGEMENT

Transperitoneal approach is preferred for better visualization. Mobilization has to be gentle and meticulous to prevent rupture of the tumor. Rupture or spill increases local recurrence rate by sixfold. Lymph nodes have to be sampled to assess the spread. The opposite kidney has to be mobilized and examined before tumor mobilization. The renal vein has to be ligated early in dissection.

A review of NWT4 showed a surgical morbidity rate of 11 percent. The most common complications were hemorrhage and small intestinal obstruction. Renal failure can occur to the tune of 15 percent in 15 year follow up in patients with bilateral Wilms' tumor.

Partial nephrectomy is advocated in solitary kidneys or bilateral tumors. Preoperative chemotherapy will be needed to shrink the tumor and facilitate partial nephrectomy. Enucleation has been tried where even partial nephrectomy was not possible. A local recurrence rate of 14 percent was reported following enucleation. Enucleation would not give adequate local tumor control if anaplasia was present (Table 42.3).

CONGENITAL MESOBLASTIC NEPHROMA

It is usually noticed at birth. They originate in the renal medulla and are of low-grade malignancy. They never metastasize but have high local recurrence rate.

FURTHER READING

1. Breslow N, Beckwith JB, Ciol M, et al. Age distribution of Wilms' tumor: Report from the National Wilms' Tumor Study. Cancer Res 1988;48:1653-57.
2. Breslow NE, Beckwith JB. Epidemiological features of Wilms' tumor: Results of the National Wilms' Tumor Study. J Natl Cancer Inst 1982;68:429-36.
3. De Kraker J, Weitzman MB, Voute PA. Preoperative strategies in the management of Wilms' tumor. Hematol Oncol Clin North Am 1995;9:1275-85.
4. Horowitz JR, Ritchet ML, Moksness J, et al. Renal salvage procedures in patients with synchronous bilateral Wilms' tumor: A report from the National Wilms' Tumor Study, 1998.
5. Koufos A, Grundy P, Morgan K, et al. Familial Wiedemann-Beckwith syndrome and a second Wilms' tumor locus both map to 11p15.5. Am J Hum Genet 1989;44:711-19.
6. Ritchey ML, Kelalis PP. Imaging of pediatric renal tumors. Current Opinions in Urology 1992;2:428-32.
7. Shamberger RC, Guthrie KA, Ritchey ML, et al. Surgery-related factors and local recurrence of Wilms' tumor in National Wilms' tumor Study 4. Ann Surg 1999;229:292-97.
8. Stiller CA, Parkin DM. International variations in the incidence of childhood renal tumors. Br J Cancer 1990;62:1026-30.

Table 42.2: National Wilms' Tumor Study Group staging system

Stage I	The tumor is limited to the kidney and is completely excised. The renal capsule has an intact outer surface. The tumor is not ruptured or manipulated for a biopsy prior to removal (fine-needle aspiration biopsies are excluded from this restriction). The vessels of the renal sinus are not involved.
Stage II	The tumor extends beyond the kidney but is completely excised. There may be regional extension of tumor (i.e. penetration of the renal capsule or extensive invasion of the renal sinus). The blood vessels outside the renal parenchyma, including those of the renal sinus, may contain tumor. Biopsy of tumor has been performed (except for fine-needle aspiration), or there is spillage of tumor before or during surgery that is confined to the flank and does not involve the peritoneal surface.
Stage III	Residual nonhematogenous tumor is present and confined to the abdomen. Any one of the following may occur: (1) Lymph nodes within the abdomen or pelvis are found to be involved by tumor (renal hilar, para-aortic or beyond). Lymph node involvement in the thorax or other extra-abdominal sites would be a criterion for stage IV. (2) The tumor penetrates through the peritoneal surface. (3) Tumor implants are found on the peritoneal surface. (4) Gross or microscopic tumor remains postoperatively (e.g. tumor cells are found at the margin of surgical resection on microscopic examination). (5) The tumor is not completely resectable because of local infiltration into vital structures. (6) Tumor spill not confined to the flank occurs either before or during surgery.
Stage IV	Hematogenous metastases (e.g. lung, liver, bone, brain) or lymph node metastases outside the abdominopelvic region are present.
Stage V	Bilateral renal involvement is present at diagnosis. An attempt should be made to stage each side according to the above criteria on the basis of the extent of disease prior to biopsy or treatment (Tables 42.2 and 42.3).

Table 42.3: Protocol for national Wilms' tumor study-v

Stage of disease	Radiotherapy	Chemotherapy
Stage I and II favorable histology	None	Regimen EE-4A*
Stage I, focal or diffuse anaplasia		
Stage III and IV, favorable histology	Yes	Regimen DD-4A †
Stage II, III, and IV, focal anaplasia		
Stage II-IV, diffuse anaplasia	Yes	Regimen l ‡
Stage I-IV, clear cell sarcoma of the kidney		
Stage I-IV, rhabdoid tumor of the kidney	Yes	Regimen RTK §

*Regimen EE-4A: pulse-intensive dactinomycin, vincristine (18 weeks)

† Regimen DD-4A: pulse-intensive dactinomycin, vincristine, doxorubicin (24 weeks)

‡ Regimen l: dactinomycin, vincristine, doxorubicin, cyclophosphamide, and etoposide (24 weeks)

§ Regimen RTK: carboplatin, etoposide and cyclophosphamide (24 weeks)

RENAL CELL CARCINOMA IN CHILDREN

It is a rare tumor that could occur in children. These tumors can develop at a very young age, from 14 months to 19 years, median range being 11.8 years.

SYMPTOMS AND SIGNS

Most patients presented with pain and hematuria with or without a palpable mass. Investigations consist of abdominal ultrasound, CT san, IV urography and renal arteriography.

TREATMENT

The treatment is radical nephrectomy. In a few cases (5%), these children can be subjected to chemotherapy or radiation therapy or both.

PROGNOSIS

Fifty percent of these children die of distant metastases within one year (range: 4 months to two years) after diagnosis. 50% may survive free of relapse at a median of 4 years (range: two to ten years) from the time of diagnosis, provided the tumor is diagnosed at an early stage.
It has been noted that
1. RCC in children is similar to its counterpart in adults,
2. RCC has a worse prognosis than Wilms' tumor except for the earliest stage,
3. Nephrectomy alone is adequate treatment for early stages,
4. Young age (less than 11 years old) may be prognostically favorable.

FURTHER READING

1. Booth CM. Renal cell carcinoma in children. Br J Surg 1996;73:313-16.
2. Brooker B. Renal cell carcinoma in children. Urology 1991;38:54-56.
3. Palmer N, Suton W. Renal cell carcinoma in children. Med Pediatr Oncol 11:91-96.
4. Young JL, Miller RW. Incidence of malignant tumor in US children. J Paediatr 1975;86:254-58.

NEUROBLASTOMA

Neuroblastoma is one of the common malignancies of the childhood. The incidence varies from 1 in 8000 to 1 in 10000 children. In Japan where children are screened at 3 weeks and 6 months using urinary homovanillic acid (HVA) and vanillyl mandelic acid (VMA) the incidence is 1 in 7000 children. Although the incidence detected has increased with screening, actual incidence of manifest disease has not gone up, and this indicates the possibility of some of these tumors undergoing spontaneous resolution.

CLINICAL PRESENTATION

The mean age at diagnosis is 2 years, 35 percent occur under 1 year and the remaining under 10 years. 50 percent occur in adrenals, 22 percent occur in mediastinum, 20 percent occur in paraspinal area. In the region of pelvis 4 percent of tumors are seen while on the neck, it is around 4 percent; 50 to 75 percent present with solitary mass. The mass may be tender and nodular. Abdominal distension, weight loss and anorexia may occur. Hypertension is noted in 25 percent of cases. This may be because of catecholamine production or renal vascular compression. Mediastinal masses compressing stellate ganglion can produce Horner's syndrome characterized by Potts's miosis and enopthalmos. Excessive catecholamine production can lead to flushing, sweating and irritability.

Paraspinal tumors that invade intervertebral foramina can give rise to cord compression leading to paraplegia, bladder and anal sphincter dysfunction and disturbances in gait. 2 percent of children present with opsomyoclonus characterized by involuntary fluttering of eyes and jerking movements of the muscles. About 50 percent of children with opsomyoclonus have small neuroblastomas or ganglioneuromas. This results from cerebellar atrophy due to immunological cross reactivity between tumor cells and cerebellar neurons. Neuroblastoma may be associated with other disorders of neural crest like Hirschsprung's disease and central hypoventilation syndrome (Ondine's curse).

Children may present with watery explosive diarrhea and hypokalemia due to the production of vasoactive intestinal peptide (VIP) by the tumor. Patients with bone marrow involvement may present with anemia.

PATHOLOGY

Macroscopically neuroblastoma is a highly vascular tumor that is often solid but occasionally cystic. It has purple gray color and is very friable. It has a pseudocapsule, which is easily ruptured. Tumor may have hemorrhagic or necrotic areas inside. The neuroblast is a small round cell without much cytoplasm. Undifferentiated tumors have closely packed small spheroid cells without any special arrangement. Rosette formation is considered an early sign of differentiation. Mature stroma rich tumors may contain cells that resemble normal ganglion cells, abundant nerve filaments and neuroblastic rosettes.

International staging is more widely accepted now since it differentiates tumors that are unilateral from tumors that cross the midline; tumors that have histologically positive nodes from those with histologically negative nodes (Table 42.4).

Table 42.4: Staging		
Evans system (CCG)	*St. Jude system (POG)*	*International staging system*
Stage I. Tumor confined to the organ or structure of origin.	*Stage A.* Complete gross resection of the primary tumor, with or without microscopic residual disease: intracavity lymph nodes not adhered to the primary tumor histologically negative; possible positive nodes adhered to the surface of or within the primary; liver free of tumor.	*Stage 1.* Localized tumor confined to the area of origin; complete gross excision, with or without microscopic residual disease; identifiable tumor histologically free of ipsilateral and contralateral lymph nodes microscopically negative.
Stage II. Tumor extending in continuity beyond the organ or structure of origin but not crossing the midline; possible involvement of regional lymph nodes on the ipsilateral side.	*Stage B.* Grossly unresected primary tumor; nodes and liver the same as in stage A.	*Stage 2A.* Unilateral tumor within complete gross excision, identifiable ipsilateral and contralateral lymph nodes microscopically negative.
		Stage 2B. Unilateral tumor with complete or incomplete gross excision, with positive ipsilateral regional lymph nodes; identifiable contralateral lymph nodes microscopically negative.
Stage III. Tumor extending in continuity beyond the midline; possible bilateral involvement of regional lymph nodes.	*Stage C.* Complete resection of primary tumor; intracavitary nodes not adhered to primary histologically positive for tumor; liver as in stage A.	*Stage 3.* Tumor infiltrating across the midline with or without regional lymph nodes involvement; or, midline tumor with bilateral lymph node involvement.
Stage IV. Remote disease involving the skeleton, bone marrow, soft tissue, and distant lymph node groups.	*Stage D.* Dissemination of disease beyond intracavitary nodes (i.e., extracavitary nodes, liver, skin, bone marrow, bone).	*Stage 4.* Dissemination of tumor to bone, bone marrow, liver, distant lymph nodes, and/or other organ (except as defined in Stage 4S).
Stage IV-S. As defined in Stage I or II, except for the presence of remote disease confined to the liver, skin, or bone marrow (without cortical bone metastases)	*Stage DS.* Infants <1 year of age with Evans Stage IV-S disease.	*Stage 4S.* Localized primary tumor as defined for Stage 1 or 2 with dissemination limited to liver, skin, and/or bone marrow.

DIAGNOSIS

Initial laboratory studies should include hemoglobin level estimation and platelet count to detect bone marrow invasion. Elevated VMA and HVA are diagnostic of neuroblastoma. HVA and VMA levels fall to normal after tumor resection and this helps in monitoring tumor recurrence. Serum neuron specific enolase greater than 200 ng/mL, serum ferritin greater than 143 ng/mL, and lactic dehydrogenase greater than 1500 u etc. signify a poorer prognosis. Meta-iodobenzyl guanidine (MIBG) scintigraphy with iodine 131 or iodine 123 will help in detecting tumor in unexpected places. It will also distinguish tumor from other tissues. The radioactive iodine-guanine complex is actively absorbed by neuroblastoma cells in nearly 80 percent of tumors. In 5 percent cases x-ray may show finely stippled calcification. CT scan will help in differentiating the mass from liver and kidney. MRI is extremely helpful in detecting intraspinal extension and defining the relationship of tumor to the vessels. Neuroblastoma has a predilection for cortical bone metastasis. A bone scan with Technetium-99m (^{99m}Tc) or MIBG will pick up most of the metastasis. Bilateral posterior iliac bone marrow aspirates and core bone marrow biopsy containing at least one cm of marrow should be obtained. Presence of malignant cells even in one site indicates bone marrow involvement.

IMMUNOLOGIC ASPECTS

Lymphocytes from children with neuroblastoma inhibit colonies of neuroblastoma in culture but not cells from other tumors. Sera from patients with progressive disease has a blocking antibody that blocks the lymphocyte mediated cytotoxic response. Operative electrocoagulation has induced immunity in experimental mice. At the moment there is no accepted immune therapy for neuroblastoma.

CYTOGENETICS

N- myc oncogene located in the distal arm of chromosome 2 is associated with rapid tumor growth and poor prognosis. It controls the expression genes responsible for cell growth and differentiation. Amplification of N-myc oncogene is an intrinsic property of certain neuroblastoma cell lines. 1p deletion and 17q gain: Deletion or loss of heterozygosity of chromosome 1p is highly predictive of poor outcome. There is a direct relation between 1p deletion and 17q gain. This results from an unbalanced translocation between the two sites. The overall 5-year survival rate was 86 percent in patients with normal 17q versus 31 percent in patients with 17q gain.

Diploidy or near tetraploidy predicts an aggressive tumor and poor outcome. Near triploidy has a favorable outcome.

THE TRK PROTO-ONCOGENE

This is expressed by a high affinity protein receptor for neurotrophin growth factor. High level of TRK expression is associated with better prognosis.

The MDR1 gene is associated with failure of chemotherapy.

The multidrug resistance associated protein (MRP): This is associated with N-myc oncogene and predictive of poor outcome.

TREATMENT

Treatment of neuroblastoma is multidisciplinary involving surgeon, oncologist and radiotherapist. Surgery may be curative in Stage 1 and 2. Overall survival of Stage 3 patients is significantly improved by complete resection of tumor. The timing of surgery does not affect survival or rate of complications. Tumors become less vascular and less friable with chemotherapy. Hence when resectability of Stage 3 tumors is in doubt, it is better to give a course of chemotherapy and wait for tumor shrinkage. The risk of nephrectomy is 25 percent in initial tumor resection compared to 9 percent in delayed resection following chemotherapy. The surgical advantage in the resection of primary tumor in Stage 4 disease is controversial. Resolution of metastasis following chemotherapy contributes to more effective survival.

Comparison of chemotherapy and surgical resection: Surgical resection of tumor in Stage 4 disease is not the mainstay of treatment especially in children with advanced disease. Common chemotherapeutic agents used are:

Cyclophosphamide, cisplatin, doxorubicin, carboplatin, and ifosfamide. Increased dosage of these drugs has improved survival in Stage 3 and 4. Marrow ablative chemoradiotherapy followed by bone marrow transplant has improved short term survival in patients with Stage 4 disease.

Radiotherapy is an important adjuvant to chemotherapy. This holds true especially for patients with intracavitary lymph nodes.

PROGNOSIS

Prognosis depends on the age of the patient, stage of disease and treatment given. In Stage 1 disease with tumor completely resected survival can be as high as 95 percent regardless of the age.

Patients above 1 year and Stage 2 disease can expect 85 percent survival with surgery alone. Patients above 1 year and Stage 3 disease can expect 50 percent survival with surgery and chemotherapy and 70 percent survival when radiotherapy is added. In disseminated Stage 4 disease in children above 1 year, survival can be as low as 10 to 30 percent. Survival in Stage 4 is 90 percent in children with favorable histology and 30 to 60 percent in children with unfavorable histology.

THE FUTURE

Radio-labeled MIBG has been used to target neuroblastoma cells.

Newer angiostatic agents like TNP-470 have been shown to cause reduction in vascularity of tumor and arrest growth of tumor in animal models. Transgenic infection of antitumor agents like interleukin-12 has been shown to improve immunity against neuroblastoma. These findings along with improvements in chemoradiotherapy may improve the future of these children.

FURTHER READING

1. Baker ME, Kirks DR, Korobkin M, et al. The association of neuroblastoma and myoclonic encephalopathy: An imaging approach. Pediatr Radiol 1985;15:184-90.
2. Bown N, Cotterill S, Lastowska M, et al. Gain of chromosome arm 17q and adverse outcome in patients with neuroblastoma. N Engl J Med 1994;340:1954-61.
3. Brodeur GM, Seeger RC, Schwab M, et al. Amplification of N-myc in untreated human neuroblastomas correlates with advanced disease stage. Science 1984;224:1121-24.
4. Castleberry RP, Kun LE, Suster JJ, et al. Radiotherapy improves the outlook for patients older than 1 year with pediatric oncology group stage C neuroblastoma. J Clin Oncol 1991;9:789-95.
5. Chan HSL, Haddad G, Thorner PS, et al. P-glycoprotein expression as a predictor of the outcome of therapy for neuroblastoma. N Engl J Med 1991;325:1608-14.
6. Gaze MN, Wheldon TE: Radiolabelled MIBG in the treatment of neuroblastoma. Eur J Cancer 1996;32:93-96.
7. Guglielmi M, De Bernardi B, Rizzo A, et al. Resection of primary tumor at diagnosis in stage IV-S neuroblastoma: Does it affect the clinical course? J Clin Oncol 1996;14:1537-44.
8. Haase GM, Wong WY, deLorimier AA, et al. Improvement in survival after excision of primary tumor in stage III neuroblastoma. J Pediatr Surg 1989;24:194-200.
9. Katzenstein HM, Bowman LC, Brodeur GM. Prognostic significance of age, MYCN oncogene amplification, tumor cell ploidy, and histology in 110 infants with stage D(S) neuroblastoma: The pediatric oncology group experience—a pediatric oncology group study. J Clin Oncol 1998;16:2007-17.
10. Labrosse EH, Com-Nouque C, Zucker JM, et al. Urinary excretion of 3-methoxy-4-hydroxy-mandelic acid and 3-methoxy-4-hydroxy-phenylacetic acid in 288 patients with neuroblastoma and related neural crest tumors. Cancer Res 1980;40:1995-2001.
11. Miller RW, Young JL Jr, Novakovic B. Childhood cancer. Cancer 1995;75(suppl):395-405.
12. Nakagawara A, Arima-Nakagawara M, Scavarda NJ, et al. Association between high levels of expression of the TRK gene and favorable outcome in human neuroblastoma. N Engl J Med 1993;328:847-54.
13. Norris MD, Bordow SB, Marshall GM, et al. Expression of the gene for multidrug resistance-associated protein and outcome in patients with neuroblastoma. N Engl J Med 1996;334:231-38.

14. Sawada T, Nakata T, Takasugi N, et al. Mass screening for neuroblastoma in infants in Japan. Lancet 1984;2:271-73.
15. Schamberger RC, Smith EI, Joshi VV, et al: The risk of nephrectomy during local control in abdominal neuroblastoma. J Pediatr Surg 1998;33:161-64.
16. Stram DO, Matthay K, O'Leary M, et al. Consolidation chemoradiotherapy and autologous bone marrow transplantation versus continued chemotherapy for metastatic neuroblastoma: A report of two concurrent children's cancer group studies. J Clin Oncol 1996;14:2417-26.
17. Wassberg E, Christofferson R. Review: Angiostatic treatment of neuroblastoma. Eur J Cancer 1997;30:2020-23.
18. Woods WG, Tuchman M, Robison LL. A population-based study of the usefulness of screening for neuroblastoma. Lancet 1996;348:1682-87.

SACROCOCCYGEAL TERATOMA

Sacrococcygeal tumors account for 47 percent of teratomas both benign and malignant. 70 percent occur in females, 48 percent are benign, 29 percent are malignant, and 23 percent have immature but non-malignant components.

There are four types:
1. Predominantly external, minimal presacral component.
2. External with significant intrapelvic component.
3. External with predominantly presacral component and extension into abdomen.
4. Entirely presacral without external presentation.

Constipation is the usual presenting symptom in Type 4. Increased urinary frequency and lower limb weakness can be the other presenting symptoms in Type 4.

During the intrauterine period these teratomas can produce a vascular steal syndrome and high output cardiac failure resulting in fetal death.

Ultrasound will pick up most of these lesions in the intrauterine period. MRI scan will delineate the anatomy better in the intrauterine period without the risk of attendant radiation.

If the lesion is more than 5 cm, a planned cesarian section is recommended.

INCIDENCE

The overall incidence is 1:40000 births. Since there is a high incidence of intrauterine death due to hydrops fetalis or massive hemorrhage into the tumor the true incidence may be much higher.

Before 2 months of age the incidence of malignancy is 10 percent in boys and 7 percent in girls. After 2 months of age the incidence increases to 67 percent in boys and 47 percent in girls.

DIAGNOSIS

Per rectal examination is the easiest way to diagnose. Ultrasound scan will differentiate between solid and cystic components.

Plain X-ray of the pelvis will show abnormal calcifications, tooth buds or incompletely formed bones.

Concave defects in the back of vertebral bodies and neural arches are highly suggestive of intraspinal extension.

CT and MRI will give details regarding involvement of other tissues and extensions of the tumor.

SERUM ALPHA-FETOPROTEIN

Serum alpha-fetoprotein is a useful tumor marker in sacrococcygeal teratoma. It is elevated in malignant teratomas disproportionate to the normal elevation found in the first few months of life. Billmire and Grosfeld reported elevated AFP levels in 100 percent of malignant lesions, 50 percent immature lesions and 6 percent of benign mature lesions·

STAGING

(Children's Cancer Study Group and Pediatric Oncology Group)

1. Complete excision with coccygectomy, negative tumor margins, tumor markers fall to normal levels postoperative, negative lymph nodes.
2. Microscopic residual tumor, lymph nodes negative. Tumor markers positive or negative.
3. Gross residual tumor or only biopsy. Retroperitoneal nodes negative or positive, tumor markers positive or negative.
4. Distant metastasis including liver (Figs 42.4 and 42.5, Plate 10).

MANAGEMENT

Intrauterine

In those cases where there is hyperdynamic circulation and vascular steal syndrome radio frequency ablation probes were placed percutaneously under ultrasound guidance into the tumor and either the tumor mass or tumor vessels were ablated. In two cases the result was good while in two others there was hemorrhage into the mass resulting in fetal loss.

Thermocoagulation of fetal sacrococcygeal teratoma also has been tried at eighteen weeks by placing an insulated electrode into the feeding vessels of the tumor at its neck and applying the electric current. Although the blood supply was reduced fetal death followed.

Extrauterine Management

Surgery is the mainstay in extrauterine management. Complete excision of the tumor is important. Sacrum is divided between the fourth and fifth pieces, tumor is removed en bloc with the last piece of sacrum and coccyx. If this is not done recurrence rate and malignancy are very high. Although the tumor is approached from the sacral area initially, abdominal exploration will be needed if there is abdominal extension.

PROGNOSIS

Prognosis is good if operated in the neonatal period since incidence of malignancy is low. In cases of benign tumors recurrence is rare. AFP has to be closely monitored to pick up recurrences early.

FURTHER READING

1. Altman RP, Randolph JG, Lily JR. Sacrococcygeal teratomas. J of Pediatric Surgery 1974;9:389.
2. Bettina W, Paek Md, et al. Radiofrequency ablation of human fetal sacrococcygeal teratoma. American Journal of Obstetrics and Gynecology 2001;184.
3. Billmire DF, Grosfeld JL. Teratomas in childhood: Analysis of 142 cases: J of Pediatric Surgery 200;21:548-51.
4. Holzgreve W, Flake AJ, Langer JC. The fetus with sacrococcygeal teratoma. The Unborn Patient, Philadelphia: WB Saunders, 1991.
5. MR imaging of fetal sacrococcygeal teratoma. Diagnosis and assessment. Avni FE - Am J Roentgenol 2002;178(1):179-83.

Tumors of the Salivary Gland

43

AR Rama Subbu

Tumors can arise in major or minor salivary glands. These tumors account for 0.5 percent to 2 percent of all head and neck tumors.

ETIOLOGY

Cigarette smoking and alcohol have not proved to be risk factors but workers in rubber, automotive and wood industries are more prone to salivary gland tumors. Ionizing radiation too is considered to be a risk factor. It is noted that in Eskimos, the incidence of both the benign and malignant salivary tumors is high, for unknown reasons. The salivary gland is broadly classified into major and minor glands, the major being the parotid, submaxillary and sublingual and the minor being the oral, nasal and paranasal sinuses which appear mainly in the upper aerodigestive tract. Most of the malignant tumors arise from the parotid gland. It is only rarely, we find malignant tumors from the other major and minor salivary glands.

PAROTID GLAND TUMORS

INCIDENCE

Benign

72.5 percent of the salivary gland tumors are benign, the commonest being the mixed parotid tumor or the pleomorphic adenoma. They are seen as a swelling of the parotid gland. They are of slow growth with minimum symptoms and become malignant after 15 to 20 years of existence. It is not unusual to see benign and malignant tumors exist in one resected specimen of the salivary gland. Pleomorphic adenoma is also seen in the minor salivary glands as painless and slow growing tumor.

Malignant

27.5 percent of the tumors of the salivary glands are malignant and the most common among them is mucoepidermoid cancer.

There is no sex difference. A tumor of the parotid in a child is more likely to be malignant than in an adult (Table 43.1).

STAGING

Malignant tumors account for 14 percent of tumors arising in the parotid gland, 12 percent of tumors arising in the submandibular gland.

Mucoepidermoid carcinoma accounts for 26 percent of minor salivary gland tumors and 74 percent of parotid tumors. Some of these are high-grade tumors, aggressive in nature and spread rapidly by local invasion and widespread metastases in sinuses, cranial nerves, blood vessels of the neck and at the base of the skull. These high-grade tumors are best treated with radical surgery, including neck dissection and postoperative radiation therapy. The low grade tumors are the commonest, and usually have a long history which can be cured by radical resection of the involved salivary gland.

Adenoid cystic carcinoma accounts for 41 percent of malignant submandibular and minor salivary gland tumors and 4 percent of malignant parotid tumors. This tumor has a propensity for perineural invasion and spreads to long distances along the nerve sheath (Table 43.2).

40 percent of cases develop metastasis in the lung and may have many years of survival. With visceral metastasis, the prognosis is poor.

Adenomas present for more than 15 years have a 9.4 percent incidence of malignant transformation. Adenocarcinoma accounts for 13 percent

Table 43.1: Clinical characteristics of benign and malignant tumors		
Salivary gland tumors	*Benign*	*Malignant*
1. Growth	Slow, Steady	Rapid
2. Pain	Absent	Occasionally present
3. Facial palsy	Absent	Diagnostic, if present
4. Tenderness	Rare	Frequent
5. Consistency	Cystic or Rubbery	Stony hard
6. Attachment	Mobile	Fixed
7. Trismus	None	May be present
8. Nodes	None	May be present

Table 43.2: Primary tumor staging of salivary gland tumors
T1: Tumor < 2 cm without extraparenchymal extension.
T2: Tumor > 2 cm but < 4 cm without extraparenchymal extension.
T3: Tumor with extraparenchymal extension without seventh nerve involvement and/or > 4 cm but < 6 cm.
T4: Tumor invades base of skull, seventh nerve and/or is > 6 cm.

malignant tumors and a high percentage of them are seen in the minor salivary gland tumors. These tumors have a spectrum of behavior from very indolent to very aggressive. Most are high grade, with a propensity for regional and distant metastasis.

TREATMENT OF THE SALIVARY GLAND TUMORS

Surgery

Surgery is the mainstay of treatment in patients with resectable salivary gland cancer. All malignant tumors of the parotid gland warrant total parotidectomy. The facial nerve should be sacrificed only for direct tumor invasion. Patients with high-grade tumors should also undergo selective neck dissection [N0] or modified or radical neck dissection [N+].

Postoperative Radiotherapy

Postoperative radiotherapy is indicated in all high-grade tumors (any histology except low-grade mucoepidermoid and acinic cell carcinoma), close surgical margins, recurrent disease, skin, bone, nerve or extraparotid involvement, positive nodes, and for gross residual or unresectable disease. Fast neutron radiation therapy has a role in patients with large, inoperable salivary gland cancers.

Chemotherapy

The role of chemotherapy is limited to those tumors that are recurrent, unresectable or metastatic. There is lack of trials with adequate number of cases and hence there is no established chemotherapy schedule. Cisplatin with 5 FU or cisplatin with doxorubicin with cyclophosphamide is given as a palliative therapy. Transient response is seen in 30 percent of cases.

Acinic cell carcinoma and squamous cell carcinoma are uncommon and account for 17 percent of the malignant salivary gland tumors. They are less aggressive and with infrequent nodal metastasis.

Mention has already been made about the pleomorphic adenoma of the parotid gland, which is essentially a benign tumor. It can become malignant in 14 percent of the parotid gland adenomas and 12 percent of the submandibular gland adenomas. The treatment is aggressive resection of the gland with the sacrifice of the facial nerve if needed.

OTHER SALIVARY GLANDS

Salivary gland tissue is located in the palate, buccal mucosa, lip, tongue, lacrimal gland, pharynx, nasal fossa, trachea and bronchi as well as in the submaxillary and sub-lingual glands. This tissue gives rise to the same spectrum of tumors discussed under parotid gland tumors (Ref. page 492).

Complete excision and en bloc dissection is the preferred treatment for malignancies of the submaxillary gland.

Complications of Surgery

1. Facial palsy
2. Auriculo-temporal syndrome

PROGNOSTIC FACTORS

1. Presence of metastasis lowers the cure rate.
2. Histologic features of higher grade of malignancy and degree of lymphatic and vascular invasion suggest poor prognosis.

REASONS FOR FAILURE

1. Undue concern for integrity of facial nerve leading to inadequate resection.
2. Ill-advised biopsies which seed tumor, lower cure rate.
3. Extensive disease at the time of presentation for treatment.

FURTHER READING

1. Braunstein E, Buchner A. Immunohistochemical study of epidermal growth factor receptor in adenoid cystic carcinoma of salivary gland origin, head and neck. 2002;24(7):632-36.
2. Capone RB, Ha PK, Westra WH, Pilkington TM, Sciubba JJ, Koch WM. Oncocytic neoplasms of the parotid gland: A 16-year institutional review. Cummings Otolaryngol Head Neck Surg. 2002;126(6):657-62.
3. Castrilli G, Fabiano A, La Torre G, et al. Expression of hMSH2 and hMLH1 proteins of the human DNA mismatch repair system in salivary gland tumors. J Oral Pathol Med 2002;31(4):234-38.
4. Locati LD, Quattrone P, Pizzi N, Fior A, Cantu G, Licitra L. Primary high-grade mucoepidermoid carcinoma of the minor salivary glands with cutaneous metastases at diagnosis. Oral Oncol 2002;38(4):401-04.
5. Maes A, Weltens C, Flamen P, Lambin P, et al. Preservation of parotid function with uncomplicated conformal radiotherapy. Radiother Oncol 2002;63(2):203-11.
6. Rosa JC, Nunes JF, Fonseca I, Cidadao A, Soares J. Hyalinizing clear cell carcinoma of salivary glands: A study of extracellular matrix. Oral Oncol 2002;38(4):364-68.
7. Wang B, Brandwein M, Gordon R, Robinson R, Urken M, Zarbo RJ. Primary salivary clear cell tumors—a diagnostic approach: A clinicopathologic and immunohistochemical study of 20 patients with clear cell carcinoma, clear cell myoepithelial carcinoma, and epithelial-myoepithelial carcin. Arch Pathol Lab Med 2002;126(6):6-16.
8. Zlotolow IM. Clinical manifestations of head and neck irradiation. Otolaryngol Head Neck Surg 2002;126(6):695-96.

Head and Neck Tumors (Tumors of Oral Cavity, Lip, Tongue, etc.)

44

AR Rama Subbu

Cancers of the upper aerodigestive tract, collectively known as head and neck cancers, arise from a multiplicity of sites. Oral cancer is one of the 10 most common cancers in the world. In India, oral cancer ranks first among all cancers in male patients and third among cancers in female patients. Oral cancer is common where people, especially villagers are habituated in betel quid chewing, bidi smoking and where alcohol and tobacco consumption is high. Thus it is a common cancer in Southeast Asia, where more than 10,000 new cases are reported every year. In India and China, the etiology, pattern of primary sites and clinical behavior are different. Survival rates in head and neck malignancies have not significantly improved over the past four decades despite the improvement in diagnosis and local management. Development of second primary tumors remains a major threat to long-term survival in patients initially cured of these tumors. Risk factors for head and neck cancers include tobacco (whether smoked, chewed or inhaled as snuff), alcohol and dietary factors, such as poor intake of proteins and vitamins.

Most head and neck cancers are squamous cell carcinomas of varying degrees of differentiation occurring in several distinct sites and linked only by common squamous histology. Squamous cell carcinoma may be the most diverse class of malignancies lumped together under one diagnostic heading. New strategies for the management of head and neck malignancies are desperately needed in the developing countries. Advances in organ preservation utilizing chemoradiation approaches and chemoprevention are beginning to offer realistic hopes for improvem ent in survival and quality of life.

ETIOLOGY AND EPIDEMIOLOGY

Approximately 90 percent of head and neck cancers occur after exposure to known carcinogens, specifically tobacco and alcohol. 50 percent of all cancers in South India where chewing betelnut is endemic are squamous cell carcinomas of oral cavity and hypopharynx. Alcohol potentiates the carcinogenic effect of tobacco. There is increasing evidence that viruses may be also an etiological factor. Infection with Epstein-Barr virus is clearly associated with nasopharyngeal carcinoma and viral oncogenes of the human papillomavirus have also been detected in head and neck cancers.

DIET

Considerable evidence suggests that vitamin A and B-carotene play a protective role in epithelial neoplasia.

OCCUPATION

Exposure to nickel refining, wood and leather working can be risk factors for adenocarcinomas of the sinonasal region.

ANATOMY OF THE ORAL CAVITY (FIG. 44.1)

The term 'cancers of head and neck' describes a diverse collection of cancers arising from a variety of anatomical sites in the upper aerodigestive tract with a varied histopathology.

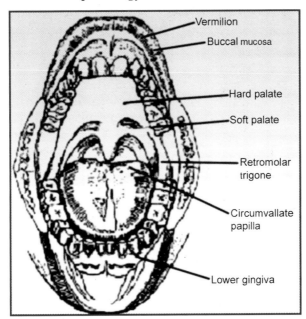

Figure 44.1: The oral cavity

THE ORAL CAVITY

The oral cavity includes the lips, buccal mucosa, anterior or oral tongue, floor of mouth, hard palate, as well as upper and lower alveolar ridges and retromolar trigone.

PHARYNX

The pharynx can be subdivided into the nasopharynx, oropharynx and hypopharynx.

LARYNX

The larynx is divided into the supraglottis, the glottis, and the subglottis.

NECK

Anatomical considerations in the treatment of cancers of head and neck must include a thorough understanding of the neural, vascular and lymphatic structures of the neck. There are 10 major groups of lymph nodes in the head and neck. They are the occipital, mastoid, parotid, submandibular, facial, submental, sublingual, retropharyngeal, anterior cervical and lateral cervical lymph nodes (Fig. 44.2).

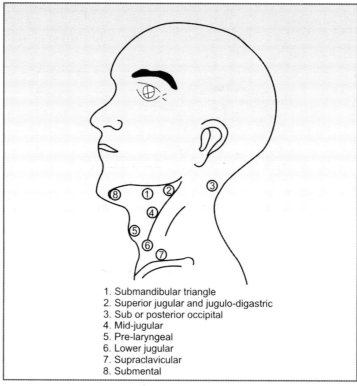

1. Submandibular triangle
2. Superior jugular and jugulo-digastric
3. Sub or posterior occipital
4. Mid-jugular
5. Pre-laryngeal
6. Lower jugular
7. Supraclavicular
8. Submental

Figure 44.2: Distribution of the cervical lymph glands

The various lymph node groups have been divided into six levels (Fig. 44.3):

Level I   It includes the submental and submandibular nodal groups.

Level II   It consists of the upper jugular or jugulodigastric lymph nodes.

Level III   It includes the middle jugular nodes (from the carotid bifurcation to the omohyoid muscle).

Level IV   It includes the lower jugular group (from the omohyoid muscle to clavicle).

Level V   It includes the posterior accessory chain and transverse cervical nodes.

Level VI   It contains the lymph nodes of anterior compartment from the hyoid bone to the suprasternal notch inferiorly.

PATHOLOGY AND CLINICAL PRESENTATION (FIGS 44.3 AND 44.4)

More than 90 percent of head and neck cancers are squamous cell carcinomas. Other fairly common tumor types include lymphoma and adenoid cystic carcinoma, both more common in oral and pharyngeal sites than in the larynx. Head and neck lymphomas seem to be occurring more frequently, possibly as a result of AIDS, organ transplant surgery and other instances in which there is immunodeficiency present in the patient.

TNM system of staging has gained wide acceptance. Patients frequently present not with the symptoms of primary disease but with the neck node

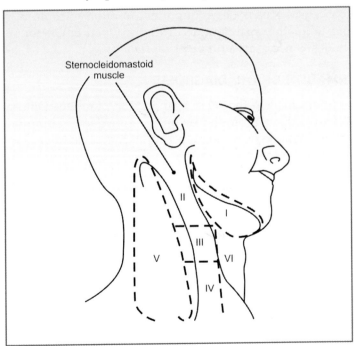

Figure 44.3: Diagram of the neck showing levels of lymph nodes

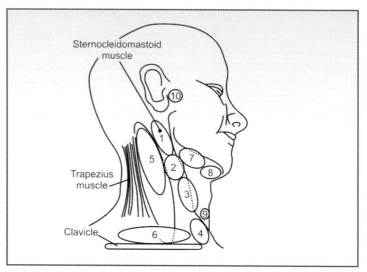

Figure 44.4: Lymphatic drainage pattern for head and neck

metastases. Features reflecting aggressive behavior include the presence of lymphatic invasion, perineural invasion, lymph node metastasis and extracapsular spread (penetration of tumor through the capsule of the involved lymph node). The presence of large or fixed node disease almost always renders the patient incurable by surgery. Fine-needle aspiration cytology of suspicious nodes is important in order to confirm the tumor stage and tailor the treatment accordingly. Open biopsy of suspicious lymph nodes is necessary at the appropriate time.

CONFIRMATION OF THE DIAGNOSIS

Staging should include thorough examination of all head and neck sites by a skilled otolaryngologist or an oral surgeon. Common clinical presentations include hoarseness from a laryngeal nodule, ulcer or vocal cord fixation. The other features are dysphagia, visible ulcer in the oral cavity, oral discomfort, nasal stuffiness or discharge. Cranial nerve palsy and facial swelling or ulceration over the cheek may be present with associated cervical lymphadenopathy. Apart from expert examination, important investigations include fine-needle aspiration biopsy of the tumor and the palpable lymph node. Chest radiography and computed tomography of chest are also indicated. In case of an 'unknown primary carcinoma', careful inspection under anesthesia together with panendoscopy should be carried out by an ENT colleague. If necessary, blind biopsy of nasopharynx, base of the tongue, tonsil or hypopharynx are all helpful. It must be remembered that a firm unilateral neck mass is cancer until proved otherwise. In an adult, 80 percent of firm neck masses represent cancer and most are cervical metastasis from squamous cell carcinoma.

STAGING

Staging criteria for cancers arising in the upper aerodigestive tract, paranasal sinuses and salivary glands have been developed by the American Joint Committee on Cancer (AJCC). The stage grouping for head and neck cancers are based on T (primary tumor), N (regional node status), and M (distant metastasis) (Table 44.1).

TNM and clinical staging of head and neck cancer (American Joint Committee on Cancer Staging is depicted in Table 44.2.

Table 44.1: TNM staging

TX	–	Primary tumor cannot be assessed
T0	–	No evidence of primary tumor
Tis	–	Carcinoma *in situ*
T1	–	Tumor < 2 cm in greatest dimension
T2	–	Tumor > 2 cm but < 4 cm
T3	–	Tumor > 4 cm
T4	–	Tumor invades adjacent structures (for example cortical bone, deep muscle of tongue, maxillary sinus, skin)
NX	–	Regional lymph nodes cannot be assessed
N0	–	No regional lymph node metastasis
N1	–	Metastasis to single ipsilateral lymph node < 3 cm
N2	–	Metastasis to single ipsilateral lymph node > 3 cm but < 6 cm, to multiple ipsilateral lymph node (none> 6 cm) or to bilateral or contralateral lymph nodes (none > 6 cm)
N2a	–	Metastasis to single ipsilateral lymph node> 3 cm but < 6 cm
N2b	–	Metastases to multiple ipsilateral lymph nodes (none > 6 cm)
N2c	–	Metastases to bilateral or contralateral lymph nodes (none > 6 cm)
N3	–	Metastasis to lymph node > 6 cm
MX	–	Presence of distant metastasis cannot be assessed
M0	–	No evidence of distant metastasis
M1	–	Distant metastasis

Table 44.2: Clinical staging

0	–	Tis N0 M0
I	–	T1N0M0
II	–	T2N0M0
III	–	T3N0M0
T1	–	T3N1M0
IV	–	T4N0-N1M0
Any T N2	–	N3 M0
Any T and N and M1		

CLINICAL MANAGEMENT

General Principles

Surgery with or without radiation therapy is the mainstay of treatment for most of the head and neck cancers. Stage I and II tumors are typically treated with a single modality, either radiation therapy or surgery. Stage III and IV tumors require a combined modality approach, typically surgery plus radiation therapy.

Surgical Principles

Wide surgical resection for primary squamous cell carcinomas of the head and neck generally can be interpreted as resection of tumor with 1 to 2 cm margins, often with frozen section control of surgical margins. When tumor is adherent to mandibular periosteum without bony erosion, a cortical or rim mandibulectomy is advisable. When mandible is invaded, segmental mandibular resection is recommended. In carcinomas of the head and neck, it is the nodal status that affects prognosis. George Crile Jr. (1962) said, "Cancer of the mouth and tongue usually kills by direct extension into or invasion of vital structures by nodal metastases." A common denominator in the treatment of head and neck cancer, is management of cervical lymph nodes. Staging of the neck for primary tumors of the oral cavity and oropharynx can be accomplished with a supraomohyoid neck dissection that encompasses the submental and submandibular triangles (level I), the upper jugular nodes (level II) and the midjugular lymph nodes (level III). Similarly, staging of the neck for primary tumors of the larynx or hypopharynx can be accomplished with a lateral neck dissection which includes the upper, mid and lower jugular nodes (levels II, III, IV). Surgical management of N1 neck is controversial. Though Crile (1906) first described radical neck dissection (RND), Mackenzie had actually already carried it out in 1900. Polya described the anatomic basis for the procedure in 1902. The present day procedure of RND differs slightly from what Crile described a century ago (Fig. 44.5).

RADICAL NECK DISSECTION

The classical RND includes removal of lymphatic and lymph nodes from the mandible above to clavicle below and from the midline inferiorly to the anterior border of trapeziums posteriorly. The block of tissue thus excised includes the sternomastoid and omohyoid muscles, the internal and external jugular veins, the accessory and greater auricular nerves, the sub-mandibular salivary gland and the tail of parotid gland and all the lymph nodes and lymphatics from the investing layer to the pre-vertebral layer of deep-fascia of the neck. RND is not indicated if: the lymph nodes are fixed to pre-vertebral fascia or muscles and remain unchanged following radiotherapy.

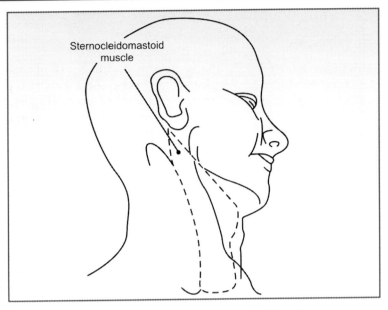

Figure 44.5: Incision for lateral neck dissection

RND is also not indicated when life expectancy is less than 6 weeks and when there is wide-spread cutaneous deposits, and evidence of distant metastases. Surgery is contraindicated if there is tethering of nodes to the carotid sheath.

Modified RND includes excision of all the lymph nodes from both anterior and posterior triangles of the neck preserving the accessory nerve, the sternocleidomastoid muscle and the internal jugular vein (Fig. 44.6).

The indications for modified RND are:

a. Well-differentiated thyroid neoplasm with nodal metastases.
b. As a prophylactic block dissection for occult secondaries.
c. In patients requiring a bilateral RND, a modified RND saving the internal jugular vein and spinal accessory nerve on one side should be performed. This procedure of modified RND has limitations and is contraindicated when the nodes are matted or fixed and when the nodes are large (more than 6 cm) or multiple. Postoperative radio-therapy is recommended if there is histological evidence of capsular invasion to reduce the chance of recurrence.

Extended RND includes excision of sub-occipital, retropharyngeal, parotid, pretracheal and upper mediastinal lymph nodes in addition to what is removed in classical RND. This type of RND is indicated in malignant lesions of the oropharynx, parotid and all those head and neck cancers where these nodes are likely to be involved.

Regional block dissections include localized resections that may be either suprahyoid or infrahyoid. These are recommended in carcinomas

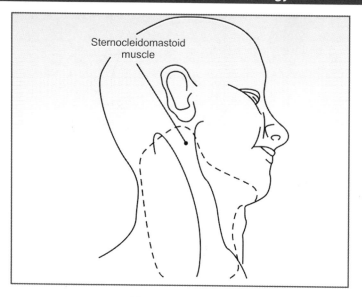

Figure 44.6: Modified radical neck dissection

of thyroid, neoplasms of major salivary glands and wide-field laryngectomy with N0 nodal status.

SKIN INCISIONS

The whole subject of RND is full of controversies and this holds true for choice of incisions as well. A number of incisions have been advocated by various authors but the popular ones are Crile's "Y" incision and MacFee's double horizontal incision (Fig. 44.7).

The basic principles of placement of incisions for RND include avoidance of incisions directly over the carotid sheath and also acute angles in the flaps to reduce the possibility of skin necrosis. Horizontal incisions are preferable for irradiated necks. The postoperative complications of RND include:
- Hemorrhage especially following carotid blow out
- Neurological deficit due to inadvertent damage to the hypoglossal or phrenic nerves and/or the sympathetic trunk
- Lymphatic fistula due to thoracic duct injury
- Airway obstruction especially following bilateral RND and Commando procedures
- Cerebral edema

PROGNOSIS

The prognosis of head and neck cancers is adversely affected by the nodal status. A review of literature reveals that five-year survival with negative

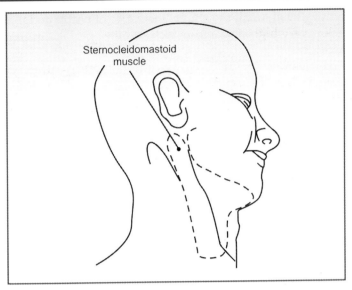

Figure 44.7: Supraomohyoid block dissection

nodes is 75 percent and this figure drops down to 49 percent, 30 percent and 13 percent respectively when one, two and three or more nodes are positive. Similarly the five year survival with involvement of upper nodes is 42 percent (above hyoid bone) whereas it is only 18 percent and 12 percent with middle and lower level positive nodes.

PRINCIPLES OF RADIATION THERAPY

Radiation therapy is an effective modality in treating local/regional disease.

Role of Radiotherapy in the management of head and neck tumors.

INDICATIONS

To eradicate occult metastasis in uninvolved areas.

To decrease the incidence of recurrence in radical neck dissections and to eradicate clinically positive nodes.

Dose: 50 Gy/25 fractions over 5 weeks is effective in controlling subclinical disease. Radiation therapy can be either preoperative or postoperative.

ELECTIVE NECK DISSECTION

Indications

Elective neck radiation is employed in tumors of the nasopharynx, base of tongue, oral segment of the tongue, the floor of the mouth, tonsil, tonsillar fossa and the pillars, the soft palate, retromolar trigone and oropharyngeal wall. In all the above, incidence of occult nodal metastasis to the neck is very high. The entire neck and the possible primary regions are covered.

For early lesions (Stage I/II), radiation therapy offers cure rates comparable to that of surgical excision.

COMBINED SURGERY AND RADIATION THERAPY

Indications

1. When there is low probability of tumor control with one particular modality.
2. When there is likelihood of gross residual disease after surgery or radiation therapy. Commonly used in T3-T4 lesions or/and N2 N3 neck nodes.
3. Selectively used for some tumors irrespective of the disease status viz. head and neck sarcomas, paranasal sinus tumors, tumors with unclear surgical margins.

COMBINATION OF SURGERY AND RADIATION THERAPY HAS TWO BASIC APPROACHES

PREOPERATIVE AND POSTOPERATIVE RADIOTHERAPY

An ideal combination would be primary surgery followed by post-operative radiation therapy, because surgery removes large bulky lesions, while radiation therapy takes care of the microscopic disease.

On the other hand, the advantages of preoperative radiation therapy would be:
1. Inoperable lesions may be converted to operable.
2. Extent of surgery may be decreased.
3. Blood supply at the time of radiation therapy is intact which is very important for effective radiation therapy.
4. Distant spread may decrease.

Tumors of the paranasal sinuses, larynx and bulky neck nodes which are on the borderline of operability can often be made operable by preoperative radiotherapy.

Tumors which infiltrate the skin, muscle and soft tissue can also benefit. The dose of radiation will be around 45-50 Gy in 25 to 28 fractions over 4 to 5 weeks.

The preoperative radiotherapy has the problem of increased morbidity and delayed wound healing.

POSTOPERATIVE RADIATION THERAPY

Indications

Positive margins at the primary macroscopic residual disease, soft tissue, skin, cartilage or bone infiltration.

Perineural invasion, lymph node metastasis of the neck, advanced primary tumors T3-T4.

The advantage of postoperative radiotherapy is that the micrometastasis may be destroyed with delayed recurrence. The disadvantages of postoperative radiation therapy would be that the distant metastases are likely to be greater and there will be decreased vascularity of tumor-bed. Radiation therapy is ideally started after 3 weeks of surgery. Radiation therapy reduces the recurrence rate to less than 5 percent.

Dose prescribed: 55 Gy to 63 Gy fractionated over 6-7 weeks.

CHEMORADIATION THERAPY

Combination of chemotherapy and radiation therapy improves local control and decreases distant metastasis thereby improving survival.

INDICATIONS

Nasopharyngeal carcinoma, advanced cancers, inoperable tumors.

Preoperative chemo-radiation therapy (2 cycles of combination chemotherapy + 40 Gy/ 20 fractions of external beam radiation therapy) may be tried initially for more locally advanced cancers. If operable surgery is followed by postoperative radiation therapy. If not chemo-radiation therapy is continued to completion. Brachytherapy application may be attempted for residual disease if any.

The acute effects of radiation include mucositis and skin erythema. The late sequelae include fibrosis, xerostomia and altered taste.

PRINCIPLES IN CHEMOTHERAPY

Chemotherapy does play a role in the palliation of recurrent or unresectable disease and has proved effective when combined with radiation for organ preservation. The head and neck tumors have unique features, as it tends to invade the deeper structures at an early stage of growth, which is responsible for a high rate of local recurrence. Chemotherapy appears to be an attractive additional therapy to the existing modalities of surgery and radiotherapy for advanced squamous cell cancers of head and neck region.

The most active agents in head and neck cancer are cisplatin or carboplatin, 5-fluorouracil, bleomycin, hydroxyurea and methotrexate.

Chemotherapy in head and neck cancer falls into 3 main categories:
1. Neoadjuvant (primary or induction) chemotherapy before surgery or radiation.
2. Maintenance (adjuvant) following definitive standard primary therapy.
3. Concomitant therapy (in combination with radiotherapy).

The principal goals of primary chemotherapy in head and neck cancers are to enhance loco-regional control, to decrease distant metastases and to improve overall survival.

"Organ preservation" is a term that means avoiding surgery at the primary site. More than 80 percent of squamous cell cancers in the head and neck regions present at the first consultation with locally advanced disease at the primary site and cervical lymph nodes.

NATURAL HISTORY AND TREATMENT OF THE SITE

Oral Cavity

Pre-cancerous lesions Leukoplakia, erythroplakia and the palatal changes associated with reverse smoking are probably important pre-cancerous conditions. A pre-cancerous lesion may be defined as a morphologically altered tissue in which cancer is more likely to occur than in its apparently normal counterpart and there is significantly increased risk of cancer. Syphilis, sideropenic dysphagia and oral sub-mucous fibrosis fall into this category. Oral lichen planus is also regarded as a possible pre-cancerous condition. The salient histological features of epithelial pre-malignancy are:

- Loss of polarity of basal cells
- Loss of cell apposition among adjacent cells
- Nuclear hyperchromatism
- Nuclear and cellular pleomorphism
- Atypical keratinisation
- Mitosis, abnormal in number, appearance or location

Oral cancer probably evolves from multiple sites from mucosa primed by carcinogens and this multi-centric origin explains the high rate of recurrence. Tumor growth and treatment affect speech and swallowing, particularly for patients with oral cavity cancers (Table 44.3).

The principles of treatment of oral cavity cancers are stage dependent. For early lesions (T1 N0, T2 N0), excision of the primary tumor with or without a unilateral or bilateral selective (supra omohyoid) neck dissection is usually the treatment of choice. Postoperative radiation therapy is indicated for close surgical margins, perineural/lymphatic/vascular invasion,

Table 44.3: Current 'T' staging of carcinoma oral cavity and tongue	
TX :	Primary tumor cannot be assessed
T0 :	No evidence of primary tumor
Tis :	Carcinoma *in situ*
T1 :	Tumor < 2 cm
T2 :	Tumor > 2 cm but < 4 cm
T3 :	Tumor > 4 cm
T4 :	Tumor invades adjacent structures

multiple positive lymph nodes and/or extra-capsular extension. For resectable advanced oral cavity tumors, combined surgery and postoperative radiation therapy is the standard treatment approach.

LIP

Squamous cell carcinoma of the lip is the most common oral cavity cancer. Most occur on the lower lip (90%). Early lesions without neck metastasis can be treated most efficiently with wide excision and closure of the defect. Neck dissection is indicated for nodal metastasis.

TONGUE

The incidence of oral cancer in India is 24.2 per 100,000 population for males and 11.2 per 100,000 population for females. The development of cancer is now believed to be a multi-step process with accumulation of many genetic abnormalities. The development of oral cancer sometimes appears clinically in its pre-malignant stage as leukoplakia, erythroplakia or both of them together. The reported average cancer transformation rates of leukoplakia vary from 0.13 percent to 36 percent with majority reports around 5 percent in 10-year follow-up. The cancer transformation rate of leukoplakia will increase with the presence of dysplasia (6 to 14 times higher), erythroplakia (4 to 7 times higher) or veracious (papillary) hyperplasia. There is a high recurrence rate of 35 percent after excision biopsy of leukoplakia.

Jin et al have reported karyotypic analysis of oral cavity squamous cell carcinomas and found that 18 percent of oral and tongue carcinomas have possible loss of tumor suppressor genes with loss of heterozygosis (LOH) mostly at 9p 23-22. Li et al also showed that 9p21 and 3p14 losses are present in 51 percent leukoplakia lesions of oral cavity. Those pre-malignant lesions with LOH had the higher risk (37%) of subsequent development of invasive squamous cell carcinoma. The p53 tumor suppressor gene overexpression is found to be an early event in the process of carcinogenesis in oral carcinoma. The over expression of p53 is mostly due to mutation. The down regulation of epithelial cellular adhesion molecules and breakdown of extra-cellular matrix are hallmarks of invasive carcinoma. In oral tumor cells,there are expressions of MMP-1 (Matrix metalloproteinase), MMP 2, MT1-MMP and TIMP-2 (enzyme tissue inhibitors of MMP) while in surrounding stoma cells there are expressions of MMP-3, MMP-9 and TIMP-1.

TREATMENT

It is a more common practice to treat Stage I and II carcinomas of the tongue with surgery alone and Stage III and IV carcinomas with combined surgery and postoperative radiotherapy.

OPTIMAL SURGICAL RESECTION FOR ADEQUATE LOCAL CONTROL

It has been shown that there is a high risk of local recurrence despite adjuvant radiotherapy for patients with positive resection margin after surgical resection of cancer of the tongue. It is important to ensure adequate initial surgical resection of the tumor rather than relying on adjuvant radiotherapy or subsequent surgical salvage for the residual tumor left behind. Histological examination of resection margins by frozen section at operation is always recommended. The surgical techniques of tumor resection vary from partial glossectomy and hemiglossectomy to subtotal and total glossectomy. Additional resection of larynx, tonsils and mandible is necessary in more advanced cancer. The tongue is a three-dimensional structure and its carcinoma spreads in three-dimensional planes. Since 96 percent tumor has local spread within 1 to 2 cm from the edge of the tumor, a clear histological resection margin could be achieved with over 95 percent confidence level for a 2 to 3 cm margin from the tumor border. This should be the optimal choice in the surgical resection of oral tongue carcinoma.

HIGH INCIDENCE OF SUB-CLINICAL NODAL METASTASIS OF EARLY TONGUE CARCINOMA

Tongue carcinoma has high propensity of nodal metastasis even in its early stage. The commonest site of nodal metastasis is ipsilateral level II and 95 percent metastatic nodes are found in the ipsilateral levels II, III and I. Contralateral nodal metastasis and contralateral nodal recurrence were found only in less than 5 percent patients. All available preoperative imaging modalities including CT scan, MRI and ultrasound guided fine-needle aspiration cytology cannot replace the role of elective neck dissection as an accurate diagnostic procedure for staging of the N0 neck.

PREDICTIVE MARKERS OF SUB-CLINICAL NODAL METASTASIS

Tumor thickness is a significant prognostic factor for nodal metastasis. The incidence of sub-clinical nodal metastasis increased with tumor thickness from 10 percent (thickness<3 mm), 36 percent (thickness > 3 mm and < 6 mm), 60 percent (thickness > 6 mm and < 9 mm) to 54 percent (thickness > 9 mm).

Adequate surgical margins are required for tongue carcinomas, and most early lesions require hemi-glossectomy. For more advanced tongue carcinomas, surgical management often includes partial glossectomy, neck dissection, and often mandibulectomy. The pull-through or lip split/paramedian mandibulectomy approaches are most commonly utilized for advanced tongue tumors. When tumor extends across the midline or involves the base of the tongue, sub-total or total glossectomy may be required. Modern reconstructive techniques, particularly free tissue transfer, have greatly improved the functional outcome in these patients. In spite of these improvements, a few of total glossectomy patients often require permanent feeding gastrostomy.

EVALUATION OF A CERVICAL LYMPH NODE IN SUSPECTED HEAD AND NECK TUMORS

Physical examination of oral cavity and pharynx reveals 90 percent of primary.

95 percent of cases can be diagnosed by FNAC.

If FNAC is plosive for SCC, the next step would be a CT scan of the head and neck regions, and oropharyngeal panendoscopy and multiple random biopsies.

If the primary still eludes the clinician, the case is treated as one of carcinoma of unknown primary. The node is treated with surgical excision and radiotherapy.

FLOOR OF MOUTH

Surgery is the treatment of choice for most patients with floor of mouth cancer. Patients with lesions greater than 2 cm in diameter should have either selective neck dissection (supra omohyoid) or irradiation of the cervical nodes. The rates of mandibular invasion increase with stages. Involvement of periosteum dictates partial thickness mandibular resection. Exploration by elevation of periosteum at the time of surgery is recommended when partial thickness mandibular resection is planned. Depending upon the site of mandibular attachment one can perform a rim (superior edge) or lingual cortical plate mandibulectomy. When there is radiological or clinical evidence of bony invasion, a segmental mandibulectomy (full thickness) should be performed. State-of-the-art reconstruction for large defects is the radial forearm free fascio-cutaneous flap. Advanced tumors with involvement of anterior mandibular arch require reconstruction with free osteocutaneous flaps (fibula, iliac crest, and scapula).

BUCCAL MUCOSA

Buccal carcinoma is an uncommon form of oral cavity carcinoma. Buccal cancers always arise in areas of leukoplakia. Stage I and II lesions are treated with radiotherapy; Stage III/IV lesions are treated by surgery with postoperative radiotherapy. The reconstruction of oral cavity in most cases of advanced buccal cancer is always a challenging one as in most cases, a through and through facial defect may occur after adequate excision of the tumor.

RETROMOLAR TRIGONE/ALVEOLAR RIDGE

The treatment of retromolar tumors is always fraught with surgical problems. Excision of the tumor with a clear 2.5 cm margin is not easy as trismus is a serious problem. Even with a split mandible, the approach is difficult. Most early tumors of the retromolar trigone or alveolar ridge can be treated with transpolar resection with rim mandibulectomy. Advanced lesions require segmental mandibulectomy followed by radiotherapy and chemotherapy. The prognosis in most cases is poor.

OROPHARYNX

The most common presenting symptom of oropharyngeal cancer is chronic sore throat and disturbances in swallowing.

Because lymphatic drainage of the oropharynx can be bilateral in all sites except lateralized oral primaries, radiation is often the first-treatment approach.

Advanced oropharyngeal tumors can be treated with combined modality treatment. Persistent disease in the neck requires comprehensive neck dissection.

TONSIL

Tonsil cancer in its early stage can be treated equally well with surgery or radiation. The advantage of surgery and postoperative radiotherapy for advanced tonsillar cancer is that both the primary site and neck receive combined modality treatment. Advanced tonsillar cancers encroaching on the mandible require composite resection. Tumors that do not invade the medial pterygoid muscle can be approached with lip split and para-median mandibulectomy (preserving the mandible, mental nerve and chin sensation) and wide local excision with neck dissection.

BASE OF THE TONGUE

The management of base of the tongue cancers is always a challenging one to the surgeon. Early tumors are best treated with external-beam radiation and advanced tumors with surgery and radiation. There are several ways to surgically approach the base of the tongue; including mandibulectomy, lateral pharyngectomy, suprahyoid and median glossectomy.

SOFT PALATE AND POSTERIOR PHARYNGEAL WALL

Both these tumors have bilateral lymphatic drainage. Radiotherapy alone is preferred in most cases. Small tumors of the soft palate and post-pharyngeal wall can be treated surgically and reconstructed with skin graft.

TREATMENT OF THE LYMPH NODES OF THE NECK

The management of the lymph nodes of the neck is important because of the high incidence of nodal metastasis. A modified anterior neck dissection is appropriate for patients with no nodal metastasis as prophylaxis. Comprehensive neck dissection by which I to V lymph nodes are removed is recommended for patients who have clinically positive nodes and who had postoperative radiotherapy. The retropharyngeal lymph nodes are often in the drainage pathway for the primaries of the oropharyngeal or hypopharyngeal wall.

The readers must note that the treatment of unresectable or recurrent neck tumors is hardly satisfactory. The mean survival rate of advanced cancer of the head and neck is less than 6 months. No therapy has proved to be effective or adequate. At the same time multimodality treatment should be attempted to reduce the tumor burden such as surgery, radiation therapy and chemotherapy.

Radiation therapy is most rewarding in combination with surgery rather than when done alone.

Local and regional recurrence can be treated with radiation or radiation with surgery. In case of nasopharyngeal tumors, a second course of radiation is found to be useful.

Combination of chemotherapy also is being tried in many centers with variable results. In case, there is widespread metastasis in initial presentation, combination chemotherapy with cisplatin and infusional fluorouracil is the commonly used therapeutic regimen.

Mostly it will depend on the patient's preference. In the case of patient with good performance status, no previous chemotherapy and minimal tumor burden, the treatment will be of benefit to the patient. With radiation and chemotherapy a group of patients will be disease-free for many years.

FOLLOW-UP

Regular 3 monthly follow-up is necessary to those patients who have undergone surgery alone or with radiotherapy during the first year. The metastasis develops in the neck glands. After the first year examination once in three months is sufficient. The peak incidence of development of secondaries is after the second year, the most of it locally or in the lungs or in the brain. Imaging modalities are necessary for confirmation of the recurrence. Chemotherapy should be tried with the intent of increasing the survival period without pain.

TUMORS OF HYPOPHARYNX

Squamous cell carcinoma of hypopharynx is an aggressive, deadly disease with a poor prognosis. The presentation is usually late and the patient has advanced disease on first consultation.

PRIMARY TUMOR STAGING OF HYPOPHARYNX CANCER

T1: Tumor limited to one sub-site of hypopharynx and < 2 cm.

T2: Tumor involves more than one subset of hypopharynx or adjacent site or measures> 2 cm but < 4 cm.

T3: Tumor measures > 4 cm or with fixation of hemilarynx

In Stage 1 and 2, the treatment is radiation therapy while in Stage 3 with locally advanced disease, total laryngectomy with radiation is the suggested treatment. It depends on the physician's and the patient's preference. In some centers, chemotherapy with radiation is attempted so that there is 'organ preservation'. The results of radical surgery with functional impairment have not increased the survival rate in hypopharyngeal cancer.

PROSTHESIS AFTER ORAL CANCER SURGERY

Quite often eradication of malignant disease by surgery leaves the patient with gross deformity. Severe functional disability and gross disfigurement result in such cases. The need for the construction of maxillofacial prosthesis has increased over the years and has become a routine procedure forming the part of the treatment for those who require replacement of anatomic parts of the face and its associated structures after surgery.

INDICATIONS FOR MAXILLOFACIAL PROSTHESIS

1. To restore esthetics and function to the patients in whom reconstructive plastic surgery is not feasible.
2. For patients who are more likely surgical risks.
3. For patients in the poor socio-economic group who cannot afford costly reconstructive surgery.

THE OBJECTIVES OF PROSTHESIS

1. Restoration of esthetics
2. Restoration of functions
3. Protection of tissues
4. Therapeutic and healing effect
5. Psychological therapy

REQUIREMENTS OF PROSTHESIS

A good prosthesis should:
1. Restore natural function to near normalcy.
2. Be life-like in appearance.
3. Be comfortable to the patient and be properly retained.
4. Be durable, strong and can be easily cleared.

Materials used for the fabrication of face-maxillary prosthesis: acrylic resins, vinyl polymers, copolymers, silicone rubber and polyurethane. Types of prostheses used after cancer surgery are:

1. An obturator
2. Prosthesis for segmental defects

It is advisable to use spectacles as an indirect mechanical retention device whenever the restoration is near the orbital cavity.

In summary, prosthesis is useful for the immediate restoration of the dissected areas for temporary protection and also in cases where reconstructive plastic surgery may not be possible.

FURTHER READING

1. American Joint Committee on Cancer. AJCC Cancer Staging Manual, 1997.
2. American Society for Head and Neck Surgery and the Society of Head and Neck Surgeons, 1996.
3. Batsakis JG. Tumors of the head and neck: Clinical and pathological considerations. Baltimore: Williams and Wilkins, 1974.
4. Batsakis JG. Surgical margins in the squamous cell carcinomas 1988;97:213-14.
5. Boyle P, Macfarkane GJ, Mc Ginn R. Primary Tumors in the Head and Neck 1990:80-138.
6. Brizel DM, Allbers M, Fisher SR. Hyperfractionated irradiation with or without concurrent chemotherapy for locally advanced head and neck cancer. N Eng J Med 1998;338:1798-1804.
7. Byres RM, Bland KL, Borlase B. Prognostic and therapeutic value of frozen section determinations in the surgical treatment of squamous carcinoma of the head and neck. Am J Surg 1978;136:525-28.
8. De Villers EM, Weidauer H, Otto H. Papillomavirus in human tongue carcinomas. Int J Cancer 1985;36;575-78.
9. Laramore GE, Scott GB. Adjuvant chemotherapy for resectable squamous cell carcinomas of the head and neck. Int J Radiat Oncol Biol Phys 1992;23:885-86.
10. Laramore GE. Radiation Therapy of Head and Neck Cancer, 1988.
11. Paz B, Cook N, Odom-Maryon T. Human Papillomavirus (HPV) in head and neck cancer 1992;51:845-50.
12. Robbins KT. Pocket Guide to Neck Dissection, 1991.
13. Sessions D, Cummngs C, Weymeller E. Nasal cavity, paranasal sinuses, and anterior cranial fossa. Mosby Year Book 1992;107-62.
14. Shanmugaratnam K, Path FRC, Sohin LH. The WHO histological classification of tumors of the upper respiratory track and ear 1993;71:2689-97.
15. Silver C. The Larynx and Hypopharynx: Atlas of Head and Neck Surgery. NY: Churchill Livingstone 1986:167-251.
16. Wynder EL, Hoffman D, Schottenfield D, Fraumen JF Jr (Eds). Cancer Epidemiology and Prevention, Philadelphia: WB Saunders 1982:277-92.

APPENDIX 15

International comparison, India and five continents—AAR (ICMR and IARC).

CANCER ORAL CAVITY TONGUE (MALE)

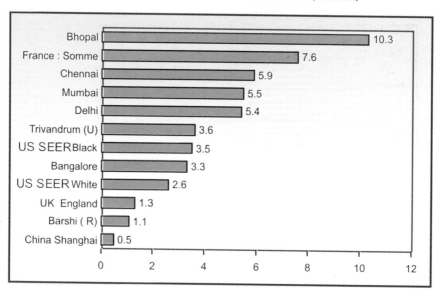

CANCER ORAL CAVITY TONGUE (FEMALE)

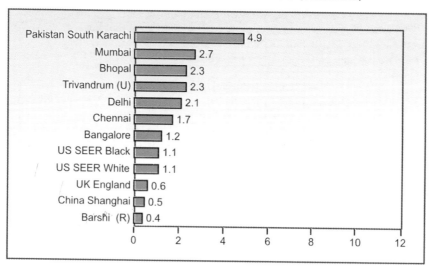

Rate per 100,000

APPENDIX 16

International comparison; India and five continents—AAR (ICMR and IARC).

CANCER ORAL CAVITY (MALE)

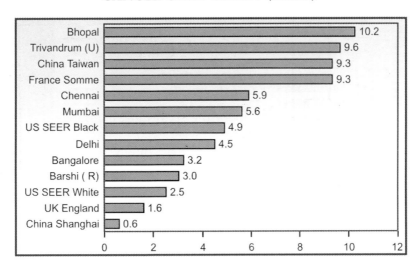

CANCER ORAL CAVITY (FEMALE)

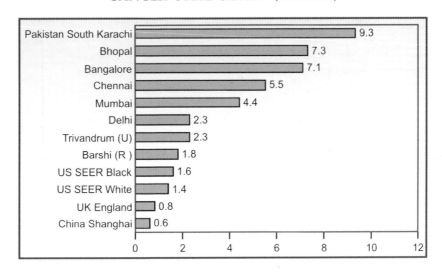

Rate per 100,000

Cancer of Head and Neck (Ear, Nose and Throat)

45

Mathew Dominic

Cancers of the head and neck are the sixth most common cancers worldwide. Although there are a variety of histological types, squamous cell carcinoma predominates among cancers of the upper aerodigestive tracts.

ETIOLOGY AND EPIDEMIOLOGY

Laryngeal and hypopharyngeal cancers are the most common head and neck squamous cell cancers in the western world. Except for post cricoid carcinoma, all other cancers in the head and neck have a male preponderance; the ratio being as high as male to female 10:1. In cancers of the larynx, cigarette smoking and alcohol consumption are the two strongest etiological factors both independently and synergistically. Cessation of smoking leads to a gradual reduction in risk by 70 percent after 10 years. Some carcinogens act on specific sites. Nickel and chromium dusts are implicated in carcinoma of the nose, paranasal sinuses, larynx and lung. Wood workers exposed to hard wood dust have a higher incidence of adeno-carcinoma of the paranasal sinuses. Children who are intro-duced to a diet of salted fish run a higher risk of developing cancer of the nasopharynx. Nitrosamine in the salted fish is suspected to be the carcinogen. Certain viruses also play an etiological role in head and neck cancers. Human Papilloma-virus (HPV), a DNA virus has been found in 15 to 62 percent of head and neck cancers using polymerase chain reaction (PCR) based analysis. Epstein-Barr virus (EBV) is associated with development of nasopharyngeal carcinoma.

Anatomical regions in head and neck can be divided into oral cavity, nasal fossa, paranasal sinuses, nasopharynx, oro-pharynx, larynx and hypopharynx.

Other head and neck structures are ears, salivary glands and cervical lymph nodes. Certain anatomists include thyroid glands too in this region.
Tumors of the oral cavity Discussed in Chapter 44.

TUMORS OF NOSE AND PARANASAL SINUSES

These are rarer sites of the head and neck cancers. They have a great variety of histological types. These tumors present late and have late nodal metastasis.

ETIOLOGY

High incidence of these tumors is seen in people working in wood industry, nickel refining and leather industry. Cancer of the maxillary sinus is common in Bantus of South Africa who use locally made snuff, which is rich in nickel and chromium.

HISTOLOGY

80 percent of the malignant tumors are squamous cell carcinoma. The rest of them are adenocarcinoma, adenoid cystic carcinoma, melanoma and sarcoma.

CLINICAL PRESENTATION

The tumor of the maxillary sinus can present in many forms, such as nasal obstruction, epistaxis, infraorbital anesthesia, toothache, facial swelling, facial pain and trismus. Ethmoidal sinus tumors can cause nasal obstruction, epistaxis, proptosis or diplopia. The examination consists of anterior and posterior rhinoscopy and nasal endoscopy with a fiberoptic endoscope.

INVESTIGATIONS

CT scan of the sinuses demonstrates presence of the tumor, its extent and the presence of erosion of the bony walls. Biopsy confirms the diagnosis and the histological type of the tumor.

CLASSIFICATION

1. Ohngren's classification
   Ohngren's line is an imaginary radiological line extending from the medial canthus of the eye to the angle of the mandible. Growths above the line have a poorer prognosis than those situated below the line.
2. Lederman's classification
   This classification uses two lines; one passing through the floors of the orbits and another through the floors of the maxillary antra dividing the nose and paranasal sinuses into:

a. superstructure   ethmoid, sphenoid, frontal sinuses and olfactory areas of the nose

b. mesostructure   maxillary sinuses and respiratory part of the nose

c. infrastructure   alveolar process

3. TMN classification

This is the currently used classification.

T classification: Maxillary sinus

T1   Tumor limited to the antral mucosa with no erosion or destruction of bone.

T2   Tumor causing bone erosion or destruction, except for posterior wall, including extension into hard palate and/or middle nasal meatus.

T3   Tumor invades any of the following: bone of posterior wall of maxillary sinus, subcutaneous tissue, skin of cheek, floor of medial wall of orbit.

T4   Tumor invades orbital contents beyond the floor or medial wall including apex and/or any of the following: cribriform plate, base of skull, nasopharynx, sphenoid sinus, frontal sinus.

TREATMENT

Both radiotherapy and surgery are required for proper control of the disease.

Cancers of the Oropharynx

Oropharynx extends from the level of the hard palate superiorly to the level of the hyoid inferiorly. Anterior limit is the anterior faucial pillar. The anterior wall consists of the base of the tongue posterior to the foramen cecum, vallecula and the lingual surface of the epiglottis. The lateral wall consists of the anterior and posterior pillars and the palatine tonsils. Roof consists of the oral surface of the soft palate and the posterior wall consists of the posterior pharyngeal wall from the level of the hard palate to the level of the hyoid.

ETIOLOGY

Tobacco is the most significant etiological factor. Consumption of alcohol, chewing of betel nut, dental sepsis, iron deficiency anemia, previous radiation, submucous fibrosis and human papillomavirus infection are the other factors which are implicated in the etiology of oropharyngeal cancers.

TUMOR TYPES

Ninety percent are squamous cell carcinoma. 8 percent are non-Hodgkin's lymphoma and the rest 2 percent are minor salivary gland tumors.

SITES

The commonest site of squamous cell carcinoma in the oropharynx is the lateral wall accounting for over 60 percent of the total tumors. 25 percent occur in the base of tongue, 10 percent in the soft palate and 5 percent in the posterior wall. 90 percent of non-Hodgkin's lymphomas occur in the lateral wall or base of tongue. Minor salivary gland tumors occur in the soft palate, lateral wall or base of tongue.

T STAGE

T1 is tumor less than 2 cm. T2 is tumor more than 2 cm but less than 4 cm. T3 is tumor more than 4 cm and T4 is when tumor invades adjacent structures.

CLINICAL FEATURES

The earliest symptom may be a sore throat. Some patients may complain of foreign body sensation in the throat. This may later progress to dysphagia. As the tumor progresses pain may be referred to the ipsilateral ear via the glossopharyngeal nerve. As the tumor spreads laterally to involve the parapharyngeal muscles there may be trismus. Sometimes the only complaint may be an enlarged lymph node in the neck. Careful examination will demonstrate the primary in the oropharynx.

EXAMINATION

Clinical examination must consist of examination of the oral cavity and oropharynx and mirror examination of the post nasal space and larynx to assess any extension to these regions. The base of tongue must be palpated as tumors in this region may not be seen on inspection but the induration may be felt on palpation.

CT and MRI are helpful in assessing the tumor and its extent.

TREATMENT

Smaller tumors may be treated by single modality of radiation or surgery. Larger tumors may require surgery followed by radiation.

MALIGNANCIES OF THE NASOPHARYNX

Nasopharyngeal malignancies can be classified as follows:

Epithelial	Nasopharyngeal carcinoma
	Adenocarcinoma
	Adenoid cystic carcinoma
Soft tissue	Fibrosarcoma
	Rhabdomyosarcoma
	Angiosarcoma

Malignant lymphomas   Non-Hodgkin's
                        Hodgkin's
   Of these the nasopharyngeal carcinoma is the most common, accounting
for 75 to 95 percent of all nasopharyngeal cancers.

NASOPHARYNGEAL CARCINOMA

Epidemiology

The Chinese and the South Koreans have a high incidence of this tumor,
ranging from 15 to 30 per 100,000. South East Asian races have a moderate
incidence of 5 to 15 per 100,000. The rest of the world including India has
a low incidence of less than 1 per 100,000. Sex ratio male to female is 2:3.
Maximum incidence of the tumor occurs between 35 and 65 years.

ETIOLOGY

Epstein-Barr virus is implicated in the etiology of nasopharyngeal
carcinomas. 90 percent of the cases have raised antibody titers to Epstein-
Barr virus antigen. Viral genome can also be identified in the tumor cells.
Environmental factors like air pollution, smoking of tobacco and opium,
nitrosamines from dry salted fish, smoke from burning incenses have all
been incriminated in the etiology of nasopharyngeal carcinoma (Figs 45.1
and 45.2).

CLINICAL FEATURES

Symptoms may be divided into four main groups:

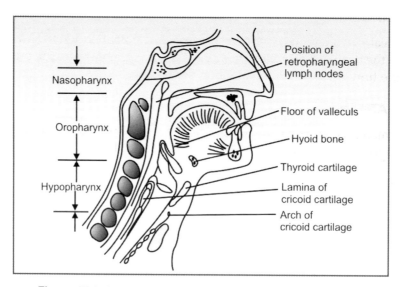

Figure 45.1: Sagittal section through upper aerodigestive tract

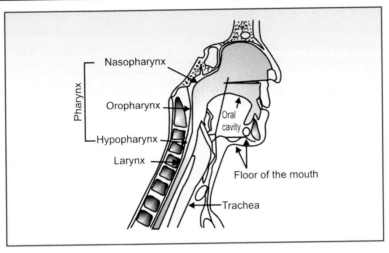

Figure 45.2: Sagittal section through nose, mouth, pharynx and larynx

1. Cervical nodal metastasis	60% of the cases have painless cervical lymph adenopathy
2. Nasal	40% have epistaxis and other nasorespiratory symptoms
3. Otological	30% have tinnitus, otalgia or deafness
4. Neurological	20% have neurological involvement. Any cranial nerve may be involved. Commonest are V, VI, IX and X.

DIAGNOSIS

Clinical examination consists of postnasal examination with mirror and with the flexible Nasopharyngoscope. CT scan demonstrates the presence of the tumor, its extent and any bony erosion.

TREATMENT

The mainstay of the treatment is radiotherapy. Chemotherapy is useful in advanced nodal disease. Surgery has only limited role.

ANATOMY OF LARYNX (FIGS 45.3 AND 45.4)

1. supraglottis
   a. epiglottis
   b. aryepiglottic fold
   c. arytenoids
   d. ventricular bands
   e. ventricles

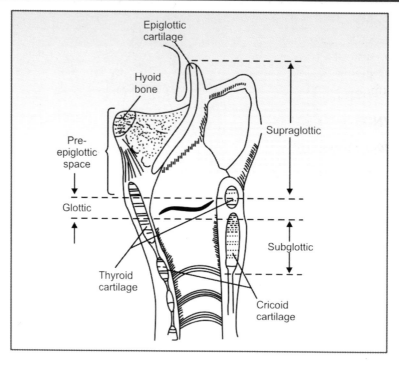

Figure 45.3: Sagittal view through the larynx

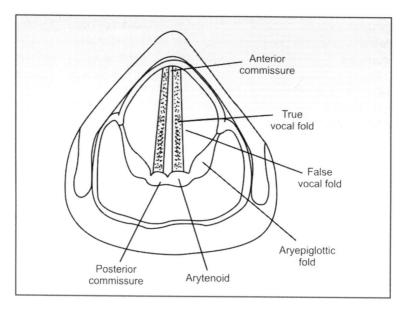

Figure 45.4: Laryngoscopic view of the larynx

2. glottis
   a. vocal cords
   b. anterior commissure
   c. posterior commissure
3. subglottis

LARYNGEAL TUMORS

Surgical Pathology

About 95 percent of laryngeal tumors are malignant and true benign tumors account for less than 5 percent of laryngeal tumors. The relative incidence of benign tumors is as follows:

Papilloma	85%
Adenoma	5%
Chondroma	5%
Miscellaneous	5%

Squamous carcinomas forms the vast majority of malignant laryngeal lesions. The relative incidence of the malignant tumors is as follows:

Squamous cell carcinoma	85%
Carcinoma *in situ*	3%
Verrucous carcinoma	3%
Undifferentiated carcinoma	5%
Adenocarcinoma	0.5%
Miscellaneous	3.5%

Approximately 90 percent of the laryngeal cancers occur in men and the peak incidence is between the age of 55 and 65 years. The cancer is more common in the lower socioeconomic group and in the urban population. Tobacco and alcohol are well-established risk factors for laryngeal cancers.

SUPRAGLOTTIC CANCER

Supraglottic cancers account for about 30 to 40 percent of the laryngeal cancers. The commonest site is the epiglottis followed by false cords and aryepiglottic folds. Supraglottic cancers may spread locally and invade adjoining areas like vallecula, base of tongue and pyriform sinus. Supraglottic growths are often silent. Hoarseness is a late symptom. Patients may present with throat pain, dysphagia, referred otalgia or cervical lymphadenopathy.

GLOTTIC CANCER

These form the majority of the laryngeal cancers comprising about 50 to 60 percent of the total. The cancer may spread locally across the anterior commissure to the opposite cord, upwards to the supraglottis or downwards to the subglottis. Glottic lesions present early with hoarseness of voice. Further growth may result in stridor and laryngeal obstruction.

EXAMINATION

Apart from routine ENT examination and general examination, specific examination would include an indirect laryngoscopy to assess the presence and extent of the tumor. This can be confirmed in the out-patient clinic with a flexible fiberoptic nasopharyngolaryngoscope. The neck is examined to evaluate the lymph node metastasis. CT scan and MRI are useful in assessing the extent of the tumor. The diagnosis is confirmed with a direct laryngoscopy and biopsy.

TREATMENT

Carcinoma *in situ*	microendoscopic removal laser excision
Small tumors of marginal zone	microendoscopic removal laser excision
T1, T2	radiation
T3	radiation or surgery
T4	surgery

TUMORS OF THE HYPOPHARYNX

Hypopharynx is the lowermost part of the pharynx. It extends from the level of the hyoid bone to the lower border of the cricoid cartilage. The hypopharynx consists of three anatomical sites:
  a. pyriform sinus
  b. post cricoid region
  c. posterior pharyngeal wall
  Almost all tumors of the hypopharynx are squamous cell carcinomas. The most common site is the pyriform sinus accounting for 50 to 75 percent of all hypopharyngeal tumors. Post cricoid region accounts for 40 percent and only 10 percent occur in the posterior pharyngeal wall. Alcohol and tobacco are the major etiological factors in hypopharyngeal carcinoma. There is a high incidence of post cricoid carcinoma in iron deficiency anemia and in Plummer Vinson syndrome. Post cricoid carcinoma is the only head and neck cancer that is more common in women than in men.

CLINICAL FEATURES

Dysphagia	may begin as a sensation of food sticking in the throat on swallowing. The dysphagia is persistent and progressive.
Pain	is lateralised to the side of the tumor. It is more on swallowing and may be referred to the ipsilateral ear.

Hoarseness　indicates extension of the tumor to the larynx.

Neck mass　75 percent of pyriform sinus tumors will have ipsilateral neck node enlargement. 5 percent will have bilateral involvement.

EXAMINATION

Indirect laryngoscopy

Neck examination

Flexible nasopharyngolaryngoscopy

ENT examination

General examination

Investigations

Barium swallow to assess lower end of the tumor

The surgeon must look for a second primary in this area. and a fine needle aspiration cytology must be done for the diagnosis of the tumor and the enlarged node, if any.

CT scan

MRI

Direct laryngoscopy　confirms the presence of the tumor

　delineates its extent

　helps in the biopsy of the tumor

Treatment

Stage I, II　radiotherapy or surgery

Stage III, IV　surgery followed by postoperative radiotherapy.

FURTHER READING

1. Helman JI. Maxillectomy. Atlas Oral Maxillofac Surg Clin North Am 1997.
2. Himi Y, Yoshizaki T, Sato K, Furukawa M. Respiratory epithelial adenomatoid hamartoma of the maxillary sinus. J Laryngol Otol 2002;317-18.
3. Jeng YM, Sung MT, Fang CL, Huang HY, Mao TL, Cheng W. Sinonasal undifferentiated carcinoma and nasopharyngeal-type undifferentiated carcinoma: Two clinically, biologically, and histopathologically distinct entities. Am J Surg Pathol 2002;26(3):371-76.
4. Omeroglu A, Petruzzelli GJ, Husain AN, Ciesla MC. Pathologic quiz case. A sinonasal mass in a 79-year-old African American woman. Arch Pathol Lab Med 2002;126(4):493-94.
5. Pignataro L, Peri A, Ottaviani F. Breast carcinoma metastatic to the ethmoid sinus: A case report. Tumor 2001;87(6):455-57.
6. Roth J, Friedlander PL, Palacios E. Primary adenocarcinoma of the maxillary sinus simulating an osteosarcoma. Ear Nose Throat J 2002;81(1):14.

LARYNX

7. Early pharyngolaryngeal carcinomas with palpable nodes. French Head and Neck Study Group (GETTEC). Am J Surg 1991.

8. Elahi A, Zheng Z, Park J, Eyring K, McCaffrey T, Lazarus P. The human OGG1 DNA repair enzyme and its association with orolaryngeal cancer risk. Carcinogenesis 2002;23(7):1229-34.

9. Jones AS, Wilde A, McRae RD, Phillips DE, Field JK, et al. The treatment of early squamous cell carcinoma of the piriform fossa. Clin Otolaryngol 1994;19(6):485-90.

10. Lang JC, Borchers J, Danahey D, Smith S, Stover DG, Agarwal, Malone JP, Schuller DE, et al. Mutational status of overexpress p16 in head and neck cancer: for germline mutation of p16/p14ARF. Int J Oncol 2002;21(2):401-08.

11. Nunez DA, West K, Wells M. Human papilloma viruses in the human hypopharynx. Clin Otolaryngol 1994;19(3):258-60.

12. Rosenfeld RM, Grundfast KM, Milmoe GJ. Occult sinus of the piriform fossa. Otolaryngol Head Neck Surg 1993;109(1):126-32.

13. Sen U, Sankaranarayanan R, Mandal S, Ramanakumar AV, Parkin DM, et al. Cancer patterns in eastern India: The first report of the Kolkata cancer registry. Int J Cancer 2002;100(1):86-91.

14. Sindwani R, Matthews TW, Thomas J, Venkatesan VM. Epithelioid leiomyosarcoma of the larynx. Head Neck 1998;20(6):563-67.

15. Wickham MH, Narula AA, Barton RP, Bradley PJ. Emergency laryngectomy. Clin Otolaryngol 1990;15(1):35-38.

APPENDIX 17

International comparison, India and five continents—AAR (ICMR and IARC)

CANCER HYPOPHARYNX (MALE)

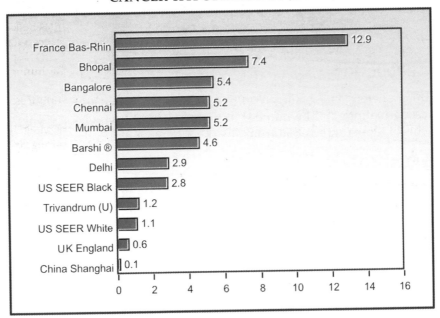

CANCER LARYNX (MALE)

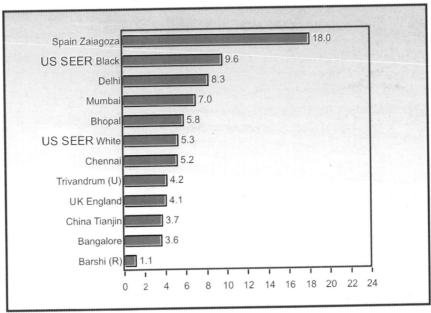

Rate per 100,000

Skin Tumors

46

Rachel Mathai, NV Seethalakshmy

INTRODUCTION

Skin is a heterogeneous organ with tissues of ectodermal and mesodermal origin. The number of tumors arising from elements of these exceeds that from any other organ in the body.

CLASSIFICATION

Skin tumors are classified on the basis of tissues of origin; namely, epithelial and mesodermal tissues. These are further classified as benign, premalignant and malignant. Epithelial tumors arise from surface epidermis, epidermal adnexal structures and melanocytes. The tumors arising from the surface epidermis are listed in (Table 46.1).

MALIGNANT TUMORS

PAGET'S DISEASE (FIG. 46.1, PLATE 11)

Paget's disease is an eczematoid intraepidermal squamous cell carcinoma occurring most frequently on the breast. Women in the 5th to 6th decades are usually affected. Rarely Paget's disease may occur on male breast. It presents as a well defined erythematous eczematous plaque on the nipple or areola.

Table 46.1: Non-melanocytic surface epidermal tumors	
Pre-malignant	*Malignant*
Various keratoses	Squamous cell carcinoma
Cutaneous horn	Paget's disease
Leukoplakia	Merkel cell carcinoma
Bowen's disease	Basal cell carcinoma
Erythroplasia of Queyrat	
Bowenoid papulosis	
Intraepidermal eyelid carcinoma	
Melanocytic tumors	
Malignant melanoma	

Plate   11

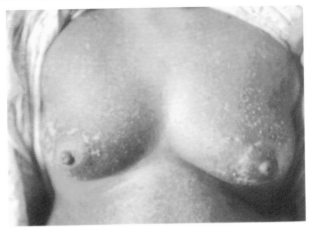

Figure 46.1: Paget's disease of the breast

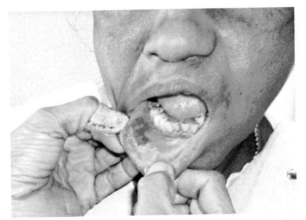

Figure 46.2: Squamous cell carcinoma of the lower lip

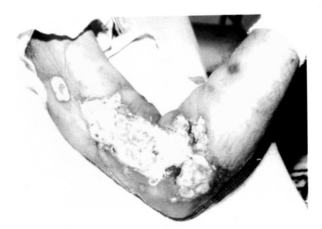

Figure 46.3: Kaposi's sarcoma

Usually one breast is affected. Extramammary Paget's disease can occur on the vulva, perianal region and scrotum. Very rarely groin or axillary areas have been involved. The lesion slowly spreads developing induration and later ulcerates. Ductal carcinoma is frequently seen. Metastasis is common. Diagnosis is established on histopathological evidence. Wide local excision is advocated.

SQUAMOUS CELL CARCINOMA (SCC) (FIG. 46.2, PLATE 11)

SCC is a malignant tumor of keratinocytes and it occurs on skin and mucosa. It is seen in the older age group with male predominance. SCC appears on a background of prior insult. Predisposing factors are chronic actinic damage, irradiation, exposure to carcinogenic chemicals, chronic inflammation in long standing ulcers and infective granulomas. SCC has been seen on chronic discoid lupus erythematosis and epidermodysplasia verruciformis (a generalized virally induced dermatosis). Patients with genetic pigmentation disorders as in albinism and xeroderma pigmentosum develop multiple SCC. Immunosuppression is another predisposing factor. There may be an increased risk for both squamous cell and basal cell carcinoma in HIV infection. Prolonged damage due to heat can cause SCC. In PUVA-treated psoriatic patients, the risk is dose dependent. Tobacco chewing is very common cause in oral mucosal carcinoma. Verrucous growth and noduloulcerative lesions are noted. Ulcers have everted edges and bleed easily. At times SCC appears as extension of a deeper situated tumor as in the case of parotid, nasal and oral mucosa. A few cases have been reported as complication of disorders like ichthyosis, epidermal nevus, porokeratosis, and congenital lymphedema.

Squamous cell carcinomas of the skin exhibit immunoreactivity for high-molecular-weight keratin and epithelial membrane antigen.

Verrucous SCC are usually seen in the oral or genital region. They are of low grade malignancy. It may be positive for HPV.

PATHOLOGY

Histopathological grading depends upon mitotic activity, degree of keratinization, presence of horn pearls and tumor demarcation. The best prognostic factors are staging, level of dermal invasion, and vertical tumor thickness.

MANAGEMENT OF SKIN CANCER

The management of skin cancer depends on the histologic nature of the tumor, the anatomic site, the underlying medical status of the patient, and whether the tumor is primary or recurrent. SCC is treated by excisional surgery, extirpation by Mohs micrographic surgery (MMS) or non-excisional approaches like electrodesiccation and curettage and cryotherapy. Radiotherapy (RT) generally is indicated when the patient's health or size or extent of the tumor precludes surgical extirpation.

BASAL CELL CARCINOMA

Basal cell carcinomas (BCC) are seen almost exclusively on hair bearing skin. They usually occur as single lesion on face in adults. Synchronous and metachronous tumors can occur. Children and young adults are affected exceptionally.

PREDISPOSING FACTORS

Most important predisposing factor is prolonged exposure of light coloured skin to strong sunlight. Basal cell carcinomas may also develop in sunlight-protected skin, in nevus sebaceous of Jadassohn, following arsenic ingestion, X-ray exposure, skin injury, venous stasis, chickenpox scars, tattoos, hair transplantation scars, and immune suppression.

Basal cell carcinomas arise from basally located cells of the epidermis and pilosebaceous units. The tumors may have solid, cystic, adenoid, keratotic, pigmented, infiltrating, and sclerosing (morphea-like) patterns. Intercellular amyloid material is seen in some cases. Immunohistochemically, the cells of basal cell carcinoma are positive for keratin (particularly low-molecular-weight type), but usually negative for EMA. More than 80 percent of basal cell carcinomas over express p53 protein.

Basal cell nevus syndrome (Gorlin's syndrome) is characterized by multiple basal cell carcinomas, palmar pits, calcification of dura, keratinous cysts of the jaws, skeletal anomalies, and occasional abnormalities of the central nervous system, mesentery, and endocrine organs.

In *linear unilateral basal cell nevus*, closely set nodules of BCC are present at birth. In *Bazex syndrome*, multiple small BCC arise on the faces of young adults or adolescents.

SPREAD AND METASTASES

Basal cell carcinoma usually grows in a slow and indolent fashion. However, if untreated, the tumor may invade the subcutaneous fat, skeletal muscle and nearby bone. Metastasis is exceptional. Lack of autonomy of cells in BCC is considered the cause for inability to metastasize. Metastases in basal cell carcinoma are more likely in the basosquamous types, in those with perineural spread, and in tumors located on sunlight protected skin.

Excisional surgery, microsurgery and cryosurgery have been used to treat circumscribed, non-infiltrating BCCs. When surgery is contraindicated, RT is an option for treating primary BCC.

MERKEL CELL CARCINOMA

Merkel cell carcinoma is an uncommon tumor occurring as a solitary painless red to bluish nodule on sun exposed skin. The origin is controversial. Divergent differentiation (neuroendocrine, squamous, adnexal and melanocytic) is seen in histology. This type of tumor is an aggressive one. Metastases can occur in the regional lymph nodes and in distant areas in 50–75 percent of the patients. Treatment involves wide excision with lymph node resection. Radiation and chemotherapy are given additionally where required.

MALIGNANT MELANOMA

Melanomas are highly malignant tumors originating from melanocytes of dermo-epidermal junction. Melanomas occur predominantly in the whites. Red and blond-haired individuals are at the greatest risk. The tumor appears in the middle aged and older individuals. The incidence of melanoma has been increasing at an alarming rate for the last 3 decades. This is attributed to behavioral changes with exposure to actinic damage. Short intense sun exposure is as risky as prolonged exposure. Hereditary predisposition is also noted. Molecular defects in tumor suppressor genes and oncogenes have been linked to melanoma. Immune status has an influencing factor in melanoma as evidenced by the occurrence in HIV infection, spontaneous regression, disease-free intervals and depigmentation. Human papillomavirus is a suspect. Melanomas appear on skin, in eyes and juxtacutaneous mucous membranes such as oral cavity, upper respiratory tract, genital and anorectal regions. On the skin, sun exposed areas are predominantly affected.

There are two major categories of melanoma—the non-tumorogenic and the tumorogenic .

In non-tumorogenic growth phase, they grow radially or horizontally. Histologically most of the cells in this lesion are located in epidermis. In microinvasion, a few of such cells are seen in papillary dermis. The cells can proliferate in the epidemics but lack metastatic capacity.

CLASSIFICATION OF MELANOMA

Four types of melanomas are recognized in this category.

Lentigo maligna melanoma (LMM, syn. Hutchinson's melanotic freckle). Lesions are seen in older age group and located on the face as brownish irregular macules, which slowly progress. The border of lesion is often impalpable and indistinct. This causes unexpected positive or close margins in resected tissue. Invasive changes are recognized when induration or discrete bluish black nodules develop. Invasive changes occur in about 5 percent of cases.

Superficial spreading melanoma (SSM, syn. Pagetoid melanoma *in situ*). This variant is seen more on intermittently exposed skin and is rare in unexposed areas. They are palpable with pronounced color variation. Depigmented area within the patch is a sign of regression. Induration, nodulation or ulceration indicates invasive changes.

Acral lentiginous melanoma (ALM): This is seen more in the colored races than in the white population. Ungual, periungual, palmar or plantar lesions appear. Overlying nail may show pigmented streaks. Uneven pigmentation, induration and ulceration are signs of invasive changes. This occurs early and the tumor has an aggressive course with poor prognosis.

Mucosal lentiginous melanoma arises in juxtacutaneous mucous membranes such as oral mucosa, nose and nasal sinuses, vagina, and anorectal mucosa.

Tumorigenic melanoma represents the vertical growth phase of melanoma. The histology shows a tumorigenic compartment adjacent to or within the confines of nontumorigenic compartment like SSM, LMM and ALM.

Nodular melanoma, by definition, contains only tumorigenic vertical phase. Clinically deeply pigmented nodules which show rapid growth, early ulceration and bleeding are characteristics of this tumor. Rarely the tumor is amelanotic. Melanoma shows reactivity for markers like S-100 protein, HMB-45 and vimentin. Metastatic melanomas from unknown foci are seen in up to 15 percent of cases in some reported series.

Metastatic malignant melanomas may be mistaken for multiple primary tumors. They may appear as satellite lesions around the primary cutaneous lesion or around the site of an affected lymph node. Distant metastases are blood or lymph borne. Diagnosis is established on histology. A helpful differentiating feature of the primary from metastatic lesion is the absence of inflammatory infiltrate and junctional activity in the latter.

There are 3 different methods of staging in melanoma. They are:
– Clark's method (levels of invasion)
– Breslow's method (Tumor thickness)
– AJCC/UICC Staging/pTNM staging.

Clark's method (level of invasion)

I. Melanoma limited to epidermis
II. Melanoma invasive infiltrating into papillary dermis
III. Melanoma reaching up to the superficial vascular plexus in the dermis
IV. Melanoma involving the reticular dermis
V. Melanoma involving the subcutaneous fat.

Breslow's method (thickness of the tumor)

I. Thickness up to < 0.75 mm
II. Thickness between 0.76 and 1.49 mm

III. Thickness between 1.50 mm and 3.9 mm

IV. Thickness above 4 mm

New AJCC staging system (2002)

Stage I: Localized

T1a or b: <1.0 mm, non-ulcerated or ulcerated

T2a: <2.0 mm, non-ulcerated

Stage II: Localized

T2b: <2.0 mm, ulcerated

T3a or b: <4.0 mm, non-ulcerated or ulcerated

T4a or b: >4.0 mm, non-ulcerated or ulcerated

Stage III: Regional metastases

N1:   1 N+

N2:   2 to 3 N+

N3:   4 N+ (or matted, in transit)

Stage IV: Distant disease

M1:   distant skin, nodes

M2:   Other, LDH

The staging of cutaneous melanoma strongly correlates with survival. Staging depends upon local, regional, or distant disease. Breslow depth of a primary melanoma is the cardinal prognostic factor for clinically localized disease. The risk of relapse and death increases with each millimeter of depth (Breslow thickness) for primary melanoma. The presence of ulceration reduces relapse-free survival by more than one-third. In patients with nodal disease, independent variables like the number of lymph nodes, the presence of ulceration of the primary tumor, and whether the nodal disease is macroscopic or microscopic affect the overall prognosis. The prognosis of patients with distant metastasis is poor, with median survivals of less than 1 year.

TREATMENT

a. Surgical excision—If the size of the tumor is less than 1 mm, 1 cm margin is enough. If the lesion is more than 1 mm then 2 cm margin should be removed.

b. Adjuvant therapy—IFN alfa-2b in high doses has been proven in three multi-institutional trials to improve prognosis after resection of the primary melanoma lesion.

c. Chemotherapy is useful in metastatic disease. Patients with distant metastatic melanoma have a median survival of about 6 months. Chemotherapeutic agents along with interferon have been useful in palliation of symptoms.

d. melanoma vaccines.

e. gene therapy.

APPENDAGE TUMORS

All cutaneous adnexa share the same origin and it is not surprising that the tumors arising from them have many features in common. But the vast majority of skin adnexal tumors differentiate only along one adnexal line, and this results in the formation of reasonably distinct types whose structure, cytochemistry, and immunohistochemistry can be correlated with those of the corresponding adnexa (hair follicle, sebaceous gland, apocrine gland, eccrine gland). However, it is not unusual to find evidence of differentiation along two or more adnexal lines in different tumors occurring in the same individual or sometimes even within the same neoplasm, whether benign or malignant. The tumors described as 'cutaneous adnexal carcinomas with divergent differentiation' are an expression of the latter phenomenon.

The tumors are not generally clinically distinctive and firm diagnosis has to be on the basis of histology.

HAIR FOLLICLE TUMORS

Trichilemmal (tricholemmal) carcinoma occurs on face and ears. The clinical course of trichilemmal carcinoma is very indolent, and the incidence of metastatic behavior is extremely low. Other malignant tumor *is malignant pilomatrixoma* (pilomatrix carcinoma).

Sebaceous Tumors

Sebaceous carcinoma is extremely rare. Those occurring in the eyelids, in caruncles, and in the orbit are much more aggressive than those located elsewhere in the skin. Some of the cases have followed irradiation therapy to the area. Sebaceous carcinoma may be seen as a component of *Muir-Torre's syndrome*. In this condition, multiple cutaneous tumors exhibiting varying degrees of sebaceous and hair follicle differentiation occur in association with multiple internal malignancies.

Malignant Tumors of Sweat Glands

Sweat gland carcinomas are diverse. These are rare tumors and comprise a minute fraction of sweat gland neoplasm. Most occur in adults.

Some sweat gland carcinomas retain morphologic features that allow them to be recognized as the malignant counterparts of the various types of sweat gland adenomas. *Malignant eccrine poroma (porocarcinoma)* is the most frequent member of this group. Most cases occur in the lower extremities, like their benign counterparts. Other distinct varieties of sweat gland carcinoma include malignant chondroid syringoma, malignant dermal cylindroma, malignant syringoma (syringoid eccrine carcinoma), malignant acrospiroma, apocrine carcinoma, mucinous (adenocystic) carcinoma and sclerosing sweat duct carcinoma. Nearly all sweat gland carcinomas exhibit immunoreactivity for cytokeratin, CEA and EMA.

FIBROUS TISSUE TUMORS

Dermatofibrosarcoma protuberans (DFSP) is a slow growing dermal spindle cell neoplasm of intermediate malignancy.

Malignant fibrous histiocytoma rarely involves dermis. Epithelioid sarcoma can occur as dermal or subcutaneous nodule.

VASCULAR TUMORS

Even though vascular tumors can be classified into benign, low grade malignant, and malignant categories, it still remains controversial.

KAPOSI'S SARCOMA (KS) (FIG. 46.3, PLATE 11)

KS is a tumor arising from endothelium of blood vessels or lymphatics affecting skin and internal organs. As the commonest initially presenting disease in HIV infected individuals, KS got worldwide attention in the early 1980s. Prior to this, KS was virtually confined to mid and sub-Sahara Africa. There is male predominance in all types of KS. Three types of KS are recognized. All have similar cutaneous lesions. Ecchymotic macules, plaques or purplish nodules progress to form large masses which on ulcerating, form fungating growths.

Sporadic KS was first described by Kaposi in 1972. This is seen in elderly males often of the East European Jew population.

Endemic KS is seen in sub-Saharan Africa and affects children and adults. As a localized form, the disease is relatively benign. In the disseminated form, lymph node and visceral involvement is seen early with fatal outcome.

HIV RELATED KS

In this form, lesions are often found on the head and the neck. KS also occurs in non-HIV related immunosuppressed patients.

TREATMENT

The extent of the disease, systemic complaints and the number of CD 4 cells are taken into account in staging the disease and planning therapy. For localized lesions cryotherapy, laser therapy, radiation, and intralesional vinblastine have been useful. For progressive disease systemic chemotherapy with vincristine, vinblastine etoposide and doxorubicin are used alone or in combination. Alpha interferon has also been used with some success. Antiretroviral therapy has a beneficial role.

ANGIOSARCOMA

Angiosarcoma is a high grade tumor of endothelial origin. Angiosarcomas of skin are classified according to the clinical setting as:
1. idiopathic (head and neck)—Occurs in elderly. Scalp, middle and upper face are common sites.
2. associated with lymphedema—Typically it occurs after longstanding lymphedema following breast surgery (Stewart-Treves syndrome). It can also occur in congenital lymphedema, and lymphedema due to filariasis.
3. post radiotherapy—Most cases arise in skin after radiotherapy for internal malignancy. Common sites are breast, chest wall and lower abdomen.
4. epithelioid angiosarcoma—Deep soft tissue is the common site of this rare tumor. Cutaneous lesions are also reported. The tumor cell looks like deposits from carcinoma or melanoma and usually requires immunohistochemistry for confirmatory diagnosis.

IHC markers are CD34 and CD31.

CUTANEOUS LYMPHOMAS

B lineage—Most lymphoblastic lymphomas of skin are of B cell lineage. Others are small lymphocytic lymphoma (SLL), immunocytoma, cutaneous follicular lymphoma, mantle cell lymphoma, plasmacytoma, diffuse large cell lymphoma and intravascular lymphoma.

In T cell lineage, T-lymphoblastic lymphoma, Mycosis fungoides, Sezary syndrome, Pagetoid reticulosis (localized form—Woringer-Kolopp lymphoma), Granulomatous slack skin, Adult T cell leukemia/lymphoma (ATLL), Peripheral T-Cell lymphoma, cutaneous CD30 + (Ki-1), Anaplastic large cell lymphomas (ALCL) are seen to be affecting skin. Angiocentric lymphoma, Hodgkin's lymphoma and granulocytic sarcoma can also involve skin.

MYCOSIS FUNGOIDES

Mycosis fungoides is the most common sub type of T cell lymphomas that arise primarily in skin. Most patients are adults/elderly. The disease has a long natural history. Patients may show non-specific scaly eruptions years before a diagnostic histopathology develops. Later the patch stage progresses to plaque, nodules and tumors. In some patients, after a long period of time, neoplasm disseminates to extracutaneous sites such as lymph nodes and viscera.

Diagnosis is established on histological basis which varies at different stages of the disease. Infiltration of the mononuclear cells of variable density in the papillary dermis extension to the epidermis is an early sign. Pautrier microabscesses refers to a discrete sharply marginated, cluster of monocytes with a characteristic halo. In the late tumor stage, large masses of infiltrate consisting of cells of pleomorphic hyperchromatic nucleus occupies the whole dermis, epidermis and subcutis.

SEZARY SYNDROME

Sezary syndrome is a generalized mature T-cell lymphoma characterized by the presence of erythroderma, lymphadenopathy and neoplastic T-lymphocytes in the blood. The behavior is more aggressive than Mycosis fungoides.

Lymphomatoid papulosis is classified as a T cell proliferation of uncertain malignant potential. The atypical lympho–proliferation which can be clonal progresses to lymphoma in some instances.

HTLV-1 Associated adult T Cell lymphoma—leukemia.

This is caused by human T cell lymphotropic type 1 (HTLV-1) retrovirus. It is transmitted through sexual contact, breastfeeding or infected blood products. Skin lesions are seen in up to 70 percent cases as widespread erythematous or purpuric papules, nodules or plaques. In the acute form of the disease which shows widespread involvement survival is for about one year. A chronic form with minimum skin involvement is also recognized.

TREATMENT

Factors which determine the nature of treatment are the age of the patient, the stage of the disease and aggressiveness. Effective therapies for CTCL include both topical and systemic therapies. Skin-directed therapy includes topical chemotherapy with such agents as carmustine (BCNU) and nitrogen mustard (NM), systemically administered psoralens activated in the skin by psoralen and ultraviolet A light (PUVA) therapy, and local and generalized superficial ionizing radiation that includes both electron-beam and X-ray therapy. Systemic therapies are photophoresis (acts both directly by killing T lymphocytes by the cytotoxic actions of UVA light/psoralen and indirectly by eliciting anti-CTCL cell immune responses), retinoids, IFN-alpha and–gamma and chemotherapy (single agent methotrexate, chlorambucil or combination chemotherapy CHOP) in advanced cases.

PARAPSORIASIS

Parapsoriasis comprises a group of uncommon disorders which have propensity to evolve into mycosis fungoides (MF).

Small plaque, large plaque and variegated types are recognized. The small plaque variety is viewed as an abortive form of lymphoma and the large plaque variety as a latent lymphoma. MF developing in patients with parapsoriasis tends to have a relatively benign course. Skin lesions are recalcitrant and inflammatory. Scaly, erythematous to brownish macules and non-indurated plaques up to about 1.5 cm in size are present on trunk and extremities. Persistent superficial dermatitis is a term often used for this. Lesions are fewer and larger in the large plaque variety. Subsequent atrophy which progresses to mottled pigmentation and telangiectasis, gives a characteristic appearance described as poikiloderma atrophicans vascular. Clinical diagnosis with supportive histopathological features call for initiating therapy. Therapeutic options are topical steroids, UVB and PUVA treatment and these are palliative measures. These appear mostly on face or scalp as alopecia boggy patches. A lesion may remain static for many years before malignant changes appear. The hair follicle shows degeneration and mucinous deposition. The hair loss is permanent. The lesion resolves with therapy for the accompanying malignancy.

PSEUDOLYMPHOMA

A wide spectrum of benign diseases is seen in the group of diseases. Persistent presence of lymphocytes and resemblance to malignant lymphoma characterize the histological findings. Differentiation from malignant lymphoma is made histologically. Drugs, arthropod bites, tattoo pigments, solar radiation, etc. are known to initiate the cellular reaction.

HISTIOCYTIC SYNDROMES

The histiocytic group of disorders result from proliferation of the cells related to the monocyte-macrophage series.

These are classified as: Langerhans cell histiocytosis (LCH) and non-Langerhans cell histiocytosis (Non-LCH). Three diseases are included in LCH. These are: 1. eosinophilic granulomas, with localized lesions in bone, affecting older children and adults, 2. Hand-Schüller-Christian disease with triad of skull defects, diabetes insipidus and exophthalmos, 3. Letterer-Siwe disease with skin and visceral involvement appearing usually below the age group of 2 years.

Skin lesions are seen as crusted or scaly papules and plaques, petechiae on scalp and other seborrheic areas like retroauricular regions, axillae and groins.

Multiple organs involvement carries a poor prognosis. Spontaneous healing which sometimes occurs suggests that LCH is a reactive disease. Corticosteroids have been found helpful in extensive diseases. Chemotherapy is indicated in generalized disease.

METASTATIC CARCINOMA OF SKIN

Metastasis to skin may be the first indication of an internal malignancy. Dissemination may take place through the lymphatic or blood stream. Alopecia neoplastica occurs as oval plaques or patches of the scalp. On the abdominal skin, umbilicus may be the commonest site. Common primary sites include breast, lung, GIT, oral cavity, kidney, pancreas and prostate.

FURTHER READING

1. Barth A, Wanek LA, Morton DL. Prognostic factors in 1,521 melanoma patients with distant metastasis. J Am Coll Surgeons 1995;181:A193.
2. Buttner P, Gabre C, Bertz J, et al. Primary cutaneous melanoma: Optimal cutoff points of tumor thickness and importance of Clarke's level for prognostic classification. Cancer 1995;75:2499.
3. Connelly JH, Evans HL. Dermatofibrosarcoma protuberans: A clinicopathological review with emphasis on fibrosarcomatous areas. Am J Surg Pathol 1992;16:921.
4. David Elder (Ed). Lever's Histopathology of Skin (8th ed). Philadelphia: Lippincott-Raven, 1997.
5. Evans HL, Baer SC. Epithelioid sarcoma: A clinicopathological and prognostic study of 26 cases. Semin Diagn Pathol 1993;10:286.
6. Jonasch E, Kumar UN, Linette GP, et al. Adjuvant high-dose interferon alfa-2b in patients with high-risk melanoma. Cancer J Sci Am 2000;6:139-45.
7. Kerschmann RL, Berger TG, Weiss LM, et al. Cutaneous presentations of lymphoma in human immunodeficiency virus disease: Predominance of T cell lineage. Arch Dermatol 1995;131:1281.
8. Kirkwood JM, Ibrahim JG, Sondak VK, et al. High- and low-dose interferon alfa-2b in high-risk melanoma: first analysis of intergroup trial E1690/S9111/C9190. J Clin Oncol 2000; 18:2444-58.
9. Kirkwood JM, Strawderman MH, Ernstoff MS, Smith TJ, Borden EC, Blum RH. Interferon alfa-2b adjuvant therapy of high-risk resected cutaneous melanoma: The Eastern Cooperative Oncology Group Trial EST 1684. J Clin Oncol 1996; 14:10-17.
10. Leffel DJ. The scientific basis of skin cancer. J Am Acad Dermatol 2000;42:18-2.
11. Lookingbill DP, Spangler N, Helm KF. Cutaneous metastases in patients with metastatic carcinoma: A retrospective study of 4020 patients. J Am Acad Dermatol 1993;29:228.
12. Nakhlen RE, Wick MR, Rocamora A, et al. Morphological diversity in malignant melanomas. Am J Clin Path 1990;93:731.
13. Ralfkiaer E. Immunohistological markers for the diagnosis of cutaneous lymphomas. Semin Diagn Pathol 1991;8:62.
14. Schwartz RA. Cutaneous metastatic disease. J Am Acad Dermatol 1995;33:161.
15. Tappero JW, Conant MA, Wolfe SF, et al. Kaposi's sarcoma: Epidemiology, pathogenesis, histology, clinical spectrum, staging criteria, and therapy. J Am Acad Dermatol 1993;28:371.
16. Tsang WYW, Chan JCK, Fletcher CDM. Recently characterized vascular tumours of skin and soft tissue. Histopathology 1991;19:489.

Musculoskeletal Tumors 47

**Narayanan Kutty Warrier, Bhagyam Nair
Mohan Kurian**

SOFT TISSUE SARCOMA

Sarcoma is a heterogeneous malignant tumor of the soft tissues of the body such as fat, muscles, nerves, tendons, blood and lymph vessels. They arise from any of the mesodermal tissues of the extremities (50%), trunk and retroperitoneum (40%) or head and neck including the orbit (10%). At times these tumors arise in the gastrointestinal tract and are called gastrointestinal stromal tumors (GISTs). Soft tissue sarcomas (STSs) are relatively rare and constitute 1 percent of all adult cancers, 15 percent of cancers of childhood and young adults. The majority of patients with soft tissue sarcoma show a better survival rate with multimodality therapy and supporting care. Five-year survival rate for early stages of STS is more than 90 percent.

Sarcomas can affect anyone, from the young to the old. In children, rhabdomyosarcoma is the commonest sarcoma-whereas in adolescents and young adults-osteogenic sarcoma and Ewing's family of tumors are the commonest.

Although STS shares a mesenchymal origin, they are a heterogeneous group of diseases. Nevertheless, they are studied and frequently treated as if they were all the same. However, recent developments suggest that a different approach may be more beneficial. STS occurs with greater frequency in patients with:
— Li-Fraumeni syndrome (P-53 mutation)
— Gardner's syndrome
— Werner's syndrome
— Tuberous sclerosis
— Basal cell nervous syndrome
—Von-Recklinghausen's disease

ETIOLOGY

The causes of STS remain obscure in the vast majority of cases. Each of the genetic and environmental factors appears to play a role in the neoplastic transformation of soft tissues into sarcoma.

Environmental exposure associated with the development of sarcomas is mainly exposure to ionizing radiation. This is most often a late effect of radiation therapy given to treat another malignancy. They are commonly seen after radiation treatment of Hodgkin's and NHL lymphoma, breast, head and neck cancers. Malignant peripheral nerve sheath tumors, angiosarcoma and other high grade unclassifiable subtypes form the majority of sarcomas. Radiation associated sarcomas arise several years after radiation and are often seen above the radiation dose of 10 Gy.

CLINICAL FEATURES

Soft tissue sarcomas can appear in different parts of the body. In the extremity, STS appears as a soft painless mass which becomes painful on rest or during exercise. This may be due to stretching or compression of the nearby structures.

In the neck, it appears as a diffuse swelling, with indefinite margins. Within the orbit, it presents with proptosis and in nasopharynx with a history of nasal discharge, and nasal obstruction. Anatomic distribution: Approximately 50 percent of STS appear in extremities and 30 percent intrabdominally. The detailed anatomic distributions: in upper extremity (14%), lower extremity (30%), visceral (15%), retroperitoneal (15%), trunk (11%), others including the orbit (14%).

Major types of STS in adults and in childrn are given in Tables 47.1 and 47.2.

PATHOLOGICAL CLASSIFICATION

A variety of histologically distinct neoplasms have been identified based on the pubertive cell of origin. However as the degree of histologic differentiation declines, it becomes increasingly difficult to determine the cellular origin. In recent times pathologists classify the soft tissue tumors based on light microscopic morphology, in conjunction with immunohisto-chemical features. Molecular genetic data have become increasingly important in the precise diagnosis of STS with overlapping morphological features. However, a much more clinically useful pathological classification is:

Malignant fibrous histiocytoma- like pattern
Pleomorphic liposarcoma
Dedifferentiated liposarcoma
Pleomorphic MPNST
Pleomorphic leiomyosarcoma
Pleomorphic RMS
Extraskeletal osteosarcoma
Hemangiopericytoma- like pattern

Table 47.1: Major types of soft tissue sarcomas in adults		
Tissue of origin	*Type of cancer*	*Usual location in the body*
Fibrous tissue	Fibrosarcoma	Arms, legs, trunk
	Malignant fibrous histiocytoma	Legs
Fat	Liposarcoma	Arms, legs, trunk
Muscle		
Striated muscle	Rhabdomyosarcoma	Arms, legs
Smooth muscle	Leiomyosarcoma	Uterus, digestive tract
Blood vessels	Hemangiosarcoma	Arms, legs, trunk
Lymph vessels	Lymphangiosarcoma	Arms
Synovial tissue (linings of joint cavities, tendon sheaths)	Synovial sarcoma	Legs
Peripheral nerves	Neurofibrosarcoma	Arms, legs, trunk
Cartilage and bone-forming tissue	Extraskeletal chondrosarcoma osteosarcoma	Legs, trunk (not involving the bone)
	Extraskeletal	Legs
	Kaposi's sarcoma	Legs, trunk

Fibrosarcoma-like pattern
  Cellular schwannoma
  Synovial sarcoma
  MPNST
Myxoid soft tissue tumors and tumor-like lesions
Round cell tumor pattern
  Ewing's sarcoma/Peripheral neuroepithelium
  RMS
  Metastatic neuroblastoma
  Desmoplastic chondrosarcoma
  Round cell liposarcoma
  Poorly differentiated synovial sarcoma
  SCOS

Malignant fibrous histiocytoma is the most common histologic type (40%) followed by liposarcoma (25%). Histologic grade of the tumor is the most important factor which determines the biologic behavior of the tumor. The grade is determined by the number of mitoses per high power field, presence of necrosis, cellular and nuclear morphology and the degree of cellularity. Gastrointestinal stromal tumors (GIST) are mesenchymal in origin and often show different histological behavior from the rest of the soft tissue tumors. Immunohistochemically they are CD_{34} positive and CD_{117} positive. They express a growth factor receptor with tyrosine kinase activity called C-kit (CD_{117}). GIST characteristically stain strongly

Table 47.2: Major types of soft tissue sarcomas in children			
Tissue of origin	*Type of cancer in the body*	*Usual location*	*Most common ages*
Muscle Striated muscle	Rhabdomyosarcoma Embryonal	Head and neck, genitourinary tract	Infant-4
	Alveolar	Arms, legs, head, and neck	Infant-19
Smooth muscle	Leiomyosarcoma	Trunk	15-19
Fibrous tissue	Fibrosarcoma	Arms and legs	15-19
Malignant	Dermatofibrosarcoma fibrous histiocytoma	Legs and trunk	15-19
Fat	Liposarcoma	Arms and legs	15-19
Blood vessels	Infantile hemangio-pericytoma	Arms, legs, trunk, head, and neck	Infant-4
Synovial tissue (linings of joint cavities, tendon sheaths)	Synovial sarcoma	Legs, arms, and trunk	15-19
Peripheral nerves	Malignant peripheral nerve sheath tumors (MPNST) (also called neurofibrosarcoma, malignant schwannomas, and neurogenic sarcomas)	Arms, legs, and trunk	15-19
Muscular nerves	Alveolar, soft tissue sarcoma	Arms and legs	Infant-19
Cartilage and bone-forming tissue	Extraskeletal myxoid chondrosarcoma	Legs	10-14
	Extraskeletal Mesenchymal	Legs	10-14

for CD_{117}. They rarely express desmin or S_{100}. By contrast leiomyosarcoma is positive for SMA and desmin but negative for KIT.

STAGING

Grade and TNM definitions

Tumor Grade (G)

GX: Grade cannot be assessed
G1: Well differentiated
G2: Moderately differentiated
G3: Poorly differentiated
G4: Undifferentiated

Primary Tumor (T)

TX: Primary tumor cannot be assessed
T0: No evidence of primary tumor
T1: Tumor 5 cm or less in greatest dimension
T1a: Superficial tumor (Superficial tumor is located exclusively above the superficial fascia without invasion of the fascia; deep tumor is located either exclusively beneath the superficial fascia, or superficial to the fascia with invasion of or through the fascia, or superficial and beneath the fascia. Retroperitoneal, mediastinal, and pelvic sarcomas are classified as deep tumors).
T1b: Deep tumor
T2: Tumor more than 5 cm in greatest dimension
T2a: Superficial tumor
T2b: Deep tumor

Regional Lymph Nodes (N)

NX: Regional lymph nodes cannot be assessed
N0: No regional lymph node metastasis
N1: Regional lymph node metastasis

Distant Metastasis (M)

MX: Distant metastasis cannot be assessed
M0: No distant metastasis
M1: Distant metastasis

Stage IA

Stage IA tumor is defined as low grade, small, superficial, and deep.
G1, T1a, N0, M0
G1, T1b, N0, M0
G2, T1a, N0, M0
G2, T1b, N0, M0

Stage IB

Stage IB tumor is defined as low grade, large, and superficial.
G1, T2a, N0, M0
G2, T2a, N0, M0

Stage IIA

Stage IIA tumor is defined as low grade, large, and deep.
G1, T2b, N0, M0
G2, T2b, N0, M0

Stage IIB

Stage IIB tumor is defined as high grade, small, superficial, and deep.
G3, T1a, N0, M0
G3, T1b, N0, M0
G4, T1a, N0, M0
G4, T1b, N0, M0

Stage IIC

Stage IIC tumor is defined as high grade, large, and superficial.
G3, T2a, N0, M0
G4, T2a, N0, M0

Stage III

Stage III tumor is defined as high grade, large, and deep.
G3, T2b, N0, M0
G4, T2b, N0, M0

Stage IV ·

Stage IV is defined as any metastasis to lymph nodes or distant sites.
Any G, any T, N1, M0
Any G, any T, N0, M1

TREATMENT

Surgery

Management of STS is essentially a multimodality approach. Surgery remains the primary treatment. Surgery is undertaken only if there is no metastasis, lymph node involvement and if the tumor can be excised with a good margin without impairment to the functions of the limb.

Stage IA, IB and IIA. Low-grade STS which comprise Grade 1 or 2 have little metastatic potential, but they may recur locally if they are inadequately treated. Surgical excision with negative tissue margins of at least 2 cm or more in all directions is the treatment of choice. Limb sparing surgery is possible in approximately 90 percent of the patients with extremity sarcoma. In 10 percent, the tumor involves the neurovascular bundle. Conservative surgical excision with preoperative or postoperative radiation is also tried. In the case of unresectable extremity low grade STS, high dose preoperative radiation therapy may be used, followed by surgical resection and postoperative radiation therapy.

Retroperitoneum, trunk and head and neck are areas where surgeons will not get adequate surgical margins. Wide margins are unusual in these sites and radiation therapy is usually advocated for trunk and head and neck STS. Surgical resection followed by postoperative radiation therapy, if negative margins cannot be obtained, also is an option in such situations. Preoperative radiation therapy is followed by maximal surgical resection. Radiation therapy is usually used to maximize local control because of the inability to obtain wide surgical margins.

Adjuvant Postoperative Therapy

The role of chemotherapy in the adjuvant setting is controversial. The benefits of adjuvant chemotherapy are not yet fully defined. Clinical trials for STS have difficulty enrolling adequate number of patients to obtain significant and generalised findings. The factors that have been identified as most important in influencing the outcome are the grade and size of the tumor. Out of 14 randomized clinical trials of adjuvant chemotherapy for STS, only two studies demonstrated a significant difference in overall survival. Results of this analysis indicated a 6 percent local relapse-free survival, 10 percent overall recurrence-free survival rate with adjuvant therapy. No significant benefit in overall survival was seen, but a small absolute benefit of 4 percent at 10 years was reported. When patients with extremely high grade STS were evaluated as a subgroup, 7 percent absolute benefit in overall survival at 10 years was observed. These studies were based on anthracycline regimens. Combination of Ifosfamide and anthracycline is not well studied, and newer combination chemotherapy also has not been analyzed in a randomized clinical trial. Recent Italian sarcoma group studies using dose intensive Ifosfamide plus epinibicin have shown statistically significant overall survival, disease free survival (DFS), freedom from local recurrence and freedom from distant metastasis. Adjuvant chemotherapy may improve relapse-free survival in carefully selected patients and can be considered for the treatment of those with tumor size >5 cm, deep tumor location and high histologic grade.

Preoperative Chemotherapy

This has been tried for patients with large high grade extremity STS. Reduction in the size of a large lesion may permit surgical resection with less morbidity and response to preoperative therapy may provide important prognostic information although this remains disputed. Preoperative chemotherapy should be considered for fit high risk patients after discussing the potential benefits and risks involved in the treatment.

Anthracycline-based chemotherapy regimen is the most studied. Combination of doxirubin 60-75 mg/m^2 or epirubicin 120 mg/m^2 plus ifosfamide 9-10 gm/m^2 or doxorubicin 20 mg/m^2/d i.v. infused continuously over 24 hours or days 1-3. Ifosfamide 2.5 gm/m^2/day i.v. infused continuously over 24 hours on days 1-3. Dicarbazine 300 mg/m^2/d IV infused continuously over 24 hours on days 1-3. MESNA 2.5 mg/m^2/d i.v. infused continuously over 24 hours on days 1-4 is given as continuous infusion. This regimen called MAID is an effective alternative regimen for Ifosfamide plus doxorubicin.

Radiation Therapy

Radiation therapy (RT) for STS is used as preoperative, postoperative or sandwich technique. Postoperative radiation is preferred, if the tumor is resected with clean surgical margin. If the tumor is bulky and unresectable and limb sparing treatment is still desired, preoperative RT is warranted. RT can be given with radical intent or palliative intent for patients refusing surgery or who have unresectable sarcoma.

Advantages of Preoperative RT

With preoperative radiation, the size of the tumor will be reduced, thus decreasing the extent of surgical resection. It also causes tumor encapsulation, thereby facilitating easier surgical removal.

Smaller radiation portals can be used as the scar and hematoma will be absent.

Disadvantages of Preoperative RT

Disadvantages of preoperative RT are delayed wound healing, and downstaging of disease.

Low grade STS, which has been excised with a negative margin is not ideally recommended for postoperative RT. The local recurrence can be re-excised effectively, followed by postoperative RT.

Guidelines for Optimal RT in STS

1. Tumor localization.
2. Muscle and compartment of involvement must be defined before the beginning of radiation therapy.
3. Patient positioning and immobilization.
   The patient must be positioned in frog leg position for optimal radiation therapy.
   Simulation.
4. Megavoltage equipment such as cobalt unit or linear accelerator (6 MV photons) is used.
5. High radiation dose.

The initial volume encompasses the tumor with complete coverage of the compartment (10 cm around high grade tumor) treated with 40-44 Gy and the second volume which cones down to tumor mass with 5 cm margin all around the mass to a dose of 54 Gy. The final volume cones on the clipped tumor with 2 cm margin to 64-74 Gy in conventional fractionation over a period of 7 to 8 weeks.

Finally 10-12 Gy can be given as interstitial therapy/electron therapy as boost.

6. Use beam shapers and beam modifiers.

CHEMOTHERAPY FOR CHILDHOOD TUMORS

Rhabdomyosarcoma

Low-risk, well-differentiated group 1 and 2 (embryonal type) at favorable sites and group III orbital tumors can be treated with vincristine and dactinomycin.

Intermediate-risk group also can be treated with vincristine, dactinomycin and cyclophosphamide.

High-risk group (all those with metastases - group IV- except patients under 10 years old who have embryonal tumors) can be administered with high doses of vincristine, dactinomycin, cyclophosphamide with hematopoietic stem-cell transplantation.

The treatment must be continued for 6 to 12 weeks. As additional treatment, resection of the primary tumor must be done except in orbital tumors.

Metastatic/Unresectable Disease

Most patients with advanced sarcoma respond poorly to currently available therapies and hence palliative treatment using the same group of drugs used in the adjuvant therapy may be used.

Recent Changes and Future Directions in Treatment for STS

Until recently STS were studied and treated as if they were all the same disease. But now it has been realised that they are heterogeneous diseases varying widely in their biological behavior. Many specific oncogenes and their protein products have been identified now and they can be effectively utilized as molecular targets. The development of maturity for GI stromal tumors may serve as an example in many aspects. Overexpression of the oncogenic product c-KIT is a frequent characteristic of GIST. Similarly in synovial sarcoma, EGFR-1 overexpression is noticed. In clear cell sarcoma of tendons, epithelial sarcoma, synovial sarcoma and malignant PNET, enhanced hepatocyte growth factor receptor signaling has been suggested to play in the etiopathogenesis of these tumors.

Farnesyl Transferase inhibitors are found to be effective in neurofibromatosis Type I and needs more study.

The future advances in sarcoma treatment can be expected to be parallel to our understanding of molecular genetics.

FURTHER READING

1. Arndt CAS, Crist WM. Common musculoskeletal tumors of childhood and Adolescence. N Engl J Med 1999;342:342-52.
2. WexlerLH, Helman LI. Rhabdomyosarcoma and undifferentiated sarcoma. In: Pizzo, Popplik, Principles and Practice of Pediatric Oncology. Philadelphia: Lippincott–Raven, 1997;799-829.

GASTROINTESTINAL STROMAL TUMORS

Gastrointestinal stromal tumor (GIST) is the most common sarcoma of GIT and it accounts for 5 percent of all sarcomas. GISTs are the most common form of mesenchymal tumor of GIT. Clinically they range from small indolent tumors curable with surgery alone to aggressive cancers. GISTs characteristically express the KIT protein, a transmembrane tyrosine kinase receptor, for stem-cell factor. Historically GISTs have been classified as either benign or malignant, with the majority of tumors diagnosed as benign. However, all GISTs have at least some malignant potential.

Until recently long term survival in patients with malignant GISTs was very rare. All patients undergo potentially curative resection of localized disease experience recurrence and salvage surgery offers minimal, if any, survival benefit. They are neither radiosensitive nor chemosensitive. Treatment with mesylate, a molecularly targeted agent that inhibits the KIT tyrosine kinase receptor leads to objective responses in the majority of GIST patients but it does not seem to be curative.

GISTs are most commonly found in the stomach (40-70%), but they can occur in all other parts of the GIT. About 20-40 percent of GISTs arise from small intestine and 5-15 percent from the colon and rectum. GISTs can also be found in the esophagus <5 percent omentum <5 percent mesentery for retroperitoneum.

GISTs characteristically stain strongly for the CD117 antigen, an epitope of the KIT- receptor, tyrosine kinase. Strong KIT expression in the absence of smooth muscle differentiation related proteins (SMA, desmin) is characteristic of GISTs.

TREATMENT

Surgery remains the standard initial treatment for nonmetabolic GISTs. These tumors are not readily amenable to RT because of organ motility and postoperatively contaminated bowel loops may relocate to remote sites. Attempts to treat malignant GISTs with systemic chemotherapy have been almost universally unsuccessful due to the frequent expression of P-glycoprotein and multidrug resistant protein 1 (MDRP 1) in GISTs.

Imatinits mesylate is a new molecule found to be effective in C-Kit positive GISTs. It is a competitive inhibitor of tyrosine kinase (KIT). Based on two studies, Imatinits is recommended for the treatment of adult patients with C-Kit positive unresectable or metastatic malignant GIST. The recommended initial dose is 400 mg to 600 mg daily with treatment maintained as long as the patient continues to benefit.

FURTHER READING

1. Dodd LG. Fine needle aspiration of gastrointestinal stromal tumors. Am J Clinic Pathol 1998;109:439-43.
2. Gibbs JF. Gastrointestinal stromal tumors. Prob Gen Surg 1999;16:107-13.
3. Masashi Yoshida. Surgical management of gastric leiomyosarcoma: evaluation of propriety of laparoscopic wedge resection. World J Surg 1997;21:440-43.

OSTEOSARCOMA

Osteosarcoma is a malignant tumor arising from bone-forming mesenchymal cells. It is the most common primary malignant tumor of bone (20%) and it can also occur in soft tissue (extraosseous). It presents with bimodal age distribution. The primary osteosarcoma is seen in young age during the period of active growth, between 15-30 years and the secondary seen in elderly (the fourth and the fifth decade). The secondary osteosarcoma is usually associated with Paget's disease, bone infarcts and prior radiation for treatment of benign conditions like aneurysmal bone cyst, simple bone cyst, osteoid osteoma or osteoblastoma. Secondary osteosarcoma can also be associated with childhood neoplasms like retinoblastoma, Wilms' tumor and neuroblastoma, and also Li-Fraumeni syndrome (P53 mutation). Osteosarcoma shows a slight male preponderance over the female (1.6:1).

CLINICAL FEATURES

These tumors usually arise in metaphysis of large long bones in adolescents, and almost half of them occur about the knee—in the distal femur or the proximal tibia. Other favored sites include the proximal humerus, the distal radius and also the upper and lower jaw. It typically presents as painful, hard, fixed and progressively enlarging mass. Symptoms are more prominent at night. Pathologic fracture is uncommon. It is rapidly growing and is aggressive in nature with high risk of local "skip" metastases and early pulmonary metastasis. Widespread metastases involving lungs, brain and bone, are associated with poor prognosis.

Risk factors are
1. prior treatment for childhood cancer with radiation therapy and/or chemotherapy.
2. hereditary retinoblastoma, Li-Fraumeni syndrome and Rothmund-Thomson syndrome.

However, most patients do not have an identifiable risk.

RADIOLOGIC FINDINGS

The radiological signs are highly characteristic.The tumor classically involves metaphysis of long bone, and is characterized by white "fluffy to cumulus" cloud like osteoblastic (bone forming) areas mixed with osteolytic areas. The lesion tends to be destructive, breaking through the cortex and rapidly elevates periosteum with subperiosteal new bone formation. The resultant formation of Codman's triangle is the deposit of new bone on the surface of the bone (Figs 47.1 and 47.2).

In recent years more reliance is placed on MRI study. It defines the tumor boundaries, the soft tissue extension to the muscles, neuromuscular tissues, and fat and nearby joint. T1 weighted MRI image of the entire long bone is taken to diagnose the presence of any skip lesions.

PATHOLOGICAL FINDINGS

Grossly they are large cortical tumors that are hard, gritty and gray-white, with or without the involvement of soft tissue. Areas of hemorrhage and cystic degeneration are often seen. Microscopically the classical lesion shows deposition of neoplastic bony matrix or osteoid surrounded by neoblastic cells. Osteosarcomas are classified according to subtypes and grades, which are determined by radiology and histology.

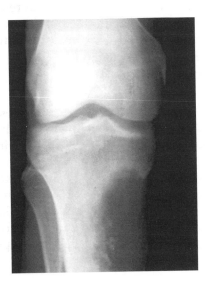

Figure 47.1: Osteosarcoma of the proximal part of the tibia. Note the Codman's triangle and 'sun ray spicules'

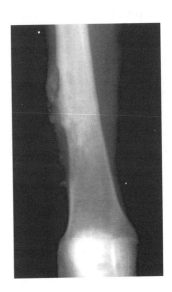

Figure 47.2: A periosteal sarcoma of the lower third of femur

HISTOLOGY AND STAGING

High grade: Conventional or cortical lesion, telangiectatic with small cell variants, chondrosarcoma with spindle cells or malignant histiocytes with giant cells (Highly aggressive secondary osteosarcoma comes in this group).

Intermediate grade: with periosteal cells.

Low grade: Intraosseous: low grade with cartilage and fibrous tissue rich, parosteal.

The prognosis of these tumors is very poor. Determination of tumor DNA content, serum lactic dehydrogenase and P-glycoprotein estimation are some of the available prognostic factors in osteosarcoma. The well-known risk factors are the loss of tumor suppressor genes p53 and Rb and the patients with Li-Fraumeni syndrome.

TREATMENT

Chemotherapy

Planned use of the chemotherapy agents, in recent times, have significantly improved the outcome of the disease, once considered fatal.

As soon as the presence of an osteosarcoma is diagnosed, immediate preoperative chemotherapy must be started and continued for 3 months before planning any ablative procedure. The rationale is to reduce the presence of micrometastases. Before starting chemotherapy, the bone marrow, renal, cardiac and liver functions must be assessed. Different multiagent protocols are used such as methotrexate and adriamycin or methotrexate and cisplatin. In the postoperative period, ifosfamide and vp 16 or ifosfamide and cisplatin are used for 35 to 40 weeks.

In case of osteosarcoma, localized to limb/with metastases, these combinations of drugs are the options available for treatment:

Methotrexate high dose with adriamycin
Adriamycin and cisplatin
Methotrexate high dose with cisplatin
Ifosfamide with cisplatin.

These drugs are given either alone or in association with surgery or radiotherapy. These treatment protocols have markedly enhanced the five-year survival rate in comparison with surgery and radiation therapy alone.

Surgery

Limb sparing (limb salvage) surgery is preferred to limb ablation as it produces better functional outcome. If tumor ablation is planned, amputation or disarticulation may be necessary in tumors of the long bones. Radical local excision and reconstruction using custom made prosthesis have recently been tried. In earlier years, the prognosis was poor with a five year survival rate of 5 percent. With the advent of chemotherapy and radiation, the survival rate has been considerably improved and is around 20 percent. If preoperative chemotherapy is tried, there may be extensive tissue necrosis. In cases where there is no soft tissue invasion, amputation is replaced by resection of the tumor with clear margins. Specially made endoprosthesis can be used with minimal discomfort in movement. Five-year survival rate with any form of treatment varies between 5 to 20 percent.

Radiation therapy may be used to augment the erasure of surgical margins in selected situations.

Prognosis

Localized osteosarcoma responding to chemotherapy has a better prognosis. Conservative surgeries and introduction of various prosthesis have markedly improved the life style of patients. Spread to other organs, such as lungs reduces the chance of survival. However multidrug combination chemotherapy and the surgical resection of pulmonary metastatic lesions have proved to be more effective in survival.

Metastatic Osteosarcoma

With more than one site of disease at diagnosis, a more intensive chemotherapy may be recommended. In addition, surgical removal of all visible tumor is also attempted.

Recurrent Osteosarcoma

Treatment depends on where the cancer recurred, what kind of treatment was given before, as well as other factors. If the cancer has come back only in the lungs, the treatment may be surgery to remove the cancer in the lungs with or without chemotherapy. If the cancer has come back in other places besides the lungs, the treatment may be combination chemotherapy.

FURTHER READING

1. Goorin AM. Osteosarcoma: Fifteen years later. N Eng J Med 1985;313:165.
2. Klein MJ. Osteosarcoma: Clinical and pathological considerations. Orthop Clin North Am 1989;320:327.
3. Lane JM, Glasser DB, Healey JH, et al. Two hundred thirty-three patients with osteosarcoma: Survival and prognostic factors. Ortho Trans 1987;11:495.
4. Unni KK, Dahlin DC. Osteosarcoma: Pathology and classification. Semin Roentgenol 1989;243:24-32.

EWING'S FAMILY OF TUMORS

Ewing's family of tumors is neoplasms, which occur most frequently during the second decade of life. They account for about 4-5 percent of all childhood and adolescent malignancies and about 10-15 percent of all bone sarcomas. They are almost equally distributed in both sexes, with a slight male preponderance (F:M 1:1.2). Ewing's tumor of the bone forms almost 60 percent of the entire Ewing's family of tumors.

This family consists of:

Ewing's tumor of the bone (otherwise called Ewing's sarcoma of the bone)

Extraosseous Ewing's tumor

Primitive neuroectodermal tumor

Askin's tumor and esthesioneuroblastomas.

Research has indicated, using immunohistochemistry, cytogenetics, and molecular markers, as well as tissue culture, that these tumors are derived from the same primordial stem cell.

CLINICAL FEATURES

The most favored sites for Ewing's tumor of the bone are the distal extremities, ribs and pelvis. Centrally located tumors, e.g. in the skull, vertebra, ribs, pelvis, as well as those that start in the proximal extremities, tend to have a less favorable prognosis. In the case of PNETs, roughly half of the tumors originate in the chest (44%), abdomen and pelvis (26%), extremities (20%), head and neck (6%). The sites of origin of extraosseous Ewing's tumors are, the trunk in about a 3rd of patients (32%), extremities (26%), head and neck (18%) and retroperitoneum (16%).

The patient usually presents with pain at the site of the tumor. Typically the diaphysis is involved in Ewing's sarcoma of the bone. A plain radiograph may show a characteristic "onion peel" appearance. Fever may be an initial presenting symptom. The patient will usually be anemic and the serum LDH (lactic dehydrogenase) levels may be elevated. In fact, high LDH levels are indicators of a poor prognosis.

PATHOLOGY

These tumors consist of small, round and basophilic cells. In Ewing's sarcoma, sometimes larger cells with lighter staining nuclei are observed to interdigitate with smaller cells with dark, hyperchromatic nuclei, giving rise to a "light cell/dark cell" pattern. The tumor cells tend to be closely packed, and show no evidence of any classical structural pattern. This feature is often helpful in differentiating Ewing's tumors from PNETs, which have typical "rosette" or trabecular patterns, are best appreciated under low power magnification. While Ewing's tumors are usually PAS (Periodic Acid Schiff) positive, immunohistochemistry based on neural markers like neuron specific enolase and S-100, are helpful in identifying the PNETs.

GENETICS

Cytogenetic studies have identified the EWS locus to be on chromosome 22, band q12. Changes involving chromosome 11 and 21 have also been implicated. The classical change in PNETs is a reciprocal translocation on the long arms of chromosomes 11 and 12. Molecular studies have shown that the presence of the MIC2 gene product, a surface protein, is expressed in most Ewing's tumor and PNET.

STAGING

EICESS (European Intergroup Co-Operative Ewing's Sarcoma Studies) allows the EWS to be staged using the rhabdomyosarcoma staging system, as shown below:
    Group I: Can be completely excised
    Group II: Microscopic residual tumor
    Group III: Gross residual tumor
    Metastatic—where tumor has spread to distant sites, most commonly, the lung/bone and bone marrow. This would constitute Group IV (using other common staging systems).

TREATMENT

An extensive hematological and biochemical work up, including LFT and LDH levels, and radioimaging of primary tumor, as well as metastases, are required as a pre-treatment evaluation of the patient. The orthopedic oncologist, medical oncologist, radiologist, and pathologist form the typical team involved in evaluation and follow up.

CHEMOTHERAPY

A multidrug regimen is used, because all patients with apparently localized disease at the time of diagnosis tend to have occult disease. The drugs used include doxorubicin and cyclophosphamide. Vincristine and dactinomycin are equally active. Ifosfamide and etoposide in combination has been found to be effective in Ewing's sarcoma.

Local tumor control is achieved using surgery and/or radiation, depending on the size, resectability of the tumor, and age of the patient. In younger patients, an attempt is made to achieve complete local control without radiation, so that future growth retardation of the bone can be avoided. Clinical trials are presently ongoing to evaluate intensified chemotherapy regimens combined with stem cell rescue (SCR).

RADIATION

Radiation therapy is the primary mode of therapy for Ewing's sarcoma as the tumor is highly radiosensitive. RT technique includes megavoltage equipment, immobilization technique for daily reproduction, and use of beam modifiers like tissue compensators, wedge filters, and individually constructed blocks. In these tumors, a shrinking field technique is used and the dose is 50-55 Gy in conventional fractionation (180-200 cgy/per day) over a period of 6 weeks. Before improved radiotherapy equipments were available to the radiologists, treatment of Ewing's sarcoma was surgery.

In case of metastatic disease, palliative dose of RT 30 Gy/10 to 12 weeks (300 cGy/per day) along with adjuvant chemotherapy is ideal.

Radiation is adjusted based on the stage, and sometimes the age of the patient. The usual regimen is to administer 5,580 cGy to the prechemotherapy tumor volume.

The intergroup Ewing's sarcoma study (IESS) recommends, for patients with gross residual disease, 4500 cGy to original disease site, plus a 1080 cGy boost to gross residual disease. No radiation is recommended for those with no evidence of microscopic residual disease.

PROGNOSIS

The prognosis is substantially better in patients with <5 percent viable tumor, as compared to those with higher volumes of residual viable disease. The French study group EW88 indicated the event free survival in the former to be 75 percent, as compared to those with 75 percent tumor (20%). The prognosis for patients with recurrent Ewing's family of tumors is poor. Patients with either local or distal recurrence have a bad prognosis. Recurrent or refractory tumors call for aggressive treatment including myeloablative regimens, with autologous or allogeneic stem cell transplantation. Radiation to bone lesions can be used to provide palliation. Pulmonary metastases should receive whole lung irradiation. New chemotherapeutic agents used in clinical trials (e.g. topotecan) should be considered in refractory cases.

FURTHER READING

1. Ambros IM, Ambros PF, Strahl S, et al. MIC 2 is a specific marker for Ewing's sarcoma and primitive neuroectodermal tumors. Evidence for a common histiogenesis of Ewing's sarcoma and Peripheral primitive neuroectodermal tumors from MIC2 expression and specific chromosome aberration. Cancer 1991;67(7):1886-93.
2. Cotterill SJ, Ahrens S, Paulussen M, et al. Prognostic factors in Ewing's tumor of bone: Analysis of 975 patients from European Intergroup Co-operative Ewing's Sarcoma Study Group. J Clin Oncol 2000;18(17):3108-14.

3. Delattre O, Zuvman T, Melot T, et al. The Ewing family of tumors- A subgroup of small round cell tumors-defined by specific chimeric transcripts. N Engl J Med 1994;331(5):294-99.
4. Raney RB, Asmar L, Newton WA, et al. Ewing's sarcoma of soft tissues in childhood: A report from the Intergroup Rhabdomyosarcoma Study. 1972-1991 J Clin Oncol 1997;15(2):574-82.

METASTATIC BONE TUMORS

Metastatic tumors of the skeleton outnumber the primary bone tumors by 25 to 1. These are mostly secondary to carcinoma of the prostate, breast, thyroid, lung or kidney. These secondary deposits occur late in the disease, but in bronchogenic carcinoma the pathological fracture through the secondary deposit may be the first symptom.

In children it is secondary to neuroblastoma, leukemia or Ewing's sarcoma.

In young adults the lesions are due to secondaries in lymphoma.

In the elderly, bone metastases are from a primary tumor of the lung, thyroid, prostate or GI tract.

The secondaries are always blood-borne and are seen in bones containing blood forming marrow as in the spine, the ribs, the skull, the pelvis and the metaphysis of the long bones like the femur and the humerus. It must be remembered that metastasis can occur in any bone and in certain cases, this may be the earliest sign of the malignant tumor.

Osteolytic	Osteoblastic
Lung	Prostate
Kidney	Breast
Thyroid	
GI Tract	

Different types of bone metastasis with different primary tumors

Osteolytic metastasis can develop from primary tumor of the lung, kidney, thyroid or GI tract, while the osteoblastic are from the prostate and breast.

The radiographic study of the suspected bone, computerized tomography and isotope bone scan are very helpful in diagnosing metastasis. A needle biopsy should be considered before an open biopsy (Figs 47.3 to 47.5)

The treatment consists of chemotherapy, hormonal manipulation and palliative radiation therapy. Internal fixation is done as a palliative procedure in the case of fracture.

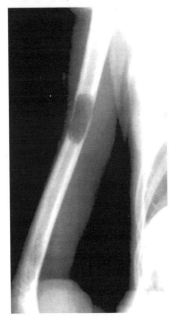

Figure 47.3: Osteolytic metastatic lesion in the body of the humerus, primary not confirmed

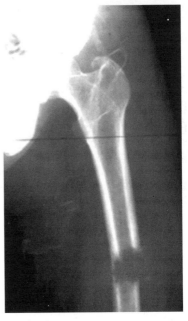

Figure 47.4: Metastatic deposit in the middle of femur with pathological fracture in a case of carcinoma of the lung

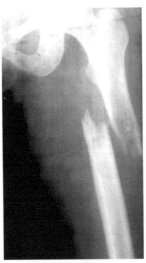

Figure 47.5: Fracture of the femur caused by metastasis from carcinoma of the breast

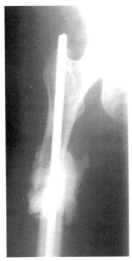

Figure 47.6: Internal fixation with an intra-medullary rod with cementation in a pathological fracture of femur

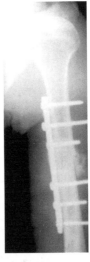

Figure 47.7: Fixation with plate and screw and bone graft with cement in a case of lung cancer

FRACTURE PROPHYLAXIS (FIGS 47.6 AND 47.7)

Biopsy, curettage or excision of some tumors requires the removal of the cortical bone. Therefore the risk of subsequent fracture is always a threat. The weakened bone can be protected with plaster cast or brace until the defect heals. Large defects are reconstructed with bone graft – cortical or fibular graft. Metastatic carcinoma or marrow cell tumors usually produce pathological fractures on trivial trauma. Hence prophylactic internal stabilization using intramedullary rods with or without cementation is an accepted form of treatment.

FURTHER READING

1. Chindia J. Osteosarcoma of the jaw bones. Oral Oncol 2001;37(7):545-47.
2. Debray MP, Geoffroy O, Laissy JP, et al. Imaging appearances of metastases from neuroendocrine tumors. Br J Radiol 2001;74(887):1065-70.
3. Odetayo OO. Pattern of bone tumors at the National Orthopaedic Hospital, Lagos Nigeria. West Afr J Med 2001;20(2):161-64.
4. Orliaguet GA, Hanafi M, Meyer PG. Limited magnetic resonance imaging in low back pain instead of plain radiographs: Experience with first 1000 cases.Clin Radiol 2001;56(11):922-25.
5. Pavlou M, Tsatsoulis A, Efstathiadou Z, Bitsis S. A study of the growth-promoting and metabolic effects of growth hormone (GH) in a patient with the "growth without GH" syndrome. Growth Horm IGF Res 2001;11(4):225-30.

Section III

Treatment of Cancer

- *Principles of Radiation Oncology*
- *Principles of Chemotherapy*
- *Novel Targeted Treatment in Oncology*
- *Stem Cell Collection in Allogenic Transplantation*
- *Hematopoietic Growth Factors*
- *Palliative Care in Cancer Patients*
- *The Care of the Cancer Patients*
- *The Nursing Care of Cancer Patients*
- *The Journey's End*

Principles of Radiation Oncology

48

Babu Zachariah

In the late 1890's both X-rays and gamma rays were discovered. Ever since scientists have been trying to harness these "mysterious" rays for the use in industry, medicine, etc. In the early part of 1900, the clinical effects of radiation on cancer were demonstrated. The injurious effects of radiation on normal tissues were also observed by the researchers. Understanding the mechanism by which radiation works on cancer cells requires a basic knowledge of radiation production and absorption as well as the biologic processes involved. Also needed is an understanding of tumor growth and normal tissue healing. Sensitivity of cells to radiation is greatly dependent on the cell cycle and the presence of oxygen. The potential for repair of radiation damage also varies considerably between tumor cells and normal cells.

THE PHYSICAL BASIS OF RADIATION ONCOLOGY

Since ionizing radiation is used to treat malignancies it is important to know the characteristics of radiation, how it is produced, how it interacts in tissues and how it can be administered effectively in treating malignancies. Ionizing radiations are either electromagnetic or particulate (Fig. 48.1).

Electromagnetic radiation consists of X-rays and gamma rays. They are like packets of energy (photons). They are part of the continuous spectrum that includes radio waves and light. The high-energy end of the spectrum comprises ionizing radiation.

IONIZING RADIATION

Particulate radiation includes electrons, protons, alpha particles, neutrons, negative pi mesons and heavy ions. At present only electrons are commonly used in radiotherapy.

X-rays are produced artificially in a device that accelerates electrons to a high energy and then suddenly stops them by

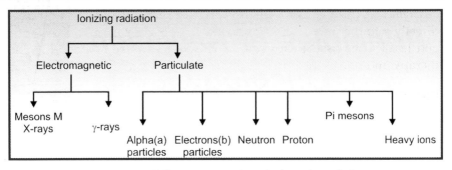

Figure 48.1: Different types of particulates in radiation

an appropriate target of tungsten or copper. Part of the stopping energy is dissipated as heat and the rest is converted into X-rays. This is the process used to produce radiation in X-ray units, accelerators and betatrons. X-rays are also produced when an orbital electron is removed from an atom. X-rays are produced when electrons from other orbitals lose energy as they cascade into the vacancies created. Such a radiation is called characteristic radiation since the radiation is characteristic of the elements from which the electrons have been removed.

Gamma rays are emitted from the nucleus of a radioactive isotope. Radioactive isotope decay occurs when an unstable nucleus gives off excess energy in the form of gamma radiation while attaining a more stable form. Radioactive decay occurs exponentially as a function of time. Half-life of a radioactive isotope represents the time needed for it to decay from a given activity to one-half of that activity. The source of radiation in a Cobalt machine is the decaying ^{60}Co isotope, which produces gamma rays. ^{60}Co has a half-life of 5.3 years.

Electrons are also produced during nuclear decay. X and gamma rays differ only in their origin. They have similar physical and biological properties. Electrons are the most useful among the particulate radiations. Electrons are negatively charged and can be accelerated to high speed in a variety of machines. Protons and neutrons are about 2000 times heavier than electrons. Since protons possess a positive charge they can also be accelerated in a machine. Colliding protons or neutrons on to an appropriate target material produces neutrons. Neutrons are neutral in charge. Alpha particles are about four times heavier and positively charged. Presently they are of no particular relevance.

Ionizing radiation can be delivered in two ways. In *teletherapy*, the radiation-producing source is at some distance from the patient. The long distance is advantageous because the dose distribution will be uniform across a given volume and it allows field shaping or dose modifying devices to be interposed between the source and the patient. In *brachytherapy* (radioactive seed implant), the radioactive sources are placed directly into the tumor site. The dose will be highest close to the sources and least in the tissues farther from the sources. A combination of teletherapy and brachytherapy is used in the treatment of many neoplasms.

BIOLOGIC BASIS OF RADIATION ONCOLOGY

Absorption of X-rays

Radiation is classified as directly or indirectly ionizing. Charged particles like electrons, protons, alpha particles and negative pi mesons are directly ionizing, provided the individual particles have sufficient kinetic energy so that they can directly disrupt the atomic structure of the absorbing tissues through which they pass and produce the chemical and biologic changes.

Electromagnetic radiations (e.g. X-rays and γ-rays) are indirectly ionizing.

The process by which X-rays are absorbed depends on the energy of the X-rays as well as the chemical composition of the absorbing material. In the energy range commonly used in radiation therapy, absorption occurs frequently by the *Compton process*, whereby a photon interacts with "a loosely bound" orbital electron of one of the atoms of the absorber (Fig. 48.2).

The photon interacts with a loosely bound planetary electron of an atom of the absorbing material. Part of the photon energy is given to the electron as kinetic energy and the photon proceeds with reduced energy, deflected from its original direction.

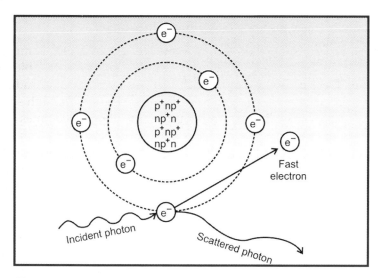

Figure 48.2: Absorption of an X-ray photon by the Compton process

Part of the photon energy is given to the electron as kinetic energy. The photon is deflected from its original direction and proceeds with reduced energy. The ejected fast electron and the scattered photons with reduced energy go on to take part in further interactions in the tissue.

The net result of this process is the production of a large number of fast moving electrons which can ionize other atoms of the absorber, break vital chemical bonds and initiate a chain of events, which is ultimately expressed in biological damage.

RADIATION-INDUCED BIOLOGIC DAMAGE

Radiation-induced cell death occurs only when certain critical targets in the cell are damaged. It is almost certain that DNA in the chromosome represents the most critical target. The nuclear membrane may be yet another target. When X-rays, gamma rays or particulate radiation is absorbed in a biologic material, it can interact directly with the critical targets in the cells leading to ionization or excitation of the target and initiation of a chain of events leading to a biological change. This is called direct action of radiation. This is the dominant process that occurs when high Linear Energy Transfer (LET) radiations such as neutrons or alpha particles are used for irradiating cells (LET is discussed later in the chapter). Radiation can also produce biologic damage by indirect action. Radiation may interact with other atoms or molecules in the cell (e.g. water) and produce free radicals which are able to diffuse far enough to reach and damage the critical targets. This is called indirect action of radiation (Fig. 48.3). The structure of DNA is shown schematically; the letters S, P, A, T, G, and C represent sugar, phosphorus, adenine, thymine, guanine, and cytosine, respectively.

Direct action: A secondary electron resulting from absorption of an X-ray photon interacts with the DNA to produce an effect.

Indirect action: The secondary electron interacts with a water molecule to produce an OH^- radical, which in turn produces the damage to the DNA. It is estimated that free radicals produced within a cylinder of radius 20 Å can damage the DNA. The indirect action is dominant for sparsely ionizing radiation such as X-rays.

A free radical is a free atom or molecule with an unpaired or odd orbital electron. It is highly reactive chemically. Let us consider the interaction of radiation with the cell, since 80 percent of the cell is composed of water. The water molecule becomes ionized.

$$H_2O \longrightarrow H_2O^+ + e^-$$

H_2O^+ is called an ion radical. An ion radical is highly reactive and has extremely short life span. The ion radical interacts with another molecule of water and produces a highly reactive hydroxyl radical (OH^-). This hydroxyl radical can diffuse a short distance and reach the critical target and damage it. Nearly 70 percent of X-ray damage to DNA is mediated

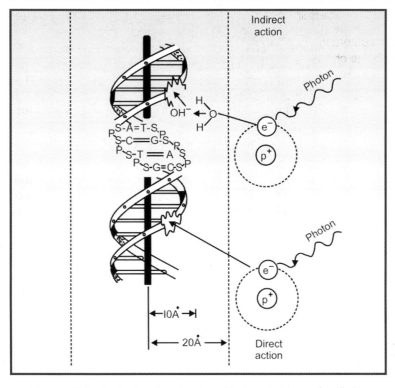

Figure 48.3: Illustrating the direct and indirect actions of radiation

through hydroxyl radical. The indirect action of radiation can be summarized as follows (Fig. 48.4).

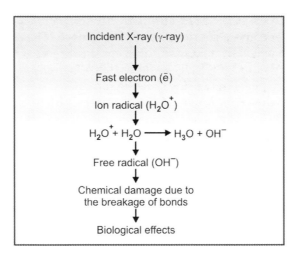

Figure 48.4: Indirect effects of radiation

It may be days, months or years between the breakage of chemical bonds and the final expression of biologic effect of radiation.

Biologic effectiveness of free radicals may be prolonged by the presence of oxygen and other electron affinic molecules. Nitro imidazoles such as metronidazole and misonidazole are examples of such electron affinic agents. Sulfhydryl molecules can scavenge free radicals and reduce their biologic effectiveness. Chemicals with sulfhydryl molecules could produce radioprotection of irradiated cells.

Ionizing radiation when passing through a biologic material produces ionization and excitation. These events tend to be localized along the track of the individual ionizing particles in a pattern characteristic of the type of radiation. The average separation of primary events along the track of ionizing particles decreases with increasing charge and mass. When photons (X-rays/gamma rays) are absorbed electrons are produced which produce ionizations, which are well separated in space. Hence, X-rays are called "sparsely ionizing" radiation. On the other hand, alpha particles which are slowly moving and heavy, produce individual ionization which are very close together. Hence, alpha particles are considered to be densely ionizing. Neutrons are of intermediate ionizing density. Linear Energy Transfer (LET) is the energy transferred per unit length of the track of radiation. Radiation of high charges and high mass have high LET. Radiation with high energy and high velocity have low LET.

If you closely study the cell survival curve (Fig. 48.5A), it has an initial slope (dotted straight line) at low doses where the surviving fraction appears to be an exponent function of dose. As the dose is increased the curve bends over and becomes progressively steeper. At very high doses, the curve tends to become straight again, i.e. the surviving fraction returns to be an exponential function of the dose again. Alpha represents the linear non-reparable component of cell kill and beta represents cell kill after some repair process has been eliminated with increasing dose. Beta represents the reparable component of cell damage. The dose, at which the two components of cell kill are equal constitutes the alpha-beta ratio.

The fraction of surviving cells is plotted on a logarithmic scale against dose on a linear scale. For densely ionizing radiations, such as low-energy neutrons, the dose-response curve is a straight line and may be characterized by one parameter, the 37 percent dose slope or D_0 For sparsely ionizing radiation such as X-rays, the dose-response curve has an initial shoulder followed by a portion which is almost straight. The curve is characterized by two parameters: the 37 percent dose slope, D_0 and the straight portion. The extrapolation number, n, is a measure of the "width" of the initial shoulder.

BASIS OF FRACTIONATION IN RADIOTHERAPY

Radiation is administered conventionally in daily fractions. The most important biologic phenomenon that influences the fractionation response

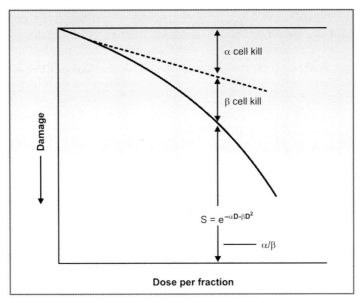

Figure 48.5A: Typical survival curves for mammalian cells exposed to radiation

to the radiation therapy is the capacity for cellular repair of sublethal damage. Each repeated fractional dose allows for cell repair of sublethal damage and is expressed as multiple shoulders in the cell survival curve (Fig. 48.5B).

Each repeated fractional dose allows for repair of sublethal damage of the cells and is expressed by the recapitulation of the shoulder of the survival curve. If 1,000 rad (10 Gy) is given as a divided fractional dose ($D_1 D_2 D_3 D_4 D_5$) of 200 rad (2 Gy) daily, it achieves a similar degree of cell kill (S on the dashed line) as 600 rad (6 Gy) given in one single exposure. The survival curve for single acute exposure to X-rays is curve A. A differential effect on therapeutic ratio between tumor cells and normal cells increases with divided or fractional doses of radiation. This is displayed by the increasing differences in the slopes of the solid lines (single dose) and dashed lines (fractional dose) *Modified from: Elkind and Whitmore (1967)*

The repair occurs rapidly. Slowly responding tumors show greater repair capacity than rapidly responding ones. Repair of sublethal injury is slower in slowly responding tumors than rapidly responding tissues. Repair is usually complete in 6-8 hours. Late responding tissues are spared more by dose fractionation than are acutely responding tissues. Most malignant tumors and proliferating normal tissues such as skin, mucosa and bone marrow fall in the acutely responding group. The clinical implication is that large dose fractions are relatively more harmful to late responding tissues. Therapeutic gain may be possible by using smaller daily fractions.

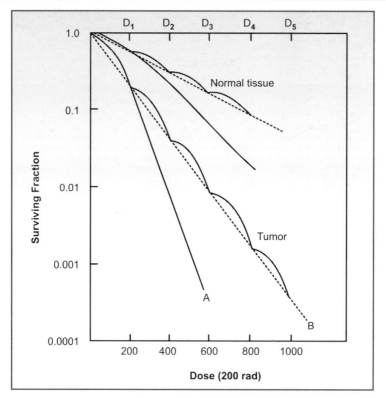

Figure 48.5B: Cell repair and fractionation effect

When radiation dose rate diminishes, significantly more cells survive a given dose of radiation. This is due to repair of sublethal damage and the proliferation of undamaged or viable cells. This effect is important in interstitial and intracavitary brachytherapy where dose rates are typically 40 cGy/hr compared to 100 cGy/min with external beam radiation. With low dose rates used in brachytherapy a higher total dose can be given over a shorter overall time due to repair and repopulation of normal tissues.

CELL CYCLE EFFECT

Radiation sensitivity of cells varies with cell age. Cells are most sensitive during mitosis and G2 phases of cell cycle (Fig. 48.6A). In the survival curve with no shoulder and the steepest slope is representing cells in the mitosis/G2 phase (Fig. 48.6B). Cells in the late "S" phase are the most resistant. The survival curve of late S phase cells is less steep and has a larger shoulder. Cells in the G1 and early 'S' phases are of intermediate sensitivity. The broken line is a calculated curve, which represents mitotic cells under hypoxia which is 2.5 times shallower than the solid line for mitotic cells which applies to an aerated condition.

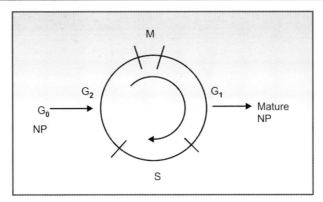

Figure 48.6A: Cell cycle age: G_0 = Resting (quiescent) cell; G = Gaps; G_1 = First gap before DNA synthesis; G_2 = Second gap before mitosis; NP = Nonproliferating (mature cells); M = Mitosis; S = DNA synthetic phase. [Modified from : Hall (1988)].

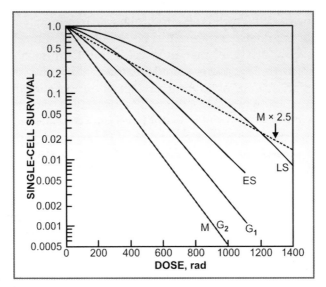

Figure 48.6B: Cell-survival curves for Chinese hamster cells at various stages of the cell cycle. For cells in mitosis and G2, the survival curve is steep and has no shoulder. For cells late in S, the curve is less steep and has a large initial shoulder. G_1 and early S are intermediate in sensitivity. The broken line is a calculated curve expected to apply to mitotic cells under hypoxia [From Sinclair WK: Radiat Res 33:620-643, 1968]

The surviving fraction is function of cell cycle age. The radiosensitivity of a cell changes as it moves through the cell cycle, being most sensitive in G_2 M.

The range of sensitivity between the most sensitive cells and the most resistant cells is of the same order of magnitude as the oxygen effect. One of the purposes of fractionation is to take advantage of the cells moving from the resistant to the sensitive phase of the cycle (*re-distribution*) during the daily fractional doses of radiation.

REPOPULATION

Both tumors and normal cells have proliferating stem cells which continue to divide during the course of fractionated radiotherapy. As normal cells die during radiotherapy the tissue responds by changing from a quiescent state to a regenerative state recruiting new cells into the cycle. This repopulation of normal tissues is beneficial since it helps to reduce the overall injury from radiation. It is more important in the early responding tissues such as skin, mucosa and bone marrow. It is less important in late responding tissues like liver and central nervous system.

Tumors also regenerate during the course of fractionated radiotherapy. Hermens and Barendsen showed exponential increase in the number of clonogens in a rat rhabdomyosarcoma after a delay equal to one volume doubling time (A cell which is able to proliferate indefinitely to produce a large clone or colony is considered to be clonogenic). It has been shown by Suit, Howes and Hunter that an increase in total dose is required for tumor control with increasing overall treatment duration.

Tumors might have proliferating clonogens during radiotherapy even when the tumor is regressing clinically. This may be due to improved oxygenation as dead tumor cells are removed from the cell pool. The tumor cell may be proliferating even more rapidly than before treatment was initiated.Tumor regeneration appears to affect the cure rate in certain cancers such as head, neck, bladder, skin and inflammatory breast cancer and melanoma.

Protraction of treatment time should be avoided if possible. If a break in treatment is necessary because of acute toxicity it should be as short as possible. Planned treatment breaks are not recommended unless they are parts of an accelerated treatment protocol. Rapidly growing tumors should be treated using a short course of therapy to avoid repopulation of the clonogenic cells.

CLINICAL ASPECTS OF RADIATION ONCOLOGY

The ability to eradicate a tumor is highly dependent on the size and radio sensitivity of the tumor. Cell killing by radiation is an exponential function of the dose. Fewer total doses are required to eradicate microscopic disease (less than 10^6 cells) compared to a kilogram of tumor cells (10^{12} cells). The radiation dose required for a given tumor control probability is dependent on tumor volume. Tumors show a wide variation in their sensitivity to radiation. The most sensitive to radiation among the tumors are lymphomas, leukemias, seminomas and dysgerminomas. The least sensitive ones are the melanomas and sarcomas.

The *radiosensitivity* and *radio resistance* are relative terms. Large tumors of "radio resistant" cells can be killed with high doses of radiation.

Normal tissues contain no or few hypoxic cells. But tumors contain at least 5-20 percent hypoxic cells. The extent to which reoxygenation occurs during the radiotherapy may help to determine the chance of eradication of these tumors.

The goal of any form of cancer therapy is to cure the cancer with minimal normal tissue complications. The *radiocurability* of a tumor depends not only on the radiosensitivity but also the normal tissue tolerance. Any tumor can be cured if given enough doses of radiation, provided the normal tissue around it is protected from radiation injury.

THERAPEUTIC RATIO

Therapeutic ratio is the ratio of normal tissue tolerance dose to the tumor lethal dose. When tumor control probability is plotted against the dose of radiation given, a sigmoid shaped curve is obtained. If normal tissue complications are plotted against radiation dose, a similar curve will be obtained (Figs 48.7 and 48.8).

These curves depict much of the art of radiotherapy. The probability of tumor control should be balanced against the probability of normal tissue complications when deciding the radiation dose and fractionation schedule. At certain dose levels, if the tumor control probability was already 90 percent there would be no therapeutic gain from dose increases, if there was already an incidence of severe complications of 5 percent or

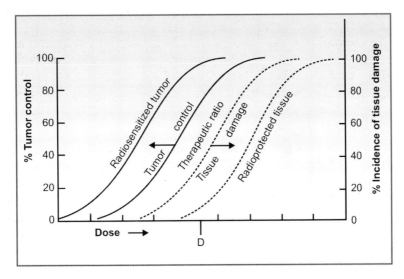

Figure 48.7: The concept of radiosensitization and radioprotection is based upon the use of agents that can displace either the tumor dose-response curve to the left or the normal tissue damage curve to the right, thereby increasing the therapeutic ratio

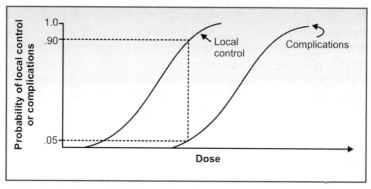

Figure 48.8: Both the probability of local tumor control and the probability of complications are a sigmoid function of dose. If the two curves are widely separated, it is possible to achieve a high rate of tumor control with a small complication rate. If the curves are closer together, as may be the case for large, resistant tumors, this favorable situation would not apply

more. Improvement in therapeutic ratio requires that the curves for tumor response and normal tissue complications be separated further. Increase in biologic effectiveness of therapy must be greater in the tumor than in normal tissues. Normal tissues should be preferentially spared if there is to be a therapeutic gain.

RADIATION RESPONSE

The response to radiation varies among different tumors. Some tumors respond very slowly, many regress quickly. Variation in radiosensitivity among tumor cells cannot be measured by the response to irradiation. Radiation response will depend on the proliferation kinetics of the malignant clonogens, programmed lifetime of terminally differentiated cells in the tumor and the rate of removal of the dead cells. Local control rate may be slightly higher for rapidly regressing tumors than for slowly regressing ones. It is not recommended to reduce radiation dose based on rapid regression of the tumor.

Slow regression of a tumor may be due to slow proliferation and cell loss kinetics of the tumor, residual stroma or treatment failure. Some tumors regress slowly even though the clonogens are completely sterilized (e.g. prostate carcinoma, teratocarcinoma of the testis, some cases of nodular sclerosing Hodgkin's disease, soft tissue sarcoma, pituitary adenoma and chordoma). A small portion of most tumors regresses slowly even though the major portion regresses quickly. Biopsy results of slowly regressing tumors could be misleading since the cells which are sterilized but still living may be histologically indistinguishable from cells with retained clonogenic capacity. Biopsy should be avoided if the tumor is continuing to regress.

Cure of a cancer is defined as removal of the risk of death invoked by the disease that was treated. *Local control* means that the tumor never returned in the area that was treated; the *response* is assessed from the change in the size of the tumor. *Complete response* (CR) means that the tumor is no longer detectable clinically. *Partial response* to therapy means more than 50 percent reduction in tumor size. Partial response in most clinical situations provides some palliation of symptoms without any impact on the duration of survival.

Radiocurability means that the tumor-normal tissue relations are such that curative doses of radiation can be applied without excessive damage to normal tissues. Carcinomas of cervix, larynx, prostate, breast, Hodgkin's disease and seminoma are some of the examples of radiocurable tumors. Curative doses for different tumor types are shown in Table 48.1.

Table 48.1: Curative doses of radiation for different tumor types

2000-3000 cGy
Seminoma
Dysgerminoma
Acute lymphocytic leukemia

3000-4000 cGy
Seminoma (bulky)
Wilms' tumor cancers
Neuroblastoma

4000-4500 cGy
Hodgkin's disease
Lymphosarcoma
Histiocytic cell sarcoma
Basal cell skin cancer

5000-6000 cGy
Lymph nodes, metastatic (N0, N1)
Squamous cell carcinoma,
cervix cancer and head and neck
cancer
Embryonal cancer
Breast cancer, ovarian cancer
medulloblastoma
Retinoblastoma
Breast cancer (excised)

6000-6500 cGy
Larynx (<1 cm)
Breast cancer (T$_1$)

7000-7500 cGy
Oral cavity (<2 cm, 2-4 cm)
Oro-naso-laryngo-pharyngeal
Breast cancer (T$_2$)
Bladder cancer
Cervix cancer
Uterine fundal cancer
Ovarian cancer
Lymph nodes, metastatic (1-3 cm)
Lung cancer (<3 cm)

8000 cGy or Above
Head and neck cancer (>4 cm)
Breast cancer (>5 cm)
Glioblastoma (glioma)
Osteogenic sarcoma (bone sarcoma)
Melanoma
Soft tissue sarcoma (>5 cm)
Thyroid cancer
Lymph nodes, metastatic (>6 cm)

Modified from Rubin P: Clinical Oncology: A Multidisciplinary Approach, 6th Ed, p 64. New York, American Cancer Society, 1983

PRINCIPLES OF CLINICAL RADIOTHERAPY

External beam radiotherapy is administered conventionally using daily dose fractions of 180-200 rads (cGy). Radiation is administered continuously usually 4-5 days a week with a 2 day weekend break. Radiation field is made covering the tumor with a margin for possible microscopic extension of cancer beyond the grossly visible tumor and taking into account the setup variation and organ movements during daily treatment. A dose of 4500-5000 cGy in 4 ½-5 weeks is needed to kill microscopic cancer cells (10^6 cells). Subsequently the field size is reduced to cover the gross tumor with a margin and the full planned dose is delivered. Additional boost dose is added in special situations (Fig. 48.9).

When deciding the tumor dose, the total tumor burden should be taken into consideration. As the tumor size increases the dose required to eradicate the tumor also increases (Table 48.2).

CONVENTIONAL FRACTIONATION

Usually radiation is administered once a day (180-200 cGy/fraction) which is considered as conventional fraction. For a curative course of therapy, radiation is continued for 6 to 8 weeks (Table 48.3).

HYPERFRACTIONATION

In this schedule of fractionation, the dose size per fraction is reduced, total dose increased and the number of dose fractions is increased. The overall treatment time is relatively unchanged because 2 fractions a day are administered. Hyperfractionation allows higher total dose to be administered within the dose tolerance of late responding normal tissues and this translates into a higher biologically effective dose to the tumor. The greater the number of dose fractions, the greater the opportunity for tumor cells to be sensitized by redistribution in the cell cycle. The cells in the radioresistant phase at the time of any given fraction administered

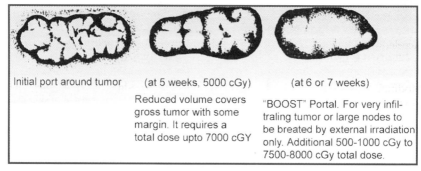

Initial port around tumor	(at 5 weeks, 5000 cGy)	(at 6 or 7 weeks)
	Reduced volume covers gross tumor with some margin. It requires a total dose upto 7000 cGY	"BOOST" Portal. For very infiltraling tumor or large nodes to be breated by external irradiation only. Additional 500-1000 cGy to 7500-8000 cGy total dose.

Figure 48.9: Shrinking field technique (Modified from Fletcher GH: Textbook of Radiotherapy, 3rd Ed, p 228. Philadelphia, Lea and Febiger, 1983)

Table 48.2: Tumor control probability correlated with radiation dose and volume of cancer

Dose	Squamous cell carcinoma of the upper respiratory and digestive tracts	Adenocarcinoma of the breast
5000 cGy*	> 90% subclinical 60% T1 lesions of nasopharynx ~50% 1-3 cm neck nodes	>90% Subclinical
6000 cGy*	~90% T1 lesions of pharynx and larynx† ~50% T3 and T4 lesions of tonsillar fossa ~90% 1-3 cm neck nodes ~70% 3-5 cm neck nodes	90% Clinically positive axillary nodes 2.5-3 cm‡
7000 cGy*	~90% T-2 lesions of tonsillar fossa and supraglottic larynx ~80% T3 and T4 lesions of tonsillar fossa	
7000-8000 cGy (8-9 wk) ⟶		65% 2-3 cm primary 30% >5 cm primary
8000-9000 cGy (8-10 wk) ⟶		56% >5 cm primary
8000-10,000 cGy (10-12 wk) ⟶		75% 5-15 cm primary

*1000 cGy in five fractions each week
† Universal experience
‡ The control rate is corrected for the percentage of nodes that would be positive histologically, had a dissection of the axilla been done.
(Fletcher GH, Shukovsky LJ: J Radiol Electrol 56:383, 1975)

Table 48.3: Various types of fractionation used in radiation therapy

Fractionation schedules: Dose-Fractionation in Radiotherapy

Type	Time	Dose	Schedule
Conventional	T	D	‖‖‖ ‖‖‖ ‖‖‖ ‖‖‖ ‖‖‖ ‖‖‖ 200 cGy/day
Hyperfractionation	T	D + d	‖‖‖ ‖‖‖ ‖‖‖ ‖‖‖ ‖‖‖ ‖‖‖ 115 cGy × 2/day
Accelerated MDF	T/$\frac{2}{3}$	D − d	‖‖‖ ‖‖‖ ‖‖‖ ‖‖‖ ‖‖‖ 150-200 cGy × 2/day
Modified Accelerated Fractionation	T	D + d	‖‖‖ ‖‖‖ ‖‖‖ ‖‖‖ ‖‖‖ ‖‖‖ Boost
Split Course	T + Rest	D	‖‖‖ ‖‖‖ REST ‖‖‖ ‖‖‖ >250 cGy/day
Hypofractionation	T − t	D − d	‖‖ ‖‖ ‖‖ ‖‖ ‖‖ 500 cGy/day

are more likely to be caught in a more sensitive phase at the time of subsequent fraction administrations. With small fractional doses, the influence of tumor cell hypoxia is reduced on two counts. Since the rationale for hyperfractionation depends on tumors behaving like acutely responding normal tissues, it is inevitable that the use of this strategy will be associated with more severe acute reactions than are associated with conventional fractionation. For hyperfractionation to be effective the α/β ratio of tumor cells must be greater than that for the dose limiting normal tissue. The nonreparable component of cell kill should be higher. (α/β represents the capacity to repair the sub-lethal damage). α/β ratio of acutely responding tissues is higher than that of late responding normal tissues. Tumors also tend to have larger α/β ratio.

Comparing conventional fractionation to hyperfractionation, several Phase III clinical trials on head and neck and bladder cancers have shown improved local control and survival favoring hyperfractionation. There was no difference in late treatment-related morbidity except for the bladder cancer study (Table 48.4).

HYPOFRACTIONATION

In this schedule the size of dose per fraction is increased. The total dose, the number of dose fractions and overall time are reduced. Most tumors have a large α/β ratio; hence it would result in a therapeutic disadvantage. Hypofractionation may be advantageous in treating tumors with a low α/β ratio. One example of such a tumor is malignant melanoma.

ACCELERATED FRACTIONATION

In this regimen the overall treatment time is reduced. The number of dose fractions, total dose, and size of dose per fraction are either unchanged or somewhat reduced, depending on the extent of overall treatment time reduction.

ACCELERATED HYPERFRACTIONATION

This is a fractionation schedule incorporating features of both accelerated fractionation and hyperfractionation. In accelerated fractionation schedules 2-3 fractions with daily fractional dose ranging from 1-3.75 Gy has been used (mostly 1.25-3.00 Gy/fractions) with at least 4-hour interval between fractions. This schedule will help prevent repopulation of tumor during therapy. Accelerated treatment regimens have produced better tumor control and improved survival in many tumors (head and neck, breast, lung, etc.) Acute reactions associated with accelerated and hyperfractionation schedules could be very severe depending on the fraction size. Late normal tissue reactions may be increased depending on the fraction size, number of fractions given daily and interfraction

Table 48.4: Clinical studies using predominantly hyperfractionation: Phase III trials

Tumor site	Patients N	Dose/ Fraction Gy	Fractions/ D/N (Time, h)	Total dose Gy	Overall time, wk	Tumor response	Complications	Reference
Head and neck; Oropharynx; T2-T3, NO-N1	356	1.15	2 (6-8)	80.5	7	5 yr LRC: 59% vs 40% (P-0.02)	More severe acute myositis in hyper-fractionation arm.	Horiot et al.
		2.0	1	70.0	7		No difference in incidence of late complications	
Head and neck; oral cavity, oropharynx, and larynx, T2-T3, NO-N1	91	1.2	2 (4-6)	79.2	6.5	2-yr LRC: 63% vs 33% (P<0.001)	More acute mucosal and skin reactions in hyperfraction arm (requiring 3-5 days) interruption in 34 pts. Similar late complication rate	Datta et al.
	85	2.0	1	66.0	6.5			
Head and neck; oropharynx; Stage III-IV	50	1.1	2 (>6)	66.0	6.5	Control of primary lesions: 84% vs 64% (P-0.02)	Earlier onset of acute reactions in hyper-fractioned arm	Pinto et al.
	48	2.0	1	70.4	6.5	Survival at 42 mos: 27% vs 8% (P=0.03)	Late complications not fully reported	

contd...

Table 48.4: contd...

Tumor site	Patients N	Dose/Fraction Gy	Fractions/D/N (Time, h)	Total dose Gy	Overall time, wk	Tumor response	Complications	Reference
Bladder; T2–T4	83	1.0	3(4)	84.0	8 (2 wk break)	CR at 6 mos 65% vs 36% (P=0.001)	Severe late reactions (intestinal obstructions, fistulae, bleeding): 12% vs 5%	Edsmyr et al.
	85	2.0	1	64.0	8 (2wk break)	5-year survival: 34% vs 22% (P=0.01)		

CR—complete response; LRC—local-regional control

Table 48.5: Comparison of various fractionations

	Conventional	Multiple daily split-course	Fractions	Hyperfractionation
Indication in tumors of growth rate	Average	Average or slow	Rapid	Slow (with large cell loss factors)
Normal tissue effects, acute	Standard	Standard	Greater	Standard or greater
Normal tissue effects, late	Standard	Greater	Standard (if complete repair of SLD occurs) or greater	Lower
Advantages	Shorter actual treatment time (fewer fractions)	Shorter actual treatment time (fewer fractions)	Destroys more tumor	(?) Lower OER with small doses; spares late damage; allows reoxygenation; allows more fractions stem cell
Disadvantages	May permit tumor repopulation	May permit tumor repopulation		Repopulating more fractions

SLD—Sublethal damage; OER—Oxygen enhancement ratio

interval. Interfraction intervals of 6 hours appear to be sufficient for repair of sublethal damage in order to reduce the late normal tissue complications. A comparison of various fractionations is shown in Table 48.5.

NORMAL TISSUE EFFECTS OF RADIATION

Normal tissues have a substantial capacity to recover from sublethal and potentially lethal damage induced by radiation. The cells may undergo several divisions before final somatic death occurs. Injury to normal tissue from radiation may be due to the radiation effect on the microvascular system and support tissues. Radiation tolerance of various organs is shown in Table 48.5. TD 5/5 represents the dose of radiation that could cause no more than 5% severe complication rate within 5 years after radiation therapy.

TD$_{50/5}$: The maximal tolerance dose—the dose to which a given population of patients is exposed under a standard set of treatment conditions resulting in a 50 percent severe complication rate within 5 years after treatment (Table 48.6).

Hemopoietic tissues are very sensitive to radiation. Among them, lymphocytes are the most sensitive component of the peripheral blood

Table 48.6: Fatal or severe morbidity following cumulative doses of radiation delivered with standard fractionation

Organ	Injury	TD (5/5*)	TD (50/5)	Whole/Partial
Bone	Aplasia, Pancytopenia	250	450	Whole
		3000	4000	Segmental
Liver	Acute and chronic hepatitis	2500	4000	Whole
		1500	2000	Whole (strip)
Stomach	Perforation, ulcer, hemorrhage	4500	5500	100 cm
Intestine	Ulcer, perforation, hemorrhage	4500	5500	400 cm
		5000	6500	100 cm
Brain	Infarction, necrosis	5000	6000	Whole
Spinal cord	Infarction, necrosis	4500	5500	10 cm
Heart	Pericarditis, pancarditis	4500	5500	60%
		7000	8000	25%
Lung	Acute and chronic pneumonitis	3000	3500	100 cm
		1500	2500	Whole
Kidney	Acute and chronic nephrosclerosis	1500	2000	Whole (strip)
		2000	2500	Whole
Fetus	Death	200	400	Whole

TD$_{5/5}$: minimal tolerance dose-the dose to which a given population of patients is exposed under a standard set of treatment conditions resulting in no more than a 5% severe complication rate within 5 years of treatment.

(Rubin P, Cooper R, Philips TL [eds]: Radiation Biology and Radiation Pathology Syllabus. Set RT1: Radiation Oncology. Chicago, American College of Radiology, 1975)

cells. No clinically significant change is seen in peripheral blood cell count during limited field fractionated external beam therapy. Most of the drop in count occurs during the 2nd and 6th week of radiotherapy. Patients who had prior or concurrent chemotherapy with radiation therapy are prone to have a decrease in peripheral blood count during radiotherapy.

Older patients are generally considered poor candidates for radiotherapy due to decreased functional reserve. Zachariah et al have reported that older patients with good performance status and fewer comorbid illness tolerate radiotherapy as well as younger patients. Hence older patients should not be denied curative radiotherapy based on age alone.

PALLIATIVE TREATMENT

A major portion of the clinical practice in radiation oncology is palliative care. Where cure is not possible, relief of uncomfortable symptoms and improvement of quality of life are the goals of therapy. Palliation is usually achieved with a short course of therapy using higher daily fractions. A typical palliative course of radiotherapy is 3000 cGy given in 10 fractions to the metastatic site. Fraction size used for palliative therapy ranges from 250 cGy to 1000 cGy.

Some clinicians give 2000 cGy in 4 or 5 courses for bone metastasis whereas a single dose of 800-1000 cGy is preferred by some others. Brain and bone are the most common sites of cancer metastasis. Very modest doses of radiation could stop bleeding from an oozing ulcerative tumor surface. Vaginal or bronchial bleeding could be stopped by a dose of 800-1000 cGy. Radiation is used as an emergency measure in spinal cord compression or superior vena cava syndrome to avoid permanent functional and circulatory compromise.

COMBINED THERAPY

Radiation may be combined with surgery or chemotherapy. In locally advanced cancer, surgery alone is inadequate to eradicate the tumor. In some situations the tumor cells may be relatively resistant to radiotherapy. In these situations debulking or grossly removing the tumor and treating the remaining tumor mass with radiotherapy will be more effective in achieving maximum tumor control. In some situations the tolerance of the tissues surrounding the tumor may be very low. Hence combination of surgery will be helpful to obtain optimal tumor control.

Radiation therapy usually fails at the center of the tumor where the concentration of tumor clonogens is largest and the cells are relatively hypoxic. Surgical resections fail because the tumor extends beyond the margins of excision infesting the contiguous tissues with microscopic foci. Radiotherapy in moderate doses is efficient in sterilizing microscopic extension beyond the visible tumor. Surgical resection is capable of removing the bulky necrotic tumor mass. These efficiencies lead to the logical combination of radiation and surgery.

The optimal sequencing of surgery and radiation should be selected depending on the clinical situation. Radiation given prior to surgery has the advantage of treating undisturbed tissues. The area irradiated may be smaller in preoperative radiotherapy compared to postoperative therapy. Technically unresectable tumors may be made resectable by preoperative radiotherapy.

Major disadvantages of preoperative radiotherapy include the lack of precise pathologic definition of the extent of the tumor and the impairment of normal tissue healing at the time of subsequent surgery.

Postoperative radiation has the disadvantage of requiring treatment of a larger area potentially contaminated by tumor cells at the time of surgery. Combined radiotherapy and surgery has the potential of improving local control of the tumor while reducing the morbidity associated with more aggressive single modality therapy.

Chemotherapy is generally used to enhance the local effects of radiotherapy or to control microscopic subclinical disease elsewhere in the body. The chemotherapeutic agents should be selected in such a way that their toxic effects are in the organs distant from the site of radiotherapy. In some situations the benefits of combining surgery, chemotherapy and radiotherapy should be explored. The combination of three modalities seems to be beneficial in inflammatory breast cancer where each discipline has a significant impact on the disease process producing an improvement in disease-free survival.

SUMMARY

Radiation therapy is an important modality used for the treatment of cancer. It has the potential of eradicating tumor either alone or in combination with surgery or chemotherapy. Radiation is used for curative as well as palliative treatments. Currently most cancers are treated using a multidisciplinary approach. A thorough understanding of the radiobiologic principles will enable us to use this modality to its maximum potential. Basic knowledge of radiotherapy enables us to select the optimum beam energy, fractionation schedule and total dose in the treatment of solid tumors. The limitation of radiation therapy due to large tumor size, presence of hypoxia, normal tissue tolerance etc. should be taken into consideration while selecting the therapeutic modality for different tumors.

The 4 R's of radiobiology are Repair, Repopulation, Reoxygenation and Redistribution. Fractionation of radiation is based on these principles. Fractionation is useful in escalating the dose without increasing the normal tissue complications. It has been shown in several tumors that increasing the dose increases the local control and hence survival of the patient. 3 dimensional conformal radiotherapy (3DCRT) and intensity modulated radiotherapy (IMRT) are being used widely now to improve local control by escalating the tumor dose and reducing the dose to the surrounding normal tissues. Chemical and biologic modifiers enhance the effect of radiotherapy. The ultimate goal in radiotherapy is to provide cure without significant complications. We are not too far from achieving this goal.

FURTHER READING

1. Allen EP. A trial of radiation dose prescription based on dose-cell survival formula. Australas 1984;28:156.
2. Ang KK, Landuyt W, Rijnders A, et al. Differences in repopulation kinectics in mouse skin, during split course multiple fractions per day or daily fractionated irradiations. Int J Radiat Oncol Biol Phys 1985;10:95-103.
3. Barendsen GW. Dose fractionation, dose rate and iso effect relationship for normal tissue response. Int J Radiol Oncol Biol Phys 1982;8:1984.
4. Barker JL, Montague ED, Peters LT. Clinical experience with irradiation of inflammatory carcinoma of the breast with and without elective chemotherapy. Cancer 1980;45:625.
5. Choi KN, Withers HR, Rotman M. Metastatic melanoma in brain; rapid treatment or large dose fractions. Cancer 1985;56:10.
6. Coutard H. Principles of X-ray therapy of malignant diseases. Lancet II 1934;1-12.
7. Elkind MM, Sutton H. X-ray damage and recovery in mammalian cells in culture. Nature 1995;184:1293.
8. Elkind MM, Swain RW, Alesco T, et al. Oxygen, nitrogen, recovery and radiation therapy. Cellular Radiation Biology. Baltimore: Williams and Wilkins 1965;442-46.
9. Gray LH, Conger AD, Ebert M, et al. The concentration of oxygen dissolved in tissues at the time of irradiation as a factor in radiotherapy. Br J Radiol 1953;26:638.
10. Hall EJ. Radiobiology for the Radiologist (2nd edn) 1978. Medical Department Harper and Row, Publishers Hagerstown, Maryland.
11. Hermens AF, Barendsen GW. Changes of cell proliferation characteristics in a rat rhabdomyosarcoma before and after X-irradiation. Euro J Cancer 1969;5:173.
12. Knee R, Field RS, Peter LJ. Concomitant boost radiotherapy for Advanced Squamous Cell Carcinoma of the head and neck, 1985.
13. Suit DH, Gallagher HS. Intact tumor cells in irradiated tissue. Arch Pathol 1964;78:648-51.
14. Suit HD, Howes AF, Hunter N. Dependence of response of a C3H mammary carcinoma to fractionated irradiation on fractionation number and intertreatment interval Radiat Res 1977;72:440.
15. Suit HD, Lindberg RD, Fletcher GH. Prognostic significance of extent of tumor regression at completion of Radiation Therapy. Radiology 1965;84:1100.
16. Thames HD, Withers HR, Peters LJ, et al. Changes in early and late radiation responses with altered dose fractionation; implications for dose survival relationships. Int J Radiat Oncol Biol Phys 1982;8:219.
17. Thomlinson RH, Gray LH. The histological structure of some human lung cancer and the possible implications for radiotherapy. Br J Cancer 1955;9:539-49.

18. Whithers HR, Thames HD, Peters LJ, et al. Normal tissue radio resistance in clinical radiotherapy. In, Fletcher GH, Nervi C, Withers HR (Eds): Biological Basis and Clinical Implications of Tumor Resistance. New York: Masson 1983;139.

19. Zachariah B. Radiotherapy for cancer patients aged 80 and older. A study of effectiveness and side effects. International J of Radiation Oncology Biology Physics 1997;39(5):1125.

20. Zachariah B, Jacob S, Gwede C, Cantor A, Patil J, Casey L, Zachariah A. Effect of fractionated regional external beam radiotherapy on peripheral blood cell count. Int J Radiation Oncology Biol Phys 2001;50(2):465-72.

Principles of Chemotherapy

49

Jame Abraham, Ramin Altaha

INTRODUCTION

Over the past 60 years treatment of cancer with chemotherapy has evolved into a mature field. Advances in the field of oncology in the fifth and sixth decades of the twentieth century have resulted in the development of curative therapeutic interventions for patients with several types of advanced solid tumors and hematological neoplasms. Over the past 25 years, advances in the field of basic science have helped the oncologists to understand the pathophysiology of the disease better and develop targeted treatments. Targeted treatment will eliminate one of the major limiting features of chemotherapy, which is the toxic effect on the normal tissues.

The effective use of cancer chemotherapy results from a comprehensive understanding of the principles of pharmacology and tumor biology along with detailed knowledge of the natural history of the disease being treated. At the same time it is very important for the physician to understand the goals and expectations of the patient and family. The selection of a particular chemotherapy plan depends on many factors. These include clinical experience, an understanding of the pharmacology of the drugs to be used, the potential for drug interactions, the likelihood of drug-resistant cells in the tumor, the physiologic status of the patient, and the presence of sanctuary sites or other unusual characteristics of the tumor that may influence the dose, schedule, or route of administration of a particular drug.

HISTORY OF CHEMOTHERAPY

Paul Ehrlich, who used *in vivo* rodent model systems to develop antibiotics, coined the term chemotherapy. George Clowes, at Roswell Park Memorial Institute in Buffalo, New York, in the early 1900s, developed inbred rodent lines bearing transplanted tumors to screen potential anticancer drugs. This *in vivo* system provided the foundation for mass screening of novel compounds. Alkylating agents, that were a product of the secret gas program of the United States in both world wars, represent the first class of chemotherapeutic drugs to be used in the clinical setting. The exposure to mustard gas in World War II caused marrow and lymphoid hypoplasia. This observation led to the use of alkylating agents in humans with hematologic neoplasms, including Hodgkin's disease and lymphocytic lymphomas, at the Yale Cancer Center in 1943. Because of the secret nature of the gas warfare program, this work was not published until 1946. The demonstration of dramatic response in advanced lymphomas with chemotherapy generated much excitement. Meanwhile Sidney Farber reported that folic acid had a significant proliferative effect on leukemic cell growth in children with lymphoblastic leukemia. This led to the discovery of folic acid analogs as cancer drugs to inhibit folate metabolism. That was the beginning of the chemotherapy era.

GUIDELINES TO USE CHEMOTHERAPY

1. Use chemotherapy only when a diagnosis of malignancy has been established histologically.
2. Determine whether the malignancy is known to respond to the treatment in a reasonable percentage of patients.
3. For patients with metastatic disease, follow objective markers of the tumor if at all possible in order to determine the response of the tumor to the chemotherapy.
4. Do not use chemotherapeutic agents unless there are proper supportive facilities available and a cooperative patient.
5. Chemotherapy should be given only under the supervision of a physician who is specially trained to the use of chemotherapy.

DRUG RESISTANCE

There are many drugs for the treatment of patients with cancer. But some patients initially respond to chemotherapy, and then fail to respond later or some patients do not respond early on. As with antibiotics, cancer cells could develop resistance against chemotherapeutic agents. There are many mechanisms of drug resistance identified. Resistance to chemotherapy can occur from random, spontaneous accumulation of somatic mutations by tumor cells. Clinical drug resistance can be due to the emergence of the resistant clones.

Chemotherapeutic agents cause apoptosis or programmed cell death. Drug resistance could be due to inactivation of apoptosis. This is mediated through multiple mechanisms.

Multiple drug resistance (MDR) refers to a phenomenon in which tumor cells become simultaneously resistant to many drugs after getting exposed to a single antineoplastic agent. Classic MDR refers to the tumor cells that are resistant to vinca alkaloids, taxanes, anthracyclines and epipodophylotoxins. The MDR1 gene is responsible for MDR phenotype. MDR1 gene expresses a glycoprotein (p-glycoprotein), which acts as an efflux pump on the cell wall which practically pumps out the drugs from the intracellular compartment.

While considering chemotherapy, it is important to consider the agents which are not cross resistant to each other. There are many clinical trials looking at the effectiveness of a variety of agents in overcoming drug resistance.

COMBINED MODALITY

Effective treatment of cancer requires a combined approach, which includes local treatment with surgery and/or radiation therapy and systemic treatment with chemotherapy. Usually the treatment is planned in a combined meeting where a pathologist explains the details of the pathology and a radiologist maps out the extent of the disease. After the diagnosis and staging of the disease, the treatment sequence is decided by a discussion between surgeons, radiation oncologists and medical oncologists.

It is critical to have effective communication between these three modalities, i.e. surgeons, radiation oncologists and medical oncologists.

Neo-adjuvant Chemotherapy

This refers to the immediate use of chemotherapy before local therapy such as surgery or radiation therapy. This is to achieve a tumor debulking with chemotherapy to increase the potential of a successful surgery or radiation therapy. Neoadjuvant chemotherapy is widely used in breast cancer, head and neck cancer, lung cancer, esophageal cancer, etc.

Adjuvant Chemotherapy

Chemotherapy given immediately after the local therapy such as surgery and/or radiation therapy is known as adjuvant chemotherapy. When a patient is given adjuvant chemotherapy, he or she may not have any gross evidence of cancer. Adjuvant chemotherapy is given to eradicate the micrometastatic disease. The majority of the patients with cancer receive some form of adjuvant systemic therapy. Studies have shown that adjuvant chemotherapy prolongs survival in testicular cancer, breast cancer, colon cancer, head and neck cancer, etc.

Palliative Chemotherapy

When chemotherapy is given to control the symptoms of the patients such as pain or shortness of breath, and not with the intention of improving survival, it is known as palliative chemotherapy. In the majority of the metastatic patients the only *Indications* for chemotherapy is palliation. While treating patients with metastatic disease it is very important to set the goals and expectations.

CLINICAL TRIALS

As in any other field in medicine, advances in oncology are made through dedicated research by many scientists from around the world. Many wonderful, highly effective treatment modalities, which evolved from a little unknown laboratory, reached the bedside, only through clinical trials. In western countries, enrolling in clinical trial for a novel treatment is very common in patients who have only limited standard treatment option. For most of the cancer medicines we are indebted to thousands of patients from all over the world, who volunteered to be part of the clinical trials.

A clinical trial, which is conducted ethically, scientifically, and with fully informed consent, is as safe as any standard treatment available. In western countries any patient without a standard treatment option is offered a clinical trial.

Clinical trial has tremendous importance in the field of oncology.

ALKYLATING AGENTS

The alkylating agents are antitumor drugs that act through the covalent bonding of alkyl groups (one or more saturated carbon atoms) to cellular molecules. Historically, the alkylating agents have played an important role in the development of cancer chemotherapy. The nitrogen mustards were the first non-hormonal agents to show significant antitumor activity in humans.

MECHANISM OF ACTION

The alkylating agents react with (or "alkylate") many electron-rich atoms in cells to form covalent bonds. With regard to their antitumor activities the most important reaction is with the DNA bases. Some alkylating agents are monofunctional and react with only one strand of DNA. Others are bifunctional and react with an atom on each of the two strands of DNA to produce a "cross-link" that covalently links the two strands of the DNA double helix. Unless repaired, this lesion will prevent the cell from replicating effectively.

COMMON TOXICITIES

Hematopoietic Toxicity

It is the usual dose-limiting toxicity for alkylating agents.

Gastrointestinal Toxicity

It frequently produces nausea and vomiting; this effect is usually not as severe as with the platinum agents.

Gonadal Toxicity

The alkylating agents can produce significant gonadal toxicity. The characteristic testicular lesion in men is depletion of germ cells without damage to the Sertoli cells. It could also cause oligospermia or aspermia but spermatogenic dysfunction is reversible in some patients. Women treated with alkylating agents may develop amenorrhea associated with a marked decrease in ovarian follicles.

Pulmonary Toxicity

Interstitial pneumonitis and fibrosis were initially reported as a consequence of busulfan but subsequently have been reported with melphalan, chlorambucil, cyclophosphamide, and BCNU. Patients can present with dyspnea and a nonproductive cough, which can progress to cyanosis, pulmonary insufficiency, and death.

ALOPECIA

Cyclophosphamide, busulfan and ifosfamide can cause alopecia.

TERATOGENICITY

All the clinically used alkylating agents are teratogenic in animal studies. Women treated with an alkylating agent during the first trimester of pregnancy may have a risk as high as 15 percent of having a malformed infant. Administration of alkylating agents during the second and third trimesters has not been associated with increased fetal malformations.

CARCINOGENESIS

The incidence of leukemia is probably approximately 5 percent. An increased frequency of solid tumors also occurs after alkylating agent therapy.

IMMUNOSUPPRESSION

All alkylating agents produce some degree of immunosuppression, but cyclophosphamide is the most immunosuppressive.

COMMONLY USED ALKYLATING AGENTS

1. Mechlorethamine (Mustargen) is a highly reactive and unstable molecule with extremely short plasma half-life in the order of 15-20

minutes; its clinical use has become limited to the four-drug MOPP regimen used to treat Hodgkin's disease and occasionally other lymphomas.

2. Chlorambucil (Leukeran) has a very narrow spectrum of activity, and is being restricted to the treatment of slowly growing lymphoid neoplasm such as CLL, Waldenstrom-macroglobulinemia and indolent NHL.

3. Melphalan (Alkeran) was used mainly in ovarian and breast cancer treatment. Now it is used mainly in the treatment of multiple myeloma.

4. Cyclophosphamide (Cytoxan) is the commonly used alkylating agent. It is used in breast cancer, leukemia, lymphoma, multiple myeloma, neuroblastoma, ovarian cancer etc.

5. Ifosfamide (Ifex) is a newer analog of cyclophosphamide and shares the same responsibility for acute sterile hemorrhagic cystitis as cyclophosphamide, which occurs in up to 10 percent of treated patients. *Indications*: Hodgkin's disease, non-Hodgkin lymphoma (NHL), sarcoma, head and neck cancer, bladder cancer and recurrent germ cell tumors.

6. Carmustine (BCNU) a lipid-soluble drug with broad tissue distribution crosses the blood-brain barrier. *Indications*: GBM (glioblastoma multiforme), brainstem glioma, medulloblastoma, astrocytoma, and ependymoma.
   Implantable BCNU-impregnated wafer (Gliadel) is used in glioblastoma multiforme, NHL, Hodgkin's disease and multiple myeloma.

7. Lomustine (CCNU) crosses the blood-brain barrier. The CNS levels approach 15-30 percent of plasma level compared to BCNU which reaches >50 percent. *Indications*: primary or metastatic brain tumors, primary or metastatic Hodgkin's disease, NHL.

8. Streptozocin (Streptozotocin) selectively concentrates on pancreatic-β-cells, presumably due to glucose moiety on the molecule. *Indications*: pancreatic islet cell cancer, carcinoid tumors.

9. Busulfan (Myleran) distributes rapidly in plasma with broad tissue penetration. Crosses the blood-brain-barrier and also crosses the placenta-barrier. *Indications*: bone marrow/ stem cell transplantation for refractory leukemias, lymphomas (high dose), CML (standard dose) in p.o. form.

10. Dacarbazine (DIC, DTIC-Dome) volume of distribution exceeds total body water content, and drug is distributed in body tissue. *Indications*: metastatic melanoma, Hodgkin's disease, soft tissue sarcoma, neuroblastoma and oligodendroglioma.

11. Thiotepa (Thioplex) is widely distributed throughout the body. *Indications*: superficial transitional cell cancer of the bladder,

controlling intracavitary effusion secondary to diffuse or localized neoplasms of the serosal cavities, breast and ovarian cancer, Hodgkin's disease, and NHL. High dose in transplant setting is used for breast and ovarian cancer.

PLATINUM COMPOUNDS

Mechanism of Action

Platinum compounds act by covalently binding to DNA with preferential binding to N-7 position in guanine and adenine. Like the alkylating agents, platinum coordination complexes form strong covalent bonds by displacement of nucleophilic atoms to form inter-strand cross-links that correlate with cytotoxicity.

Common side effects: With cisplatin the dose limiting toxicity is nephrotoxicity (vigorous hydration), neurotoxicity and ototoxicity (check auditory acuity). But for carboplatin the dose limiting toxicity is myelosuppression, but nephrotoxicity and neuro-toxicity are significantly less than that of cisplatin.

Commonly used platinum compounds:
1. Cisplatin (Platinol)
   It is commonly used in testicular, ovarian, bladder, head and neck cancer, small and non-small cell lung cancer, and esophageal cancer.
2. Carboplatin (Paraplatin): Dose of carboplatin is usually calculated to a target area under the curve (AUC) based on the GFR.
   Calvert formula is used to calculate the dose: Total dose (mg)= (target AUC) × (GFR+25).
   Target AUC is usually between 5-7 mg/ml/min for previously untreated patient.

Indications: ovarian cancer, germ cell tumor, head and neck cancer, bladder cancer, and small and non-small lung cancer.

ANTIMETABOLITES AND ANTIFOLATES

Aminopterin was the first antimetabolite and antifolate analog used to induce remission in children with acute leukemia in the 1940s. Aminopterin has since been replaced by methotrexate, the 4-amino, 10-methyl analog of folic acid.

MECHANISM OF ACTION

Antimetabolites function by either competing with normal metabolites for the catalytic or regulatory site of a key enzyme or substituting for a metabolite that is normally incorporated into an important molecule, e.g. DNA or RNA.

Because most antimetabolites interfere with nucleic acid synthesis (rather than preformed nucleic acid, like alkylating agents), they have little, if any, effect on cells in G_0 and usually exhibit maximum activity during S-phase.

Folic acid analogs inhibit dihydrofolate reductase (dhfr). Methotrexate is the only folic acid analog in current clinical use. dhfr is responsible for the generation of reduced folates, which are essential for nucleic acid synthesis. Also inhibition of dhfr blocks the production of a reduced folate coenzyme that participates with thymidylate synthetase in conversion of 2-deoxyuridylate to thymidylate and so inhibits thymidylate synthesis, which leads to interruption of DNA synthesis.

Commonly used antimetabolites and antifolates:

1. *Methotrexate (MTX):* The toxicity of MTX depends mostly on the duration of exposure rather than the peak level, but the toxicity does not occur until the peak level reaches certain level, irrespective of the exposure duration. By checking daily MTX-level and dose adjustment depending on renal function, a useful therapeutic level with least toxicity could be achieved. Leucovorin could be used to decrease the toxicity to the normal tissue due to MTX.

   High dose MTX with leucovorin rescue is used in primary CNS lymphoma, meningeal leukemia and carcinomatous meningitis. Other diseases are osteogenic sarcoma, ALL, lymphoma, and head and neck cancer. MTX as a single agent is curative in gestational trophoblastic carcinoma.

2. *Hydroxyurea*: It is an antimetabolite cell cycle specific analog of urea with activity in the S-phase. Oral absorption is rapid and nearly complete with a bioavailability close to 80 percent. *Indications*: CML, essential thrombocytosis, polycythemia vera, AML in blast crisis. Dose limiting toxicity: myelosuppression.

3. *5-Fluorouracil (5-FU):* It is an analog to both uracil and thymidine. Phosphorylation of 5-FU to 5-Fluorouridine triphosphate (5-FUTP) allows its incorporation into RNA, which disrupts processing of mRNA and rRNA. 5-FU is also converted to 5-Fluorouridine monophosphate (5-FdUMP), which irreversibly inhibits thymidylate synthetase and leads to thymidine depletion and ceasing of DNA synthesis. These two mechanisms of cytotoxicity allow 5-FU to be active throughout the cell cycle and not just in S-phase.

   5-FU is given intravenously because of variable and erratic GI-absorption. *Indications*: adjuvant and metastatic setting of colorectal and breast cancer, ovarian cancer, head and neck cancer.

   Dose limiting toxicity: myelosuppression, mucositis, and hand-foot syndrome.

4. *Capecitabine (Xeloda):* It is an oral prodrug that is converted to 5-FU in the liver. The conversion requires thymidine phosphorylase, an

enzyme with higher level in many human carcinomas than in normal tissue.

Indications: metastatic breast cancer resistant to anthracycline or taxane-based chemotherapy regimen.

Dose limiting toxicity: diarrhea, hand-foot syndrome.

5. *Cytarabine (Cytosine Arabinoside, Ara-C)*: In the cell the active form of the drug, Ara-CTP competitively inhibits binding of dCTP to DNA polymerase, which arrests DNA synthesis. Also incorporation of Ara-CTP in DNA causes defective ligation or incomplete synthesis of DNA.

   Indications: AML induction chemotherapy. Because Ara-C destroys only cycling cells through S-phase and many leukemic cells are in G_0, hence Ara-C must be administered for a larger period of time (5 to 7 days) to allow maximum cells to enter the S-phase. Intrathecal Ara-C is used in prophylaxis and treatment of leptomeningeal carcinomatosis secondary to leukemia or lymphoma.

   Dose limiting toxicity: myelosuppression.

6. *Gemcitabine (Gemzar)*: It is structurally similar to Ara-C and it is a cytidine analog.

   Indications: Approved for advanced pancreatic cancer. Gemcitabine has shown activity in a variety of solid tumors such as breast cancer, non-small cell lung cancer, head and neck cancer, bladder, colon, and ovarian cancer.

   Dose limiting toxicity: myelosuppression.

7. *6-Mercaptopurine (6-MP) and 6-Thioguanine (6-TG)*: The concomitant administration of allopurinol, an inhibitor of xanthine oxidase used to prevent tumor lysis syndrome may increase the toxicity of 6-MP. The dose of 6-MP therefore should be reduced by 75 percent, no dose reduction is needed for 6-TG because of different metabolism pathway. *Indications*: leukemia.

   Dose limiting toxicity: myelosuppression.

8. *Pentostatin (Nipent)*: It is an adenosine analog produced by a species of streptomyces. It is a powerful inhibitor of adenosine deaminase (ADA). *Indications*: hairy cell leukemia, also active in cutaneous T-cell lymphoma and in CLL.

   Dose limiting toxicity: myelosuppression, immunosuppression.

9. *Fludarabine (Fludara)*: It is an adenosine analog that is resistant to deamination by adenosine deaminase (ADA) and has antitumor activity against both dividing and resting cells.

   Indications: CLL.

   Dose limiting toxicity: myelosuppression, immunosuppression.

10. *Cladribine (Leustatin)*: It is an adenosine analog with high specificity for lymphoid cells, with antitumor activity against both dividing and resting cells. *Indications*: hairy cell leukemia, CLL, low grade NHL.

    Dose limiting toxicity: myelosuppression.

ANTITUMOR ANTIBIOTICS AND ANTHRACYCLINES

The antitumor antibiotics, actinomycin D, anthracyclines, bleomycin, mitomycin C and mithramycin are a structurally diverse group of compounds all derived from the species of streptomyces.

COMMONLY USED ANTHRACYCLINES

1. *Doxorubicin (Adriamycin)*: It is the most commonly used anthracycline. Mechanism of action
    a. It intercalates into DNA resulting in inhibition of DNA synthesis and function.
    b. It inhibits transcription through inhibition of DNA-dependent RNA-polymerase.
    c. It inhibits topoisomerase II and leads to DNA strand breaks.
    d. It leads to the formation of toxic oxygen-free radicals and results in single and double stranded DNA-breaks.
       Indications: breast cancer, ovarian cancer, Hodgkin's disease and NHL.
       Dose limiting toxicity: myelosuppression, cardiotoxicity. It can cause dilated cardiomyopathy and congestive heart failure when the cumulative dose exceeds 400 mg/m^2.
2. *Doxil (Doxorubicin liposome)*: Liposomal encapsulation of doxorubicin is protected from chemical and enzymatic degradation. It penetrates the tumor tissue and then doxorubicin is released.
   Indications: Metastatic ovarian cancer and AIDS related Kaposi's sarcoma.
3. *Daunorubicin (Daunomycin)*: It is a cell-cycle nonspecific agent.
   Indications: AML, AML-remission, induction and relapse.
   Dose limiting toxicity: myelosuppression, cardiotoxicity.
4. *Daunorubicin liposome (Daunoxome)*: It is liposomal encapsulation of daunorubicin.
   Indications: HIV-associated advanced Kaposi's sarcoma.
5. *Idarubicin (Idamycin)*: It is anthracycline glycoside analog of daunorubicin.
   Indications: AML, ALL, CML in blast crisis and MDS.
   Dose limiting toxicity: myelosuppression, cardiotoxicity.
6. *Bleomycin (Blenoxane)*: Cytotoxic effect results in the generation of activated oxygen-free radicals, which result in single and double strand-DNA breaks.
   Indications: germ cell tumors, Hodgkin's disease, NHL, head and neck cancer.
   Dose limiting toxicity: pulmonary fibrosis, if a decrease in DLCO > 15 percent the drug should be immediately stopped.
7. *Mitomycin-C (Mitomycin)*: It activates oxygen free radicals, acts as an alkylating agent to cross-link DNA, resulting in inhibition of DNA-synthesis and function.

Indications: gastric, pancreatic, superficial bladder and cervical cancer, and head and neck cancer in combination with radiation.

Dose limiting toxicity: myelosuppression, hemolytic-uremic-syndrome, interstitial pneumonitis, hepatic veno-occlusive disease.

TOPOISOMERASE- I INHIBITORS

1. *Topotecan (Hycamtin)*: It is a topoisomerase I inhibitor which prevents the ligation of DNA after it has been cleaved by topoisomerase I. Topotecan is a semisynthetic derivative of camptothecin, an alkaloid extract from the camptotheca acuminata tree.
   Indications: FDA approved it for patients with advanced ovarian cancer not responding to platinum-based chemotherapy, AML and small cell lung cancer.
   Dose limiting toxicity: myelosuppression.
2. *Irinotecan (Camptosar, CPT 11)*: It is a topoisomerase I inhibitor, parent form is inactive and needs to be converted to its active metabolites. It is a cell cycle nonspecific drug with activity in all phases.
   Indications:
   i. Colorectal cancer This drug is approved in colorectal cancer; in combination with 5-FU and leucovorin as first line treatment of patients with metastatic colorectal cancer.
      Irinotecan is also approved as a single agent for second line treatment of patients with metastatic colorectal cancer not responding to 5-FU based chemotherapy.
   ii. Non-small cell lung cancer.
      Dose limiting toxicity: myelosuppression and diarrhea.

TOPOISOMERASE-II INHIBITOR

Etoposide (VP-16): It is a semisynthetic derivative of podophyllotoxin. It can induce strand breaks in DNA, an effect that is likely to be mediated by its interaction with topoisomerase II.

Indications: small and non-small cell lung cancer, germ cell tumor, NHL, relapsed Hodgkin's disease, gastric cancer, high dose chemotherapy in bone marrow transplant setting.

Dose limiting toxicity: myelosuppression.

VINCA ALKALOIDS

Extracts of the periwinkle plant, long believed in folklore to have medicinal value, led to the isolation of two active alkaloid anticancer compounds, vincristine and vinblastine. Vincristine and vinblastine act as microtubule stabilizers by preventing the microtubule polymerization; this leads to the arrest of cells in metaphase with subsequent cell lysis.

1. *Vincristine (Oncovorin)*
   Indications: ALL, Hodgkin's disease, NHL.
   The dose limiting toxicity: neurotoxicity but myelosuppression is infrequent with conventional doses.
2. *Vinblastine (Velban)*:
   Indications: Hodgkin's disease, NHL, testicular cancer.
   The dose limiting toxicity: myelosuppression with less neurotoxicity.
3. *Vinorelbine (Navelbine)*: It is a semisynthetic alkaloid derived from vinblastine. It is cell cycle specific with activity in mitotic phase. It has relatively high specificity for mitotic microtubules with lower affinity for axonal microtubules.
   Indications: breast cancer, ovarian cancer, Hodgkin's disease, non-small cell lung cancer.
   Dose limiting toxicity: myelosuppression with less neurotoxicity than other vinca alkaloids.

TAXANES

Taxanes are microtubule-stabilizing agent. Unlike vinca alkaloids that inhibit microtubule polymerization; taxanes interfere with mitosis by blocking the cell cycle at the G_2 or M-phase by promoting microtubule polymerization.

1. *Paclitaxel (Taxol): Indications*: ovarian cancer, breast cancer, non-small cell lung cancer, head and neck cancer and AIDS related Kaposi's sarcoma.
   Dose limiting toxicity: myelosuppression, neurotoxicity. Hypersensitivity reaction may be caused by the drug itself or the vehicle in which it is formulated, Cremophor EL.
   Premedication should be administered, dexamethasone-12 and 6 hours prior to administration of H_1 and H_2 blocker.
2. *Docetaxel (Taxotere): Indications*: locally advanced or metastatic breast cancer that has progressed or relapsed with anthracycline based chemotherapy. Taxotere has also activity in non-small cell lung cancer, ovarian cancer, etc.
   Dose limiting toxicity: myelosuppression. (Peripheral neuropathy is less commonly observed than with Taxol). Premedication consists of oral steroids 3 days prior to the administration of taxotere to reduce hypersensitivity reaction and to reduce the severity of fluid retention.

HORMONAL AGENTS

Selective estrogen receptor modulators (SERM):
1. *Tamoxifen (Nolvadex)*: It is a nonsteroidal antiestrogen with weak estrogen agonist effect. It competes with estrogen for binding to estrogen receptor (ER).

Indications:

1. adjuvant therapy in axillary node-negative, ER positive breast cancer following surgical resection,
2. adjuvant therapy in axillary node-positive, ER positive breast cancer in postmenopausal women following surgical resection,
3. metastatic (ER-positive) breast cancer in women and men,
4. chemoprevention for women at high risk for breast cancer.
   Side effects: hot flushes, weight gain, deep venous thrombosis, pulmonary embolism, vaginal discharge, vaginal bleeding and endometrial cancer.

2. *Raloxifene:* It is another estrogen receptor modulator (SERM). This agent has antiestrogen effects, similar to those of tamoxifen, on the breast and uterus but has estrogenic effects on the cardiovascular system and bone. Raloxifene has no stimulatory effect on the endometrium (unlike tamoxifen).
   Indications: prevention of osteoporosis. It is being studied in postmenopausal women for prevention of breast cancer.
   Side effects: hot flushes, leg cramps and deep venous thrombosis.

AROMATASE INHIBITORS

In postmenopausal women, aromatase inhibitors act by blocking the synthesis of estrogen by inhibiting the conversion of adrenal androgens to estrogens.

Most common toxicities: mild musculoskeletal pain, arthralgias and hot flushes. Thromboembolic events are rarely observed.

1. *Anastrozole (Arimidex):* It is a nonsteroidal aromatase inhibitor approved for use in the treatment of advanced breast cancer in postmenopausal women.
2. *Letrozole (Femara):* It is a nonsteroidal aromatase inhibitor with the same mechanism of action as that of anastrozole.
   Indications: second line hormonal treatment of postmenopausal women.
3. *Exemestane (Aromisin):* It is a steroidal aromatase inactivator, that permanently binds to and irreversibly inactivates aromatase.
   Indications: advanced breast cancer in postmenopausal women whose disease progressed following tamoxifen therapy.

LHRH AGONISTS

Administration of LHRH agonists leads to initial release of FSH and LH followed by suppression of gonadotropin secretion as a result of desensitization of the pituitary to gonadotropin-releasing hormone. This eventually leads to decreased secretion of LH and FSH from the pituitary gland resulting in castration levels of testosterone after 1-2 weeks of therapy.

1. *Leuprolide (Lupron):* It is a luteinizing hormone-releasing hormone (LHRH) agonist.
   Indications: advanced prostate cancer, neoadjuvant therapy of early stage prostate cancer.
   Toxicity: hot flushes, impotence and gynecomastia.
2. *Goserelin (Zoladex)*: It is an LHRH-agonist.
   Indications: advanced prostate cancer.
   Toxicity: hot flushes, decreased libido, impotence, and gynecomastia.

Tumor flare may occur in 20 percent of patients (same as Lupron) usually within the first 2 weeks of starting therapy. The patient may experience increased bone pain, urinary retention or back pain with spinal cord compression symptoms. Pretreating the patients with an antiestrogen agent such as flutamide may prevent these.

NON-STEROIDAL ANTI-ANDROGENS

Flutamide (Eulexin): It is a nonsteroidal, anti-androgen agent, that binds to androgen receptor and inhibits androgen uptake as well as inhibits androgen binding in nucleus in androgen sensitive prostate cancer cell.
Indications: locally confined stage B2-C prostate cancer, stage D2 metastatic prostate cancer.

Toxicity: hot flushes, decreased libido, impotence, gynecomastia.

OTHERS

Estramustine (Emcyt): a conjugate of nitrogen mustard and estradiol phosphate. It is active against ER-positive and ER-negative tumor cells, and inhibits microtubule polymerization by binding it to microtubule-associated proteins (MAPs) but has no alkylating activity.

Indications: hormone refractory metastatic prostate cancer.

Toxicity: nausea, vomiting, gynecomastia and diarrhea.

FURTHER READING

1. Abraham and Allegra. Bethesda Handbook of Clinical Oncology. Philadelphia: Lippincott Williams and Wilkins 2001;558-634.
2. Adjei AA, Haluska P, Dy GK. Novel pharmacological agents in clinical development for solid tumors. Expert Opin Investig Drugs 2001;10(12):2059-88.
3. Bennett C, Waters T, Stinson T, Almagor O, Pavletic Z, Tarantolo S, Bishop M. Valuing clinical strategies early in development: A cost analysis of allogenic peripheral blood stem cell transplantation. Bone Marrow Transplant 1999;24(5):555-60.
4. Bensinger WI, Clift R, Martin P, Appelbaum FR, Demirer T, Gooley T, Lilleby K, Rowley S, Sanders J, Storb R, Buckner CD. Allogenic peripheral blood stem cell transplantation in patients with advanced hematologic malignancies: A retrospective comparison with marrow transplantation. Blood 1996;1;88(7):2794-800.

5. Bredeson C, Malcolm J, Davis M, Bence-Bruckler I, Kearns B, Huebsch L. Cost analysis of the introduction of PBPC for autologous transplantation: Effect of switching from bone marrow (BM) to peripheral blood progenitor cells (PBPC). Bone Marrow Transplant 1997;20(10):889-96.

6. Casciato and Lowitz. Manual of Clinical Oncology, Lippincott Williams and Wilkins's, Philadelphia, 2000.

7. Champlin R, Khouri I, Kornblau S, Marini F, Anderlini P, Ueno NT, Molldrem J, Giralt S. Allogenic hematopoietic transplantation as adoptive immunotherapy. Induction of graft-versus-malignancy as primary therapy. Hematol Oncol Clin North Am 1999;13(5):1041-57.

8. Childs R, Epperson D, Bahceci E, Clave E, Barrett J. Molecular remission of chronic myeloid leukemia following a non-myeloablative allogenic peripheral blood stem cell transplant: in vivo and in vitro evidence for a graft-versus-leukemia effect. Br J Haematol 1999;107(2):396-400.

9. Cragg GM. Paclitaxel (Taxol): A success story with valuable lessons for natural product drug discovery and development. Med Res Rev 1998;18(5):315-31.

10. DeVita, Hellman, Rosenberg: Cancer. Principles and Practice of Oncology (6th ed). Philadelphia: Lippincott Williams and Wilkins, 1997.

11. Dillman RO. Monoclonal antibody therapy for lymphoma. Cancer Pract 2001;9(2):71-80.

12. Ferrara JL, Levy R, Chao NJ. Pathophysiologic mechanisms of acute graft-vs.-host disease. Biol Blood Marrow Transplant 1999;5(6):347-56.

13. Fojo T. Cancer, DNA repair mechanisms, and resistance to chemotherapy. J Natl Cancer Inst 2001;3;93(19):1434-36.

14. Henslee-Downey PJ, Gluckman E. Allogenic transplantation from donors other than HLA-identical siblings. Hematol Oncol Clin North Am 1999;13(5):1017-39.

15. Huston JS, George AJ. Engineered antibodies take center stage. Hum Antibodies 2001;10(3,4):127-42.

16. Kantarjian H, Sawyers C, Hochhaus A. Hematologic and cytogenetic responses to imatinib mesylate in chronic myelogenous leukemia. N Engl J Med 2002;346(9):645-52.

17. Lacombe D, Fumoleau P. The EORTC and drug development. Eur J Cancer 2002;38(Suppl 4):19-23.

18. Lazarus HM, Rowlings PA, Zhang MJ, Vose JM, Armitage JO, Bierman PJ, Gajewski JL, Gale RP, Keating A, Klein JP, Miller CB, Phillips GL, Reece DE, Sobocinski KA, van Besien K, Horowitz MM. Autotransplants for Hodgkin's disease in patients never achieving remission: A report from the Autologous Blood and Marrow Transplant Registry. J Clin Oncol 1999;17(2):534-45.

19. Lee SJ, Weller E, Alyea EP, Ritz J, Soiffer RJ. Efficacy and costs of granulocyte colony-stimulating factor in allogenic T-cell depleted bone marrow transplantation. Blood 1998;15;92(8):2725-29.

20. Leonard DS, Hill AD, Kelly L, et al. Anti-human epidermal growth factor receptor 2 monoclonal antibody therapy for breast cancer. Br J Surg 2002;89(3):262-71.

21. Lokich J. Phase I clinical trial of weekly combined topotecan and irinotecan. Cancer Center of Boston, Massachusetts 02120, USA. Am J Clin Oncol 2001;24(4):336-40.

22. Nabhan C, Rosen ST. Conceptual aspects of combining rituximab and Campath-1H in the treatment of chronic lymphocytic leukemia. Semin Oncol 2002;29(1 Suppl 2):75-80.

23. O'Dwyer ME, Druker BJ. Chronic myelogenous leukaemia—new therapeutic principles. J Intern Med 2001;250(1):3-9.

24. Pavletic ZS, Bishop MR, Tarantolo SR, et al. A hematopoietic recovery after allogenic blood stem-cell transplantation compared with bone marrow transplantation in patients with hematologic malignancies. J Clin Oncol 1997;15(4):1608-16.

25. Popplewell L, Forman SJ. Allogenic hematopoietic stem cell transplantation for acute leukemia, chronic leukemia, and myelodysplasia. Hematol Oncol Clin North Am 1999;13(5):987-1015.

26. Przepiorka D, Smith TL, Folloder J, Khouri I, Ueno NT, Mehra R, Korbling M, Huh YO, Giralt S, Gajewski J, Donato M, Cleary K, Claxton D, Braunschweig I, van Besien K, Anderson BS, Anderlini P, Champlin R. Risk factors for acute graft-versus-host disease after allogenic blood stem cell transplantation. Blood 1999;15;94(4):1465-70.

27. Rosenberg: Principles and Practice of the Biologic Therapy of Cancer (3rd ed). Philadelphia: Lippincott Williams and Wilkins, 2000.

28. Savage DG, Antman KH. Imatinib mesylate—A new oral targeted therapy. N Engl J Med 2002;346(9):683-93.

29. Stadler WM, Ratain MJ. Development of target-based antineoplastic agents. Invest New Drugs 2000;18(1):7-16.

30. Tan AR, Swain SM. Novel agents: clinical trial design. Semin Oncol 2001;28:148-53.

31. Umemura S, Sakamoto G, Sasano H, et al. Evaluation of HER2 status: for the treatment of metastatic breast cancers by humanized anti-HER2 Monoclonal antibody (trastuzumab). Breast Cancer 2001;8(4):316-20.

32. Walke DW, Han C, Shaw J, et al. A In vivo drug target discovery: Identifying the best targets from the genome. Curr Opin Bio Technol 2001;12(6):626-31.

Novel Targeted Treatment in Oncology

50

Jame Abraham, Ramin Altaha

The traditional chemotherapeutic agents are like blind bombs, because they destroy cancer cells and normal tissue cells almost with the same intensity. Only in a few cases, the toxicity to normal tissues can be avoided, such as, administration of leucovorin with methotrexate or 5-FU. Narrow therapeutic index of chemotherapeutic agents is still a challenging problem for oncologists.

Over the past 30 years, our understanding of the fundamental biology of the disease has increased significantly. These discoveries in cancer biology opened new doors to fight the growth and proliferation of cancer cells in a targeted form. Novel treatments can target specific signaling pathways such as tyrosine kinase pathway (e.g. imatinib mesylate or gleevecä) or certain growth factor receptors (e.g. trastuzumab or herceptinä) and destroy the malignant cells in a selective way without harming normal cells. This area is advancing rapidly with the discovery of new drugs and moving the field of oncology to an era of smart bombs instead of blind bombs.

Reduction in significant side effects to normal tissues will be the main advantage of these targeted drugs. Most of the medications developed in this category do not cause nausea, vomiting, loss of hair, myelosuppression or significant immunosuppression. These drugs could be given to patients for a very long time. The emerging concept is that, cancer is a chronic disease like hypertension or rheumatoid arthritis, so patients should be on a lifelong maintenance treatment.

Another exciting area of rapid advancement is the completion of the Human Genome Project. Now we have new insights into the genetic causes of the diseases. This opens a completely new world of genomic classification of disease, tailoring the treatment based on the specific gene expression and developments in pharmaco-genomics.

Some tumors with similar microscopic appearance may have totally different clinical outcome. This could be clearly predicted by the totally different gene expression pattern of the tumors. Genomic and proteomic analysis of the human tissue can identify the molecular constellation of tumors and show us, what genes are over-expressed in which tumor and what abnormal protein may be responsible for the abnormal growth and proliferation. The most frequently and excessively expressed genes or proteins can be attacked with tailored inhibitors.

Many monoclonal antibodies or other targeted agents are at different stages of development. They can selectively modulate or eliminate the defective part and result in the arrest of malignant cell cycles. However the transformation of normal cells to malignant cells *in vivo*, the growth, the proliferation and the metastatic potential of these cells constitute a complicated process, which cannot be fully understood only with the identification of the gene and protein constellation of the malignant cells. There is no doubt that the future of cancer therapy will be directed in this way. The results are promising but many questions are still open.

MONOCLONAL ANTIBODIES

In 1975 for the first time the technique of producing monoclonal antibody was described by Kohler and Milstein, for which they won the 1984 Nobel Prize. They fused antibody-producing plasma cells of a mouse with cancer cells and hence they produced multiple copies of a single specific antibody called monoclonal antibody. In theory a monoclonal antibody can bind to cancer-specific antigens and the immune system would destroy the cancer cells. Mice-derived antibodies are strongly immunogenic and the human immune system develops antibodies against these foreign proteins and inactivate them. New techniques are now producing chimeric antibodies with mostly human components, which modify the human immune response.

Monoclonal antibodies are excellent tools to attack targeted areas in the cells. Rituximab is an anti-CD 20 antibody, FDA-approved and used for large B-cell non-Hodgkin's lymphoma. Trastuzumab is an antibody against human epidermal growth factor, which is overexpressed in 30 percent of breast cancer cells. Many other monoclonal antibodies, such as, anti-VEGF (vascular endothelial growth factor) with antiangiogenesis activities are under investigation.

Some of the epidermal growth factor receptor (EGFR) inhibitors in clinical trials include ZD 1839 (Iressaä), which is an orally bioavailable compound. This is found to be effective in many tumors including, colorectal cancer, lung cancer, breast cancer and ovarian cancer. Another monoclonal antibody against epidermal growth factor receptor (EGFR) is IMC 225 which is found to be active in refractory head and neck tumors and the clinical trials are still going on.

SIGNAL-TRANSDUCTION INHIBITORS (STI'S)

Each growth factor binds to its cell surface receptor and causes its activation. This triggers the transmission of growth signals to the interior of the cells through a multiple complicated tyrosine kinase pathway. Blocking of this pathway could be an effective way of stopping the cell division. Many tyrosine kinase inhibitors are undergoing clinical trials.

The FDA has approved imatinib or gleevecä (STI-571) for the therapy of chronic myeloid leukemia (CML). Imatinib is an inhibitor of bcr-abl tyrosine kinase, an abnormal gene product formed by translocation of chromosomes (9; 22 Philadelphia chromosome). Studies have shown that it could be effective in more than 95 percent of the patients with CML and cause molecular eradication of the disease in 60 percent of the patients. These results are as good or even better than the bone marrow transplantation studies. Imatinib has no or minimal side effects compared to any chemotherapy. Patients could be maintained on this medicine for many months.

Imatinib is also active against tumors with overexpression of c-kit or PDGF (platelet derived growth factor). Recent studies have shown it could cure patients with gastrointestinal stromal tumor (GIST), which was considered a fatal condition before.

Some of the targeted agents approved by the Food and Drug Administration (FDA) of the US are mentioned here:

NOVEL TARGETED AGENTS

1. *Rituximab (Rituxan™):* It is a genetically designed chimeric anti-CD20 monoclonal antibody and is the first antibody approved by FDA to fight malignant B-cells. CD20 is expressed on almost all B-cells of NHL but it is not found on bone marrow stem cells, pre B-cells or normal plasma cells. The antibody is an IgG1 kappa immunoglobulin, which binds to CD20 and mediates cell lysis.
   Indications: relapsed or refractory low grade or follicular NHL.
   Toxicity: infusion-related symptoms: fever, chills, flushing, hypotension, bronchospasm, angioedema, nausea (it usually occurs within 30 minutes to 2 hours after initiation of first infusion and usually resolves upon slowing or stopping the infusion, but incidence decreases with subsequent infusions), arrhythmia, chest pain (particularly in patients with preexisting heart disease), development of human anti-chimeric antibodies (HACA), etc.
2. *Alemtuzumab (Campath-1H™):* It is humanized IgG1, anti-CD52 monoclonal antibody. CD52 is highly expressed on the surface of B and T lymphocytes, a majority of monocytes, macrophages, NK-cells and a minority of granulocytes. After binding to target cells an antibody-mediated leukemic cell lysis occurs.

Indications: B-CLL, which failed with alkylating agents and fludarabine Campath is being used also in a phase trial in promyelocytic leukemias as well as NHLs. It has been used to purge bone marrow prior to allogenic bone marrow transplantation.

Side effects: The treatment is associated with reactivation of herpes simplex, oral candidiasis, *Pneumocystis carinii* pneumonia (PCP), cytomegalovirus pneumonitis, pulmonary aspergillosis and disseminated tuberculosis.

Prophylaxis therapy against PCP and herpes virus infection is recommended upon the initiation of the therapy and at least for 2 months following the last dose or until CD4 count = 200 cells/µl. CD4 and CD8 lymphocyte counts may not return to baseline level for more than one year.

3. *Gemtuzumab ozogamicin (Myelotarg™)*: CD33 is found on many myeloid leukemic blasts and leukemic progenitor cells (>80% in AML-cells); CD33 is also present on myelo-monocytic and erythroid progenitor cells. Myelotarg is an antibody against CD33 antigen, and cell death occurs after the antibody-antigen complex binds to the DNA (internalization of complex) and results in double strand break.

   Indications: AML (CD33-positive) in first relapse, who are 60 years old and not a candidate for cytotoxic chemotherapy.

   Toxicity: infusion related symptoms, fever, chills, dyspnea and hypotension likely to occur during 24 hours after administration. Severe myelosuppression may occur at recommended dosage.

4. *Imatinib (Gleevec™, STI 571)*: Signal transduction inhibitor 571 (STI 571) is a tyrosine kinase inhibitor, which selectively inhibits bcr/abl tyrosine kinase, and so inhibits the proliferation of cell lines expressing the abnormal gene product bcr/abl found on Philadelphia chromosome in CML. STI 571 also inhibits tyrosine kinase for platelet derived growth factor (PDGF) and c-kit.

   Indications: STI 571 is approved for CML in blast crisis, accelerated phase or in chronic phase after failure of interferon-alpha therapy: very recently Gleevec also has been approved for gastrointestinal stromal tumors (GIST).

   Toxicity: fluid retention, neutropenia with median duration of 2-3 weeks, thrombocytopenia with median duration of 3-4 weeks.

5. *Trastuzumab (Herceptin™)*: It is a monoclonal antibody, which binds to the extracellular domain of the human epidermal growth factor receptor 2 protein (HER2/neu) and mediates cytotoxic effect. Approximately 25-30 percent of all breast cancers overexpress HER2/neu, these tumors are mostly ER/PR negative, aggressive and tend to recur more frequently.

   Indications: metastatic breast cancer.

   Toxicity: CHF in association with Herceptin may be severe; extreme caution should be used in patients with preexisting cardiac condition and/or in combination with anthracyclines.

6. *Tretinoin (ATRA)*: All-trans-retinoic-acids (ATRA) are vitamin A derivatives, and induce terminal differentiation of leukemic promyelocytic cells in patients with acute promyelocytic leukemia (APL). APL is associated with reciprocal chromosomal translocation 15 and 17, t(15; 17); this translocation is highly specific for APL. The breakpoint on chromosome 17 occurs within retinoic-acid-receptor-alpha (RARA), whereas the break on chromosome 15 occurs within PML-gene. The translocation results in a fusion PML-RARA gene and produces a protein, which acts as a dominant negative compound, responsible for differentiation arrest at the level of promyelocyte.

By binding oral ATRA to this complex PML-RARA protein is released and results in active transcription and maturation of promyelocytes.

Toxicity: vitamin A toxicity like headache, dryness of skin, mucosa, fever.

Retinoic acid syndrome: can be dose limiting, occurs in 25 percent of patients; severe cases result in death, characterized by diffuse pulmonary infiltrate and pleura effusion on chest X-ray, prompt high dose corticosteroid treatment.

7. *Zevalin*™ *(ibritumomab tiuxetan)*: It was approved by FDA in February 2002, and is a novel treatment regimen for one type of non-Hodgkin's lymphoma (NHL). Zevalin™ is a combination of a monoclonal antibody and a radioactive chemical. Zevalin, must be used along with Rituxan, an already approved biotechnology product for the disease—low-grade B-cell NHL. It is approved for patients who have not responded to standard chemotherapy treatments or to the use of Rituxan alone. The Zevalin therapeutic regimen is administered in two parts. The patients first receive Rituxan followed by a form of Zevalin with a low dose of radioactive chemical for screening purposes. If patients' tumors are properly targeted with this procedure, they receive Rituxan again with a form of Zevalin that has a different radioactive chemical that can provide a treatment benefit. Studies have shown an overall response rate of 74 to 80 percent. The duration of response was approximately 2 months longer with the Zevalin therapeutic regimen, although it is too early to say whether it will allow patients to live longer than Rituxan therapy does.

CONCLUSION

The treatment of cancer is moving to a new and exciting era. With the rapid development in molecular biology and the evolution of the human genome project, treating all cancer patients with specific targeted treatments or combinations of targeted medications is not that far.

Recognition of targeted agents is just the beginning, and many questions like the following need to be answered:

1. What is the impact of single pathway or protein blocking of the oncogene with regard to future tumor behavior?
2. What is the response of the normal tissue to these agents?
3. What is the best time to administer these agents and the combination of which cytotoxic agents may enhance their therapeutic effect?

COMMONLY USED CHEMOTHERAPEUTIC AGENTS

- Alkylating agents
  - Altretamine
  - Busulfan
  - Chlorambucil
  - Cyclophosphamide
  - Ifosfamide
  - Mechlorethamine
  - Melphalan
  - Procarbazine
  - Streptozocin
  - Temozolomide
  - Thiotepa
  - Carmustine
  - Lomustine
- Anthracycline antitumor antibiotic agents
  - Daunorubicin
  - Doxorubicin
  - Epirubicin
  - Idarubicin
- Anti-angiogenic agents
  - Thalidomide
- Antifolate agents
  - Methotrexate
- Antihelminthic
  - Levamisole
- Antimetabolite agents
  - 5-Fluorouracil
  - 6-Thioguanine
  - Capecitabine
  - Cladribine
  - Cytarabine
  - Floxuridine
  - Fludarabine
  - Gemcitabine
  - Hydroxyurea
  - Mercaptopurine
  - Pentostatin

- Antineoplastic arsenical compound
  - Arsenic trioxide
- Antitumor antibiotics
  - Bleomycin
  - Dactinomycin
  - Mitomycin C
  - Plicamycin
- Aromatase inhibitors
  - Aminoglutethimide
  - Anastrazole
  - Exemestane
  - Letrozole
- Atypical alkylators
  - Carboplatin
  - Cisplatin
  - Dacarbazine
- Biologic molecules
  - Denileukin Diflitox
- Biologic response modifiers (cytokines)
  - Interferon – alpha
  - Interferon – gamma
  - Interleukin – 2
  - Oprelvekin
  - Sargramostim
- Cytoprotectant
  - Amifostine
- Hematopoietic growth factors
  - Erythropoietin
  - Filgrastim
  - Sargramostim
- Immunostimulant-vaccine
  - Bacillus Calmette-Guérin
- Iron-chelating
  - Dexrazoxane
- LHRH agonists
  - Buserelin
  - Goserelin acetate
  - Leuprolide acetate
- Monoclonal antibodies
  - Gemtuzumab ozogamicin
  - Rituximab
  - Trastuzumab
- Natural enzymes
  - L-asparaginase
  - Pegaspargase

- Nonsteroidal antiandrogens
  - Bicalutamide
  - Flutamide
- Nonsteroidal antiestrogens
  - Tamoxifen
  - Toremifene
- Organic bisphosphonates
  - Pamidronate
  - Zoledronate
- Platelet aggregation inhibitor
  - Anagrelide
- Retinoids
  - Bexarotene
  - Isretinoin
  - Tretinoin
- Somatostatin analog
  - Octreotide
- Steroidal progestational
  - Medroxyprogesterone
  - Megestrol acetate
- Synthetic steroidal androgen
  - Fluoxymesterone
- Taxane molecule
  - Docetaxel
  - Paclitaxel
- Topoisomerase I inhibitor
  - Irinotecan
  - Topotecan
- Topoisomerase II inhibitor
  - Etoposide
  - Teniposide
- Thiol uroprotectant
  - Mesna
- Tubulin polymerization inhibitor
  - Estramustine
  - Vinblastine
  - Vincristine
  - Vinorelbine

STEM CELL TRANSPLANTATION

Hematopoietic stem cell transplantation (HSCT) is an effective treatment for leukemia, several other malignant and non-malignant conditions, and for selective solid tumors. Worldwide, about 30,000 autologous and 17,000 allogenic stem cell transplants were performed in 1997.

RATIONALE OF STEM CELL TRANSPLANTATION

- Both lymphoid and myeloid cells are derived from a single pleuripotent stem cell that is capable of both self-renewal and differentiation.
- Many malignancies exhibit a steep dose-response relationship to chemotherapy or radiotherapy, but the dose limiting toxicity for most of the chemotherapeutic agents is myelosuppression.
- Dose intensity and marrow rescue with infusion of hematopoietic stem cells, obtained either from the peripheral blood or from the bone marrow, are the primary biologic rationale of autologous hematopoietic stem cell transplantation.
- High dose chemotherapy rarely eradicates malignancy completely.
- The therapeutic benefit in allogenic hematopoietic stem cell transplantation is largely due to the immune mediated graft versus malignancy effect.
- In hematopoietic disorders, the HSCT replaces the defective clone with a normal stem cell (e.g. leukemia) or replaces a missing hematopoietic or lymphoid component in disorders such as aplastic anemia or severe combined immune deficiency (SCID) (Table 50.1).

TYPES OF TRANSPLANTATION

- Autologous:
  - Patient's own bone marrow or peripheral blood stem cells (PBSC) are collected before the administration of high dose chemotherapy (HDCT).
- Allogenic:
  - Stem cells can be collected from
    i. Matched, related—HLA identical sibling of the patient.
    ii. Partially matched sibling or parent of the patient.
  - Matched unrelated donor is selected through a search of the computer files of various international registries, including National Marrow Donor Program (NMDP).
  - Bone marrow, PBSC or umbilical cord blood may be used as a stem cell source.
- Syngenic:
  - Marrow or peripheral blood stem cells are collected from an identical twin.

ALLOGENIC TRANSPLANTATION

Donor Selection

The success of allogenic transplantation depends on the degree of donor-recipient matching at the Human leukocyte antigen (HLA) or major histocompatibility (MHC) locus. Genes encoding for HLA are located on chromosome 6 and they are codominantly expressed. HLA Class I antigens are A, B and C and Class II antigens are DP, DQ and DR. Even when a

Table 50.1: Indications for hematopoietic stem cell transplantation

Malignant	Nonmalignant	Congenital
Acute myeloid leukemia	Aplastic anemia	Immunodeficiencies
Acute lymphocytic leukemia	Paroxysmal nocturnal hemoglobinuria (PNH)	Hematologic defects
Chronic myeloid leukemia		Mucopolysaccharidoses
Non-Hodgkin's lymphoma	Myelodysplastic syndrome	Mucolipidoses
Hodgkin's lymphoma		Other lysosomal diseases
Multiple myeloma		
Hairy cell leukemia		
Chronic lymphocytic leukemia		

donor-recipient pair is related and completely genotypically matched for HLA, the incidence of GVHD in allogenic transplant is about 50 percent.

Histoincompatibility can cause increased incidence of:
1. Graft versus host disease (GVHD)
2. Graft failure
3. Graft rejection

The types of donors:
a. Related donor:
   - The probability of HLA–identity between any two given siblings is 25 percent.
   - In the USA the chance of having an HLA-matched sibling is about 35 percent.
   - HLA typing is done on blood samples from the patient and the donor.
   - Both serological and molecular methods are used for HLA typing.
   - For allogenic transplantation the most important HLA antigens are
   - Class I (A, B) and Class II (DRB1).
   - Most transplant centers prefer a 6/6 match or a minimum of 5/6 match.
b. Unrelated donor: If the patient has no donors in the family
   - A search can be done in the National Marrow Donation Program (NMDP).
   - About 20-30 percent of the searches through the NMDP result in transplant.
   - The median time to transplant from the initiation of search is 208 days.
   - The phone number of NMDP is 1 800 627 7692.
   - Because of the high incidence of GVHD, the mortality and morbidity associated with matched unrelated transplant can be high.

FURTHER READING (SEE PAGE 601 TO 603)

Stem Cell Collection in Allogenic Transplantation

51

Jame Abraham, Ramin Altaha

I. Peripheral blood stem cell (PBSC) collection
Stem cells can be mobilized to the periphery by growth factors and collected through an apheresis procedure.
- Usually GCSF 5-16 mcg/kg subcutaneously, once a day is given for 5 days.
- Stem cells are collected through an apheresis procedure on day 5 or 6.
- Stem cell dose varies with protocol (2-8 $\times 10^6$ cells per kg of CD^{34+} cells).
- This is increasingly becoming the most preferred mode of stem cell collection.

II. Bone marrow harvest
- The marrow can be aspirated from the posterior iliac crest through multiple aspirations while the donor is under general anesthesia.
- Usually a marrow of 10-15 ml/kg of the donor weight is aspirated.
- Complications of the donors are anemia, bone pain and neuropathies.
- Life threatening complications occur only in 0.27 percent of the procedures.

T CELL DEPLETION

- It is done to decrease the incidence of GVHD.
- Complete depletion of T cells increases the risk of relapse and graft rejection.
- Selective depletion is the commonly accepted mode.
- It is commonly done with monoclonal antibodies with or without complement.
- Magnetic beads coated with monoclonal antibodies are used.

STAGES OF ALLOGENIC TRANSPLANTATION

   I. Conditioning
  II. Transplantation phase
 III. Post-transplant phase (supportive care)

Conditioning

Conditioning regimens are used for 2 main purposes:
   a. Immunosuppression of the recipient to prevent graft rejection and allow engraftment.
   b. Eradication of malignant disease or an abnormal cell population.
   Conditioning regimens are chosen according to the particular clinical situation, the disease under treatment, the age and health of the patient, and the source of stem cells (Table 51.1).

Transplantation Phase

After the conditioning regimen, the patient receives stem cells as an intravenous infusion. Usually this is a well-tolerated procedure. The day of transplant is considered as day 0.

Engraftment: The rate of engraftment depends on the source of stem cells, use of hematopoietic growth factor and choice of prophylaxis against GVHD. Most rapid engraftment is seen in SCT, where granulocyte recovery occurs by day 10-12. This is accelerated by the use of filgrastim (G-CSF) or sargramostim (GM-CSF) after the transplant.

Post Transplant Phase

Most important events in the post transplant period are multiple complications including mucositis, nausea, vomiting, infection, hemorrhage, GVHD, graft failure and relapse of the disease. Supportive care, prevention of GVHD and graft failure are the major consideration of this period.
   a. Supportive care: Patients require intensive supportive care during this period for several complications including:
     1. Infectious complications
     2. Hematologic complications
     3. Other complications

Table 51.1: Commonly used regimens
Total body irradiation (TBI) and high dose cyclophosphamide
Busulfan and high dose cyclophosphamide
TBI and anti-thyomcyte globulin (ATG)
Cyclophosphamide and total lymphoid irradiation (TLI)

1. Among the infections, cytomegalovirus infection is a very serious complication.
   - It is the major cause of morbidity and mortality.
   - 5-10 percent of death in post transplant period is due to CMV interstitial pneumonia.
   - Pneumonia usually occurs 7-10 weeks after transplantation.
   - CMV infection is treated with ganciclovir 5 mg/kg/bd for 3 weeks, and IV immunoglobulin (IVIG).
2. Hematologic complications
   - All patients require both red cell and platelet transfusions for 3-4 weeks, and then intermittently for months.
   - All blood products should be a) irradiated to prevent GVHD and b) filtered to prevent CMV infection and febrile reaction.
   - Platelet count is usually kept at more than 10,000-20,000 cells/mm^3.
3. Other complications
   - Mucositis can occur.
   - Hemorrhagic cystitis may develop.
   - Can be due to cyclophosphamide or viruses like Adenovirus and BK virus.
   - Veno-occlusive disease (VOD) of the liver occurs in 20-30 percent.
   - Clinical features of VOD are right upper quadrant pain, hepatomegaly, jaundice and ascites.
   - Treatment is supportive care.

GRAFT-VERSUS-HOST DISEASE (GVHD)

- Immunologically competent donor T-lymphocytes react against recipient tissues, which leads to GVHD.
- Acute GVHD is usually seen before 100 days and chronic GVHD, after 100 days.
- It is seen in about 40-80 percent of the allogenic transplantation.
- The incidence of GVHD increases with age.
- Clinical manifestations are usually seen in liver, GI tract and skin.

MANAGEMENT OF GVHD

Commonly used agents for prophylaxis
- T-cell depletion of the donor cells
- Prednisone
- Cyclosporine
- Methotrexate
- Antithymocyte globulin (ATG)
- Tacrolimus (FK 506)
- Azathioprine
- Mycophenolate mofetil

TREATMENT

- Methylprednisone 1-2 mg/kg/day in divided doses (30-50% will respond)
- ATG 30 mg/kg/day IV (25-30% response)
- Cyclosporin 5 mg/kg/day PO
- Mycophenolate mofetil 500-1000 mg/day PO
- PUVA therapy for skin GVHD

CHRONIC GRAFT-VERSUS-HOST DISEASE (CGVHD)

- It occurs usually after day 100.
- The pathology of CGVHD is different from acute GVHD.
- The diagnosis is made by clinical presentation.
- The management is the same as acute GVHD.

GRAFT-VERSUS-LEUKEMIA (GVL)

- The major challenge is to separate the adverse effects of GVHD from the beneficial effects of GVL.
- The allogenic transplantation with T-cell depleted bone marrow has increased relapse risk.
- The greatest GVL effect is seen in CML, intermediate in AML and the least in ALL.
- GVL occurs more in recipients of mismatched family or unrelated donors, less in HLA identical sibling.

AUTOLOGOUS STEM CELL TRANSPLANTATION

Usually PBSC are collected through an apheresis procedure. Bone marrow harvest is rarely used in autologous transplantation due to concerns about tumor cell contamination.

Prior to the apheresis, the patient receives two or more cycles of chemotherapy with growth factors for cytoreduction and mobilization of the stem cells.

Since autologous stem cells can be potentially contaminated with malignant cells (gene marking studies showed that relapse could be from infused marrow in AML), different purging methods are extensively studied. After collecting, the autologous stem cells are stored in dimethyl sulfoxide (DMSO).

Conditioning regimens are meant for cytoreduction and mobilization of the stem cells.

The hematological and infectious complications during transplant and post transplant phases are similar to those of allogenic transplantation. Mucositis can be severe in autologous transplantation. GVHD and VOD are not that common.

FUTURE DIRECTIONS

Non-myeloablative Transplantation

- It is the conventional myeloablative transplant.
- It causes high morbidity and mortality.
- It can be used only in young patients without comorbid conditions.
- In non-myeloablative transplant, the conditioning regimen is designated not to eradicate the malignancy, but rather to produce immunosuppression to achieve engraftment and development of graft versus malignancy effect.
- Encouraging results are reported in CML, CLL and renal cell carcinoma.
- At present it is an active area of research.
    1. Donor lymphocyte infusion (DLI)   The infusions of lymphocytes obtained from the original donor, represent a new approach for treating patients who have relapsed after an allogenic transplantation. The purpose of DLI is to use the graft versus leukemia effect from the T cells of the donor.
        - In patients who relapsed after allogenic transplantation, DLI induces complete remission in 70 percent of CML, 30 percent of AML and 30 percent of MDS patients.
        - DLI is associated with GVHD in 90 percent of the patients who achieved remission.
    2. Cord blood transplantation (CBT)   CBT is an active area of research. Cord blood is collected most commonly after placenta delivery from uterus. However cord blood collection while placenta is in uterus, also has been done.

There is very low incidence of GVHD with CBT, despite detectable maternal cells in cord blood (1 in 10,000 to 100,000). There is no difference in cell numbers with vaginal delivery versus cesarean sections.

FURTHER READING (SEE PAGE 601 TO 603)

Hematopoietic Growth Factors

52

Shirley George

One of the significant problems of chemotherapy in cancer is the deleterious effects of the drugs on the bone marrow and the reduction of all three cell lineages namely white and red blood cells, and platelets. Occasionally the reduction can be sudden and severe that life-threatening emergencies can occur. The function of the totipotent hematopoietic stem cells is inhibited and the patient will show evidence of progressive pallor and dyspnea (anemia), fever with intercurrent infections (leucopenia) and bleeding diathesis (thrombocytopenia).

It is noted that there is a regulatory molecule known as hematopoietic growth factor which controls the differentiation and maturation of the cell lineages, and the release of the functional neutrophils into the peripheral blood. Efforts to develop these factors in the laboratory were successful and a few molecules are already there in clinical practice. The use of these hematopoietic growth factors (HGF) has had a considerable impact on cancer management in recent years. Its role has to be assessed in optimizing cancer chemotherapy at different levels of dose intensity namely the standard dose and high dose chemotherapy. The most widely utilized class of HGF has the ability to reduce the duration and severity of neutropenia, and more recently, other cytopenia after myelo-suppressive chemotherapy has been applied in many different types of cancer.

BIOLOGICAL PROPERTIES OF HGF

HGF are glycoprotein hormones of low molecular weight which regulate hematopoietic progenitor cell proliferation and differentiation but also act on the activation and survival of mature blood cells. Their genes, chromosomal location and many associated receptor molecules have been identified and the recombinant proteins of these factors have revolutionized experimental and clinical hematology. Among hematopoietic stimulatory hormones, four groups have been identified, namely granulo-cyte colony-stimulating factor (G-CSF) and granulocytic macrophage colony-stimulating factor (GM-CSF), erythrocyte growth factor and platelet growth factor. Among them colony-stimulating factors (CSF), the G-CSF and GM-CSF are most important. While predominantly acting on less mature progenitor cells, they can influence many functions of mature blood cells. They also affect T cells, fibroblasts, macrophages and endo-thelial cells which represent the major natural sources of HGF upon inflammatory or antigenic challenge.

At present two drugs are available in the group of G-CSF Filgrastim (Neupogen, Roche, India) and sargramostim. GM-CSF Filgrastim is a specific molecule for growth of myeloid cells, sargramostim stimulates the growth of myeloid cells and also monocytes and eosinophils.

GRANULOCYTE COLONY STIMULATING FACTOR

G-CSF is produced by monocytes, endothelial cells and fibroblasts. *In vitro*, G-CSF induces specific colony growth of granulocyte lineage and acts synergistically on the committed stem cells and hence neutrophil recovery is fast.

The capacity of G-CSF to increase bone marrow cellularity and peripheral blood neutrophil count in chemotherapy-induced neutropenia has been established. Tolerance of G-CSF is usually good, with only occasional occurrence of bone pain or mild fever. It is probably the best clinically tolerated of all myeloid HGF and is widely utilized in cancer chemotherapy in both developed and developing countries.

INDICATIONS

For Prophylaxis

1. In patients with high dose chemotherapy.
2. In patients who may develop intercurrent infections with history of febrile neutropenia.
3. In patients who have undergone extensive radiation.
4. In patients with open wound, tissue infection and poor immune response.

Dose and the mode of administration: Neupogen 0.5 MU (5 µg/kg per day) either s.c. or i.v. for 1 week.

For Therapy in Established Neutropenic Patients

Group 1
1. To reduce the duration of neutropenia.
2. To control the refractory febrile neutropenia during the period of neutropenia.
3. In elderly patients after induction therapy for AML.

Neupogen 5 μg/kg/day either s.c. or i.v for 6 consecutive days till the absolute neutrophil count (ANC) reaches 1000/cmm.

Group 2

Neupogen 10 μg/kg/day either s.c. or i.v. for peripheral blood cell mobilization or after bone marrow transplantation.

1. For peripheral blood stem mobilization before transplantation.
2. Treatment of MDS.
3. Allogenic and autologous bone marrow transplantation.

In neutropenia, the therapy is discontinued when the ANC reaches 1000/cmm.

GM-CSF-Sargramostim can be used *in vivo* as adjunct to cytotoxic drug treatment, in marrow infiltration, and marrow failure. GM-CSF and G-CSF are used to treat myelosuppression after chemotherapy and for hematopoietic reconstitution after high dose chemotherapy. They can shorten neutropenia and reduce the incidence and severity of infections and other cytopenia-associated problems.

GM-CSF associated toxicity is tolerable, and side effects are usually mild, mostly consisting of fever, bone pain and weakness. Another adverse effect is dyspnea which is seen in certain patients with elevated granulocyte counts; this effect might be due to the accumulation of activated neutrophils in the lung during the phase of leukocyte recovery.

GM-CSF is frequently used in breast cancer chemotherapy. Two major North American randomized trials on the effects of HDC and SCT in high risk primary and metastatic breast cancer, use subcutaneous (s.c.) GM-CSF for hematopoietic reconstitution at a dose of 5 mg/kg/d until an absolute neutrophil count (ANC) of 1,000/mL is achieved. When G-CSF is used instead of GM-CSF, dose and target ANC are usually similar.

Erythrocytic Growth Factor (Epoetin)

Indication of the use of epoetin is anemia that develops during antineoplastic therapy due to marrow failure. It is not uncommon to find a patient with hemoglobin less than 4 gm/dl. The cause of the anemia is multifactorial and one of them is due to reduced epoetin production.

Therapeutic Dose

Commercially epoetin is produced by recombinant DNA technique and it has the same amino acid composition as naturally occurring epoetin. The dose is 600 i.u./kg 3 times a week. Most of the patients respond well to this dose and the hemoglobin rises to 8 g/dl in 2 weeks time.

The drug is non-immunogenic and relatively harmless. Some of the patients develop fever, arthralgia and gastric upset like nausea and vomiting.

Platelet Growth Factor

It is not uncommon to find life threatening bleeding developing in persons with antineoplastic chemotherapy. The platelet can drop to very low levels so that bleeding takes place from different mucosal surfaces like gums, nose and GI tract. Transfusion with platelet fraction is one form of therapy but to produce a sustained rise in platelets, drugs like thrombopoietin or oprelevekin (Neumega) has to be used. The latter is nearly homologous to naturally present interleukin II. It promotes stem cell proliferation and induces megakaryocytic maturation. Neumega has received FDA approval and is used in cases of thrombocytopenia after anticancer chemotherapy.

One of the most important recent discoveries in HGFs has been the identification functional characterization and clinical introduction of thrombopoietin (TPO). According to these investigations, TPO supports the growth and differentiation of megakaryocytic progenitors *in vitro* and *in vivo*. The predominant site of TPO production is the liver. Regulation of TPO serum levels seems to depend on the degradation of circulating TPO by platelets.

Despite these limitations, areas of potential clinical benefit have been identified. Pegylated recombinant human megakaryocytic growth and development factor (PEGrHuMGDF, a chemical modification of TPO) was tested in patients with advanced cancer before chemotherapy. A dose of 0.03 to 1.0 mg/kg was given daily s.c. for up to 10 days or until a target platelet count was reached. Counts peaked between days 12 and 18 and remained above $450 \times 10^9/L$ for up to 3 weeks. The dose-dependent increase in platelet counts ceased after stopping the drug. Alterations in white blood cell count, hematocrit or major toxicities were not observed. Platelets examined at the time of peak platelet counts were morphologically and functionally normal. The high potency and low toxicity of a TPO derivative in this seminal study indicate that it may also be useful for the management of thrombocytopenia in chemotherapy.

ADAPTED FROM AMERICAN SOCIETY OF CLINICAL ONCOLOGY-RECOMMENDATIONS FOR THE USE OF HEMATOPOIETIC COLONY STIMULATING FACTORS; GROWTH GUIDELINES FOR THE USE OF GF FACTORS (1996)

Guidelines for Primary Prophylactic CSF Administration

General Circumstances

Primary prophylactic administration of colony-stimulating factors (CSFs) was shown to reduce the incidence of febrile neutropenia by approximately 50 percent in the three major randomized trials in adults in which the incidence of febrile neutropenia was greater than 40 percent in the control group. The value of primary CSF administration has not been clearly established in cases where severe myelosuppression is encountered.

It is recommended that primary administration of CSFs be reserved for patients expected to experience febrile neutropenia. Thus, in general, for previously untreated patients receiving chemotherapy regimens, initial use of CSFs should not be considered routinely.

Special Circumstances

Clinicians may occasionally be faced with patients who might benefit from a relatively non-myelosuppressive chemotherapy but have potential risk factors for febrile neutropenia or infection because of bone marrow compromise or comorbidity. It is possible that primary CSF administration may be exceptionally warranted in patients at higher risk for chemotherapy-induced infectious complications even though the data supporting such use are not conclusive. Such risk factors might include preexisting neutropenia due to disease, extensive prior radiation containing large amount of bone marrow; a history of recurrent febrile neutropenia while receiving earlier chemotherapy of similar or lesser dose-intensity; or conditions potentially enhancing the risk of serious infection, e.g. poor performance status and more advanced cancer, decreased immune function, open wound, or already active tissue infections. This is not meant to be an all inclusive list; it is anticipated that, depending on the unique features of the clinical situation, there will be instances when the administration of a CSF will be appropriate in spite of the uses recommended in other guidelines.

1996 Recommendation

Note, however, that the Special Circumstances section 1994 was amended; specifically, "poor performance status and more advanced cancer" were added to the list of conditions potentially enhancing the risk of serious infection.

Guidelines for Secondary Prophylactic CSF Administration

There is evidence that CSF administration can decrease the probability of febrile neutropenia in subsequent cycles of chemotherapy after a documented occurrence in an earlier cycle. Even if febrile neutropenia has not occurred, the use of CSFs may be considered if prolonged neutropenia is causing excessive dose reduction or delay in chemotherapy. However, in the absence of clinical data supporting maintenance of chemotherapy dose-intensity, physicians should consider chemotherapy dose reduction as an alternative to the use of CSFs.

Guidelines for CSF Therapy in Afebrile Patients

There are inadequate data to detemine whether patients with neutropenia without fever will benefit clinically from the initiation of CSF at the time neutropenia is diagnosed; intervention with a CSF in afebrile neutropenic patients is not recommended.

Febrile Patients

For the majority of patients with febrile neutropenia, the available data do not clearly support the routine initiation of CSFs as adjuncts to antibiotic therapy. However, certain febrile, neutropenic patients may have prognostic factors that are predictive of clinical deterioration, such as pneumonia, hypotension, multiorgan dysfunction (sepsis syndrome), or fungal infection. The use of CSFs together with antibiotics may be reasonable in such high-risk patients, even though the benefits of administration under these circumstances have not been definitively proved.

Guidelines for Use of CSFs to Increase Chemotherapy Dose-intensity

Outside the clinical trials, there is little justification for the use of CSFs to increase chemotherapy dose-intensity. In a setting where clinical research demonstrates that dose-intensity therapy not requiring progenitor-cell support produces improvement in disease control, CSFs should be used when these therapies are expected to produce significant rates of febrile neutropenia (e.g. in 40% of patients).

Guidelines for Use of CSF as Adjuncts to Progenitor-cell Transplantation

CSFs can successfully shorten the period of neutropenia and reduce infectious complications in patients undergoing high-dose cytotoxic therapy with autologous bone marrow transplantation (BMT). Available data suggest the potential for similar benefits after allogeneic BMT, but these data remain less conclusive, and the routine use of CSFs following allogeneic transplantation cannot be strongly encouraged at the present time. Until further trials are performed to determine specifically the value of CSF administration after high-dose chemotherapy and peripheral-blood progenitor-cell (PBPC) transplantation, CSF use in this setting seems reasonable. There also may be role for the CSFs in assisting in the recovery of patients who experience delayed or inadequate neutrophil engraftment following progenitor-cell transplantation. Available evidence indicates that the CSFs are effective in mobilizing PBPC for transplantation. The same dose, routes, and schedules of CSF administration mentioned in the Guidelines for CSF Dosing and Route of Administration and Guidelines for Initiation and Duration of CSF Administration should be used in the transplantation setting.

It is noted that the CSFs are effective in mobilizing autologous PBPC for transplantation which leads to an earlier hematopoietic recovery than autologous BMT. Trials have demonstrated the value of CSF administration after high-dose chemotherapy and PBPC transplantation. There also may be a role for the CSFs in assisting in the recovery of patients who experience delayed or inadequate neutrophil engraftment following progenitor-cell transplantation.

CSFs can be routinely recommended as adjuncts to allogeneic and autologous progenitor-cell transplantation, both for mobilization of PBPC and as a means to speed up hematopoietic reconstitution following BMT or PBPC transplantation. Administration of a CSF in case of engraftment failure is warranted.

Guidelines for Use of CSF Patients with Myeloid Leukemia and MDS

Acute myeloid leukemia   There is evidence from several studies that CSF administration can achieve a modest decrease in the duration of neutropenia when begun shortly after the completion of acute myeloid leukemia (AML) induction therapy, but beneficial CSF effects on such end points as duration of hospitalization, incidence of severe infection, complete response rates, and long-term outcome have yet to be completely determined, necessitating caution in the use of CSFs in this setting. CSFs given either before and/or concurrently with chemotherapy for 'priming' effects cannot be recommended outside a clinical trial. Potential concerns include inhibition of chemotherapeutic activity and enhancement of toxicity.

There is evidence from several studies, most of them conducted in older patients, that CSF administration can achieve modest decreases in the duration of neutropenia, accompanied in some but not all studies by an amelioration of infectious complications, when begun shortly after the completion of AML induction therapy. There has been no consistent improvement in complete response rates and long-term outcome after two years. It does not appear to cause any harm from CSF administration when given after completion of induction chemotherapy.

Recommendation: Primary administration of a CSF can be used after completion of induction chemotherapy in patients above 55 years of age. Although there are fewer data, it is likely that the results showing shortening of the duration of neutropenia may apply to younger patients as well. CSFs given either before and/or concurrently with chemotherapy for priming effects still cannot be recommended outside a clinical trial.

Myelodysplastic syndrome   CSFs can increase the absolute neutrophil count in neutropenic patients with myelodysplastic syndromes (MDS). Data supporting the routine long-term continuous use of CSFs in these patients are lacking. Intermittent administration of CSFs may be considered in a subset of patients with severe neutropenia and recurrent infection.

Guidelines for Use of CSF in Patients Receiving Concurrent Chemotherapy and Irradiation

CSFs should be avoided in patients receiving concomitant chemotherapy and radiation therapy.

Guidelines for Use of CSF in the Pediatric Population

In the absence of conclusive data, the guidelines recommended for adults are generally applicable to the patients in pediatric age group. However, optimal CSF doses have yet to be determined. Further clinical research into the use of these factors in support of chemotherapy and progenitor-cell transplantation in the pediatric age group should be given high priority.

Guidelines for CSF Dosing and Route of Administration

In adults, the recommended CSF doses are 5 mg/kg/m^2/d of granulocyte CSF (G-CSF; neupogen) or 250 mg/kg/m^2/d of granulocyte-macrophage CSF (GM-CSF: sargramostim). These agents can be administered subcutaneously or intravenously as clinically indicated. CSF dose escalation is not advised. The available data suggest that rounding the dose to the nearest vial size may enhance patient convenience and reduce costs without clinical detriment.

Guidelines for Initiation and Duration of CSF Administration

Existing clinical data suggest that starting G-CSF or GM-CSF between 24 and 72 hours subsequent to chemotherapy may provide optimal neutrophil recovery. Continuing the CSF until the occurrence of an absolute neutrophil count (ANC) of 10,000/mm^3 after the neutrophil nadir, as specified in the G-CSF package, is known to be safe and effective. However, a shorter duration of administration that is sufficient to achieve clinically adequate neutrophil recovery is a reasonable alternative, considering issues like patient's convenience and cost.

FURTHER READING

1. Berends FJ, Kazemier G, Bonjer HJ, et al. Subcutaneous metastases after laparoscopic colectomy. Lancet 1994;344:58 (letter).
2. Cirocco WC, Schwartzman A, Golub RW. Abdominal wall recurrence after laparoscopic colectomy for colon cancer. Surgery 1994;116:842-46.
3. Dobronte Z, Wittman T, Karacsony G. Rapid development of malignant metastases in the abdominal wall after laparoscopy. Endoscopy 1978;10:1277-87.
4. Nduka CC, Monson JRT, Menzies-Gow N, et al. Abdominal wall metastases following laparoscopy. Br J Surg 1994;81:648-51.
5. Wilson JP, Hoffman GC, Baker JW, et al. Laparoscopic-assisted colectomy. Initial experience. Ann Surg 1994;219:732-43.

Palliative Care in Cancer Patients

53

Venugopala Rao Tanneru

INTRODUCTION

At least a million people in India are in pain with cancer. For patients at the end of life, maximizing the quality of life rather than postponing of death is the first priority of terminal care. In this context, symptoms that cause disability and suffering must be considered as medical emergencies and managed aggressively by frequent elicitation, continuous reassessment and individualized treatment. The relief of distressing symptoms at the end of life should not be withheld out of reluctance to use appropriate medications and procedures.

Palliative care is a branch of modern medicine aimed at improving the quality of life of people living with incurable diseases. It offers a pain-free life rather than a prolonged and painful life. Since this involves a 'holistic approach' to the patient and family, the palliative care team should take the patient's socioeconomic, cultural and spiritual status into consideration.

Towards the end of the 20th century, many centers for the terminal care of patients have been started. In the UK St. Christopher Hospital is the first of its kind. Dame Saunders, the pioneer in this field introduced the concept of 'hospice' which is meant for managing terminally ill patients. It stands midway between home and a regular hospital. The original hospice concept has evolved greatly and is now giving service to patients with incurable diseases both in hospitals and in the local community.

Traditional hospices are probably not the best mode of delivery of palliative care in countries like India. Issues of cost effectiveness and cultural factors, including strong family ties very often make traditional hospices not very appealing in the Indian situation. The first hospice called Shanthi Avedan Ashram was opened in Mumbai in 1984. The following two decades saw few initiatives in this direction. But, over the last nine years, there has been exceptionally rapid development of community based palliative care services in the southern state of Kerala. Certain districts in Kerala now have good quality palliative care services which cover more than 50 percent of the need. This can be compared with the facilities available in the West.

ROLE OF PHYSICIANS IN PALLIATIVE CARE

Caring for patients at the terminal stage requires the same skill of eliciting history, clinical examination and careful diagnosis. Communication skills are vitally important. This involves good teamwork, with the physician taking a major role in the team.

The physician and the palliative care team must identify, understand and relieve the patient's suffering. The suffering may include physical, psychological, social or spiritual distress. The caregiver of these patients must serve as a facilitator and as a ray of hope. They must reassure the patient that care will be continued throughout the final stages of their lives.

COMPONENTS OF PALLIATIVE CARE

For patients who need terminal care, maximizing the quality of life, rather than postponing death is the first priority. Added to the physical debility, the patient is troubled by emotional problems. He is worried about the intensity of pain he has to suffer. The future of his family is a major concern to him. The emotional problems are closely entwined with the social and financial problems. The treatment either curative or palliative often adds to the financial burden of the family. Families go into debt, and it would weigh heavily in the patient's mind. For an average patient in India, 'non medical' issues like worry about the future of the family top the list of problems. But it is important that, symptoms that cause disability and suffering must be considered and managed.

The relief of distressing symptoms, for example, pain at the end of life should not be held out of reluctance to use appropriate medication and techniques. The common problems are:
- Pain
- Fatigue
- Dyspnea
- Vomiting
- Constipation
- Delirium and agitation
- Issues related to nutrition and hydration
- Fungating ulcers/fistula

Pain is an important problem next to fatigue in incidence. Up to 75 percent of patients dying of cancer experience pain. Pain is undertreated at the terminal stage, because of the improper approach to evaluation, interpretation and application of various techniques.

Pain is often excruciating, occupying every moment of the patient's life. Most of this pain is unnecessary as medical science today has the better know-how to address it effectively.

Chronic pain, as different from acute pain, does not serve any purpose and needs to be tackled aggressively.

MECHANISM OF PAIN

The peripheral nerve endings (nociceptor) transmits the pain impulse to the dorsal horn of the spinal cord, where it gets modified before onward transmission to the brain.

One of the things that we now understand about pain is that pain is self-perpetuating. Untreated pain causes worsening of the pain day by day, by:
- sensitization of the nociceptors by mediators of inflammation,
- recruitment of silent or sleepy nociceptors,
- sensitization of the dorsal horn of the spinal cord,
- recruitment of adjacent spinal segments and
- skeletal muscle spasm induced by the painful stimulus that adds a muscular component to the pain.

Pain relief is not something to be reserved for the last few days of life; treatment of pain should start when the pain starts. It is universally recognized now that pain should be prevented rather than treated and that in all continuous pains, pain relief must be a continuous process.

TYPES OF PAIN

Basically there are two types of pain, namely nociceptive and neurogenic pain.

Nociceptive Pain

This term can be defined as a centripetal message reporting tissue damage that is conveyed via a specific afferent system within the CNS. Signals travel through dorsal horns of the spinal cord via ascending pathway to multiple associative modulating tracts in the brainstem, midbrain and cortex.

Tumor growth and metastatic spread are the immediate causes of noci-perception where the inflammation of the surrounding tissues plays a major role, through mediators and tissue substances (prostaglandins, substance P., etc.).

Most cancer pain syndromes are primarily of this nociceptive type. The source of this type of pain may include skin, mucosa, bones, joints, ligaments, muscles, lymph nodes, internal organs and the region showing inflammatory and/or ischemic changes.

It has been established that most of this pain can be controlled through a simple protocol called World Health Organization analgesic ladder.

Chronic cancer pain may be related to the tumor progression in 62 percent of cases or tumor treatment in another 25 percent or may be preexisting chronic pain in 10 percent unrelated to the tumor.

Pain due to cancer is often managed on a cooperative basis between the general practitioner, oncology and radiotherapy departments and the pain clinic. The specific role of pain clinics is to provide pain-relieving procedures; most patients benefit from the combination of these procedures.

Neurogenic Pain

This term suggests a heterogeneous group of pain symptoms in which somatosensory (nociceptive) afferents play a minor role at the most.

A careful search for symptoms of sensory and/or motor deficit in the affected region will confirm tentative diagnosis or support attribute to nerve roots, plexuses, segments and/or the peripheral system.

Chronic cancer pain may be related to the tumor progression in 62 percent of cases, or tumor treatment in another 25 percent or pre-existing chronic pain in 10 percent unrelated to the tumor.

MANAGEMENT OF PAIN

Pain is not just a physical sensation, it is also an emotional experience. While managing cancer pain we must consider the following points.

The patient must be relieved of his pain.

The goal of the treatment is to improve the quality of life, rather than pain relief only.

Management includes a combination of physical, emotional, social, spiritual and economic problems.

INTENSITY OF PAIN

There are no objective criteria for measuring the intensity of pain. Simplified scales are used to document initial findings and course of therapy (Figs 53.1 and 53.2).

Verbal five-point scale
    0. No pain
    1. Mild pain
    2. Moderate pain
    3. Severe pain
    4. Excruciating pain

0 – 1 – 2 – 3 – 4 – 5 – 6 – 7 – 8 – 9 – 10

Figure 53.1: Analog numeric scale showing intensity of pain

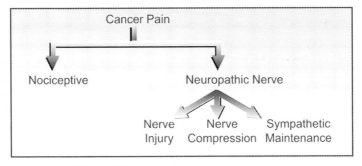

Figure 53.2: Classification of cancer pain

There is a 100 mm scale with one end zero (no pain), and the other end 100 (worst pain imaginable) with increments of 10 mm (Fig. 53.3).

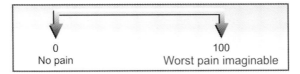

Figure 53.3: VAS (Visual analog scale)

PHARMACOLOGICAL TREATMENT

Oral Administration

Basically symptomatic pain therapy begins with oral drug administration and is continued as long-term oral medication unless special conditions contraindicate such a regimen. The World Health Organization (WHO) Three-step Analgesic Ladder has revolutionized the treatment of cancer pain all over the world. It involves the use of oral drug therapy by the clock, depending on the duration of the action of the drug (Fig. 53.4).

Non-opioid analgesics have been established as basic (step I) pain therapeutics on the basis of high levels of antinociceptive efficacy. Their favorable pharmacokinetics with hour-long effective level maintenance subsequent to oral and rectal administration and minimum CNS (central) effects in normal dosage ranges makes them ideal analgesics. Slow-release preparations are preferred as soon as a stable situation is achieved (Table 53.1).

Most non-steroidal anti-inflammatory drugs (NSAIDs) are used in the long term by mouth to treat cancer pain. These substances are contraindicated in patients with gastroduodenal ulceration.

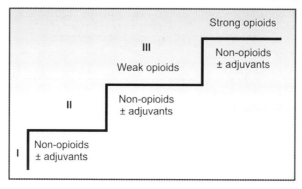

Figure 53.4: WHO 3-step analgesic ladder

Table 53.1		
Drug	Dose	Interval
Aspirin	500-1000 mg	4-6 hrs.
Ibuprofen	200-400 mg	6-8 hrs.
Diclofenac	25-50 mg	6-8 hrs.
Naproxen	250-500 mg	8-12 hrs.

Common side effects of NSAIDs:
- Gastritis
- Platelet dysfunction
- Renal failure
- Allergic manifestations, e.g. bronchospasm

Step II: Weak opioids agonist (low potency central analgesic).

If step I by itself is inadequate to control the pain step II involves the addition of a weak opioid. The commonly available drugs in our country, the recommended dose and the required frequency of administration are given below:

Drug	Frequency in hours
Codeine 30-60 mg	4
Dextropropoxyphene 65 mg	6-8
(This is available in combination with paracetamol)	
Tramadol 50-100 mg	6-8

Tramadol is more potent but more expensive. Weak opioids have a special place in our country because of limited availability of oral morphine.

Step III: Strong agonist and partial agonist opioids.

When step II drugs are inadequate to treat pain, step III involves continuing the step I drugs, stopping the weak opioids and adding a strong opioid.

Oral morphine is the mainstay of the treatment of severe cancer pain. Contrary to popular belief, oral morphine (when used for opioid-sensitive pain, with dose titrated to the degree of pain relief) does not cause addiction or respiratory depression. An overdose causes side effects like drowsiness, delirium and myoclonus. The usual starting dose is 5-10 mg 4 hourly. As required the dose is increased by 50 percent every 1-2 days, till the desired effect is reached. Recently fentanyl patches have been made available in India for the management of cancer pain, but are too expensive for the routine use.

The common side effects:
- Constipation can be troublesome and needs adjuvant therapy with laxatives, for example, bisacodyl.
- Vomiting is experienced by one-third of the patients in the first few days and they require anti-emetics.
- Urinary hesitancy occurs in a small percentage of patients.

MANAGEMENT OF NEUROPATHIC PAIN

The mainstay in the treatment of neuropathic pain is the use of two groups of drugs, anticonvulsants and antidepressants. Antidepressants are well tolerated and they form the first line drug. The usual drugs in these groups are:

Tricyclic antidepressants
    Amitryptilene   —   25-75 mg at bed time
    Doxepin   —   25-75 mg at bed time
    Imipramine   —   25-75 mg at bed time
    Venlafaxine   —   37.5-75 mg at bed time
Anticonvulsants
    Carbamazepine   —   200-400 mg 8 hourly
    Sodium valproate —   up to 1200 mg daily
    Gebapentin   —   300-1200 mg daily

Anticonvulsants act by membrane stabilization. It is possible that sodium valproate also works by GABA enhancement. Tricyclic antidepressants act on the descending inhibitory pathways by preventing re-uptake of serotonin and nor-epinephrine thus increasing the concentration of these inhibitory neurotransmitters at the synapses.

When these two first-line drugs are inadequate to control neuropathic pain, there are several other options. One is the oral administration of local anesthetic agents like meaxiletine. An intravenous dose of lignocaine 2-3 mg/kg can be used as a therapeutic trial. If it succeeds in achieving analgesia for more than 20 minutes (a short-lived analgesia could be used because of placebo effect) the patient can be started on oral maxiletine on a regular basis.

Pain clinics in India being few, it is not uncommon to see patients presenting with long-standing excruciating pain. The concept of WHO analgesic ladder, needs to be modified in such situations. In some centers, titrated i.v. bolus dose of 1.5 mg morphine every 10 minutes, till the patient either gets pain relief or becomes drowsy, is becoming popular.

Role of intravenous barbiturates and corticosteroids in pain relief:

Barbiturates have been advocated to manage dying patients who have inadequate analgesia or uncontrolled symptoms. Intravenous thiopentone titrated to a level of sedation was the approach advocated in a series of 17 terminally ill patients. But generally the need for such sedation is an exception rather than the rule.

Corticosteroids: Steroids are of particular value in nerve compression pain and in pain of elevated intracranial tension. They may be administered systematically but when feasible, local drug delivery (epidural) has advantages. Dexamethasone is the preferred agent for systematic administration and triamcinolone for epidural injection.

Other agents: Ketamine, the NMDA receptor antagonist is now being commonly used for the management of neuropathic pain. The drug can be used orally, sublingually or subcutaneously in doses which do not cause much sedation.

Amantidine, an anti-Parkinson and anti-viral drug also has been shown to cause NMDA antagonism and has been seen to alleviate pain related to nerve injury. The usual dose is 100-200 mg at bed time.

Gabapentin and lamogrigine are two newer anticonvulsants, which may be helpful in neuropathic pain resistant to conventional treatment. Gabapentin is believed to be useful in managing post-herpetic neuralgia. Lamotrigine has to be given at doses of 50 mg at bed time. Every week the dose can be increased by 50 mg a day.

SPECIALIZED THERAPIES FOR PAIN RELIEF

Ninety percent of cancer pain can be managed through proper use of WHO ladder. If severe, persistent pain does not respond to analgesic drug, or if the side effects of the drug are not tolerated, the physician should consider changing analgesics and changing the route of administration. A trial of an adjuvant drug together with opioids and non-opioids would be appropriate.

Specialized therapeutic approaches described here are meant only to give practitioners a general idea of how to judge their practicability in a given situation. As a rule, the use of these methods entails specialists, special equipment and special training. This chapter briefly summarizes their specific pain-relieving effects and typical indications in cancer therapy as a basis for interdisciplinary consultation.

LOCAL AND REGIONAL ANESTHESIA

Local and regional analgesia used in peripheral or spinal nerve blocks have become an important clinical tool of intraoperative and postoperative pain therapy with the introduction of well-tolerated, long-acting local anesthetic and catheter technique facilitating continuous medication. Several controlled studies support the use of intravenous, subcutaneous, intrapleural and epidural local anesthetics in the management of patients with somatic, visceral and neuropathic pain. Intravenous lignocaine should be considered in some refractory cases especially in neuropathic pain.

Intrapleural local anesthetics have been used for the management of chronic cancer pain from tumor infiltration of the liver, through a sub-cutaneously, tunneled intrapleural catheter for a long term.

Epidural local anesthetics are used to manage patients with localized pain syndrome, usually below the umbilicus. Intermittent and continuous epidural infusions of local anesthetics have been used to manage the chronic pain associated with metastatic disease, involving sacral and lumbosacral plexus. This method consists of infusing a local anesthetic, through a subcutaneous infusion pump or Oomiya reservoir connected to a catheter placed in epidural space.

SPINAL OPIOID ADMINISTRATION

Spinal opioid administration is the introduction of opioids (preservative free) directly into the lumbar or thoracic spinal region. The two routes of delivery are distinguished by their relation to the dura mater, the envelope of the connective tissue surrounding the spinal cord. Epidural adminis-tration places the therapeutic substance in the epidural space—the loose connective tissue around the dura. Intrathecal administration refers to delivery by injection through the dura mater into the cerebrospinal fluid. The opiate receptors in the central nervous system are the site of action of the opioid analgesics.

IMPLANTABLE SYSTEMS

A variety of subcutaneous ports and complete systems are now available for continuous opioid delivery. The systems include a functioning reservoir and an energy source for the proper functioning of the pump, obviating the need for external pumps suitable for intrathecal administration only.

EXTERNAL PUMPS WITH ELECTRIC OR MECHANICAL DRIVE (SYRINGE DRIVER)

These pumps are as a rule easy to operate, dependable, simple in design and somewhat less accurate and flexible than electronic systems as far as dosage is concerned. Varying infusion rate and solution concentration sets the dosage. A bolus dose function usually provided for such a setup is completely adequate in a stable clinical situation.

PATIENT-CONTROLLED ANALGESIA (PCA)

This signifies parenteral or spinal administration of analgesics in which patients can control themselves by means of electronically controlled programmable pump systems. The basic assumption is that the analgesic dose required to control a given pain is subject to considerable individual variation. This method is now practiced widely in the UK and US clinics. It is a safe and effective pain control method that allows patients a high degree of self-determination. In cancer pain management, the value of PCA systems is seen mainly in individual dosage determination, especially during periods of route changeover (e.g. from oral to parenteral to spinal).

PCA or syringe driver is indicated in persistent nausea and vomiting, swallowing difficulty, intestinal obstruction and severe weakness. There are advantages in this PCA or syringe driver technique. It permits good symptom control, avoiding repeated injections. The patient can wear his garments and there is mobility in his daily chores. Mixture of drugs is possible and different sites like shoulder, thigh and abdomen can be used to place the syringe driver safely. The physician has to assess the symptoms frequently and adjust the therapy once in 24 hours especially towards the end of life.

NERVE BLOCKS

Lack of response to pharmacological management and/or unacceptable adverse effects are a major indication for nerve blocking technique for pain due to malignancy.

The common nerve blocks that are useful in the cancer pain management are:
- Peripheral
- Extradural
- Intrathecal
- Autonomic
  - Cervical ganglion block
  - Stellate ganglion block
  - Lumbar sympathectomy
  - Celiac plexus block

Peripheral nerve blocks are used both diagnostically to localize the nerve distribution and therapeutically to interrupt pain transmission within the nerve distribution. It is useful in patients who have pain in the chest, abdomen and head. These techniques are most useful in patients with somatic pain; an example is Gasserian ganglion block for craniofacial pain, intercostal block for chest wall infiltration. In patients who respond to a local anesthetic block, neurolytic blockade with either phenol or alcohol may provide prolonged relief. This procedure is done under fluoroscopic control or CT localization to accurately interrupt the individual nerve transmission.

Epidural and intrathecal neurolytic blocks have been used to manage patients with advanced disease whose pain is unilateral in the chest or abdomen, or central in the perineum.

A review of a large number of alcohol subarachnoid blocks reports an average of 60 percent good relief, 21 percent fair and 18 percent poor. The mean duration is between 2 weeks and 3 months. Patients should be warned that with this procedure, a few of them might develop motor paresis, and bladder dysfunction, especially incontinence.

AUTONOMIC NERVE BLOCKS

The most commonly used sympathetic block is that of the celiac ganglion for pain due to abdominal malignancy including cancer of pancreas, stomach, liver, gall bladder, colon, etc. Celiac plexus block is successful in 70 percent to 85 percent of patients so treated.

Technique: Using CT monitoring or fluoroscopic control, after placement of the needle, 25 mg of absolute alcohol mixed with local anesthetic and contrast is injected. Bilateral needle placement has been reported to provide the best results. The major side effect of this procedure is transient hypotension.

Stellate ganglion block may sometimes be useful for pain in the face, upper neck, ear and the intracranial area. The complications with this technique limit the use.

OTHER PALLIATIVE MEASURES FOR TERMINAL CANCER

Nausea and Vomiting

This is a common and distressing symptom. The management of nausea may be maximized by round the clock dosing. The act of vomiting is controlled by the vomiting center, the respiratory, the vasomotor centers and the vagus innervation of the gastrointestinal tract (Table 53.2).

The 'vomiting center' may be stimulated by four different sources of afferent input.

1. Afferent vagal fibers and splanchnic fibers from gastrointestinal viscera stimulated by biliary or gastrointestinal distension, mucosal or peritoneal irritation.
2. Vestibular system stimulated by motion or infection. These fibers have high concentration of histamine, muscuranic (cholinergic) receptors.
3. Higher central nerve system center.

Table 53.2: Antiemetics

Drugs	Dose	Route
Antihistamine and Anticholinergics		
Scopolamine patch	1.5 mg every three days	Patch
Diphenhydramine	25-50 mg every 4-6 hours	PO, i.m.,i.v.
Promethazine	25 mg every 4-6 hours	PO. i.m.
Meclizine	25-50 mg every 24 hours	PO
Dopamine Anatgonists		
Metoclopramide	10-20 mg every 6 hours	PO
	0.5-2.0 mg per kg 6-8 hours	i.v.
Droperidol	1-2.5 mg every 4-6 hours	i.v.
Promethazine	25 mg 4-6 hours	PO, i.m.
Procloperzine	5-10 mg 4-6 hours	PO, i.m.
Serotonin 5-HT$_3$ antagonists		
Ondansterone	0.15 mg/kg 15 minutes before Chemotherapy Or 4-8 mg IV single dose 6 hourly	i.v.
Granisetrone	8 mg twice	PO
	Or 10 mcg/kg once	i.v.
Corticosteroids		
Dexamethasone	6-10 mg	Orally or i.v.

4. Chemoreceptor trigger zone (CTZ) located in the area of postrema of the medulla. This area may have chemoreceptors that may be stimulated by drugs, toxins, chemotherapeutic agents, hypoxia, uremia, acidosis and radiation therapy. This area is rich in serotonin 5-HT$_3$ and dopamine D$_2$ receptors.

Nasogastric suction may provide rapid relief for vomiting associated with gastroparesis or gastric outlet obstruction, but should only be used as a temporary measure in an acute emergency. Increased intracranial pressure may cause vomiting and may be relieved with high dose corticosteroids, or palliative cranial radiation. Cannabinoids, like Dronabinol 2.5-20 mg orally every 4-6 hours, have also been found to be helpful in the management of nausea and vomiting.

CONSTIPATION

This is one common problem in the care of terminal illness. The causes may be frequent use of opioids, poor dietary intake, and restricted physical activity. Constipation is an easily treatable cause of significant discomfort and distress. This may be prevented or relieved if patients can increase their intake of dietary fiber and fluids. Simple methods such as privacy, undisturbed toilet time, bedside commode, etc. may be important for some patients (Table 53.3).

Table 53.3: Pharmacological management of constipation

Drug	Dose
1. Stimulants:	
Bisacodyl	5-15 mg orally at bedtime or 10-20 mg rectally
Senna	5-15 mg orally at bedtime 3 times per day
2. Osmotic laxatives	
Lactulose	15-60 mg orally 1-3 times per day
Sorbitol	15-60 ml orally 1-3 times per day
Other interventions	
Glycerine suppositories	
Enemas of saline or tap water	
Digital disimpaction	

For a patient taking opioids, anticipation and prevention of constipation is important. A prophylactic bowel regimen of stool softener and stimulants (bisacodyl or senna) should be started when opioid treatment begins; lactulose, sorbitol, magnesium citrate and enema can be added as and when needed.

DELIRIUM AND AGITATION

Many patients of terminal illness due to cancer die in a state of delirium with disturbance of consciousness and change in cognition. This is manifested by illusion, hallucinations, disturbance of sleep cycle, psychomotor disturbance and mood disturbance. A few of these are reversible. Identification of such cases and correction of the underlining causes are important so that the appropriate drug and its dosage of psychoactive medication can be chosen. Careful attention to patient safety and non-pharmacological strategies may be useful to prevent minor delirium. Delirium at the last stage of life is distressing to patients and the family and requires treatment.

When the cause is not identified, it may be treated symptomatically with neuroleptics and benzodiazipines. Haloperidol 1-10 mg orally, s.c., i.m. or i.v. twice or thrice a day is used commonly. The problem with this drug is significant extrapyramidal adverse effects. Thiorodzine and disperidone may be helpful in delirium but they are available orally only. As an adjuvant to neuroleptics, benzodiazipines such as lorazepam 0.5-2 mg orally, sublingual, subcutaneous or i.v. 4-6 hrs. may be useful when anxiety is also associated with delirium.

When delirium is refractory to treatment and remains intolerable, sedation may be required, and midazolam 0.5-5 mg every hour s.c. or i.v. In certain cases, barbiturates can be used.

PARANEOPLASTIC SYNDROMES (SEE CHAPTER 10)

The term 'paraneoplasia' has been coined to denote the remote effects of malignancy that cannot be attributed either to direct invasion or metastatic lesions or may be the first sign of malignancy seen in 15 percent of patients. These may often be considered to be due to aberrant hormonal or metabolic effects not associated with malignant tissues.

The effects may be due to:
1. those initiated by tumor products (e.g. carcinoid syndrome) or due to destruction of normal tissue by tumor (e.g. hypercalcemia due to osteolytic metastasis).
2. unknown mechanisms, such as unidentified tumor products.

The most common cancer associated with paraneoplastic syndrome is small cell cancer of the lung.

PSYCHOSOCIAL AND SPIRITUAL CARE

Most people with advanced diseases are in need of social, emotional and very often, spiritual (religious or non-religious) support. Gently assessing how the patients feel about their disease and situation can shed light on their needs and distress. How the patient interprets his disease and its symptoms may be a cause of suffering in itself. Being able to take decisions in one's life is an important factor for maintaining dignity for most people. This will be possible only if the healthcare professional provides the patient and family with as much information as they want, in a way they can understand. This process takes time and issues often need to be discussed further and clarified as more information is imparted.

A fairly good number of patients want to know about their illness. Many patients who have been denied this knowledge have difficulty in understanding why they are deteriorating. Many of them show intense emotional distress characterized by irritability, anger, depression, etc.

Physicians are often caught up in a potential 'conspiracy of silence' situation with the family insisting on concealing the truth from the patient. The common argument is "Do not tell him the diagnosis or the prognosis because he would not be able to cope with it. We know him better than you do." This can be an awkward situation. The family needs to know that the physician has understood their concerns of not wanting to cause any more hurt to the patient. They also need to know that the doctor accepts that some patients use denial as a way of coping. But it would be unwise for the clinical staff to be untruthful if the patient wants to know the truth and was asking direct questions, because of the inevitable breakdown in trust that this could cause.

The patient in pain and physical discomfort very often finds life intolerable because of the agony afflicting both baby and mind. The inability to maintain one's integrity on the face of severe crisis leads to intense suffering encompassing the whole being. Incurable diseases can cause the disintegration of not just the body, but the whole being. The disintegration and ensuing suffering is the result of the patient's alienation from oneself and from the outside world. The distress resulting from this process is often called 'spiritual pain'.

Exploring the patient's insight and addressing the informational needs are part of the basics of psychosocial and spiritual support. The process invariably needs different skills and requires a lot of time. It is this need to see the patient as a whole and address problems of different nature and magnitude which makes palliative care the job for a team rather than an individual.

FURTHER READING

1. Foley KM. The treatment of cancer pain. N Eng J Med 1985; 313:84-95.
2. Koshy RC, Rhodes D, Devi S, et al. Cancer Pain Management in Developing Countries: A mosaic of Complex Issues resulting in Inadequate Analgesia. Supportive Care in Cancer 1998;6:430-37.
3. Pandey M, Krishnan Nair M, Paul Sebastian. Advances in Oncology (vol.1) Pain relief in cancer patients, Delhi: Jaypee Brothers 2000.
4. World Health Organization. Cancer Pain Relief. World Health Organization, Geneva, 1986.

The Care of the Cancer Patients

54

J Samuel

The care of the cancer patients during the period of investigations, surgery, radiotherapy and multiple courses of chemotherapy forms an important part of the learning process of medical students, physicians and nurses. Tending to the needs of such patients requires round the clock commitment, whether it be physical, emotional or spiritual. It is all the more important, when in a joint consultation of the oncologist and the radiotherapist, a decision has been taken to stop all curative treatment as it would serve no useful purpose. It is imperative at this stage to plan to make the final days of the patient as painless, comfortable and meaningful as far as possible.

The oncologists treating patients with cancer cannot be unmindful of the severe strain the patient undergoes daily in his life. It is a tremendous emotional impact on the person when he realizes that he has been stricken with cancer. During the early days of the disease, it is necessary that the patient is made aware of the existence of such a disease in his body and to assure him that with modern modalities of treatment, cancer can be cured or controlled. One must of course try to understand the personality of the patient, the strength of his mind, religious beliefs, and social resources and then decide to break the news. In Indian conditions, the family is informed first and the oncologist must prepare himself to inform the patient in a gentle and compassionate way. As soon as he or she comes to know about the diagnosis, a pall of gloom and helplessness will envelop the hapless individual. In spite of the fact that there are new modalities for early detection, better surgical procedures, modern chemotherapy and radiotherapy, to the Indian patient, the term 'cancer' implies severe suffering and inevitable, slow death. In the modern context, this is not true. By proper planning of the treatment protocol, many oncologists believe that cancer can be controlled in the same way as hypertension or rheumatoid arthritis. This is true in the western world and other developed countries in Asia but in the Indian subcontinent, the financial constraints of the patient and his family, limit the chemotherapy or radiotherapy schedule offered to him by the oncologist. Other diseases, even though they can cause death, do not evoke the same anxiety as cancer. 'The term cancer has a threatening and destroying connotation.' (William A. Greene). Cardiac, pulmonary, cerebral and renal diseases, even though life threatening, are thought of as old age-related diseases and the expected end in aging. In the case of serious trauma or battlefield injuries, the person either gets well with modern medical care or dies soon. These deaths too are tragic. The physician and the nurses must not fail to appreciate the common psychological stress and the anxiety experienced by the patient and his dear ones like his wife and children during every waking hour.

This understanding is crucial for the degree of comfort as the patient goes through the different treatment modalities such as surgery, chemotherapy and radiation. In most cases, the medical staff must learn to recognize the patient's own attitude to the disease and his attitude to life and death. A few of the patients face the pain and inevitable end as their fate and succumb to it with equanimity, while others become rebellious asking God why they are made to suffer in such a way. It has a lot to do with the social beliefs, social resources, religious affiliation, family support and financial status.

The second important group in this team in the care of the cancer patients comprises the nurses, specially trained in oncology services. Next to the oncologists, the role of the nurses is seminal. In fact during the primary acute form of treatment as in surgery, radiotherapy and chemotherapy, their services are invaluable. They are the most visible and consistent members of the team. In Western countries, with excellent home nurse services, the nurse is concerned not only with the care of the patient, but also with the prevention of cancer. She advises relatives of patients who have familial types of cancer to have early consultations and investigations. It must be understood that the nurses are speaking to healthy persons and care must be taken not to cause any undue anxiety to them. Special attention must be paid to the members of the family with a cluster of cancers. Wherever the regular home nursing services are not available the hospital nurse should find time during her busy schedule in the wards, to tell the close relatives about the possibility for inheritance of cancer. There are clusters of cancer families in India too, as Li-Fraumeni families or limited range cancers as in hereditary colon, stomach, breast and ovary. The nurse should also teach the women to examine the breast when abnormal mass or pain develops in that area. Regular classes must be conducted for women in primary health care centers, and they should be reminded to report to the doctor if there is any menstrual irregularity, bleeding between the periods, pain in the lower abdomen, etc. The language used in these discussions should be the local dialect. Difficulty in swallowing, vomiting, loss of appetite, change of voice, chronic cough with blood stained sputum, chronic ulcer in the mouth, change in the size of a skin mole, blood stained motion, etc. should also be reported to the doctor as they are the early symptoms of aerodigestive tract tumors, skin tumors, etc. The relatives should be warned against smoking cigarettes and bidis, chewing 'pan' or drinking spurious alcohol. The rationale of these discussions is to make the relatives aware of such conditions and attempt to meet the family physicians early if such symptoms develop in them.

The nurses actively participate during the intensive period of therapy. It is the nurse's role to help the patient to make independent decisions and thus accept the surgeon's plan for surgery and tolerate the painful aftermath of mutilating operations. She helps them to return to the optimum level of activities. She also must maintain proper intravenous medication, keep watch over the fluid and metabolic needs, proper care for any stoma in fecal diversion, and many such day to day needs. Gastrostomy is not usually done, but if there is a case with gastrostomy, the nurse should see that it does not slip out as reintroduction is painful and causes hemorrhage from the side of the stoma. The skin around the gastrostomy tube may get inflamed and ulcerated and must be carefully cleaned and protected with Zinc cream. If there is a tracheostomy, suction must be done through the inner tube with aseptic precautions. The inner tube is taken out and cleaned with sodium bicarbonate solution, boiled and put back once in 4 hours. If a portex-cuffed tube is used, the tube is deflated once in 2 hours for 3 minutes. In hot humid conditions, a wet gauze is kept over the tracheostomy tube. If this is not done regularly, the sputum can get attached to the side of the inner tube producing extensive crusting leading to stridor and respiratory distress.

Once the chemotherapy schedule is started, they have to be alert to the problem of nausea, vomiting, diarrhea and fever with chills, early signs of marrow depression and loss of hair. Women patients with beautiful long hair often feel devastated by the loss of the hair and even a trained counselor may find it difficult to console them.

Sometimes the chemotherapy schedule may last weeks and months. A few drugs have to be stopped suddenly due to life-threatening toxicity while others will be continued for years as they are found to suppress metastasis. The team consisting of the oncologist, nursing staff and family members work closely as the oncologists make important decisions and determine the different modalities of treatment. The family members share the patient's fear and anxiety with love and tenderness during the treatment, but the nurse's role is important. It complements the medical care. She cares for the physical needs of the patient such as, feeding, and dispensation of drugs. It must not be forgotten that the nurses are the visible part of the team who are available day and night in the service of the patient. They are also concerned with advising the family members to mobilize the resources and also suggest names of funding organizations which many offer financial aid.

The responsibilities of the oncology nurse increase during the post-therapy period. The nurse must help the patient to return to their normal life and to adapt to the changed body situations. The patients must be helped in such a way that they can live with an uncertain future. She can lessen the patient's burden by trying to get jobs for his wife or children through cancer societies.

A good number of patients take advice from a doctor dealing in alternative medicine. The oncologist is often weighed down by the ethical dilemma between respecting the competence or wisdom of the patient's choice and protecting a vulnerable individual from making a wrong choice. Why do so many people choose alternative therapy? There is no simple answer. Many current alternative cancer treatments are based on the principles of holistic medicine, and often allow patients to be more involved in their care than is typical of conventional cancer therapy. Some patients seek alternative cancer therapy because of the degree of support they obtain in the therapeutic alliance with their Ayurvedic physician who is more personal and kind. Others are probably looking for hope and optimism they do not find in the existing hospitals in the cities.

WHAT TO TELL THE PATIENTS?

There is no universally accepted policy on what to tell the patient and the relatives and when. The right to know is the fundamental right of man in a civilized society but care must be taken about the way in which the information is given. There is no place in medicine where proper communicative skills are so essential as in dealing with cancer patients. After a cystoscopic examination, it is not fair for the urologist to come out of the theater and tell the son that his father has carcinoma of the bladder. A wiser approach is to tell him that the things are not looking well and both the clinician and the son must wait for the histological confirmation. Once the clinician receives the histology report and his fears have come true, he has to share with the patient the gravity of the condition and the course of the disease and the different treatments that are offered. It is a continuous dialogue and the process of imparting information can be verbal and nonverbal. The way it is expressed should be tempered with compassion and understanding after planning in advance. A few of the patients may react in a strange way. It is reported that relatively unstable persons have even attempted to commit suicide the very night they were told they had cancer. The patients can be given truthful, practical, and specific information about the nature of the disease progression, associated problems, emotional ramifications and treatment options. A few would like to know about the type of treatment and whether the end would be painful. They may seek for approximation of time of death. It is almost impossible to forecast the time of death. Inaccurate and oblique information can leave the patient feeling bewildered and insecure and anxious about what to expect. Communication of such a serious nature frequently takes several interviews. The anxious patient must be given adequate time to integrate the information in a logical and correct sequence. Answers have to be repeated several times so that the patient is clear in his mind about the course of action to be taken by the oncologist. Honest disclosure is essential in dealing with the relatives of the patient suffering from cancer. A few patients learn to live their life, whatever that remains, courageously without being paralyzed by fear or anxiety. Some of them even though courageous, at times, break down and weep at their sad plight. A large number of them have difficulty in adjusting to the fatal disease that interferes with the movements, breathing, eating, defecation and micturition. The next most distressing aspect is the loss of secondary sexual organs like the genitals and breast. For example loss of the eyes or a limb with cancer, would tell upon their work. They will be worried the income they will have to forgo and eventually distressed about the family and his dear ones. Some of them are concerned about their looks. Once the disease starts spreading inside the patient's body, it becomes very evident with regard to his physique and looks. He starts losing weight considerably, loses the color and texture of the skin. The chemotherapy makes him irritable, and causes uncontrollable retching and vomiting. Most of the time, the chemotherapy is so distressing that the patient may refuse to go to the clinic for the following cycle. It is the duty of the oncologist and his dear ones to make him understand not to give up in the middle of the treatment. A gentle touch, a loving embrace, and a soothing word will go a long way in cheering him up. In fact, these patients should be treated as infants with care and concern during the anxious and difficult days. There may be sleepless nights, even two to three nights in a row, due to pain, discomfort or fear that the end may come at any moment. To many, it is a grueling experience. Somebody dear to him should sit with him, hold his hands and reassure him that the members of the family too share his anxiety. Some pleasant conversation about the happy occasion, which will bring happy memories of good old days, is quite desirable. It is noted that in the Indian practice of surgical oncology, a few of the patients refuse surgery due to the fear of postoperative pain, morbidity, mortality and mutilation. Occasionally this reaction may be due to his fear about what his friend or neighbor went through during surgery and his painful death. Colostomy, urinary diversion, jejunostomy and such stomal diversions are abhorrent to the Indian mind. "I don't want my motion coming through my skin" is the usual reaction of many. The problem is that once the patient is discharged, there is none to give them proper care even though his family may be more than willing to be of service. Even the patients willing for surgery may refuse radiation because of the long period of treatment and its indefiniteness in the cure. Almost all patients accept chemotherapy with a sense of relief.

The next aspect is the availability of economic resources. Unfortunately in a country like India, the resources are meager. There is neither any social security scheme nor universal medical insurance. The country cannot afford to look after their ill people due to serious financial constraints and most of them are pushed beyond the edge of penury.

The patient is anxious about his work and his family. One question many of them ask, is it infective? Will my son or daughter develop this cancer after some years?" Religious belief and help from a guru or a priest or a trained social worker will appreciably alleviate the patient's psychological distress. Most of them are concerned about their ability to earn a livelihood and keep the family from poverty and also bear the cost of the treatment. The cancer treatment is expensive and it is obvious that the lower income group can ill afford it. Many accept the pain and death associated with cancer as destined by God-something beyond the understanding of ordinary mortals.

FIVE RECOGNIZED PHASES IN A PERSON WITH CANCER

The adult cancer patients go through 5 recognized phases even though one merges with the other imperceptibly.

1. The phase of disbelief
2. The phase of anger and resentment
3. The phase of bargaining with God
4. The phase of acceptance
5. The phase of peaceful death

The first phase is the phase of disbelief. The diagnosis of cancer is a death-knell to the patient and he travels along the lonely road of pain and anxiety with muffled drums of death closely behind him. The news that a child in the family has developed acute leukemia will hit all the members in the family with a sense of helplessness and disbelief. They rush from place to place in search of a cure but in most cases it is only palliative. In a few cases of leukemia and lymphoma a 'cure' can be achieved, provided the patient is taken to a center where multidisciplinary treatment is available. So also in the case of a breadwinner in the family, stricken with cancer. The first phase, namely that of disbelief, is a natural phenomenon. One tends to convince oneself that cancer can develop in another person or a neighbor, but never really in 'me'. When the doctor, the wife or the children slowly break the news about his condition, it never registers in his mind. 'The medical tests may be wrong' is the first reaction and he wishes to see another doctor for a second opinion. In India, many seek the help of a doctor practicing indigenous medicine who may agree with the patient that there is no cancer within him. It is not unusual that valuable time is lost by the patient's state of disbelief. Once the pain and other symptoms of cancer get worse, he would realize that after all he too is a victim of the dreaded disease.

Once the realization takes over, the next is the phase of anger and resentment. "Why does it have to be me? What wrong have I done to deserve this punishment from God?" Thoughts about one's future life, new projects undertaken, about education of the children or the marriage of the daughter, bewilder him. The patient gets angry and irritable, loses his temper for the slightest and most trivial reasons. His anger is against the creator. He refuses to pray, refuses to visit the temple, mosque or church. He knows that his fight is futile against God. It is a difficult time for the dear ones, the doctor and the nurses when the patient also starts doubting about God's fairness in dealing with people. Innocent children die of leukemia or cerebral tumors. Is He a just God? As days go by, he reconciles himself to the fact that he too is a victim of cancer, probably due to reasons beyond his control. The oncologist, family members and nurses must understand that this is a passing phase and very soon the patient will accept the reality. It is also noticed that it is during this phase, one or two of the patients may attempt to commit suicide due to frustration, pain and anger. We must try to understand that this is a passing phase and sooner or later, the patient will come to terms with the situation.

The next phase is the attempt of the patient and relatives to bargain with God. The patient promises that he would lead a life without sin, stop imbibing alcohol and control his sexual transgression. He also decides to keep good relationship with his relatives and friends. He further promises to pay gifts to the temple, mosque or church, if God could heal his cancer. He plans to visit temples for atonement of his sins. He attempts to reduce Brahma or the Creator to the worldly level of a good bank manager. From this stage, he moves to the most difficult phase in his life, the stage of depression. He finds that cancer is destroying his body slowly while his cognitive powers are normal. There is no escape from the inevitable end. He sees the painful death in front of him. He realizes that neither God nor man can help him. The pain and other symptoms get intolerable. There is considerable change in his physical appearance namely loss of weight, loss of hair, particularly after chemotherapy. There is change in his skin color; it looks darker and husky. The patient feels depressed about the sins of commissions and omissions, unfulfilled dreams and hopes, and failures in life due to carelessness and negligence. It is at this stage that the nurses in the palliative care hospitals can offer words of compassion, tenderness and love. They must spend time with the patient, try to answer the questions with great care and kindness. The nurses must never try to introduce concepts of death and life after death which are not acceptable to the patient's own religion. Any attempt to bring in new religious ideas will only confuse the patient. The counseling team and the nursing staff must understand the beliefs in Hinduism, Islam and Christianity about death and the dying.

The next phase is the phase of acceptance. All the emotional battles have been fought and lost. His anger, disbelief and fear have exhausted him. The pain is almost continuous. He wants to escape from the agony of pain. He is waiting for the end in a calm and peaceful state of mind. This is the time, the nurses must speak of death as a great emancipator from life. A surgeon who had a massive gastric bleeding became unconscious and after a few minutes regained consciousness. His words were as follows, " I found myself by the side of a cool pool with still water, I was lying quietly on a grassy slope. There were trees nearby and I saw pink flowers like apple blossoms falling around me. All was so peaceful. In fact I have never experienced this kind of peace in all my life. But suddenly, I found my daughter walking across water, stretching her small hands and picking me up. I slowly got up. Suddenly I became conscious." The surgeon further adds " I was sorry, I came back to this wretched world of envy, petty quarrels and endless struggle."

In a strange way, it is a case of giving up in a positive manner. In 'Charaka Samhitha', the author distinguishes between two types of death, namely the timely death and the untimely death. Death that takes place before the normal span of life belongs to the untimely type of death and death from cancer is an example of untimely death. In case the disease is incurable, the physician must give the patient proper guidance and direct his mind to the other world. Charaka further instructs the physician to advise the patient regarding prayers and worship so as to develop calmness of mind. In chapter 56, the concept of death and life after death that is accepted in four great religions in India namely Buddhism, Hinduism, Islam and Christianity shall be discussed.

FURTHER READING

1. Barber JM, Booth DM, King JA, Chakraverty S. A nurse led peripherally inserted central catheter line insertion service is effective with radiological support. Clin Radiol 2002;57(5):352-54.
2. Bird C. Supporting patients with fungating breast wounds. Prof Nurse 2000;15(10):649-52.
3. Boyle DA, Schulmeister L, Lajeunesse JD, Anderson RW. Medication misadventure in cancer care. Semin Oncol Nurs 2002;18(2):109-20.
4. Chelf JH, Deshler AM, Thiemann KM, Dose AM, Quella SK. Learning and support preferences of adult patients with cancer at a comprehensive cancer center. Oncol Nurs Forum 2002;29(5):863-67.
5. Edwards M, Miller C. Improving psychosocial assessment in oncology. Prof Nurse 2001;16(7):1223-26.
6. Faull C, Hirsch C. Symptom management in palliative care. Prof Nurse 2000;16(1):840-43.

7. Fletcher K, Painter V. Building a dream: creating an oncology day/evening hospital. Can J Nurs Leadersh 2002;15(2):10-13.

8. Given B, Given CW, McCorkle R, Kozachik S, Cimprich B. Pain and fatigue management: Results of a nursing randomized clinical trial. Oncol Nurs Forum 2002;29(6):949-56.

9. Higginson IJ, Wilkinson S. Nurses: enabling patients with cancer to die at home. Br J Community Nurs 2002;7(5):240-44.

10. Levenson D. Advanced practice nurses lengthen survival of elderly cancer patients. Rep Med Guide Outcomes Res 2001;12(5):5-7.

11. Murphy A, Holcombe C. Effects of early discharge following breast surgery. Prof Nurse 2001;16(5):1087-90.

12. Ohizumi Y, Tamai Y, Imamiya S, Akiba T. Complications following re-irradiation for head and neck cancer. Am J Otolaryngol 2002;23(4):215-21.

13. Porock D, Nikoletti S, Kristjanson L. Management of radiation skin reactions: literature review and clinical application. Plast Surg Nurs 1999Winter;19(4):185-92, 223; quiz 191-92.

14. Rawl SM, Given BA, Given CW, Champion VL, Kozachik SL, Intervention to improve psychological functioning for newly diagnosed patients with cancer. Oncol Nurs Forum 2002;16.

15. Scherbring M. Effect of caregiver perception of preparedness on burden in an oncology population. Oncol Nurs Forum 2002;29(6):E70-76.

16. Shannon-Dorcy K. Nursing implications of mylotarg: A novel antibody-targeted chemotherapy for CD33+ acute myeloid leukemia in first relapse. Oncol Nurs Forum 2002;29(4):E52-59.

17. Swenson CJ. Ethical issues in pain management. Semin Oncol Nurs 2002;18(2):135-42.

18. Thain C, Wyatt D. A review of a multiprofessional cancer course. Eur J Cancer Care (Engl) 2002;11(2):82-90.

The Nursing Care of Cancer Patients

55

M Thomas

NURSING CARE—GENERAL PRINCIPLES

As mentioned earlier, the most visible member of the oncology team is the nurse and she must be familiar with the different problems that face the patient. The prime duty is to provide physical and psychological comfort and a sense of hope. The nurse must be careful not to cause undue worry to the patient and relatives. It is her duty to protect the patient from complications such as pre- and postoperative hazards, drug allergy and problems that occur as the treatment progresses. The nurse should teach the patient and the relatives skills like the care of the colostomy, catheter drainage, tracheostomy tube and nasogastric feeding. This is undertaken to give the patient reasonable independence. These objectives are achieved by spending time with the patient and relatives and teaching them each technique with care and clarifying their doubts and fears. The patient must also be given an idea about general healthcare and the availability of drugs and equipment like catheters and colostomy bags from stoma care centers in India. All through the days spent in hospital, the patient must be given the opportunity for developing a close human relationship with the nursing staff. He must be made to accept that the nurses' suggestions are helpful and can be trusted. In this ambience of trust and goodwill, the patient can take correct decisions regarding the treatment. The feeling of loneliness, anger and frustration can also be reduced as days go by.

INVESTIGATIONS BEFORE SURGERY

In the modern era, it is understood that a battery of investigations is made to arrive at a correct diagnosis. Some of them are simple and some others difficult and risky. The nurse must see that the investigations are done at the proper time and the results collected. Certain tests are done in the morning on empty stomach and it is the duty of the nurse to be explicit in describing the time and the duration of the test. Ultrasound of abdomen is done on an empty stomach while that of pelvis is done with full bladder. CT scans are also done on empty stomach. In case, an endoscopy biopsy is carried out, there must be a close watch over the patient. It has been mentioned that duodenal perforation has taken place after an upper abdominal endoscopy and similarly colonic perforation after a total colonoscopy. In case of fine-needle aspiration, hematoma can develop at the site of aspiration and in CT guided biopsy, intra-abdominal bleeding can occur. After every procedure, either major or minor, the nurse has a duty to check the pulse, respiration, and blood pressure and the general condition of the patient. If she feels that something amiss has occurred, no time should be lost in informing the doctor on duty.

THE NURSE IN THE SURGICAL WARD

It is universally known that most of the patients are worried about surgery and its aftermath. They are anxious about the change in the appearance after head and neck surgery, particularly excision of the mandible and maxilla. Women undergo severe emotional trauma after simple or radical mastectomy. Amputation of the penis in carcinoma of the penis can be a devastating experience in young men. The patient has to be helped to work through the grief of amputation of the limbs in cases of osteosarcoma and such long bone tumors. It is the duty of the nurse to give adequate comfort and sympathy the previous night so that he can be courageous as he is moved to the operation theater. The patient should be apprised of pain in the postoperative period and must be assured that analgesics will be given during the postoperative period to relieve him of pain.

RADIATION THERAPY

Radiation therapy too can cause a lot of problems to the patient, particularly if the skin care is neglected. Serious and troublesome radiation dermatitis can develop. The nurse should help the patient to deal with anorexia, nausea, vomiting or diarrhea by drugs, diet management and diversional therapy. The ward nurse should accompany the sick patient to the radiation room and should be available by the side of the bed when he returns after radiation.

CHEMOTHERAPY

The last 5 decades of the 20th century have seen a rapid progress in the use of drugs in the treatment of cancer and considerable research has taken place in many centers of the world. Most of the new drugs are available in Indian markets also. Unlike antimicrobial agents which inhibit the growth of microbes without causing damage to the normal human cells, anticancer drugs cause damage to both the cancer cells and the normal human cells as there is not much difference between the metabolic pattern of tumor cell and normal cell. The nurses should know the role of the common groups of drugs namely plant alkaloid, alkylating agents, antimetabolites and antibiotics. She must also note that these drugs have inherent cytotoxic action on normal, rapidly dividing cells. Nausea, vomiting, loss of appetite, diarrhea, alopecia and marrow depression are the common effects of these drugs. It is not unusual that the patients suffer from very distressing nausea and vomiting and may refuse further chemotherapy cycles. It is the nurse's duty to enthuse the patient to continue the therapy for the control of the tumor. Oral ulcers and pruritus are also troublesome and the patient is taught to keep the mouth clean and the skin around the anus, foreskin and the groins clean. She must teach the patient plans to maintain nutrition by taking smaller feeds at regular intervals in times of distressing anorexia.

SPECIFIC NURSING CARE IN CANCER IN DIFFERENT SYSTEMS

Alimentary Tract Cancer —Tumors of Colon and Rectum

Colorectal tumors are on the increase and in case, the investigations have proved that the patient is carrying a malignant colonic tumor, surgery may be contemplated. In a large number of cases, colorectal or colo-anal anastomosis with staplers is done avoiding colostomy. But in a few cases, colostomy is done when distal rectum and anus are removed, to protect a distal colocolic anastomosis, as an outlet for obstructed distal colon and to divert the fecal material from a distal segment with inflammatory colonic lesion. If colostomy is necessary, the nurse must reinforce the physician's explanations and help the patient toward a realistic view of his situation. Naturally, the patient resists colostomy but in certain cases, colostomy is essential to maintain life. The surgeon may choose the left iliac fossa or the upper epigastrium for colostomy. The care of the colostomy is a burden to the patient and the nursing staff. It would be advisable to introduce such a patient to another person who has made correct adjustment with colostomy. That individual must be willing to answer specific questions and doubts of the patient. The nurse should show a colostomy bag with the straps and allow the patient to put it on the abdominal wall where it fits well, so that the surgeon could plan the site of colostomy.

In the early postoperative period the colostomy will not function well. It would take 3 to 5 days for the optimum drainage through the colostomy and by a week's time, the colostomy bag must be fitted. There are 2 types of colostomy bags available in India, the disposable one made of plastic and the non-disposable one made of rubber. The patient can choose what is suitable in his home and the work area. Do not forget that the straps of the colostomy bag are fitted around an abdominal wall, which is sore, by recent surgery. The nurses must be vigilant to detect the complication of colostomy like bleeding from the edges of the wound, prolapse of the mucosa or even the whole thickness of colon and internal strangulation, which will express itself as intestinal obstruction. Stricture can occur at the stoma after a few weeks. It is the duty of the staff to help the patient with colostomy to return to independence and back home. An intelligent person can look after the colostomy reasonably well. Younger persons can go back to their place of work. In India, many colostomy patients find it difficult to have gainful employment mostly due to the lack of confidence and fear of social ostracization. Health workers must encourage them to go out and try to do some form of job. There are inherent problems in different sites of colostomy. The cecostomy or transverse colostomy can rarely be regulated easily due to the fluid state of the feces. Even with a well fitting colostomy bag, with karya gum seal, the feces can be seen soiling the skin and the clothes. One major problem the patient faces is the selection of food. Certain foods have a laxative effect. Diarrhea can be troublesome and the patient must learn to deal with this problem by restricting the diet. He also must be taught about proper skin care and the correct use of appliances. The patient would soon identify those foodstuffs, which produce loose motion and learns to avoid them. In case of constipation, particularly in sigmoid colostomy, the problem can most often be controlled by irrigation that is begun when bowel activity is reestablished.

POSTOPERATIVE CARE

During the postoperative period, every effort is taken to make the patient comfortable. The patient should be taught the ways to manage colostomy. It is necessary to establish a regular bowel evacuation pattern. The best way to achieve this is by colonic irrigation of 300 to 500 cc of warm water introduced into the stoma using enema tubing and a large syringe. The irrigation can be done once in 3 days. If there is troublesome diarrhea, the diet pattern should be adjusted so that the patient avoids food with laxative effect. In India food like wheat products such as chapathis, gruel and ragi have a tendency to bind the bowel. Bananas and certain vegetables are non-laxative in nature and can be used. Disposable colostomy bag with karya gum skin paste is used once the patient returns home. There are stoma societies in India in different cities and the nurse should introduce them to these societies. The enemas and later even the colostomy bag can be omitted once control is achieved. A dressing can be used over the stoma as he goes to his workplace. It must be understood that there can be problems which the patient has to face, such as diarrhea, constipation, fecal leakage, odor, skin irritation, narrowing of stoma and delayed healing of perineum.

LUNG CANCER

It is the duty of all health workers and nurses to prevent carcinoma of the lung by exhorting all those who come in contact with them to stop this pernicious habit of smoking. In the early postoperative period, the patient experiences pain and discomfort while breathing. He would require regular pulmonary toilet and oxygen support. A well-trained physiotherapist must take the responsibility of teaching the postoperative chest movement. During radiation therapy, adequate nutrition is necessary and care must also be taken to avoid radiation necrosis of the chest wall, trachea and esophagus. After discharge from the hospital, the physiotherapist should teach shoulder exercises and posture. Help is necessary to modify the regimen of rest and work as needed. Extra care must be taken by the patient to protect him from respiratory infections.

FEMALE GENITAL TRACT MALIGNANCIES

The health workers should take time to teach women, particularly those from villages, wholesome personal hygiene. Pap smears yearly or every other year after the age of 40 is an accepted way to detect early cancer of the cervix. As the cancer progresses, the nursing staff have an added responsibility as they have to deal with ascites, leg edema, anorexia, insomnia, malaise, constipation, pain, depression and vaginal hemorrhage. A few of the patients may undergo extensive resection in tumor debunking and may end with colostomy and ileal bladder. The patient must be taught to handle these stomas with bags and other appliances. One difficult problem the nurses have to deal with is the vesicovaginal fistula developed as a consequence of cervical tumor. The tumor can infiltrate into the posterior surface of the bladder and later develop necrosis producing a vesical fistula. Catheter drainage has to be instituted and the vagina is kept as much dry as possible with dry sterile pad. Excoriation of the introitus must be prevented by regular changing of pads.

GENITOURINARY CANCER

The general population should be advised that both in the occurrence of macroscopic and microscopic hematuria, the patient must immediately seek medical advice. It is not uncommon for a malignant mass in the kidney or bladder to bleed once and then bleed only after several weeks. Any symptoms of urinary obstruction should be referred to a urologist for investigation for bladder, prostate or bladder neck, and malignant tumors. In total bladder resection, the nursing staff should be alert in early detection of rectal injury, abdominal distension due to ileus, weakness of the lower limbs due to neuropraxia of the perineal nerves and superficial wound injury.

Management of ileal bladder or sigma rectal bladder has the inherent problem with frequency and dysuria. In the west most of the total bladder resections have continent diversion of urine with less psychological trauma to the patient.

SKIN CANCER

The ideal way to prevent skin cancers is to protect skin from prolonged irritation - sunrays, ultraviolet or ionizing rays, and from chemical irritants. Changes in the size and color of moles and satellite moles near the original moles require scrutiny. Persistent sores can turn malignant in the course of years.

HEAD AND NECK CANCERS

Every oral lesion such as ulcer, the mucosal trauma with ragged teeth, change in the color and texture of the oral mucosa, etc. should be examined and referred to a surgical oncologist. Irritable, unproductive cough and hoarseness may be the first symptom of cancer of the pharynx, hypopharynx and larynx.

The following preoperative care is necessary for a smooth postoperative period. Preoperative care includes:
1. With the heavy smoker, a program to improve pulmonary function.
2. With the alcoholic, a program to improve nutrition.
3. Devising a means of postoperative communication.
4. Teaching the patient the skills he will need postoperatively.
5. Plan for teaching speech therapy with the team, if laryngectomy is done.
6. Postoperative care.

In case of oral surgery when mandible is resected there is obvious facial deformity. The nursing staff should help him to tide over the psychological crisis of deformity. There may be drooling of saliva along the corner of the mouth. There is malocclusion of the jaws making normal bite impossible. A few may find it difficult to drink fluids and they must be encouraged to use straw for drinking. In case there is partial or total glossectomy, the patient should have pencil and paper available for communication and no i.v. drip is planned in the writing arm. A bell is useful to get the help of the nursing staff. Tracheostomy, if present, needs special care. The whole appliance can slip off unless it is firmly tied across the neck. The inner tube should be taken out and cleaned and boiled in sodium bicarbonate solution once in 6 hours to prevent encrustation of dried mucus within the tube. The tracheostomy wound can get bigger and mucus may escape through the wound soiling the shirt and the skin at the suprasternal notch. After laryngectomy, the speech therapist should plan for early speech therapy. In some countries, electrolarynx is used if esophageal speech is impossible.

BREAST CANCER

It is found that at least 5 percent of breast tumors occur in closely related individuals, like mother and daughter, among sisters or nieces. Hence the nurse should teach all women particularly, those in this susceptible group to do self-examination of the breast.

The nurses in the oncology services should listen with compassion, to the patient's expressions of fear, anger and grief over the loss of her breast. She may not be able to express these feelings to the physician.

Care after mastectomy:

a. Avoid injections in the arm on the operative side.
b. Set up an exercise regimen to maintain full range of motion in the shoulder.
c. Help the patient to deal with depression by interpreting her grief as a normal, self-limiting response to the loss of an important organ which gives the correct profile to the human body.

CONVALESCENCE AND REHABILITATION

Different types of breast prostheses must be shown to the patient. Encourage her to accept breast reconstruction. The patient must be informed where to purchase one and how to care for it. The patient should be advised to be responsive to the prescribed drug regimen.

Care of the skin at the area of surgery is the duty of the nurse. Firm bandaging with crepe bandage can reduce the unpleasant swelling of the arm.

LEUKEMIA

The last 3 decades have seen a rapid increase in the number of acute lymphoblastic leukemia in school-going children and adolescents and acute myeloid leukemia in married men and women and older people.

When the patient is a child, the social worker should help the family maintain reasonable protection from infection, normal activity, and adequate intake of nutritious food.

1. Accept anger and rebellion from the patient. The family set reasonable limits to its expression.
2. See that the children with alopecia have wigs or caps.
3. Pre-schooler
   a. Explain procedures done at the time and proceed firmly.
   b. Help mothers devise ways of increasing the child's food consumption.
4. School age child
   a. Encourage participation in all reasonable activities in the school.
   b. Organize a support group for the child in the family.

5. Adolescent
   a. Allow discussion of feelings and fears.
   b. Help the child adhere to the medication regimen and accept necessary physical limitations.
6. Young adult
   a. Reinforce establishment of reasonable goals.
   b. Recognize own limitations in counseling.
7. Older person with chronic leukemia
   a. Help modify daily routine.
   b. Teach reasonable protection against infection.
   c. Allay unreasonable fear.

FURTHER READING (SEE PAGE 649-650)

The Journey's End 56

J Samuel

THE JOURNEY'S END

Finally the journey's end has been reached. All the therapeutic regimens have been attempted and the patient is in the terminal stage of malignancy. In India, in the principal cities, there are hospices to look after these types of patients. The oncologist and nursing staff are fully aware that in these hospitals, the patients are admitted when the last stage of malignancy has reached and when further treatment is of no help. The patient is kept free of pain till his death. In most cases, he accepts the finality of illness. Very soon he realizes that he has only a few weeks left before death. These hospices are usually little away from the main city limits and there is no hustle seen as in acute cancer wards. The oncologists visit their patients once in a week but general practitioners and the nursing staff undertake the actual care of the patient in these centers. The terminal care is an extension to active therapeutic regimen and the nursing staff is alert to the needs of the patient in terms of control of pain. Drugs to relieve pain particularly analgesics including different types of NSAIDs, morphine, etc. are used regularly to relieve pain. Morphine is used either in oral or injectable forms: the former is more widely used (In India, special permission from the Drug Controller is necessary to get morphine or pethidine to prevent its misuse). Certain hospices use the treatment schedule known as pethidine on demand. In this form the patient is allowed to take intravenous pethidine as and when he chooses. Self-loaded syringe with 50 mg of pethidine is available and after each use, the empty syringe is discarded and the nurse keeps a new loaded syringe with the drug. In the present context of medical care in India, a large number of patients seek help from an alternative therapy mainly Ayurvedic form of treatment before entering a hospice or a palliative care center. It is believed by most Indians that the Ayurvedic system has the special blessing of God and it is far less expensive. A prevalent concept is that the gods have transferred to humans, especially those who have spent long years in prayer, the precise treatment of different maladies including cancer.

Communication with a dying patient is a difficult but ongoing process. New problems can arise in the terminal stage of cancer. New questions and concerns will arise over a period of time. What is the end like? Where I am going after death? Is there a life after death? etc. These are the questions, which the palliative care personnel have to answer. Theological fantasies may not be of any use to the patients unless it carries with it sound logical explanations. Only the intelligent among them will ask these questions and they want intelligent answers. We have attempted to give the perceptions of the theologians in the prominent religions in India, on these questions in the later part of this chapter. In the present Indian ambience the family members take an active part in bringing solace and comfort to the patient. Dear ones find time to be at the side of the patient consoling him, feeding him and they never make him feel lonely while some others are consoled spiritually by the philosophy of 'Karma'. It is a well known fact that the patients differ in their levels of endurance. Some of them tolerate pain and even welcome pain as retribution for the mistakes they have committed, most of them being imaginary. They can accommodate themselves to the variations in the degree of pain and weakness often associated with cancer. A gentle touch, a loving embrace, and a soothing word will go a long way in cheering him up. In fact, these patients should be treated as infants with care and concern during the anxious and difficult days. There may be sleepless nights, may be two to three nights in a row and it may be due to pain, discomfort or fear that the end may come at any moment. To many it is a grueling experience. There is no harm in giving these patients hypnotic drugs so that they have good night rest. Somebody dear to him should sit with him, hold his hands and reassure him that they all love him and care for him. As the disease progresses, he slips into a state of unconsciousness and later stupor and slowly sinks into death and eternal peace.

CONCEPT OF HOPE IN A DYING PATIENT IN DIFFERENT FAITHS IN INDIA

In the following pages, there is an attempt to highlight the thoughts of death and dying that are prevalent in the major religions in India namely Buddhism, Christianity, Hinduism and Islam.

The authors make no claim that it is the universally accepted theological ideas in different religions but these interpretations about death and dying are not far from the known concepts in each religion.

"The clear light, ground luminosity manifest at the time of death."
— *Sogyal Rinpoche*
Death and dying: The Buddhist approach
R.Chogyal, The Hermitage, Delhi

Buddhism is practiced in many countries in the world especially in Asia. There are several million followers of this faith in India and the neighboring countries. This reformist faith has its origin from the teaching and life of Gautama Buddha born in 540 BC in Bihar in the northern part of India. It is a religion of nonviolence, penance, self-control of emotions and total renunciation from all the pleasures of flesh. It is a faith of deep compassion and continuous search by the mind for enlightenment. The cause of both physical and mental pain in the world, according to Buddha, is the human craving for power, wealth and satisfaction of his lust. He taught his disciples that renunciation of material wealth and carnal pleasures is essential for the peace and well being of a person. Lord Buddha's main attempt was to guide his followers to the path of peace and nonviolence so that their life will be free of pain. He constantly reminded his followers that the cause of maladies in the universe is man's selfishness and his continuous struggle for wealth and physical power. To him, the destruction of nature in any form adds to the sum total of human misery. He wanted mankind to think of nature as his mother and constantly advised men to love all the creatures of nature as his or her brothers and sisters.

In Buddhism, there is some clear conception about death. It maintains that death is the beginning of another life. It has a similarity to Hindu thoughts. Buddhists too believe that in case, the mind cannot attain the state of final enlightenment, the person is reborn to begin the sequence of one more cycle of reincarnation. According to Buddhist scholars, the Mind and God are one and each human being a part of the infinite God in the finite form of Mind. All Buddhists during their lifetime train themselves in death meditation, read poems written by sages to inspire them in this meditation. They study about the occult materials which prophesy the untimely death and practice Yoga and self renunciation that would save them from the advent of untimely death. The Buddhist writers speak about the time between life and death and they call it 'Bardo' (interval). Immediately after death, according to Buddhist scholars, there are 3 Bardos: 1) the painful death Bardo, 2) the luminous Bardo of Dharma, 3) the Karmic Bardo of attaining final enlightenment. In fact the three Bardos express themselves after clinical death, a thought which can be accepted by modern men only with skepticism.

After clinical death, the soul retains consciousness in another form. The liberation can only take place if the soul is fully aware of the magnificent revelation of the cosmic power. In case, the mind has not attained the final revelation, the person is reborn to begin the sequence of life again.

Lastly, the Buddhist thoughts reinforce the Hindu concept that the permanence of the external world is inevitably joined to the permanence of the internal world and hence harmony with the external world is necessary to the development of the internal world. The concept of hell is absent in Buddhism as the soul which is a part of the Infinite cannot be tortured in hell. Budhists believe that by repeated cycles of lives, the soul gets purified. In Buddhism, the man is reborn as another man and he is given yet another chance to absolve himself of his previous misdeeds in life while in Hinduism, he may not be given the human form. Buddhism teaches about the immortality of the soul, as the mind of man, which is part of cosmic power, is immortal and there is life after the physical death. This gives hope to the people dying of cancer but never gives a plausible answer for the cause of pain. In fact, no religion attempts to offer an answer to the question, Why am I chosen to suffer this agonizing pain of cancer.

The Hindu perspective of death

"Both you and I have passed through many births
You know them not, I know it all."

— *Bhagavath Gita*

Lord Yama, "You will have all the riches of the world; soldiers, elephants and
horses; mighty countries to rule; do not ask me the secret of death."

Nachiketa, " I know all these are temporal, what is eternal is immortality."

Lord Yama, " You have been born from the elements of nature and to the very
elements you will return."

— *Kathopanishad*

We are conscious that it is almost impossible to expound the magnificent perceptions of physical pain, suffering and death propounded by the great Indian sages for the last 5000 years in a few pages. There are constraints of space in this chapter on death and dying. The readers are requested to kindly bear with us in this short discussion.

Every mortal goes through the cycle of pain, suffering and death in life as destined by God. There is only difference of degree in suffering. The pain a person suffers, to some philosophers is an illusion, as time is also an illusion. The philosophical conception of time is a mere appearance, so too pain and suffering. It is only a grand delusion that there is physical pain. The term 'Maya' is very frequently used in explaining what is happening around us. The physical sense of happiness, joy, pain and death is unreal and it is only a delusion of the finite mind like a dream as the whole universe is an illusion. There is nothing real, nothing permanent except the creator. All the rest are an unreal sensory perception of the external finite world. Another explanation of physical pain is the attempt by God to make human beings more pure in life as the goldsmith melts gold to increase its purity. God tests the power of Dharma in man and measures his depth of faith as he travels along the hard road of suffering. In the case of those who trust the creator and do not move away from the path of Dharma and accept all that happens to them as God's will, their souls get purified. This absolute trust in God can break the cycle of life and death, supersede merit and sin and lead to salvation in the Absolute. Still there is a third explanation of pain. Men who have strayed into a world of Adharma and strayed away from the spiritual perceptions of Dharma will suffer the agonies of pain as part of Karma. God has given each mortal freedom of action either good or bad and the absolute does not interfere in this freedom. In Hinduism however the idea of death and what follows are somewhat more complex and subtle. Hindus believe that all of us are finite forms of an infinite consciousness, a greater reality. Where Christianity preaches that man is a body that possesses a soul, Hindus believe that man is a soul contained within a human body. Ancient religions in Egypt, Babylon and Asia Minor and Persia believed that the soul has no separate existence without the body and probably that was the reason, why the kings and queens of Egypt were kept as mummies. It was the philosophers among Aryans in India who postulated the theory that the soul is independent of the physical body and this soul can neither be created nor destroyed and is part of the cosmic power. Another fascinating thought the Hindu thinkers postulated was, the soul is immortal; there is a state of preexistence of the soul. It means that the soul, which has left one mortal form on earth, enters the body of a newborn completing one cycle. To a Hindu, death denotes the instance in space and time when the soul leaves the body that housed it. What happens after death is determined by the life that preceded it and the law of cause and effect is deemed to be cyclical which is never ending. Hindus believe that every action has a resultant effect and that every effect produces yet another reaction. More importantly, it is believed that a soul's future is determined by the manner of its earthly conduct or Karma, as it is known. If the soul has led a pure and pious life in its mortal form, it is said to have attained the highest state of consciousness, and upon death merges with the infinite consciousness. Otherwise it is reborn again in animal or human form, and given a chance to redeem itself. This process of rebirth and renewal is cyclical, until the soul has attained the highest form of consciousness and ultimately joins the cosmic power. The notion of an eternal soul coupled with the powerful concept of reincarnation reduces physical death to nothing more than a stepping stone to a long journey in which the soul takes on many guises until it reaches a state of enlightenment. From a practical counseling point of view, the Hindu philosophy on life and death could be used to assuage the fears of those facing imminent death as it promises rebirth and accommodates the irrepressible human need to remain immortal.

Finally, it is the universal truth that God or Brahma is pure spirit and the universe and matter are entirely dependent on Him. They exit with the will of God. He can manipulate the lives of the mortals and systems within the universe the way he pleases and likes. That is how the creation, preservation and dissolution occur in the materialist world. The souls are also spiritual in the original nature and they are encased in the subtle material bodies. This togetherness is seen from the beginning of time and cannot be said to have ceased. The souls with their earthly finite bodies go on transmigrating into gross bodies until they discover the true spiritual bodies. The relation between God and soul is mere reflection. God is Bimba (archetype) and soul is Prathibimba (prototype). The reflection is similar to its entity entirely reflected and souls are dependent on the Infinite. In short God and soul are spiritual in their nature. Souls are akin to God and the very essence of life lies in closeness to Brahma, the creator. The Absolute is the creator and the other is His creation and at the same time a part of the creator. As the creator is immortal, the part in the mortal man is also immortal.

CHRISTIAN PERSPECTIVES ON CARING FOR THE TERMINALLY SICK

Dr. Alex Mathew, PhD (Psych)

That death is real and it is only a moment away at any given time is hard to concede. There is hardly any preparation for the leaving. Here we want to look at ways in which we may lend strength and serenity to the dying. Where death is imminent, getting the dying person to pass on in poise, peace and hope is the onus of the living.

Often we are struck, not knowing what to say to the dying and what to do. Not because we do not care, but more because we are confused. This again is because we have very little understanding of death. We see death as the end of life. Therefore we have precious little to offer to the departing.

The Christian understanding of death, offers a distinct awareness of it as a splendid continuation of life into eternity. Persons getting prepared to care for the dying need to know and believe this fact besides other details of the mission at hand. Otherwise one may be facing a pointed question, 'Who is it that darkens counsel?'S'(Bible,Old Testament, Job 38:2).

There are three significant areas that the caregiver should be scrupulously informed of:(one) death itself, (two) the dying person and (three) his own duty.

Understanding Death and Continuation of Life

That death is part of life is undisputed. Life entails death. To understand death life itself needs to be understood more clearly. Among the patients dying of cancer, there are Christians too. From the childhood they were taught to believe in the fatherhood of God the creator and the brotherhood of men. Most of them believe that, Christ is the son of God and He is LIFE, authenticated by the unequivocal statement that, "am the resurrection and life".

Another cardinal thought in Christian philosophy is, " God so loved the world, He gave His only begotten son, so that whoever believeth in him shall not perish but have an eternal life."

To enjoy the quality of life, we must virtually put to death the past, and live in complete harmony with God's children and God's creations. There is a new life in this new identity. There is continuation of life beyond physical death in that identification with God's immortality. For a Christian approaching death, this offers great comfort and assurance. Are we going behind a screen, the screen of death?

It may need a little more explanation. God's time is not bound by the human concept of time and space. It is the same yesterday, today and tomorrow, which means it is eternal. When we understand this truth, we realize that death at any time in a human is part of an eternal process in the eyes of our Creator.

Another aspect we must learn to understand is the eternal love of God to mankind. A German philosopher standing by the death bed of his son told his wife in agony, " Nothing takes place in the universe without the knowledge of God and you must believe that the loving God knows what is happening to our son."

All this points to the fact that clinical death is just a point of change in life, never an end. It is only a passing on to a different realm of existence from mortality to immortality. The dear ones could rejoice in this change, in the mode of existence, from the physical to the heavenly life.

The Dying Person

The mental and spiritual conditions of the terminally sick and dying person are only imaginable. Let us take a look at some of the very obvious reactions, it produces in them.

The large looming question of "why?" generates a mixture of rebellion and self-pity. "There is no justification whatsoever for this sickness, especially at this point in my life." "Why me and why now?" Every sick person has the right to ask that question, but the truth is, there is no answer to any "why" in life. 'Why' is God's prerogative. God is kind, loving and merciful. It is the duty of the counselor to generate this faith in everyone, especially those nearing the end. Self-pity is worse than the physical ravages of the sickness itself. Logical and rationalized explanations does not serve any purpose in offering solace. Trust in a loving God who suffers along with the dying person, must come to the person as an irrefutable fact of life. The helper must have the mystical experience of this important fact.

The Helper

The terminally sick person looks for acceptance in a tangible form. From the face and body movements of the helper, the sick person gets messages either of love and acceptance or intolerance and rejection. The helper must never divulge irritation, distaste or annoyance at the person or the task at hand, which may be unpleasnt at times. At this point, the suffering person looks for tangible evidence of acceptance through physical touch. Therefore do not restrict touch to the minimum required for physical help procedures. An act of loving, reaching out and maintaining a soothing physical contact is of great importance in most instances. A tender pat, a caring rub or holding hands can be immensely reassuring.

The helping here is an act of love with the helper constrained by the love of God, reaching out to comfort those who are in pain, doubt, rebellion, suffering and self-pity.

The prerequisite here is that the helper must be a person experiencing the comfort from God so that he/she in turn can comfort all others who are in need of it. He brings in no other private agenda of personal gains into the ministry of comforting. One cardinal point for the helper to remember is the fact that he represents God and His comfort to the dying person, as he ministers to the needs of this hapless sufferer. This is an awesome responsibility and a unique privilege of a God-fearing Christian.

Without going into unnecessary details, some desirable qualities of a helper are listed below.

He should be:

1. a person who is familiar with gross pain and who can recognize the varying hue of suffering: a person with empathy or a fellow feeling for others in suffering.
2. one who is delicately sensitive to the pain and who can discern even the unexpressed needs of the person in suffering.
3. one who would respect the personality of the sufferer, offering only validation through every act of service.
4. a person able to keep confidence and help to maintain the dignity of life, even in exasperating circumstances.

LIFE AND DEATH: A MUSLIM PERSPECTIVE

> *It is hope and not despair.*
>
> — *M.Salaudeen Madani*
> *Imam, Juma Masjid, Cochin, India*

We are born in this world without anyone's permission and leave likewise. The interval between birth and death is what we term as life. But life does not end with death. There is a land beyond, the glorious and majestic heaven. Life is not a meaningless interlude on earth. It has a direction and a purpose. The purpose is to reach the presence of Allah, the merciful and compassionate. The entry to an immortal life in heaven is the success and divine purpose of human life.

"All will taste the painful death. The reward of your life is given on the last day of your life on earth. The escape from the torment of hell and the entry into the eternal precincts of heaven is the victory of life on earth. The earthly life is full of deceit and tragedies." (Holy Koran 3:185). The Holy book further entreats you. "Thou mortal man, you are walking along a land of trials and tribulations to the mighty presence of Allah, the merciful. You will meet him in heaven and thou shalt be judged in His presence for your good and bad deeds" (Holy Koran 84:6). Man is destined to live and work in the fields that have been given freely by Allah, the merciful and the harvest is available in heaven. You shall reap what you sow. Prophet Muhammad (S) has said this world is the field to cultivate the seeds of good things for the next world. "Truth, honesty, justice, practice of virtue, purity, forgiveness, kind care for orphans and widows, good and kind thoughts, etc. should be the seeds that you sow. The good seed that you have sowed may be damaged by the weeds of evil seeds, and by prayer and good and wholesome life you must prevent the growth of weeds in the land given to you by God."

Every true believer must be grateful to God for all the good things and mercies you enjoy. At the same time, do not despair when sad events overtake you. Life is a mixture of good and bad things. Illness, physical pain and death may occur amongst the members of your family and only God can save you from these earthly tragedies." It is only God the compassionate who can save you from the perils of illness and tragedies." (Holy Koran 6:28). As a believer has said, there is none to prevent what you have been given and none to give what God has prevented from reaching you. "A person who trusts in Allah, the merciful, may have illness, pain, mental anguish, loss of dear ones in the earthly sojourn and this is a chance for him to receive forgiveness from God if he does not lose his faith." (Bukhari).

The history of Islam is full of sufferings of the faithful prophets who preached the mercy and kindness of God. They did not waver or lose faith in the creator as they believed and trusted. It is not unusual to hear about people attempting to commit suicide as they go through a life of severe pain as in cancer and such incurable diseases. None has the right to destroy a life given freely and by the kindness of Allah, the merciful. The attempt or even the thought of killing oneself is a mortal sin. "All you can pray is to give life as long as it is graceful and also pray for death by the mercy of Allah, the merciful." (Bukhari). Each person on earth is given a specific period of life. As soon as the time expires, you are destined to leave. Death is your constant companion and so close to you as the straps of your footwear. It is the wish of God that none of his creation must leave this world in sin but with hope and faith in a new heaven and a new eternal life. The suffering of Job is a good example of what faithful people go through in this temporal world and when it was known that he had lost everything God came to his rescue. As long as you have life in you, you can crave for God's forgiveness. As the Prophet has said, even if a flicker of life exists in your throat, you can pray for his forgiveness. The merciful God will forgive you and take you to heaven as partakers of eternal life.

FURTHER READING

1. Chochinov HM. Dignity-conserving care—a new model for palliative care: Helping the patient feel valued. JAMA 2002;287(17):2253-60.
2. Dendaas NR. Prognostication in advanced cancer: Nurses' perceptions of the dying process. Oncol Nurs Forum 2002;29(3):493-99.
3. Edmonds P, Karlsen S, Khan S, Addington-Hall J. A comparison of the palliative care needs of patients dying from chronic respiratory diseases and lung cancer. Palliat Med 2001;15(4):287-95.
4. Hall P, Schroder C, Weaver L. The last 48 hours of life in long-term care: A focused chart audit. J Am Geriatr Soc 2002;50(3):501-06.
5. Heedman PA, Strang P. Symptom assessment in advanced palliative home care for cancer patients using the ESAS: Clinical aspects. Anticancer Res 2001;21(6A):4077-82.
6. McGarry RC, Song G, des Rosiers P, Timmerman R. Observation-only management of early stage, medically inoperable lung cancer: poor outcome. Chest 2002;121(4):1155-58.
7. McGrath P. End-of-life care for hematological malignancies: The 'technological imperative' and palliative care. J Palliat Care 2002 Spring;18(1):39-47.
8. McQuellon RP, Cowan MA. Turning toward death together: Conversation in mortal time. Am J Hosp Palliat Care 2000;17(5):312-18.
9. Mok E, Chan F, Chan V, Yeung E. Perception of empowerment by family caregivers of patients with a terminal illness in Hong Kong. Int J Palliat Nurs 2002;8(3):137-45.
10. Tang ST. Influencing factors of place of death among home care patients with cancer in Taiwan. Cancer Nurse 2002;25(2):158-66.
11. Variables influencing end-of-life care in children and adolescents with cancer. J Pediatr Hematol Oncol 2001;23(8):481-86.
12. Walton O, Weinstein SM. Sedation for comfort at end of life. Curr Pain Headache Rep 2002;6(3):197-201.

Index